GYNECOLOGY

PRINCIPLES AND
PRACTICE

ROBERT W. KISTNER, M.D.

Assistant Clinical Professor of Obstetrics and Gynecology,
Harvard Medical School
Senior Gynecologist and Obstetrician, Boston Hospital for Women
(formerly Free Hospital for Women) and Boston Lying-in Hospital,
Boston, Massachusetts

GYNECOLOGY

PRINCIPLES AND

PRACTICE

SECOND EDITION

YEAR BOOK MEDICAL PUBLISHERS · INC.

35 EAST WACKER DRIVE · CHICAGO

Reprinted, October 1965
Reprinted, May 1969
Second Edition, 1971
Reprinted, September 1971
Reprinted, September 1972
Reprinted, October 1973

Library of Congress Catalog Card Number: 74-125802
International Standard Book Number: 0-8151-5080-6

Preface to Second Edition

THE REMARKABLE ADVANCES which have occurred in the field of gynecology since the publication of the first edition of this book in 1964 are evidenced by the extensive changes which were required to update this edition. The same general format of the earlier volume has been followed and, in keeping with the general philosophy expressed previously, every effort has been made to present succinctly those facts and concepts which will aid the student and clinician to understand basic anatomic and physiologic principles. Only then is it possible to appreciate pathologic variations, apply proper diagnostic methods and suggest proper therapy.

For this edition, each chapter has been thoroughly revised and many have been completely rewritten. References have been updated and new illustrations added. Dr. C. T. Griffiths has rejuvenated the chapter on the cervix and, on the basis of his wide experience in the carcinoma in situ clinic of the Boston Hospital for Women, has imparted a new visage to the sequential relationship between premalignant and malignant lesions. Doctor Griffiths has also updated the chapter on the ovary, particularly the chemotherapeutic management of ovarian carcinoma. His observations are not based solely on a review of published reports but represent conclusions based on extensive personal experience as Chief of Chemotherapy at the Boston Hospital for Women.

Dr. Donald P. Goldstein has expanded and rewritten the former section on hydatidiform mole and choriocarcinoma. This subject has been afforded a full chapter in this edition because of the vast research in chemotherapeutic aspects and because of the fantastic improvement in prognosis for patients having this disease. In gynecologic cancer, two major advances have occurred during the past decade: (1) the use of methotrexate and actinomycin-D in choriocarcinoma and (2) synthetic progestins in metastatic endometrial carcinoma. Doctor Goldstein has had extensive experience in the field of chorionic tumors and has established a regional center in Boston for the treatment of these diseases. He brings to this edition the most up-to-date regimens of therapy. I have similarly detailed the specific aspects of management of metastatic endometrial carcinoma and have expanded my previous observations on the effects of progestational agents on hyperplasia and carcinoma in situ of the endometrium.

Material revisions have been made in the sections related to the central nervous system and reproductive function and in the genetic aspects of gynecologic disorders. I am indebted to Drs. John F. Crigler, Park S. Gerald and Daniel D. Federman for revising the chapter on cytogenetics, to Dr. Martin B. Levine for revising the section on radiation therapy of carcinoma of the cervix and to Dr. John Twaddle for his radiographic illustrations.

The past decade might well be described as the "years of the Pill." Surgical innovations have been sparse in the gynecologic field, not even one uterus or ovary having been transplanted. But momentous strides have been taken in endocrinologic aspects and, whereas in the first edition I reported early success in ovulation suppression and induction, detailed information is now available. In order to present this in an orderly fashion, the chapter on Infertility, Habitual Abortion and Specific Endocrine Disorders has been subdivided into three separate chapters, thus affording adequate consideration of each topic. In addition, a new chapter on Conception Control has been added, reviewing previous methods and detailing aspects of oral contraception and the intrauterine devices.

The use of steroid substances (estrogens, progestins, androgens, corticoids) in gynecologic practice is another major advance of the decade. Research in this field has been rapid—almost too rapid. The student, the generalist and even the specialist have been engulfed by these events. I have rewritten the chapter on Steroid Therapy in order to give the reader a simplified, sequential summary of the important events between 1960 and 1970. An effort has been made to apply steroid therapy to clinical problems in a logical fashion rather than on stereotyped impressions. This approach is illustrated in another new chapter, Management of the Menopause.

The first edition of GYNECOLOGY, PRINCIPLES AND PRACTICE was not intended to serve as an atlas of gynecologic surgery. Nor is the second edition. However, hormonal aspects of therapy, because of their newness, received extensive consideration in the first edition and therefore may have been unduly emphasized. An effort has been made in this edition to secure an improved balance by the inclusion of specific operative procedures. This is particularly emphasized in the completely rewritten chapter on Endometriosis.

My gratitude is due the numerous colleagues who have made this book possible. First and foremost, Dr. George V. Smith, Emeritus Professor of Gynecology, Harvard Medical School, and former Surgeon-in-Chief at the Free Hospital for Women (now Parkway Division, Boston Hospital for Women), corrected the entire manuscript and made innumerable revisions, suggestions and corrections. Dr. Olive W. Smith, former head of the Fearing Laboratory, offered valuable suggestions in revising the chapter on Steroid Therapy. I am indebted to the writings of Drs. Kenneth J. Ryan, Joseph J. Barlow, William J. Dignam, Virenda B. Mahesh and Joseph W. Goldzieher, whose stellar and original contributions are quoted liberally.

In writing this volume, I have unavoidably drawn from my more recent articles which appeared in the *American Journal of Obstetrics and Gynecology, Clinical Obstetrics and Gynecology, Progress in Infertility* and *Fertility and Sterility.* The courtesy extended by these periodicals is herein acknowledged.

Sincere appreciation is accorded Drs. Robert L. Ehrmann and John M. Craig for their skill and patience in taking the photomicrographs and to Richard W. St. Clair and Joan Price for their precise preparation; also to Drs. Donald J. Woodruff and Ralph C. Benson for permitting us to use their excellent illustrations, and to Mrs. Edith Tagrin for her continued excellent work with additional drawings for this edition. I also acknowledge a deep indebtedness to my secretaries, Mrs. Linda Angelico, Miss Jean Mackey and Mrs. Marlene Goldman, whose indefatigable efforts served immeasurably to lighten the burden of authorship.

ROBERT W. KISTNER

Preface to First Edition

THIS WORK is designed both as a textbook and as a general reference book of gynecology to meet the needs of undergraduate medical students, young practitioners of gynecology and specialists in this field. The format of each chapter is similar, the purpose being to provide a uniform and organized approach to the understanding of multiple disease processes of each organ of the female genital tract. Thus, in each chapter the embryology, anatomy and histology are correlated with specific malformations. Morphologic variations are correlated with physiologic alterations. Recent advances in the diagnosis and therapy of infectious processes are described in detail. Particular emphasis has been given to the relationship of premalignant to malignant neoplasms, and methods for the prophylaxis of certain tumors are suggested. Because of the importance and increasing incidence of endometriosis a separate chapter on this disease is included. Particular emphasis has been placed on hormonal therapy, and details of management outlined.

Because of my interest in the practical endocrinologic aspects of gynecology, a chapter is devoted to steroid therapy. In this chapter an attempt is made to obviate many of the difficulties of administration associated with the new synthetic preparations. I have included (1) a brief résumé of basic steroid chemistry, (2) a summation of the pharmacology and physiology of androgens, estrogens and progesterone, together with a similar discussion of the synthetic progestins and (3) a discussion of proved and proposed indications for the use of these steroids, with specific contraindications and optimum dosage.

The observations and opinions expressed in this text summarize the sum and substance of the teaching and practice at the Free Hospital for Women during the past 15 years. This hospital was opened on November 2, 1875, and has been in continuous operation since that time. It is the only remaining specialty hospital in the United States whose primary objective is the diagnosis and treatment of medical and surgical diseases of the female.

The Free Hospital for Women became internationally known because of the *Textbook of Gynecology* written by Dr. William P. Graves, formerly Professor of Gynecology at Harvard Medical School. Although the fourth and last edition of Graves' textbook appeared in 1928, since that time a multiplicity of original and important contributions has been published by the members of the staff. Outstanding among these have been the innumerable works of Drs. George and Olive Smith concerning the measurement and metabolism of ovarian steroids and gonadotropic hormones during the menstrual cycle, the period of conception and subsequent pregnancy. During the years 1938 through 1957 Drs. John Rock and Arthur T. Hertig accomplished their monumental studies on the earliest stages of human growth following fertilization. From 1928 through 1958 Doctor Rock directed intensive study and research projects relating to the etiologic factors in infertility. The pathogenesis of carcinoma in situ of the cervix and its relationship to invasive carcinoma have undergone thorough investigation and evaluation by Drs. Paul Younge, Arthur T. Hertig and Donald G. MacKay. During the past seven years the synthetic progestational agents have been subjected to extensive clinical investigation in specific gynecologic disorders such as endometriosis and endometrial carcinoma.

In preparing a work of this type, material must be gathered not only from the author's personal experience, but to a still greater extent from the work of others. I have, therefore, attempted to include the important observations of numerous authors who have published data concerning the clinical material at the Free Hospital for Women. From the great number of publications consulted there have been several to which I have had frequent recourse, both for new material and for corroboration of personal observations. I must, therefore, express a general acknowledgment of indebtedness to Drs. George and Olive Smith, Arthur T. Hertig, Christopher J. Duncan, Paul A. Younge, Donald G. MacKay and John Rock. I have also drawn on the writings of the late Joe V. Meigs and Langdon Parsons, both former residents at the Free Hospital for Women. In writing the sections on the relationship of endocrinology to gynecology I have received the greatest assistance from the excellent works, *Endocrine and Metabolic Aspects of Gynecology* by Joseph Rogers, *Human Endocrinology* by Herbert S. Kupperman, and *The Endocrinology of Reproduction,* edited by Joseph T. Velardo. The reader is referred to these publications for additional and specific details.

I am indebted to Mrs. Edith Tagrin for the excellent illustrations and to Mr. Leo Goodman and Dr. Robert Ehrmann for the photomicrographs. Dr. Arthur T. Hertig and Dr. Hazel M. Gore have also kindly given permission to reproduce many of their excellent photomicrographs previously published in *Tumors of the Female Sex Organs,* published by the Armed Forces Institute of Pathology. The student is advised to refer to these fascicles for a complete survey of the pathology of tumors of the female genital tract.

I also wish to acknowledge a deep indebtedness to the tireless fingers and indefatigable efforts of my secretaries, Mrs. Ann Gregory Metzger, Mrs. Constance M. Rakoske, Mrs. Linda Angelico and Mrs. Rachel Markiewicz. Valuable assistance has been given to me by the Administrator of the Free Hospital for Women, Miss Lillian Grahn. Finally, the courtesies of the staff of Year Book Medical Publishers have made the final preparation of this manuscript a pleasant task.

ROBERT W. KISTNER

Table of Contents

1. **Introduction** **1**
   The History 2
   The Physical Examination 5
   The Pelvic Examination 7

2. **The Vulva** **17**
   General Considerations 17
   Embryology 18
   Anatomy and Histology 20
   Malformations 27
   Physiologic Alterations 30
   Vulvar Injuries 31
   Venereal Diseases 33
      Syphilis 33
      Gonorrhea 35
      Chancroid (Soft Chancre) 36
      Lymphopathia Venereum (Lymphogranuloma Inguinale) 37
      Granuloma Inguinale 37
   Pruritus Vulvae 38
      Local Causes of Pruritus Vulvae 40
      Systemic Causes of Pruritus 50
   Skin Diseases 51
   Benign Neoplasms 55
   Malignant Neoplasms 58
      Carcinoma 60
      Other Vulvar Malignancies 65

3. **The Vagina** **70**
   Embryology 70
   Anatomy and Histology 72
   Malformations 75
   Physiologic Alterations 76
      Cytology 78
   Leukorrhea 79
      Trichomoniasis 80

Moniliasis 83

Nonspecific Vaginitis 86

Senescent Vaginitis 87

Chronic Cervicitis 88

Gonorrheal Vaginitis 88

Vaginal Relaxation 89

Benign Neoplasms 93

Premalignant Neoplasms 95

Carcinoma In Situ 95

Malignant Neoplasms 96

Carcinoma 96

Sarcoma 101

4. The Cervix. *Revised by* C. THOMAS GRIFFITHS, M.D., *Assistant Professor of Obstetrics and Gynecology, Harvard Medical School* . . **103**

Embryology 103

Anatomy 104

Histology 105

Physiology 109

Physiologic Alterations 110

Squamous Metaplasia 112

Squamous Epithelization 114

Pathologic Alterations 114

Inflammation 114

Acute Cervicitis 115

Chronic Cervicitis 116

Keratinization 116

Diagnostic and Minor Surgical Procedures 117

Biopsy of the Cervix 117

Cauterization of the Cervix 119

Benign Neoplasms 121

Cervical Polyps 121

Endometriosis 122

Papillomas 122

Malignant Neoplasms 124

Squamous Cell Carcinoma 124

Premalignant Neoplasia 127

Detection of Early Cervical Neoplasms 141

Invasive Cancer 145

Pathology 145

Clinical Staging of Cervical Cancer 148

Symptoms and Diagnosis 151

Treatment 152

Cervical Cancer in Pregnancy 164

Cervical Cancer Complicating Procidentia 165

Recurrent and Advanced Cervical Carcinoma 166

Adenocarcinoma of the Cervix 167

5. **The Uterine Corpus** **172**
General Considerations 172
Anatomy 173
Embryology 182
Menstruation 183
Hormonal Aspects of Menstruation 186
Dating the Endometrium 194
Systemic Changes Associated with the Menstrual Cycle 208
Uterine Retrodisplacement 212
Infections 217
Postabortal Infection 217
Tuberculosis 220
Benign Neoplasms 220
Adenomyosis 221
Leiomyoma 226
Endolymphatic Stromal Myosis 242
Endometrial Polyps 244
Endometrial Hyperplasia 247
Premalignant Neoplasms 253
Carcinoma In Situ 253
Malignant Neoplasms 257
Adenocarcinoma 257
Sarcoma 272

6. **The Oviduct** **281**
Anatomy and Histology 281
Embryology 285
Correlation of Structure and Function 286
Inflammation 288
Surface Extension—Gonorrhea 288
Puerperal or Postabortal Salpingitis 294
Tuberculosis 296
Physiologic Salpingitis 301
Nontuberculous Granulomatous Salpingitis 303
Tubal Ectopic Pregnancy 304
Diagnosis 304
Fertility After Ectopic Pregnancy 310
Combined Intra- and Extrauterine Pregnancies 311
Salpingitis Isthmica Nodosa 311
Benign Neoplasms 314
Malignant Neoplasms 315
Primary Carcinoma 315
Sarcoma 320
Carcinoma Metastatic to the Oviduct 320

7. **The Ovary.** *Revised by* C. THOMAS GRIFFITHS, M.D., *Assistant Professor of Obstetrics and Gynecology, Harvard Medical School* . . **323**
Embryology 323

Anatomy 325

Histology 328

Ovulation and Corpus Luteum Formation 329

Follicular Atresia 330

The Postmenopausal Ovary 331

Vestigial Remnants 331

Ovarian Neoplasms 331

Symptomatology and Diagnosis 335

Differential Diagnosis 339

Non-neoplastic Cysts of Graafian Follicle Origin 344

Cystic Structures Derived from the Normally Ruptured
Follicle 347

Cystomas (of Germinal Epithelial Origin) 349

Simple Serous Cystoma 351

Serous Cystadenoma 353

Papillary Serous Cystadenocarcinoma 355

Mucinous Cystadenoma and Cystadenocarcinoma 355

Cystadenofibroma, Benign and Malignant 361

Endometrioid Carcinoma 363

Carcinoma of the Ovary 365

Treatment 369

Chemotherapy 373

Gonadal Stromal Tumors 378

Granulosa-Theca Cell Tumors 378

Arrhenoblastoma 387

Gynandroblastoma 389

Germ Cell Tumors 392

Dysgerminoma 392

Benign Cystic Teratoma (Dermoid Cyst) 396

Primary Choriocarcinoma 402

Malignant Teratoma 403

Teratocarcinoma 404

Congenital Rest Tumors 405

Adrenal Rest Tumor 405

Mesometanephric Rest Tumor 407

Brenner Tumor 409

Hilus Cell Tumor 411

Nonintrinsic Connective Tissue Tumors 412

Fibroma 412

Fibrosarcoma 414

Metastatic Tumors 414

Krukenberg's Tumor 414

Secondary Ovarian Cancer from Pelvic Organs 416

Sclerocystic Ovarian Disease (Stein-Leventhal) 416

Etiology 419

Studies of Steroid Biosynthesis 420

Diagnostic Measures 422

Adrenocortical and Ovarian Suppression Studies 422

Adrenocortical and Ovarian Stimulation Tests 423

Treatment 423

Effects of Clomiphene 424

8. **Endometriosis** **432**

Histogenesis 432

Pathology 435

Clinical Features 441

Incidence 441

Symptoms 441

Correlation with Infertility 442

Diagnosis 443

Treatment 444

Prophylaxis 444

Observation and Analgesia 445

Suppression of Ovulation 446

Surgical Treatment 451

Complications 455

9. **Infertility** **458**

General Considerations 458

Clinical Management 460

Study of the Male Partner 461

Study of the Female Partner 464

The Cervical Factor 474

The Uterine Factor 476

The Tubal Factor 478

The Ovarian Factor 482

Endometriosis 494

Adrenal Factors 494

Thyroid Factors 495

10. **Habitual Abortion** **500**

General Considerations and Management 500

Psychosomatic Aspects 502

Chronic Disease and Nutritional Disorders 503

Immunologic Factors 504

Hormonal Aspects 505

Anatomic Defects 517

11. **Hydatidiform Mole and Choriocarcinoma.** *Revised by*
DONALD P. GOLDSTEIN, *Director, New England Trophoblastic Disease Center; Associate in Obstetrics and Gynecology, Harvard Medical School* **527**

Hydatidiform Mole 527

Prophylactic Chemotherapy 537

Invasive Mole (Chorioadenoma Destruens) 538

Choriocarcinoma 541

12. Endocrine Disorders **545**

Premature Onset of the Menses 546

    Constitutional Sexual Precocity 548

    Premature Menstruation Due to Organic Causes 551

Delayed Menarche 556

    Constitutional Delay in Menarche 557

    Hypogonadotropism 558

    Hypogonadism 558

Scant or Absent Menstruation 559

    Oligomenorrhea 559

    Primary Amenorrhea 560

    Secondary Amenorrhea 563

    Evalutaion of the Patient with Amenorrhea 567

    Treatment of Amenorrhea 569

Dysfunctional Uterine Bleeding 573

    History and Physical Examination 573

    Bleeding Associated with Ovulation 578

    Premenstrual Staining 578

    Normal Bleeding at Less than Usual Intervals 579

    Normal Bleeding at More than Usual Intervals 580

    Profuse or Prolonged Bleeding at Normal Intervals

        (Hypermenorrhea) 580

    Irregular Shedding of the Endometrium 582

    Constant or Intermittent Bleeding 582

Dysmenorrhea 584

Adrenogenital Syndrome 588

    Diagnosis of Adrenogenital Syndrome 594

    Treatment 596

Pituitary and Hypothalamus 598

    Cushing's Disease 598

    Simmonds' Disease 602

    Sheehan's Syndrome 603

Hirsutism 608

    Etiology 610

    Diagnosis 612

    Treatment 614

13. Steroid Therapy **618**

General Considerations 618

Biosynthesis of Steroids 620

    Formation of Androgens 622

    Formation of Progesterone 627

    Formation of Estrogens 631

    Measurement of Estrogens 634

Estrogen Therapy 636

Androgen Therapy 642

Progestational Therapy 647

Proved Indications for the Use of Progestins 649
Proposed Indications for the Use of Progestins 652

14. The Menopause **658**
Estrogens 658
Osteoporosis 661
Therapy of the Menopause 662
Psychotherapy 662
Symptomatic Therapy 663
Hormonal Regimens During Premenopause 663
Therapeutic Regimens During Postmenopause 664
Vasomotor Symptoms 665
Progesterone 667
Androgen 667
Combined Androgen-Estrogen 668

15. Conception Control **670**
Condoms 671
Coitus Interruptus 671
Rhythm Method 672
Vaginal Spermicides 672
Vaginal Diaphragms with Spermicides 672
Intrauterine Contraceptive Devices 673
Oral and Injectable Contraceptives 677
Combined Formulations 679
Control by Injections 682
Sequential Formulations 683
Estrogens and Non-Steroidal Antifertility Agents 687
Side-Effects 688
Effects of Contraceptives on Subsequent Pregnancy 688
Postpartum Use of Oral Contraceptives 689
Effects of Contraceptives on the Menopause 689
Thyroid and Adrenal Glands 690
Vascular Disturbances 690
Thrombophlebitis and Pulmonary Embolism 690
Cerebrovascular Accidents 693
Hypertension 694
Migraine 694
Hepatic Effects 695
Diabetes 696
Fibroids 698
Breast Changes 699
Relation of Oral Contraceptives to Secondary Amenorrhea and
Infertility 699
Cancer 700
Contraindications and Cautions in the Use of Oral
Contraceptives 702

16. **Cytogenetics** **705**
    General Considerations 705
    Chromosome Patterns; Gametogenesis 709
    Chromosomal Abnormalities 719
        Gonadal Dysgenesis (Turner's Syndrome) 719
        Seminiferous Tubule Dysgenesis (Klinefelter's Syndrome) . . . 724
        Triple-X Chromosome Pattern 726
        Tetra-X Chromosome Pattern 727
        XXXY Pattern 727
        Mosaicism 727
        Translocation 728
        Deletion 729
        The XY Female 731
        Mongolism (21-Trisomy) 734
        Edward's Syndrome (18-Trisomy) 737
        Bartholin-Patau Syndrome (13-Trisomy) 737
        Deletion Syndromes 737
        Spontaneous Abortions 738
        Miscellaneous Abnormalities 739
    Prophylaxis 741
    Clinical Aspects of Chromosome Determinations 743

Index **748**

CHAPTER 1

Introduction

THE SPECIALTY OF gynecology has rapidly expanded during the past two decades to encompass disciplines of surgical, medical, endocrinologic and obstetric endeavor. Prior to this time gynecology remained subservient to the field of general surgery—a stepchild with but limited possibilities in both clinical and laboratory investigation. The union of gynecology with obstetrics brought about an awareness of the all-inclusive problem of "femaleness," together with a reawakening of interest in basic scientific principles of human reproduction. It is now not sufficient for the physician to limit his scope to the surgical aspects of pelvic disorders since extirpation, although simple and expedient, may seriously alter the reproductive capacity and physiologic standards of the female.

It is imperative, therefore, that medical students and residents appreciate the intimate relationships between metabolic disorders or aberrations of endocrine function and the genital tract. The importance of psychosomatic influences on the behavior of woman must be recognized and the intimate correlation of pregnancy, delivery and the puerperium with both structure and function must be emphasized. An attempt will be made in this text to bring into clear focus the basic anatomic, physiologic and pathologic facets of most gynecologic disorders and, perhaps more important, each of these will be considered as alterations of femaleness. Therapy to preserve, restore or improve this desideratum will be outlined.

A word of caution regarding the intimacy of gynecology is perhaps in order for the beginner. Many of the problems which bring the patient to the physician center about subjects or body areas that she would rather forget than discuss. The patient who visits her physician frequently for respiratory or intestinal ailments is likely to neglect a vulvar lesion which may be, or develop into, cancer. The gynecologist must at the outset be both sympathetic and understanding but tactfully capable of eliciting details which might be omitted purposely by the patient. He must be an attentive and interested listener and, in addition, should retain a reassuring and indulgent attitude. A brief explanation of the causes of symptoms together with logical reasons for the performance of diagnostic tests or surgery will help to diminish or dispel fears and misconceptions of most patients. Numerous visits are occasioned by cancerophobia and many more by episodes of vague, fleeting pain for which no explanation is evident. It is in such situations that much may be accomplished by reassurance and frank discussion.

1

The History

Good history-taking is probably more closely related to the art than to the science of medicine. Yet it is important that a methodical approach be utilized so that important omissions may be avoided. A printed form, while sometimes cumbersome and at times inadequate, will serve this purpose in most instances and is essential for the student.

The chief complaint should be stated in the exact words of the patient, and its duration should be included. The present illness which follows is merely an expansion of the chief complaint. The account presents a chronologic sequence of events from the onset of illness up to the time of examination. It is not sufficient, however, merely to list such all-inclusive phrases as "irregular periods," "flowing on and off" or "trouble with periods." The clinician should determine the exact dates of the last normal menstrual period and the previous period. Bleeding intermenstrually should be described as to time of occurrence, duration and the presence or absence of pain and/or clots. It will often be found that the abnormal bleeding complained of is simply staining due to endometrial breakdown at the time of ovulation. Similarly, the skips and delays in periods at the time of menopause may be easily explained on the basis of irregularities in ovulation. Bleeding postcoitally or after a douche suggests a cervical polyp or malignancy. Postmenopausal bleeding is caused by malignancy of the cervix, uterine corpus or ovary in about one half of all patients. Exacting detail in the description of bleeding is therefore most important.

Frequently a diagnosis is suggested by the first few sentences of the chief complaint. This may be misleading since "snap" diagnoses are likely to result. Subsequent complaints are glossed over or a careful review of other systems is not completed. Should the physical and pelvic examination be equally sketchy, the gynecologist often becomes the victim of embarrassing "surprises" at the operating table. A common situation is the discovery of carcinoma or diverticulitis of the sigmoid colon when a fibroid or left ovarian mass was expected. The era of the master surgical technician has passed, and for the complete and successful treatment of the patient a combination of judgment, reason, skill and humanity is desirable. An unnecessary operation by the most adept surgeon may still result in death from infection, pulmonary embolism or unrecognized cardiac disease.

Previous hospitalizations are of interest, especially if pelvic surgery has been performed or radium and/or x-ray has been administered. The location of the hospital, the name of the surgeon and the date of surgery should be noted and a transcript of the patient's chart obtained. This will avoid misinterpretation of what the patient says was done or what was removed.

The past history merits consideration because of its bearing on the choice of anesthesia and on the advisability of certain surgical procedures. Obviously a patient with chronic bronchitis and a persistent cough should not be hurried to the hospital for an operation to cure stress incontinence until her pulmonary difficulties have improved. A simple check list of serious infectious, pulmonary, cardiac and renal diseases seems adequate in most cases, with elaboration when necessary.

The family history is recorded primarily to determine the incidence of diseases such as diabetes, cancer (especially breast), hypertension or coronary occlusion. Occasionally, important entities such as a familial polyposis will be discovered in this fashion.

A history of the patient's social background is important. It should include her birthplace, national descent, religion, occupation and previous marriages, if any. The age, occupation, religion and health of the husband should also be obtained.

The systems review should include all pregnancies, listed in order by year, with the length of gestation, type of delivery, fetal weight and complications, if any. Long periods of infertility, either primary or secondary, suggest endometriosis or pelvic inflammatory disease. In the patient who has been pregnant five or six times in the same number of years there may be a history of pelvic pain, sacral backache, dyspareunia and vaginal discharge. This suggests a diagnosis of "married women's complaint" and is usually causally related to a uterine retroversion with pelvic vascular congestion and a diseased cervix.

The dates and normality of the last and previous menstrual periods should be accurately recorded. If this is neglected, intrauterine pregnancies, tubal pregnancies and threatened or incomplete abortions will not be given serious consideration in the differential diagnosis. On occasion, the patient will deliberately falsify a recent period or neglect to describe its true length or character. A careful pelvic examination and visualization of the cervix will usually aid the examiner in recognizing these deceptions.

Pain associated with the menstrual flow should be classified as to site, duration, intensity and nature. Midline, suprapubic, first day (or 24 hours before flow), dull, crampy pain is characteristic of primary (idiopathic) dysmenorrhea. The pain of endometriosis is, by contrast, sharp, aching, constant, lateral or deep in the pelvis around the rectum and seems to get progressively worse month after month. Pain on defecation or dyspareunia suggests cul-de-sac or rectosigmoid endometriosis or possibly blood or pus in the pelvic cavity due to ectopic pregnancy or pelvic inflammation.

The review of systems is frequently of aid in establishing a gynecologic diagnosis or in the elimination of bowel or urinary tract disease. The proximity of bladder, uterus and rectosigmoid and the inability of most patients to pinpoint their symptoms make this survey worthwhile.

The usual data regarding age of onset, interval and duration of menstrual periods are necessary requisites of every gynecologic history. The age of onset of the menses will vary, depending on climate and genetic background. In the United States the first period usually occurs between ages 11 and 16, the average about 13. The clinician should not become alarmed, however, if menses occur two years earlier or later than the extremes mentioned above. Thus it has been noted that Jewesses menstruate sooner than gentiles, and brunettes usually start about a year or so before blondes. Vaginal bleeding occurring in a child of 6 or 8 should, however, be investigated with the same thoroughness as amenorrhea in a girl of 20. An extensive endocrinologic survey is not indicated for primary amenorrhea before age 18.

An interval of 28 days between periods is time-honored but not exact, and in normal women the interval will vary between 26 and 32 days. The singular characteristic of menstrual (i.e., postovulatory) bleeding is rhythmicity. This distinguishes it from the marked irregular flowing of anovulatory origin. Patients who have maintained rhythmic cycles of 21 days, 35 days or even 60 days should not be considered abnormal, although they cannot be called "average."

The average duration of menstruation is between three and four days with an average blood loss of 25–70 cc. A good deal of variation is noted in both of these variables since some normal women bleed for one or two days and others six to seven days, with extremes of blood loss from 10 to 200 cc. The presence of clots may mean the absence of a fibrinolysin (found normally in menstrual discharge), suggesting that the bleeding is anovulatory. Or it may mean that the vascular breakdown in the endometrium is so rapid that whatever fibrinolysin is present is unable to maintain the fluidity of blood, so that clotting occurs.

Vaginal discharge may be due to infection, malignancy, foreign bodies or trauma. Therefore, inquiries should be made about its color, consistency and the presence of blood. Pessaries and certain douche solutions may be irritating to the vaginal mucosa and should be thought of as possible etiologic factors. Bloody mucoid discharge occurring postmenopausally may be due to carcinoma of the endometrium or cervix. However, occasionally it will be due to prolonged use of estrogens, and cessation of this medication results in cure. A list of all medications the patient is presently taking or has received in the recent past should be noted. Broad-spectrum antibiotics frequently cause monilial vaginitis, vaginal discharge and pruritus, and their use should be determined.

The general health is investigated. Symptoms such as nausea, anorexia, lassitude and low-grade temperature elevation may be due to pulmonary or genital tuberculosis. Weight loss, dizziness and anemia with crampy right lower quadrant pain suggest cancer of the right colon or cecum. The finding of a large leiomyoma, while spectacular to the student, may be misleading. Generalized symptoms, such as those just noted, are not common with most gynecologic maladies and one must not be content to explain all symptoms on the basis of one gross abnormality. The cardiorespiratory, gastrointestinal, urinary and neuromuscular systems should be carefully investigated. Particular attention should be given to symptoms such as diminished appetite, change in bowel habits, alternating diarrhea and constipation, blood mixed with stool, tenesmus or pain with bowel movements or change in the stool diameter. The gynecologist encounters sigmoid or rectal carcinoma all too often during surgery for a suspected ovarian cyst or myoma. Attention to such symptoms will permit the correct diagnosis to be made before surgery.

Symptoms which arise from the urinary tract merit detailed discussion since there is frequently a correlation with the gynecologic complaint. Stress incontinence, or loss of urine while coughing, sneezing, laughing, etc., should be differentiated from urge incontinence since the former may require surgical correction whereas the latter may be treated by simple bladder irrigations or urinary antiseptics. Dysuria, frequency and nocturia suggest bladder infections but may be secondary to radium or x-ray treatments. If urinary frequency occurs, it is important to know whether there are associated polyuria and polydipsia since these may be the first symptoms of early diabetes. If there are associated itching and vulvitis, diabetes should be strongly suspected. A common complaint of a bride is that of dysuria and frequency—honeymoon cystitis. The details of the history are sufficient to make the diagnosis.

Further inquiry is also made regarding allergies or sensitivities to drugs, antibiotics and anesthetic agents as well as previous thromboembolic disease.

The Physical Examination

A complete physical examination is performed when the patient is seen for the first time. This includes gross inspection of head and neck and palpation of the thyroid gland, supraclavicular areas and superficial lymph nodes. One should particularly note the patency of the nasal airway, irregularities or nodules in the thyroid and the presence of supraclavicular nodes or masses.

The gynecologist should include a thorough examination of the breasts not only at the first visit but at subsequent visits (if the interval exceeds three months). Inspection of the breasts should be done first with the patient sitting erect with her arms at her sides and then with the arms raised. This maneuver will frequently outline asymmetry or fixation of the nipple or fixed masses under or adjacent to the areola. The supraclavicular areas and the axillae are then palpated with the patient sitting erect. An adequate examination of the axilla can be performed only if the pectoral muscles are relaxed. This is accomplished by supporting the patient's arm in slight abduction and palpating the axilla with the finger-tips. Particular attention should be given to the apex of the axilla and the undersurface of the pectoralis major muscle. A systematic examination of the breasts is then performed in both the erect and supine positions. Masses in the breast are best determined by palpation with the flat surface rather than the tips of the fingers. The whole extent of the breast, as it lies relatively flattened out and balanced on the chest wall, should be systematically palpated. The medial portion is examined first with the patient's arm raised. This flattens the pectoral muscles under the breast, and the examiner's fingers trace a series of transverse lines across the breast from the nipple line to the sternum. Palpation of the lateral portion of the breast is then performed with the patient's arm at her side. The ducts and nipples should be compressed, and if bloody secretion is obtained it is submitted to cytologic examination. Cloudy fluid may be expressed from the nipples of parous women many years after pregnancy and is of no significance. A very common finding is thickening in the upper outer quadrant of the breast; if present, this is noted and repeated observations suggested. It should be borne in mind that the breast normally presents fine nodularity on palpation. During periods of engorgement (especially premenstrually) this nodularity may be accentuated almost to the point of simulating a dominant lump. Differentiation between tumor and such physiologic change is difficult. Usually, with care in palpation and re-examination at a different time in the menstrual cycle a definite decision can be reached. About 65 per cent of all cancers of the breast occur in this quadrant, and this area should therefore be given particular attention.

All discrete masses or dominant lumps are excised in the operating room, a frozen section made and appropriate therapy performed. It has not been our practice to aspirate large cysts and perform cytology on the contents. Cancer in the wall of the cyst exists often enough to warrant complete excision of the entire mass rather than simple removal of its contents. In the average clinic about 60 per cent of patients who are seen because of breast symptomatology will have cystic disease or mastitis, 20 per cent will have cancer, 15 per cent fibroadenomas and the remaining 5 per cent, fat necrosis, tuberculosis or lipoma. The differential diagnosis of masses in the breast may be aided by the use of mammography although the report of the radiologist should be tempered by clinical experience and judgment.

The examination of the abdomen is begun by inspection, noting the presence of scars, striae, distention, dilated veins and umbilical eversion. The patient is then asked to lift her head and cough; this will delineate hernias or diastasis recti. Systematic palpation of the viscera is performed to determine abnormalities of liver, gallbladder, spleen and kidneys. Palpation of the liver is best accomplished with the patient supine, her head and shoulders slightly elevated by pillows. The examiner should stand at the patient's right side, place his left hand under the patient's right flank, pressing gently upward with it, and then place the right hand gently but firmly on the abdominal wall. As the patient takes a deep breath the right hand is moved downward and as the diaphragm descends the liver is carried down and its margin and consistency may be noted. Hepatic enlargement, especially if irregular or nodular, suggests a primary bowel tumor rather than a cancer of the uterus or ovary. An enlarged or tense gallbladder may be similarly palpated. Hydrops of the gallbladder may be confused with acute appendicitis since the tip of the distended gallbladder may extend into the right lower quadrant and since symptoms of nausea and vomiting are frequently associated. The spleen is best palpated by placing the right hand flat with the abdominal wall just at the left costal margin; as the patient inspires, the spleen descends and is palpable if enlarged. The cecum, right colon and sigmoid colon are similarly palpated. The first clue in the diagnosis of diverticulitis of the sigmoid may be obtained at this time if there is tenderness deep in the left lower quadrant. In symmetrical midline tumors, regardless of consistency, consideration should be given to the possibility of an intrauterine pregnancy or a distended bladder. Catheterization will reveal the true nature of the latter, but early pregnancy, especially if coincident with other masses such as fibroids or ovarian cysts, is often difficult to diagnose unless constantly kept in mind. Ovarian cysts may usually be differentiated from ascites by percussion, since with large cysts one usually finds areas of dullness over the cyst with tympany in the flanks. With ascites, the small intestine usually floats anteriorly and is tympanitic whereas the dullness is found laterally.

The costovertebral angles and flanks should also be carefully evaluated in the gynecologic patient since renal and ureteral lesions frequently cause symptoms which the patient interprets as "female trouble." Firm pressure exerted by the index finger in the angle between the spine and the twelfth rib will elicit inflammatory kidney processes which otherwise might go undetected. The procedure for palpating the kidneys is similar to that for palpating the liver.

Both groins are inspected and palpated. Enlargement of the superficial inguinal nodes may be associated with venereal disease (syphilis, granuloma inguinale, chancroid, lymphopathia venereum) and varying degrees of ulceration, so-called "buboes," may be revealed.

Cancer of the vulva or lower vagina, acute nongonorrheal vulvitis, tuberculosis or occasionally superficial infections of the skin of the thigh may all cause inguinal lymphadenopathy. Other causes are plantar or lower extremity melanomas, thigh vaccination and acute bartholinitis. We have recently seen a patient whose chief complaint was a unilateral, firm, 4-cm. inguinal mass. Review of the past history revealed that the right eye had been enucleated five years previously for a melanosarcoma; on excision the inguinal mass was found to be microscopically similar to the primary lesion in the eye. Hodgkin's disease and systemic illnesses characterized by generalized lymphadenopathy should also be considered. In many thin, asthenic females, firm, discrete, mobile inguinal nodes are palpable without apparent cause and need no further investigation. The patient should again be asked to raise her head and cough and careful examination performed for detection of inguinal and femoral hernias. Frequently no cause can be found for a complaint of an "aching soreness" in the lower abdomen until the patient is asked to stand and cough or to exert intra-abdominal pressure. Examination below Poupart's ligament may often reveal a femoral hernia.

The extremities are examined for edema, ulceration, scars of previous surgery and varicose veins. Bilateral edema may be caused by increased intrapelvic pressure from a pregnancy, an old phlebitis or a lymphatic obstruction due to postpartum phlegmasia alba dolens as well as to excess intake of salt. However, it may just as well be due to impaired nutrition associated with low serum albumin, carcinoma of the ovary with ascites or to cardiac failure or chronic nephritis. Its cause bears investigation. Unilateral edema may follow postpartum or postoperative deep phlebothrombosis. Bilateral edema of the extremities is occasionally congenital and occurs without venous or lymphatic obstruction (Milroy's disease). Ulceration of the legs suggests peripheral vascular disease due to venous stasis or diabetes. Varicose veins or scars of previous vein ligation or stripping should be adequate warning to initiate prophylaxis against thromboembolic disease if surgery is contemplated.

It is well for the gynecologist, as well as the student, to stop at this point and consider the differential diagnosis suggested by the history and the general physical examination. In most gynecologic diseases the history, if accurately given and carefully taken, will narrow down the possibilities to three or four conditions. The general physical examination may further reduce this to two or three, or it may suggest that the original complaint may arise from another organ system. If this is so, appropriate x-rays, endoscopy and laboratory procedures should be performed. This will avoid the embarrassment of operating on patients with unsuspected colonic or bladder carcinoma, diverticulitis, renal tumors, pelvic kidneys and ulcerative colitis.

The Pelvic Examination

This is the most important part of the armamentarium of the gynecologist—the ability to see, to palpate and, most of all, to interpret abnormal findings of the female genitalia. Frequently these findings will adequately explain the symptoms of the patient. Often, however, they will bear no relationship and one should not fall into the trap of *post hoc, ergo propter hoc* reasoning at this juncture. Occasionally the pelvic examination will be normal but laboratory procedures such as cytologic examination will aid in diagnosis.

The pelvic examination should be carried out with the patient on an examining table with the legs supported and adequately abducted (Fig. 1–1). The table should be equipped with a movable backrest so that the head may be raised slightly, permitting better relaxation of abdominal muscles. Examinations in bed are difficult and may lead to erroneous interpretations. The buttocks should extend just beyond the edge of the table. Good light is essential. The patient is instructed to urinate just before the examination, since a full bladder may be mistaken for a pregnant uterus or an ovarian cyst. If symptoms suggest urinary tract disease, the bladder is emptied by catheterization or a midstream "catch" specimen is obtained. Although routine enemas are not advised, a full rectum makes the pelvic examination difficult and inconclusive. A clean lower bowel is especially important if the examiner wishes to palpate the rectovaginal septum and uterosacral ligaments, since solid fecal particles may simulate masses and nodularity. If there is any doubt, an enema should be given and the patient re-examined.

A speculum is inserted without lubrication and a small amount of secretion is obtained from the cervix by aspiration or forceps technique and submitted to cytologic examination. Cervical scrapings are routinely performed since malignant cells are occasionally found in this specimen but not in the aspirate. At the Boston Hospital for Women better correlation

Fig. 1–1.—Position for pelvic examination. The patient is placed on the table so that the buttocks extend just beyond the edge of the table. The legs are supported in stirrups and are adequately abducted.

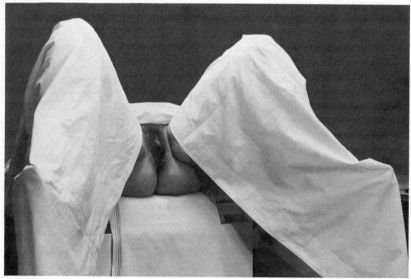

has been obtained between biopsies and cervical aspirations and scrapings than between biopsies and vaginal pool aspirations. This could conceivably be due to poor technique in aspirating the pool in the posterior vagina.

Some mention should be made of the technique of speculum examination. The gynecologist should attempt to use the speculum best adapted for a particular patient and he is aided in this by the variety of instruments available. The one used most commonly is the Graves speculum which has a posterior blade approximately 4½ in. long and 1¼ in. wide at its tip. This speculum is available in lengths varying from 3½ to 5 in. and widths from ¾ to 1¼ in. The posterior blade of the Graves speculum is usually about ¼ in. longer than the anterior blade so as to fit into the longer posterior vaginal wall. In some patients, however, when the cervix lies posteriorly or there is a large cystocele, it is advantageous to have a longer anterior blade. The ordinary speculum may then be rotated, or a modified Graves speculum with a longer anterior blade used. The Pederson speculum is narrower and flatter and may be used to advantage in nulliparous patients or when the vagina is contracted by senescence, scars or radiation. In children a Kelly cystoscope is an ideal instrument for visualization of the vagina.

Before insertion, the speculum should be warmed by holding it under warm water and it should be adequately lubricated unless it is being used for cytologic aspiration. Slight pressure is then exerted on the posterior vaginal wall and perineum by the index and middle finger of the left hand, and care is taken to keep the blades away from the sensitive periurethral area. The speculum should be angled when inserted, so that its greatest width is in the anteroposterior diameter of the vagina (Fig. 1–2). It is then rotated as it is passed along the posterior vaginal wall, and as the tip

Fig. 1–2.—Insertion of speculum. The posterior vaginal wall is depressed by slight pressure with the index finger of the left hand. The speculum is angled to conform to the anteroposterior diameter of the vagina. Care is taken to avoid the periurethral area.

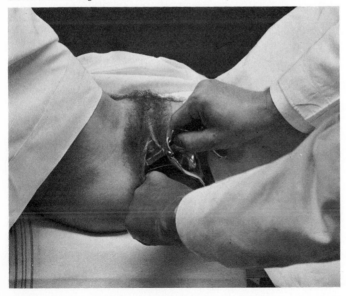

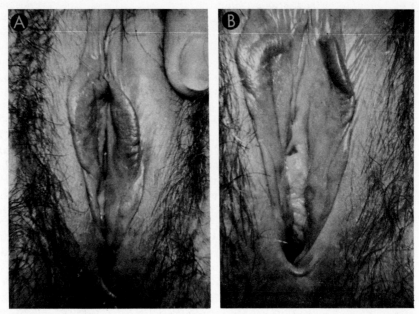

Fig. 1-3.—A, normal vulva of multiparous patient. The outer margins of the labia majora are covered with hair, and a slight degree of gaping of the labia minora permits exposure of the introitus. **B,** labia majora are displaced laterally to show clitoris, which labia minora join anteriorly. The urethral orifice is seen just above a slight relaxation of the anterior vaginal wall. Vaginal orifice is at lowermost portion of labia minora.

reaches the cervix the anterior blade is elevated by pressure on the lever under the lateral screw. When the proper exposure has been obtained the lateral set screw is adjusted. If increased vision in the anteroposterior field is desired, the central set screw may be loosened and the blades separated. When the speculum is removed only the lateral screw should be released, allowing the tips of the blades to fall together. The central screw should not be loosened since, in so doing, vaginal mucosa may be pinched between the lateral aspects of the blades.

Before proceeding to the examination of the vagina and cervix the examiner should methodically inspect the external genitalia. The general features are illustrated in Figure 1-3. A good sequence is to start with the labia majora and minora, noting the size as well as the presence of edema, inflammation, ulceration, crusting, deformity, discoloration or atrophy. Dilated veins, nevi and melanomas are obvious. Evidence of recent trauma, as by rape, should be recorded. Secretions should be examined microscopically and by culture, if indicated. The labia minora should be followed to their junction in the prepuce over the clitoris and enlargement or adhesions noted. Enlargement of the clitoris should alert the examiner to search for other stigmata of virilism and the possibility of an adrenal tumor. At this point the mons veneris and pubic hair distribution are observed for pediculosis and dermatitis. The thumb and index finger of the right hand separate the labia minora as shown in Figure 1-5, exposing the vestibule with the vaginal and urethral openings as well as those of the periurethral (Skene's) and vulvovaginal (Bartholin's) glands. At this point the patient may be asked to strain down or cough. This will delineate pelvic floor relaxation and urinary incontinence. The index finger of the gloved (left) hand is then inserted gently under the urethra and it is compressed toward the external orifice. A purulent exudate suggests gonorrhea and should be stained and cultured. The urethral orifice should be observed also for polyps, prolapse of the mucosa, ulceration or caruncle. The index finger may then be rotated and the ducts of the periurethral glands stripped. The vulvovaginal glands should be sought for, placing the index finger in the vagina and the thumb on the perineal skin. Normally they are not palpable, but undue tenderness, swelling or fluctuation suggests Bartholin's cyst or abscess. At this time the posterior commissure and perineal body may be inspected and palpated. The condition of previous episiotomies should be noted as well as small dimples which indicate the presence of vaginoperineal or vaginorectal fistulas. The integrity of the levator ani muscle may be tested but this is better done by a later combined rectovaginal examination.

Attention is next given to the condition of the hymen. In young adolescents one commonly finds the ring intact but with a small opening which may admit the index finger. Occasionally the tissue is extremely fibrotic and even the smallest finger cannot be inserted. In parous women the hymen may be in excellent condition, depending on the rigors of delivery and the technique of the obstetrician. Usually, however, it is absent in its lower third but remnants (the carunculae myrtiformes) are found anteriorly. In postmenopausal virgins the hymen is frequently tight and contracted so that even the passage of a small glass tube is impossible. Hematomas and fresh lacerations may indicate recent attempts at rape.

The examination of the internal genitalia requires a minimum amount of equipment, which is both inexpensive and simple to use. Figure 1–4 illustrates a typical arrangement used in our clinic.

The internal examination is begun by introducing first one and then two

Fig. 1–4.—Typical arrangement of the basic instruments and supplies for an adequate gynecologic examination. Bottles left to right: alcohol, Alkalol, Schiller's solution, Oxycel. Jars contain gauze pledgets and cotton balls. Tampons are at right of jars. Three Graves and one Pederson specula are at far left. Then, in order, tube and aspiration bulb for cytology, cotton-tipped metal applicators, cervical tenaculum, uterine sound, endometrial curet, thumb forceps (long), three cervical dilators sizes 11–16, three nasal-tip cauteries, lubricating jelly. A cervical biopsy punch (extra long) is shown below the jars.

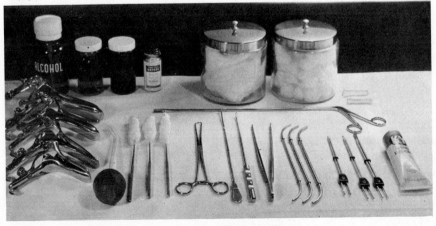

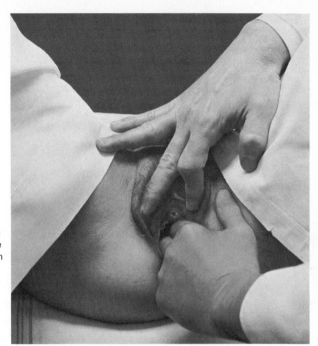

Fig. 1–5.—Method of beginning the internal examination. The labia majora and minora are held apart with the fingers of the right hand and first one and then two fingers of the left hand are gently inserted along the posterior vaginal wall.

fingers of the left hand along the posterior vaginal wall (Fig. 1–5). The reason for a right-handed examiner to use his left hand for the internal examination is twofold: it allows freedom of the right hand for forceps, biopsy instruments, cautery, insufflator, etc., and it allows the more trained hand to palpate the pelvic viscera through the abdomen after they have been lifted into position by the left hand. Specifically then, the fingers elevate and support the uterus and adnexae while the external hand is used to determine the anatomic details of these structures. In addition, any abnormalities of the vagina are noted and the size, shape and consistency of the cervix is determined, as is the patency of its external os. The cervix may then be moved laterally; if pain results, it suggests the presence of an inflammatory process. A widely patulous, soft cervix is usually found in patients with an inevitable or incomplete abortion, whereas a widely patulous, firm cervix may be palpable around a protruding leiomyoma or pedunculated adenomyoma. Cervical polyps are easily palpable as movable, soft, fleshy projections, whereas stony hardness is characteristic of carcinoma.

The vaginal fingers may note at the outset a third-degree uterine retroversion as they advance toward the posterior cul-de-sac, or nodularity and scarring of the uterosacral ligaments may suggest the presence of endometriosis.

The normal position of the uterus is one of anteversion with some anteflexion of the corpus on the cervix. To palpate the uterus, the simplest method is to place the two vaginal fingers under the cervix and elevate it and the uterine corpus toward the abdominal wall (Fig. 1–6). The external

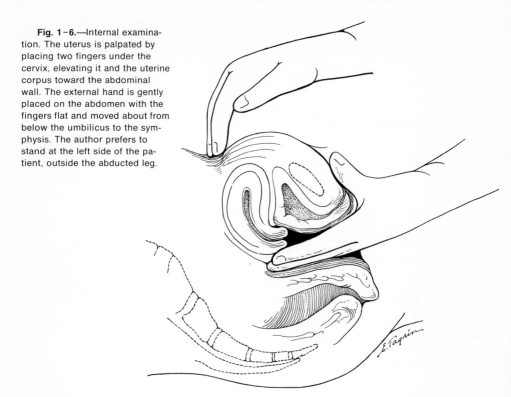

Fig. 1–6.—Internal examination. The uterus is palpated by placing two fingers under the cervix, elevating it and the uterine corpus toward the abdominal wall. The external hand is gently placed on the abdomen with the fingers flat and moved about from below the umbilicus to the symphysis. The author prefers to stand at the left side of the patient, outside the abducted leg.

hand is gently placed on the abdomen with the fingers flat and is moved about from below the umbilicus to the symphysis. Intermittent pressure on the uterus between the fingers of both hands will yield information as to size, shape and consistency. Ballottement between the two hands yields important information regarding mobility.

The left adnexal area is usually examined next. This is accomplished by moving the vaginal fingers to the left of the cervix so that they occupy the lateral and uppermost part of the vagina (Fig. 1–7). If the patient is cooperative, the vaginal fingers can actually be placed under the posterior portion of the broad ligament. On the left side the ovary is frequently underneath the sigmoid colon so that abdominal palpation must begin rather high. By a series of caudad displacements the hand is brought over the ovary, which can usually be palpated between the two hands. The vaginal fingers usually serve only to support the ovary while the external hand palpates for size, shape and mobility. The oviduct is usually not palpable in its normal state. The right ovary is palpated in the same fashion; however, if it is not easily felt, the examiner should change hands and place the right hand in the vagina. The natural curvature of the right hand sometimes makes it easier to outline the right adnexae.

In performing the internal examination it is important to bear in mind several points. (1) Always begin gently, usually with the insertion of one well-lubricated finger along the posterior vagina. (2) Gradually insinuate two fingers under the cervix. (3) Apply the abdominal hand easily, slowly

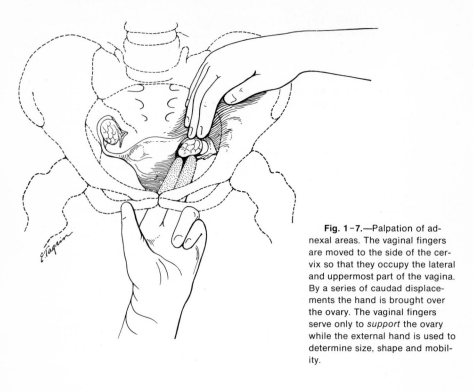

Fig. 1–7.—Palpation of ad-nexal areas. The vaginal fingers are moved to the side of the cer-vix so that they occupy the lateral and uppermost part of the vagina. By a series of caudad displace-ments the hand is brought over the ovary. The vaginal fingers serve only to *support* the ovary while the external hand is used to determine size, shape and mobil-ity.

Fig. 1–8.—Method of internal pelvic examination. To obtain additional length, the left foot may be placed on a small stool, the left elbow rested against the knee and the pelvic floor then invaginated by firm pressure.

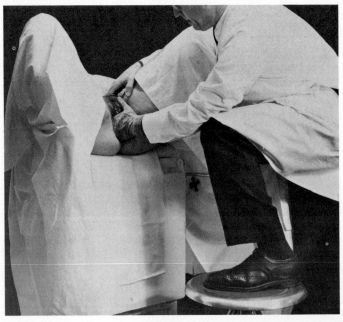

and keep it in motion. (4) Never apply force or use abrupt motion, since the initial reflex resistance will then actually increase and examination will become impossible. (5) Always examine the painful side last. (6) Employ reassuring discussion with the patient and have her breathe through her mouth during the examination to aid in securing relaxation.

Students are frequently discouraged about their inability to palpate the ovaries or masses in the sides of the pelvis, feeling that they cannot reach them. If the fingers are somewhat shorter than normal, or if a mass seems high up, additional length may be obtained by placing the left foot on a small stool, resting the left elbow against the knee and then invaginating the pelvic floor by firm pressure (Fig. 1–8). Another method is to place the middle finger in the rectum and the index finger in the vagina (Fig. 1–9). This will enable the examiner to reach almost 1 in. higher into the pelvis and is of inestimable value in differentiating left-sided ovarian cysts from diverticulitis or thickening of the sigmoid colon. Before withdrawal of the vaginal fingers an attempt should be made to palpate the ureters through the anterior vaginal wall. Unusual degrees of tenderness or thickening suggest inflammatory or neoplastic processes.

In describing the findings, it is important to bear in mind that all observers will not interpret the palpatory findings in the same way. Therefore, it is better to give accurate or estimated measurements in centimeters rather than in terms of fruit, eggs or balls of various sizes. This need not be carried *ad absurdum,* however, and if both ovaries are normal in all respects it is simpler to report "sides of the pelvis negative." Abnormal masses should

Fig. 1–9.—Combined vaginorectal examination enables the examiner to reach almost 1 in. higher into the pelvis. Thickening of the rectovaginal septum, cul-de-sac nodules, fixed uterine retroversion and involvement of the broad ligaments by tumor are more accurately outlined by this method.

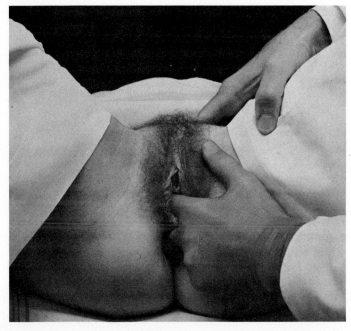

be described as to size, shape, consistency, mobility, position and whether or not they are tender.

The speculum examination is performed utilizing the technique previously described. The vaginal mucosa is inspected as the speculum is introduced, with observation made of the amount of rugation or the presence of discharge. Primary diseases of the vagina (excluding simple vaginitis) are not too common, but one should look for congenital abnormalities such as vaginal septa, double vaginas, double cervixes and Gartner duct cysts. The cervix is then brought into view and the light adjusted so that the entire portio epithelium is visible. A cotton-tipped applicator is dipped in Alkalol (an alkaline, saline solution which dissolves mucus) and the cervix is liberally swabbed. The entire area is then dried with a second applicator, and a third is used to apply Schiller's solution to the cervix and upper vagina. (Schiller's solution: 1 part iodine, 2 parts potassium iodide to 300 part of water.) The normal stratified squamous epithelium of the vagina and portio vaginalis of the cervix is rich in glycogen and stains dark brown with Schiller's solution. Abnormal squamous epithelium (whether it be acutely inflamed, leukoplakia, leukoparakeratosis, carcinoma in situ or carcinoma) does not stain. The endocervical cells also do not stain, so that an obvious erosion (really an ectropion of endocervical cells) must be differentiated from a true "Schiller-positive" or nonstaining area of squamous epithelium. We routinely do a biopsy of all Schiller-positive areas, preferably at the junction of the staining and non-staining areas. Biopsy is also done on all erosions prior to cauterization—reasons for which will be given in the chapter on the cervix.

After the cervix has been studied, a uterine sound is passed through the cervical os to determine the length of the uterine cavity. This is of particular value if the position and the size of the uterus are not definitely determined at the time of bimanual examination. The sound should be passed gently and not forced, since perforation may occur without undue pressure. In postmenopausal women it is especially important to know whether or not the cervical canal is patent. If it is closed, steps to open it should be taken since endometrial carcinoma would not give the usual early symptom of bleeding in this instance.

The vaginorectal examination is performed as previously described. Its importance lies in the fact that, by gaining extra depth, lesions of the posterior cul-de-sac, uterosacral ligaments and rectovaginal septum will become obvious. Frequently a uterus in fixed third-degree retroversion can be outlined only by this method. This examinaton is followed by a thorough digital examination of the anus and rectum. The fact that about one half of the malignancies of the rectosigmoid may be palpated by careful digital exploration is adequate reason for making this part of the examination an integral step in the gynecologic survey. A guaiac test for blood in the stool should be a routine in every rectal examination. If blood was noted in the examination of the vagina, the glove should be changed before performing the rectal examination.

CHAPTER 2

The Vulva

General Considerations

THE VULVA, or external female genitalia, includes the following structures: labia majora, labia minora, clitoris, vestibule, hymen, vestibular bulbs, mons veneris, urethral meatus, vulvovaginal glands and periurethral gland ducts. The outer portion of the vulva is covered by somewhat altered skin which contains hair follicles and sweat and sebaceous glands. This is modified on the inner surface so that the inner portions of the labia minora are moist and do not contain hair follicles. The vulva serves as the entrance to the vagina and, in the normal state, covers and protects the urethral orifice. The labia have specific importance in the process of urination since it has been found that, following vulvectomy, uncontrolled "spraying" is a common complaint.

The anatomic location of the vulva predisposes its structures to unusual and occasionally rare disorders. At the same time, systemic diseases such as diabetes, anemia, Addison's disease and gout may manifest themselves first by vulvar changes and complaints therefrom. The importance of venereal diseases as a major cause of symptomatology from these structures is obvious, and each will be considered in detail in this chapter. Since a good portion of the vulvar area may be properly classified as skin, it is at once evident that any specific cutaneous disease may occur here, but because of certain variations diagnosis may be difficult or even impossible. Difficulty in diagnosis is aggravated by the tendency of the patient to procrastinate and to utilize self-medication when the lesion involves the genitalia. Patient delay is of extreme importance when the disease is malignant since carcinoma involving these structures has a poor prognosis unless discovered early. Of equal importance in this problem is the responsibility of the physician. Numerous studies have shown that "physician delay" may actually exceed "patient delay" by many months.

Success in the diagnosis and treatment of lesions of the vulva will be forthcoming only if the physician investigates completely all possible etiologic factors and performs a meticulous examination. A thorough interview should determine the exact site and duration of specific complaints as well as generalized symptoms. Inquiry should be made about diarrhea or discharge, applications of lotions, medications or soaps, systemic medications, contraceptives, sexual habits, clothing changes and, of major importance, events which might be causative in producing mental stress, worry or anxiety. The examiner should scrutinize closely the oral mucosa, fingernails, scalp and pubic hair as part of the gynecologic examination. It is not sufficient to allay symptoms, since recurrence is commonplace. Therefore, the cause of the disorder must be found and specific therapy instituted.

Embryology

In the female, as in the male, the external genitalia develop in connection with the genital tubercle, a conical prominence caudal to the umbilical cord. This tubercle appears in the 8 mm. embryo (5 weeks)* as a simple protrusion (Fig. 2–1) and later is noted to present a groove along its caudal surface—the urethral groove. The urethra is subsequently formed from this groove. The genital tubercle becomes clearly defined as a phallus in the 16–18 mm. embryo (6–7 weeks), whereas the specific external genitalia of either male or female type are formed in the 40 mm. embryo (10 weeks).

The cloacal membrane is an epithelial structure located in the ventral portion of the embryo caudal to the genital tubercle. This membrane consists of an inner (cephalic) layer of entodermal cells and an outer (caudal) layer of ectodermal cells. When the cloacal membrane perforates about the twelfth week the openings of the urethra, vagina and anus are clearly visible. The rudimentary external genitalia appear about the sixth week of

Fig. 2–1.—Schematic representation of 9 mm. human embryo in frontal section to show anatomic relations of the genital tubercle. (After Kollman.)

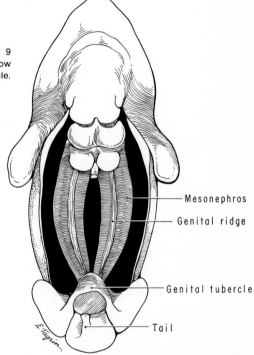

Mesonephros

Genital ridge

Genital tubercle

Tail

*Measurements correspond to values of F. P. Mall, and ages are "ovulation age," or two weeks less than menstrual age.

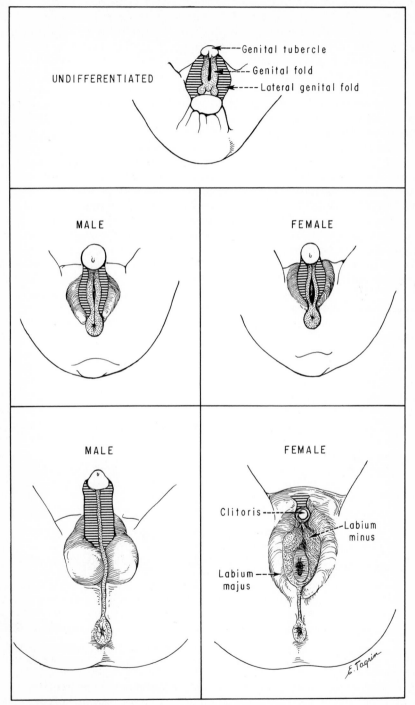

Fig. 2-2.—Schematic drawing to show the homologous development of the external genitalia from the undifferentiated state.

embryonic life as swellings on either side of the cloacal membrane. These swellings later project to form the genital folds which extend cephalad to join the genital tubercle (Fig. 2–2). The genital folds become the labia minora and the clitoris is derived from the genital tubercle. The labia majora develop from swellings at the outer sides of the genital folds (lateral genital folds). These lateral genital folds join cephalad to form the genital eminence or mons veneris, whereas caudad they curve medially to form the posterior commissure. About the fifth or sixth month a secondary upgrowth of tissue around the clitoris forms a fold or hood about it, the preputium clitoridis or prepuce.

When the cloaca becomes divided into a dorsal and ventral segment by the downgrowth of a septum, which grows mainly from mesoderm, two compartments are formed. The ventral portion constitutes the urogenital sinus and is bounded at its lower end by the cloacal membrane. The wolffian ducts are imbedded in this mesoderm of the downgrowing septum on either side and later become implanted in the septum. When division is complete they open into the urogenital sinus. Above the site of their implantation the urogenital sinus dilates to become the urinary bladder. The dorsal segment formed by the aforementioned downgrowth of mesoderm (sometimes called the urorectal fold) differentiates into the rectum. Thus, at this stage of development (12–14 mm. embryo) both rectum and bladder are continuous with the urogenital sinus which is closed at its lower end by the cloacal membrane (Fig. 2–3). Bartholin's glands appear as outgrowths from the walls of the urogenital sinus.

At the site where the solid müllerian ducts join the sinus the hymen is ultimately formed. As these solid masses of cells at the termination of the müllerian ducts proliferate, vaginal bulbs form which grow downward along the posterior wall of the sinus. They increase in size and press against the walls of the sinus, invaginating it, so that the upper part of the sinus becomes gradually shortened. In this manner, the openings of the ducts of Bartholin's glands are brought close to the hymenal margin. Later the solid vagina, thus formed, breaks down in the center and, at the site where its cavity opens into the sinus, the hymenal orifice is formed. The remainder of the urogenital sinus in front of the hymen forms the vestibule. Fig. 2–4 illustrates the definitive female genital system.

Anatomy and Histology

Labia Majora.—The skin covering the labia majora is thick, contains many sebaceous and sweat glands and is covered by hair, except along the lower part of the inner aspect. The extent of the glandular development is pronounced and accounts for the frequency of sebaceous retention cysts and hair follicle infections in this region. On the inner aspect of the labia majora, the sebaceous glands empty directly on the skin surface and are less numerous. The skin is made up of typical stratified squamous epithelium with moderate keratosis and a well-vascularized dermis (Fig. 2–5). Involuntary muscle fibers, or dartos, are present but are much less developed than in the corresponding tissue, the scrotum, of the male. A large amount of fatty tissue is usually present, situated in lobules separated by

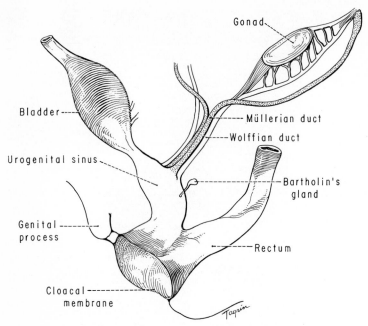

Fig. 2–3.—Schematic drawing of the undifferentiated genital system of the 12–14 mm. embryo. (After Arey.)

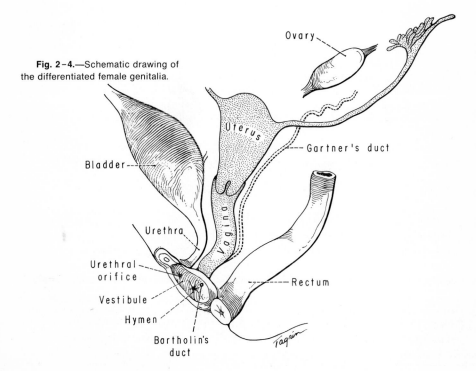

Fig. 2–4.—Schematic drawing of the differentiated female genitalia.

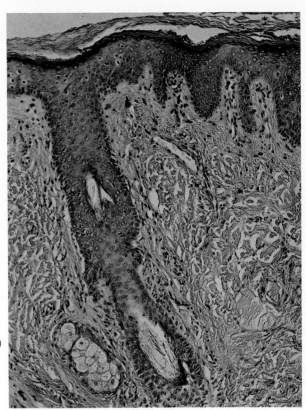

Fig. 2–5.—Photomicrograph of labium majus, showing normal histology.

elastic and connective tissue fibers. This elastic connective tissue forms a well-defined sac with an inner opening pointing toward the inguinal region. It is at this point that the round ligament enters the labium from each side, its fibers disintegrating and passing into the fibroelastic sac just described.

The labia majora form the lateral extent of the vulva. These folds continue cephalad toward the lower abdomen and fuse in the midline as the anterior commissure or mons pubis. The union of the labia majora caudally is known as the posterior commissure and is the lowermost extent of the vulva (Fig. 2–6).

The blood supply of the labia majora is derived from the internal pudendal artery through the posterior labial branch and also from a small branch of the obturator artery. The veins have approximately the same source but also communicate with the vesicovaginal plexus and the inferior hemorrhoidal veins. The nerve supply is from multiple sources. The pudendal nerve, derived from the second to fourth sacral nerves, gives off the perineal branch from which the posterior labial nerve arises. The latter innervates the labia majora and the lateral portion of the urethral triangle. In addition, adjunctive supply is afforded by the ilioinguinal, internal branch of the genitocrural and the genital branch of the lesser

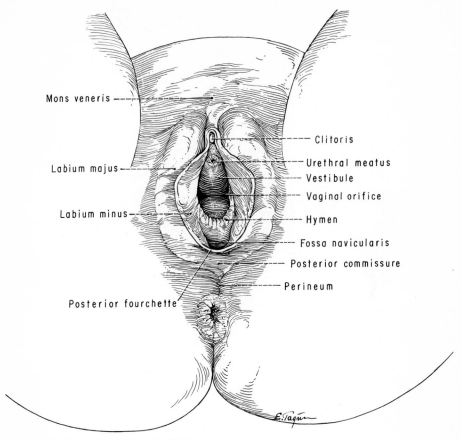

Mons veneris

Labium majus

Labium minus

Posterior fourchette

Clitoris

Urethral meatus

Vestibule

Vaginal orifice

Hymen

Fossa navicularis

Posterior commissure

Perineum

Fig. 2–6.—External genitalia of the female.

sciatic (posterior femoral cutaneous). The nerve supply of the perineum and vulva is shown in Figure 2–7.

Labia Minora.—The labia minora consist of two cutaneous folds which are usually concealed by the majora. In certain instances they may be greatly hypertrophied and project beyond the majora. They lie directly approximate to each other with a convex free border and extend caudad from the prepuce of the clitoris to join the labia majora as they terminate in the posterior fourchette. Between this fourchette and the hymenal ring is a curved depression, the fossa navicularis (see Fig. 2–6). The labia minora are reduplications of skin and not mucosa, although some pathologists have classified the labia minora and vagina as "mucous membrane" and the labia majora as skin. However, mucus is not secreted from either the vagina or the labia minora.

The skin of the labia minora contains abundant pigment and blood vessels. Microscopically the stratified squamous epithelium is characterized by minimal keratinization, but the rete ridges are numerous and prominent. The dermis is made up of connective tissue fibers with numer-

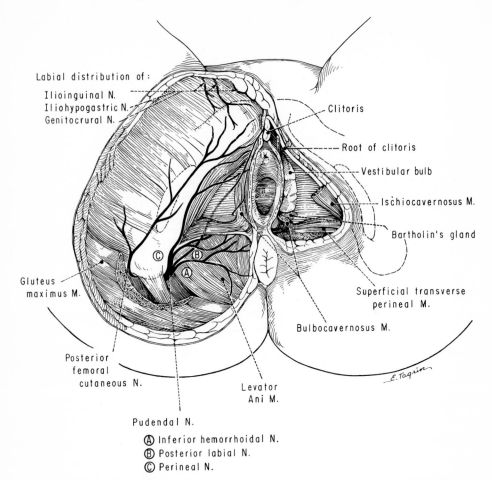

Labial distribution of:
Ilioinguinal N.
Iliohypogastric N.
Genitocrural N.

Clitoris

Root of clitoris

Vestibular bulb

Ischiocavernosus M.

Bartholin's gland

Superficial transverse perineal M.

Bulbocavernosus M.

Gluteus maximus M.

Posterior femoral cutaneous N.

Levator Ani M.

Pudendal N.
Ⓐ Inferior hemorrhoidal N.
Ⓑ Posterior labial N.
Ⓒ Perineal N.

Fig. 2-7.—The nerve supply of the vulva is represented at left. At the right, the ischiocavernosus and bulbocavernosus muscles have been reflected to show the anatomy of the clitoris and vestibular bulbs.

ous bundles of elastic tissue and blood vessels but with minimal fatty tissue. Sweat glands and hair follicles are usually absent but sebaceous glands are abundant (Fig. 2-8). As mentioned, the prepuce of the clitoris is continuous with the labia minora and is histologically similar except for its extreme vascularity. The blood supply is derived from the labial vessels, as previously described, and from the dorsal artery to the clitoris which is a terminal branch of the internal pudendal artery. The nerve supply is the same as that of the labia majora.

The labia minora may become enlarged following prolonged manipulation or masturbation so that, even in virginal women, they may project beyond the majora. Immediately preceding and during coitus they become moist and lubricated with secretions from the vulvovaginal and sebaceous glands.

Clitoris.—This structure is composed of two roots which traverse the

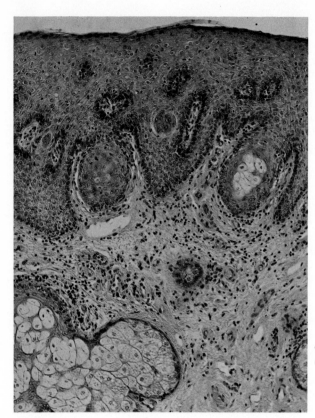

Fig. 2-8.—Photomicrograph of labium minus, showing normal histology.

pubic rami to unite beneath the symphysis in the clitoridean body. The body terminates in the upper portion of the vestibule as the glans. The roots and body are covered by overlying muscle, but the glans is exposed. Figure 2-7 illustrates the relationship of the root of the clitoris to the overlying ischiocavernosus muscle. The roots, or crura, are 3-4 cm. long in the flaccid state but in erection are 4.5-5 cm. long. The body is 2.5-3 cm. in length and is surrounded by a connective tissue capsule of fibroelastic tissue termed the clitoridean fascia. The covering of the glans is modified cutaneous tissue, not mucosa. Unlike the penis, the glans clitoridis contains no corpus spongiosum and does not possess as much erectile tissue.

The function of the clitoris seems to be that of a "nerve-center" for coitus. Prior to contact, sexual stimulation causes vascular engorgement and enlargement, so that when the penis is inserted the clitoris becomes particularly sensitive to the to-and-fro motion of the shaft. Orgasm in the female may be brought about by this stimulation even in the absence of the vagina and consists of an interrelated reflex resulting in forceful contractions of both voluntary and involuntary musculature of the pelvis and pelvic viscera. After the process of orgasm has been experienced and a conditioned reflex established, the presence of the clitoris is not absolutely necessary. Women who have had simple or radical vulvectomy with excision of the clitoris are capable of experiencing orgasm.

The arteries of the clitoris arise from the internal pudendal artery. The veins correspond to the arteries, except for the large dorsal vein of the clitoris which runs beneath the arcuate ligament of the symphysis through a small notch and communicates with the pelvic veins.

Vestibular Bulbs.—These correspond to the corpus spongiosum of the male and consist of truncated masses of erectile tissue placed on either side of the vaginal orifice. They are situated above the inferior fascia of the pelvic diaphragm and below the bulbocavernosus muscles (Fig. 2-7). The anterior ends taper to join the bulb of the opposite side in the pars intermedia, whereas the posterior surfaces are in contact with Bartholin's glands.

Hymen.—This is an irregular, membranous fold of varying thickness which partially occludes the vaginal orifice. It extends from the floor of the urethra to the fossa navicularis and may be complete (imperforate), totally absent, incomplete, or cribriform in type. The hymen may be avulsed by examination, trauma, surgery or coitus. Usually irregular remnants persist, forming a fleshy fringe about the vaginal opening (the carunculae myrtiformes).

Vestibule.—The vestibule is an elliptical space which is situated just inside the labia minora and extends from the glans clitoridis to the posterior side of the hymenal ring. The orifices of the urethra, vagina and vulvovaginal gland ducts open into the vestibule (Fig. 2-6).

Mons Veneris.—The mons veneris is the most cephalad portion of the vulva (Fig. 2-6) and consists of an accumulation of subcutaneous fat in excess amount in a rounded pad overlying the symphysis pubis. It is covered by pubic hair and the skin is similar to that of the labia majora. The fat pad characteristically remains even after marked inanition and weight loss. The typical female escutcheon of hair over the mons is triangular in shape and usually does not extend upward along the abdomen although there is much variation in this respect, depending on racial and familial traits.

Urethral Meatus.—This structure, the orifice of the urethra, is situated just caudad to the glans clitoridis and may be visualized by separating the labia minora. It has a cleftlike appearance with slightly raised lateral margins and is the uppermost structure of the vestibule (Fig. 2-6).

Periurethral Gland Ducts.—These ducts are the external orifices of the periurethral (Skene's) glands which are situated beneath the urethral floor. The orifices are extremely small, yet are usually grossly visible crypts just lateral to and somewhat posterior to the urethral orifice. These glands arise, as do the mucous glands which empty into the distal urethra, from the urethral mucosa itself and are histologically similar. They are stated to be the rudimentary homologue of the prostate gland in the male and are commonly involved by the gonococcus, in which case pus may be expressed from the openings.

Vulvovaginal Glands.—These structures, known commonly as Bartholin's glands, are the homologue of the bulbourethral glands in the male. They are racemose in type and secrete mucus, particularly during sexual stimulation. Situated at each side of the vaginal orifice, below the hymen, the glands are normally small and can be palpated only in rather thin women or if enlarged by inflammation or tumor. The duct openings are in the posterior introitus. Rapid growth occurs at puberty and shrinkage occurs after menopause. Microscopically, the glands show a single layer of high columnar epithelium in the alveoli but the duct is lined by transitional epithelium except for a short invagination of stratified squamous epithelium at the orifice.

Malformations

Congenital malformations of the vulva are rare but do occur in association with the stigmata of female hermaphroditism, hypospadias or incomplete cloacal separations. Complete absence (aplasia) of the vulva occasionally accompanies rudimentary internal genitalia and resembles the secondary atrophy of senility. The labia majora may show some differentiation but are flattened and contain little fat and practically no hair follicles. The labia minora are present, the clitoris rudimentary and the perineal body short.

Vulvar atresia may occur but is usually incomplete and consists of partial agglutination of the labia with stenosis of the introitus and occasionally an imperforate hymen. Vulvar duplication may occur along with duplication of the vagina, cervix and uterus. Vulvar fusion has recently been described in the newborn following the administration of certain progestational agents to the mother during the first 12 weeks of gestation (see Chapter 10).

Hymen.—The hymen is often involved in developmental defects, the most common types being the (1) imperforate, (2) septate, (3) fenestrate and (4) cribriform. An imperforate hymen is usually unnoticed until the menarche, at which time menstrual blood accumulates behind the membrane with resultant hematocolpos and hematometra. Blood may rarely be forced into the peritoneal cavity, giving rise to the signs and symptoms of peritonitis. The diagnosis is usually obvious by inspection, a bluish, bulging

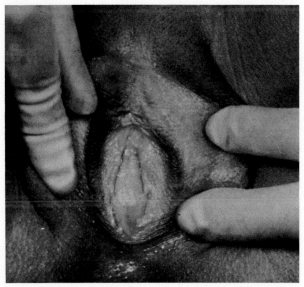

Fig. 2–9.—Imperforate hymen.

membrane presenting at the introitus (Fig. 2–9). Rectal examination will reveal a distended vagina and an enlarged uterus (occasionally the size of a 12–14 week gestation). This condition should be treated in the operating room by a generous cruciate incision, or by excising a portion of the hymen. Further surgery or exploration is not warranted at this time.

A rigid hymen is frequently seen as a cause for dyspareunia. This may be due to the presence of an excess amount of tough, fibrous tissue or to the presence of multiple small orifices, none of which is large enough to admit the penis. Although both of these types may be helped by gradual dilatation, surgical correction is preferable. A hymenectomy is a simple procedure, necessitates hospitalization for only a day or so and the results are immediate and permanent.

Clitoris.—The most common abnormality of the clitoris is not really a malformation but an enlargement seen in association with hermaphroditism. The latter condition may be due to adrenal hyperplasia or tumor, gonadal dysgenesis or unknown causes. Arrhenoblastoma or hilus cell tumor of the ovary may also cause enlargement of the clitoris.

In this complex problem of sex identification and intersexuality certain criteria are necessary for proper diagnosis and therapy. This has been aided by simple laboratory methods which determine chromosomal sex. At present three methods are available: (1) observation of nuclei in a smear from the vaginal or oral mucosa (distinctive sex chromatin usually near the inner surface of the nuclear membrane) identifies the chromosomal female; (2) study of neutrophils in a blood smear (in chromosomal females about 2–3 per cent of neutrophils have an accessory nuclear lobule); (3) determination of epidermal nuclei in a skin biopsy (in chromosomal females the typical sex chromatin occurs in from two-thirds to three-fourths of the nuclei). (See chapter on cytogenetics.)

Hermaphroditism is present when there is lack of correlation in the four basic morphologic criteria, that is, sex chromosome pattern, gonad structure, external genital morphology and internal genital morphology. True hermaphroditism exists only when both male and female elements are present in the gonad. Ambisexual individuals with male gonads only are properly termed male hermaphrodites, whereas ambisexual individuals with female gonads only are termed female hermaphrodites. The prefix "pseudo" is redundant if classification according to this scheme is used.

Enlargement of the clitoris has been noted in all varieties. Thus in mixed gonadal dysgenesis, as exemplified in Turner's syndrome (ovarian agenesis), the patient usually has normal female external genitalia and is therefore reared as a girl. The chromosomal pattern, however, usually is male and in a few of these patients enlargement of the clitoris has been reported. It has been theorized that this chromosomal male, because of an inadequate male gonad, has been feminized during intrauterine gestation by environmental factors such as high maternal estrogen. Experiments by Jost and others have demonstrated the dominance of female developmental patterns, so that all genital structures will be female unless an adequate male gonad is present. Such patterns may be altered by excessive endogenous or exogenous androgens.

In female hermaphroditism with virilization the chromosomal pattern is female and the gonad is an ovary. The virilization (enlarged clitoris to form a phallus, fusion of scrotolabial folds, hirsutism) is apparently due to deficient secretion of corticoids by the fascicular zone of the adrenal cortex. Subsequent increased ACTH stimulates the reticular layer of the adrenal to become hyperplastic, with secretion of large amounts of virilizing steroids. This process may begin during the intrauterine phase so that at birth abnormalities of varying degree may be present. The use of cortisone in the prepuberal period has permitted feminization, ovulation and menstruation to occur. Surgical correction of the external genital defects will usually restore their functional capacity.

A few patients have been classified as female hermaphrodites without virilization. There has usually been a penile urethra or simple hypospadias with fusion of the scrotolabial folds. The cause of this malformation is unknown, since there is not an excess of androgenic secretion present. The use of androgens or androgen-like substances (synthetic progestogens) in the treatment of the mother during the early phases of pregnancy has been suggested as being etiologic in some cases.

Male hermaphroditism may be classified into major groups depending on the external genitalia. The chromosomal sex is male and the gonad is basically a testis. In one group, however, the gonad contains many Sertoli cells, which apparently secrete estrogen so that at puberty the feminine sex characteristics develop. Ovulation and menstruation, of course, do not occur but vulvar formation is usually normal and the patient is reared as a female and presents herself for examination because of primary amenorrhea. Removal of the gonads (because of the possibility of later malignancy) results in a fall of urinary estrogens and 17-ketosteroids and a rise in urinary gonadotropin. These patients should continue to live as females. (See testicular feminization in Chapter 16, Cytogenetics.)

In the second group of male hermaphrodites the external genitalia are not so definite and all variations from normal male to that of a small phallus with fused scrotolabial folds may be seen. The chromosome pattern is male, as is the gonad. Feminization does not occur since estrogen is not secreted in demonstrable amounts.

Urethra.—Malformations of the urethra include stenosis, diverticula and hypospadias. Mild degrees of stenosis are fairly common and usually cause no symptoms. In some patients there may be tenesmus and recurrent cystitis from urinary retention. Urethral dilatation and treatment of the cystitis are attended by marked relief. Diverticula may be regarded as an abnormality resulting from incomplete development of the urethrovaginal septum. There may be single or multiple outpouchings of the urethra along its caudal surface but without connection with the vagina. The diagnosis is made by expressing urine or occasionally pus by firm pressure on the diverticulum. Treatment should be surgical excision. Hypospadias also results from an incomplete separation of the urethra from the vagina, with a resultant congenital urethrovaginal fistula. It may be looked on embryologically as an arrest in the normal development of the urethra in which the posterior (ventral) aspect is incomplete. Thus, in the female, an opening persists between the urethra and the vagina. (Epispadias is extremely rare and refers to the urethral orifice being anterior (ventral) to its normal position, e.g., clitoral, subsymphyseal or complete, as in bladder exstrophy). Treatment in hypospadias (or epispadias) is surgical.

Physiologic Alterations

The vulvar skin represents a surface area which is sensitive to many systemic alterations and diseases and may be the site of the first cutaneous manifestation of such conditions. The most commonly encountered diseases are diabetes, uremia, blood dyscrasias, specific vitamin deficiencies and certain circulatory disturbances.

Diabetes.—Many diabetic patients have a certain amount of stress incontinence, resulting in urine of high sugar content constantly wetting the vulva. This predisposes the area to the growth of fungi, yeasts and bacteria. Obesity with concomitant intertrigo aggravates this situation. An additional important factor is the nicotinic acid and riboflavin deficiencies so often associated with abnormal carbohydrate metabolism. Such an avitaminosis may result in vulvar edema with itching, scratching and ulceration. The labia characteristically have a dusky red color, occasionally purplish (Fig. 2–10). Any patient who complains of vulvar pruritus should be suspected of having diabetes mellitus, and adequate diagnostic measures must be performed. At the Boston Hospital for Women such patients are screened by means of a two-hour postprandial blood sugar determination. Treatment should aim at correction of the metabolic imbalance plus specific measures for the vulvitis.

Uremia.—The "urea frost" of the oral mucosa is occasionally seen also on the vulva in patients with long-standing uremia. The labial surfaces are covered with a gray membrane, with encrustations of urea and uric acid. Superficial areas of ulceration and necrosis may be identified. Treatment is supportive, consisting of correction of the elevated urea level and dehydration, local cleanliness and administration of vitamins.

Blood Dyscrasias.—Leukemia, aplastic anemia and agranulocytosis may

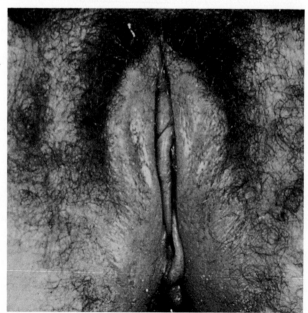

Fig. 2–10.—Diabetic vulvitis.

cause rather typical vulvar ulceration. These ulcers are deep, well-demarcated, oval lesions covered usually with a thin, gray membrane. Such lesions have been found following administration of drugs which result in depressed bone marrow function (e.g., methotrexate) and, if death does not ensue, they heal spontaneously following removal of the drug. In pernicious anemia, vulvar ulceration and hyperpigmentation may be part of the generalized tissue devitalization and hypovitaminosis so characteristic of that disease.

Vitamin Deficiencies.—Many vulvar lesions unfortunately are quickly camouflaged by scratching, local medications or secondary infection. This is particularly true of vitamin deficiency states affecting the vulva, so that primary diagnosis becomes difficult. Deficiency of thiamine is probably the most common, but riboflavin lack may favor monilial growth and pellagra may be associated with infected vulvar ulcerations. Specific cases of vulvar "eczema" have responded well to pyridoxine, whereas some patients with psoriasis have noted temporary improvement following vitamin D therapy. Administration of vitamin B complex will occasionally result in dramatic improvement in lichen planus, and the theoretical implication of vitamin A deficiency in the etiology of leukoplakia has received wide publicity but is not borne out in clinical practice.

Circulatory Disturbances.—These are most commonly evident as edema, varicose veins and simple hypertrophy. Because of the loose connective tissue of the labia majora, marked edema may be found in generalized anasarca, portal obstruction or pelvic tumors. A severe edema may be associated with inflammatory conditions such as a chancre or may follow prolonged scratching. The chronic edema of filariasis found especially in oriental countries and due to an infection with Filaria sanguinis is considered to be due to blockage of lymphatic return, excessive intercourse and a racial predisposition to skin hypertrophy. Varicose veins are especially prominent during the last trimester of pregnancy in association with hemorrhoids and leg varicosities. The patient may complain of burning, itching and a feeling of heaviness in the vulva. Relief is accomplished by placing pressure against the vulva in the form of a sanitary napkin or foam rubber held in place by a T-binder or girdle. Rest with the legs and hips elevated should be taken frequently during the day. Occasionally surgical excision or injection with sclerosing solutions is necessary for relief. During the puerperium the veins usually become smaller and asymptomatic. Rarely a telangiectatic angioma may produce unilateral vulvar swelling.

Simple hypertrophy of the labia minora is said to occur when they project more than 4–5 cm. from their attachment. Such an enlargement is usually symmetrical and is thought to be due to masturbation or repeated sexual excitement with resultant chronic hyperemia. There is usually an associated hypersecretion of the sebaceous glands, giving the surface a moist and glistening appearance. It is found more often in the Negress, in whom it may merely represent a racial tendency.

Vulvar Injuries

Accidental Injuries.—The usual injury is a hematoma, brought about by a blow to the vulvar area, particularly if there are large varices, or by falling astride some object, with resultant damage to the vestibular bulbs or to the veins of the clitoris. Minor contusions may be treated by cold compresses and pressure. A large hematoma should be evacuated and packed, and antibiotics should be administered. Inspecton should be done carefully to determine whether the urethra, bladder or rectum has been injured. Fatal perforations into the peritoneal cavity, intestine and bladder have been reported. The vascular trauma in vulvar injuries is usually venous, so that hemostasis may usually be secured by evacuation of the hematoma and firm packing. Individual ligation of small vessels is not necessary unless arterial bleeding is encountered. The venous pressure in the vulva may be reduced somewhat by elevating both hips on pillows, and the swelling may be reduced by application of cold compresses or ice.

Coital Injuries.—Minor injuries about the hymen are so constantly associated with coitus that they may be termed "physiologic." They are usually superficial lacerations at either side of the posterior commissure. Injuries following rape, however, may be extensive and occasionally fatal. Profuse hemorrhage may result from tears of the clitoris or posterior fourchette or from hymenal avulsion. If the hymen is thick and nonyielding, lacerations of the perineum into the rectum may occur.

Treatment consists of surgical repair and supportive measures. The clinician should make complete notes of his findings at the time of the first examination. Microscopic search for spermatozoa and smears and cultures for gonorrhea should be made and recorded, since such cases are frequently investigated in criminal court. Although bleeding may be severe enough to necessitate transfusion, treatment is simple and such lacerations usually heal without scarring. The possibility that syphilis and gonorrhea have been contracted at this time must be considered and prophylactic therapy given.

Obstetric Injuries.—Physiologic injuries occurring at the time of delivery include obliteration of the hymenal folds by the passage of the fetal head, abrasions and minor tears of the vestibule, periurethral area and perineum. Occasionally, however, complete perineal lacerations with division of the anal sphincter occur. All such tears should be debrided and repaired by primary suture at the time of delivery.

Vulvar hematomas may occur following rapid spontaneous delivery or difficult forceps rotations. Large varicose veins seem to be a predisposing factor and should be ligated or excised just prior to delivery. If the hematoma is small and not extending, it may be treated by elevation of the hips and application of cold compresses. Large hematomas may extend retroperitoneally and be palpable above Poupart's ligament. These should be widely incised, packed and a contralateral vaginal pack inserted together with placement of a tight T-binder. Blood transfusions and antibiotics are useful as adjunctive therapy. Only rarely can the bleeding vessel be found for ligation, and even if it is, the packing should be placed as described.

X-ray Injuries.—The vulvar structures do not tolerate x-ray therapy well. In certain instances the reaction has been extreme, with marked erythema, edema, ulceration and scarring. Although x-ray may be used occasionally as a palliative procedure for extensive vulvar carcinoma, its use for benign conditions such as neurodermatitis or lichen sclerosus is not without hazard.

Venereal Diseases

SYPHILIS

The primary lesion, or chancre, may occur on the vulva, in the vagina or on the cervix. Since the lesion is painless, the symptoms are so minimal that usually the chancre is not noticed by the patient. Although there may be some edema, bleeding and discharge are rare so that healing usually takes place in five to eight weeks without treatment. The chancre usually appears three or four weeks after exposure and is an oval ulcer with sharp edges, a surface that exudes serum and induration of the tissue surrounding it. More than one may be present. There is no clinical feature that will distinguish this ulcer from other types, and inguinal adenopathy may occur bilaterally, as with other venereal diseases. The so-called "hard chancre" of syphilis may occasionally be soft and the "soft chancre" of chancroid may be hard, so that this differential point is not adequate. If secondary infection occurs, the ulceration may become extensive with increased discharge, pain and swelling. The old dictum that any genital lesion should be suspected of being syphilis until proved otherwise still pertains. An equally valid rule of thumb is to suspect primary syphilis if there is an indolent painless lesion that fails to heal in two weeks, irrespective of the part of the body involved.

Secondary syphilis is manifested by a generalized reaction with sore throat, headache, malaise, fever and a macular or papular rash covering the body. Mucous patches on the mouth and vulva (condylomata lata) may be present. The vulvar patches are elevated, broad, flat lesions which may coalesce to form a large papillomatous mass (Fig. 2–11). Similar lesions

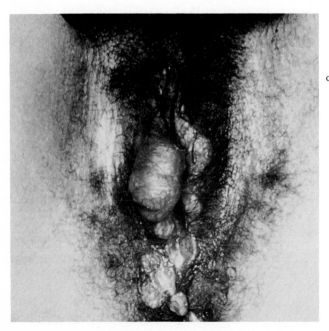

Fig. 2–11.—Condylomata lata of vulva due to syphilis.

may be present in the groin and under the breast. Again, there is no absolute distinguishing feature.

The tertiary lesion, or gumma, may occur on the vulva as a nodular ulcerative lesion. Occasionally it becomes secondarily infected, with the development of marked pain, tenderness, edema and lymphadenopathy.

The diagnosis of syphilis is made by dark-field examination of the secretions from the primary or secondary lesions and by serologic tests. Repeated dark-field examinations are frequently necessary since Treponema pallidum must be distinguished from other spiral organisms found on the genitalia, such as T. genitalis, T. calligyrum, Borrelia refringens and B. phagedenis.

A newer dark-field procedure, lymph node puncture, has been given high acclaim by both military and civilian syphilologists. This consists of removal by syringe and needle of a little tissue secretion of an enlarged lymph node and examining it by dark-field technic. Lymph node puncture is a specific procedure since usually no organism resembling Treponema pallidum is found in lymph nodes.

Early dark-field diagnosis may be facilitated by centrifuging pus from the chancre in a capillary tube for 10 minutes at 1000 rpm, then examining the supernatant fluid. This technic offers the earliest and often only means of diagnosis of the intra-urethral or intra-cervical chancre which may be masked by gonorrhea. This is especially important in this penicillin era since both diseases are effectively treated by one drug.

When the chancre first appears only 25 per cent of patients have a positive reaction to the serologic test; at the beginning of the second week approximately 50 per cent become seropositive; this increases to 75 per cent at the beginning of the third week, and by the fourth week all patients who have syphilis will have positive reactions.

There has been general acceptance of the "triple test plan" for the serologic diagnosis of syphilis. This was designed to differentiate patients having biologic false positive reactions from latent syphilitics. The Venereal Disease Research Laboratory (VDRL) flocculation test is used as a preliminary screening procedure for patients with neither history nor clinical history of syphilitic infection. A nonreactive result is accepted as evidence for the absence of syphilis while reactive or weakly positive serums are subjected to the Reiter protein complement-fixation test (RPCF). A positive RPCF is considered evidence for past or present infection with T. pallidum while a nonreactive result necessitates the performance of a T. pallidum immobilization test (TPI). A reactive TPI test indicates past or present infection; a nonreactive TPI test signifies a biologic false positive reaction.

Since the reaction to the blood test during secondary syphilis is always positive, any patient who has a sore throat that persists over two weeks should have serology performed. Any persistent rash, irrespective of its apparent nonsyphilitic nature, should be investigated for possible luetic etiology before initiating therapy.

Penicillin is the optimum treatment in infectious syphilis and is usually administered as procaine penicillin G in oil with 2 per cent aluminum monostearate. A total of 4,800,000 units is given in three injections over six to eight days (first injection 2,400,000 units; second and third injections 1,200,000 units each, given in the upper outer quadrant of the buttock).

Patients with primary or secondary syphilis in whom there is a history of severe sensitivity to pencillin or in whom such sensitivity develops during treatment may be given tetracycline, chlortetracycline or oxytetracycline by the oral route. The schedule should be as follows: Tetracycline, 2 Gm. daily in divided doses of 500 mg. four times daily over a period of 15 days for a total of 30 Gm. Erythromycin, 2 Gm. daily in divided doses of 500 mg. four times daily over a period of 10 days for a total of 20 Gm.

Post-treatment quantitative tests should be obtained monthly for six to nine months and every three months thereafter for a total observation period of two years. A satisfactory outcome can be predicted fairly confidently if the post-treatment serologic tests show progressively lower titers during the observation period.

Gonorrhea

If the gonococcus affects the vulva, it usually does so by lodging in the periurethral or Bartholin's glands. However, acute purulent bartholinitis may also be secondary to trauma or irritation by sanitary napkins or may follow invasion by pathogenic organisms from the vulvar skin (staphylococci) or bowel (Escherichia coli, Aerobacter aerogenes). A gonorrheal abscess of Bartholin's gland is characterized by a discrete, spherical, soft, fluctuant, exquisitely tender mass located lateral to and near the posterior fourchette. The treatment of such an abscess before rupture consists of application of local heat until fluctuation occurs, then simple incision and the insertion of a small wick or rubber dam to maintain drainage.

Symptoms of early gonococcal infection include dysuria due to acute urethritis, vaginal discharge and dyspareunia. The discharge is yellow and flows freely from involved structures. Occasionally the cervix is involved, and an acute purulent cervicitis is present.

The diagnosis of gonorrhea in the female is more difficult than in the male. During the acute phase a positive smear from the urethral and cervical discharge is reliable. As the infection becomes less acute, the smear becomes unreliable and cultures are necessary to confirm the diagnosis. Specimens of pus for cultures should be taken from the urethra, periurethral glands or cervix, not the vagina. Furthermore, the use of any lubricant on the speculum or gloves will kill whatever gonococci may be in the specimen. A good rule to follow is not to use any lubricant when taking a specimen from the vagina for culture, but particularly when it is being taken for gonococci.

Another question frequently raised concerns the examination and culture-taking during the menstrual flow. There is evidence that gonococci may be found with greater ease at this time. The female who contacts a male patient with gonorrhea should be examined as soon as possible. The practice of having these patients return after menstruation is to be deplored as unscientific and permits a potentially infected person to spread the infection further.

To date, smears and cultures are the only method of laboratory confirmation of gonorrhea. Complement-fixation tests are not reliable. However, in 1959 Deacon described a fluorescent antibody test for the detection of gonococci. Fluorescent antibody (FA) tests are of two types, direct and indirect. In direct FA tests, a fluorescein dye is conjugated with a specific globulin (antibody) against the organism to be tested. A smear or spread contains the organism to be identified. After the slide is flooded with the fluorescein-tagged globulin specific for the organism suspected, union between the globulin and the surface antigen of the organism occurs. Thus, when the slide is examined under ultraviolet light, the organism glows or fluoresces, proving gonorrhea is present.

Penicillin is still the drug of choice for the treatment of gonorrhea. However, ignorance about the disease and failure to make progress in its control have resulted in wide variations in dosages used and types of penicillin employed. Optimum treatment is as follows: A single intramuscular injection of 4.8 million units of Bicillin P.A.B. (disposable) containing 2.4 million units of aqueous procaine penicillin G and 2.4 million units of aqueous benzathine penicillin G. This should be given by deep intramuscular injection into the upper, outer quadrant of the buttocks.

If the use of penicillin is contraindicated, recourse to a number of effective antibiotics is available. Tetracycline (500 mg.), demethylchlortetracycline (300 mg.), erythromycin (500 mg.) or oleandomycin (500 mg.) given orally in divided doses every four to six hours (3 Gm. total) will give satisfactory results in most uncomplicated cases.

Serologic tests for syphilis should be obtained at the time of treatment and again at four to six months after treatment. Test for cure, if done at all, should consist of cultures. A patient sensitive to penicillin will have just as serious and intense a reaction to a small dosage of penicillin as to a larger dosage. Although anaphylactoid penicillin reactions are rare, at least among veneral disease clinic patients (3 per 10,000 with no fatalities), no physician should attempt treatment of patients with penicillin without having immediately at hand the equipment and drugs indicated for such an emergent and potentially fatal event.

CHANCROID (SOFT CHANCRE)

This is an ulcerative vulvar lesion, a venereal infection transmitted by coitus and caused by Ducrey's bacillus Haemophilus ducreyi. The lesion appears first as a papule or ulcer anywhere on the vulva. It has a sharply demarcated edge with an irregular contour without surrounding induration. There may be marked vulvar edema with enlargement of the inguinal glands. Suppuration of these nodes frequently occurs with skin ulceration (buboes). Diagnosis is made by identification of Ducrey's bacillus in smears or scrapings from the ulcer. Care in collecting and preparing the material is of utmost importance. All necrotic tissue and exudate should be removed. The specimen should be taken with a short wire applicator or the sterile flat end of a toothpick and "dug out" from under the undermined borders of the ulcer. After fixing by heat it is stained with Unna-Pappenheim solution with the Barritt modification. The organisms stain bright red, the pus cells blue-green. Haemophilus ducreyi is a gram-negative, short, thick rod with rounded ends. Dark-field examination will exclude syphilis. An intradermal skin test (Greenblatt and Sanderson) is available in which the result is read as positive if a 7 mm. papule or pustule with a surrounding erythema of more than 14 mm. occurs after injection of 0.1 cc. of antigen. Treatment consists of local cleanliness and soaks with aqueous Zephiran chloride (1:1,000) or potassium permanganate (1:5,000). Intermittent cleansing with pHisoHex (3 per cent) and water and sitz baths should be complemented by the administration of sulfisoxazole (Gantrisin) (1 Gm. four times daily for 10 days) or streptomycin (1 Gm. daily intramuscularly for 10 days). In the event of poor response or sensitivity, treatment may be carried out with tetracycline or oxytetracycline, 250 mg. given four times daily for seven days.

Lymphopathia Venereum
(Lymphogranuloma Inguinale)

This is a venereal infection, spread by coitus, believed to be caused by a filtrable virus; it begins as a papule, pustule or small ulcer after an incubation period of only a few days. The initial lesion quickly disappears and is followed by suppurative inguinal adenitis. The nodes undergo necrosis and abscess formation with ulceration, fibrosis and scarring. The lymphatic obstruction may produce elephantiasis of the vulva. Typical of the disease is a lymphatic extension of infection to the perirectal regions with proctitis, colitis and subsequent fibrosis and rectal stricture. Occasionally an ulcerative process is predominant, with extensive vulvar destruction.

The diagnosis is made by the Frei test (0.1 cc. of antigen injected intradermally in the forearm). A positive result is indicated by a papule 0.5–2.0 cm. in diameter surrounded by a circular reddened area occurring in 48–72 hours. The reaction may be negative, however, during the first two to three weeks of the disease.

Oxytetracycline (250 mg. four times daily for two weeks) or a sulfonamide mixture containing equal parts of sulfamerazine, sulfamethazine and sulfadiazene (1 Gm. four times daily) are effective therapeutic measures. A good rule is to continue treatment for as long a period of time after clinical healing has taken place as it took to heal the lesions. Surgical measures may occasionally be needed for later complications of the disease. Vulvectomy for severe deformity or colostomy for rectal strictures will at times be necessary.

Granuloma Inguinale

This is a chronic granulomatous disease, spread by coitus, found especially among Negroes in the tropics or southern sections of the United States, and characterized by a severe ulcerative tendency. The etiologic agent is the organism known as the Donovan body which some observers believe to be of protozoal nature. The disease begins as a small papular lesion on the labium minus or groin. After a few weeks this becomes a serpiginous ulcer which is characteristically superficial. A "pseudobubo" or subcutaneous inguinal granuloma may occur which is not an adenitis as found in gonorrhea or chancroid. The diagnosis is made by demonstrating Donovan's bodies by Wright's or Giemsa stain from scrapings or biopsies of the lesion. The tetracycline group, chloramphenicol and streptomycin are effective in the treatment of granuloma inguinale. The broad spectrum antibiotics are given by mouth in a dosage of 500 mg. every 6 hours. Dura-

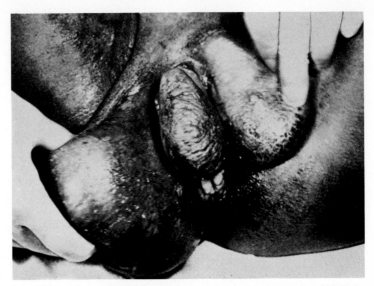

Fig. 2–12.—Severe edema and vulvar distortion due to granuloma inguinale.

tion of treatment depends upon the extensiveness of the lesions and the speed of healing. In patients with large granulomatous areas, treatment should be continued for four to six weeks. Because of its ototoxicity and the frequency of development of drug resistance, streptomycin should be reserved for treatment of small lesions of relatively recent onset.

Twenty grams of streptomycin, administered intramuscularly 1 Gm. every 6 hours for five days, is usually adequate. All of the broad spectrum antibiotics may cause nausea, vomiting and diarrhea. Chloramphenicol is the most dangerous since it may cause serious or even fatal blood dyscrasias, including aplastic anemia. Repeated hematologic observation, once or twice weekly, is essential if chloramphenicol is used. Vestibular disturbances may result from the use of streptomycin, and repeated otologic examination is imperative in patients being treated with this antibiotic. In some patients striking edema and distortion of the vulva occur, resulting in the massive proportions seen in Figure 2–12. In such cases vulvectomy may be carried out after a preliminary course of chloramphenicol or streptomycin therapy. In view of recent publications implicating the origin of some cases of vulvar carcinoma in chronic granulomatous lesions, such treatment is not only definitive but prophylactic as well.

Pruritus Vulvae

Pruritus vulvae is a symptom and not a diagnosis, the word "pruritus" being derived from the Latin *prurire*—to itch. The cause for this distressing symptom is often obscure and difficult to determine. It has been estimated that in about 10 per cent of patients seen in private gynecologic practice this is the chief complaint.

The neural mechanisms for the perception of itching are poorly understood, but it has been suggested that these impulses follow somatic pain fibers. The sensation of itching is therefore a subpain response mediated through the lateral spinothalamic tracts. This explains the absence of itching in patients who have had a chordotomy. Psychiatrists have pointed out that the central mediation of anger, resentment and eroticism may be exhibited in certain areas of the skin, such as the vulva in the female or the perianal area in the male. The persistence of the stimulus leads to scratching, trauma and visible damage, thus setting up a vicious cycle. Pathologic changes in the skin, such as hyperkeratosis, rete ridge hyperplasia and inflammatory changes in the dermis, may be produced experimentally in animals simply by scratching the same skin area repeatedly for a sufficiently long period.

The individual response and the choice of location are intimately allied with the patient's intrapsychic problem, leading to the complexity of the itch-scratch reflex. The intolerable, weak "pain" which is called "itch" is frequently so unpleasant that the patient tries to convert it to a strong pain by scratching. Itching disappears when strong pain is substituted, and such pain is often more endurable, at least temporarily, than the unpleasant sensation of itching. Examples of this are commonplace. Frequently women will, after years of vulvar scratching, resort to stiff brushes to convert itch to pain. Such trauma to the skin prevents natural healing and is followed by other effects which prolong the dermatitis.

Thus it is often impossible for the clinician to determine whether the gross vulvar changes he sees are due to prolonged scratching or the itching is due to primary skin disease. Biopsy is the only method of making an ac-

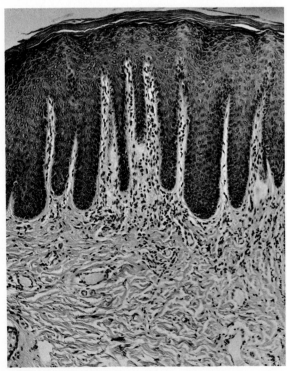

Fig. 2-13.—Photomicrograph showing the characteristics of neurodermatitis (nonspecific vulvitis).

curate diagnosis. Figure 2–13 illustrates the typical pattern, with hyper-keratosis, rete ridge elongation and lymphocytic infiltration of the dermis.

ETIOLOGY.—Two general classifications of pruritus vulvae may be employed: (1) local genital tract causes and (2) systemic causes. In the first group may be included (a) trichomonas vulvovaginitis, (b) fungous vulvovaginitis, (c) nonspecific bacterial vulvovaginitis, (d) senile vul-vovaginitis, (e) contact or atopic vulvitis, (f) atrophic and lichenified hyper-trophic vulvitis, (g) leukoplakia, (h) carcinoma. The second group includes (a) diabetes mellitus, (b) drug sensitivity and allergy, (c) chemical irritants, (d) skin diseases—herpes, intertrigo, lichen planus, psoriasis and urticaria, (e) vitamin deficiencies, especially vitamin A and the B complex vitamins, (f) diseases due to animal parasites—pediculosis and scabies, (g) systemic diseases—anemia, leukemia, hepatitis (with or without jaundice) and tuberculosis, (h) neurogenic dermatitis.

DIAGNOSIS.—This will be aided by a meticulous history, careful exami-nation and selected laboratory studies. The important features of the history are the intensity and duration of pruritus, the relationship to menses, associated leukorrhea or bleeding and previous allergic or derma-tologic episodes. Examination should include a careful survey of skin lesions elsewhere as well as inguinal lymphadenopathy. The local lesion should be examined in good light and its general and specific character-istics noted. Fissuring, ulceration, bleeding, scratch marks, thickening and discoloration are important signs. In addition, inspection of the urethra, periurethral glands, vagina, cervix, anus and Bartholin's glands should be made.

Selected laboratory tests of importance are: (1) a complete blood study for anemia or blood dyscrasia, (2) urinalysis for diabetes, (3) hanging-drop preparations of vaginal discharge for trichomoniasis and fungous diseases, (4) cultures for nonspecific bacterial infections, (5) cytologic studies for cancer, (6) serologic and antigen studies for venereal disease, (7) blood chemistries for uremia and diabetes, (8) biopsy for chronic vulvitis, leuko-plakia and cancer.

TREATMENT.—This will be considered in detail for each of the specific vulvar diseases.

LOCAL CAUSES OF PRURITUS VULVAE

Trichomoniasis.—This is usually evidenced as a vaginitis, but the thin, frothy, yellow-green discharge often may cause vulvar itching. The vagina is reddened and inflamed, with a granular or strawberry-like appearance. Diagnosis is made by placing a drop of the discharge on a warm slide to which warm normal saline is added and noting motile T. vaginalis. Treat-ment consists of (1) the re-establishment of vaginal acidity (to about pH 4.5) with lactic acid douches and (2) the use of a trichomonacide. Flagyl, an oral trichomonacide, has given excellent results and appears to be the most effective agent in trichomoniasis, particularly in the recurrent and resistant types. This specific disease will be considered in more detail in the chapter on the vagina.

Fungous Vulvitis.—The vulvar area harbors numerous fungi as sapro-phytes, and under conditions of lowered general resistance, increased heat, friction or excessive perspiration these may become virulent pathogens. Predisposing causes to this transformation are pregnancy and diabetes, and the finding of a fungous vulvitis should be sufficient to alert the clinician to the possibility of the diabetic state. The most common forms are tinea cruris and moniliasis.

Tinea cruris is characterized by superficial, pale pink to bright red lesions with well-defined scaly borders. By a process of coalescence the adjacent vulvar skin, thighs and pubis may become involved. Following periods of scratching or maceration, the process may resemble a weeping type of eczema. Tinea cruris is caused by a specific fungus, Epidermophyton inguinale, and the diagnosis may be made by microscopic examination of the scales, by direct gram stain or by culture on Sabouraud's maltose agar. Direct mycologic examination of scales, hairs and scrapings is facilitated by preparing the specimens without heating in an aqueous solution of 0.1 per cent aminol and 0.2 per cent basic fuchsin. Treatment depends on the degree of associated inflammation. If the area is edematous and oozing it should be dried by applications of calamine lotion, saturated solution of aluminum acetate or 1–2 per cent silver nitrate. After this, any one of the various fungicidal ointments (undecylenic acid, 3 per cent salicylic acid or 5 per cent sulfur) may be used.

Moniliasis is caused by the most common saprophyte of the normal vagina and vulva, Candida (Monilia) albicans. The lesion begins as a reddish papule which later becomes vesicular. After these rupture, a moist, red mucous membrane remains. Secondary infection is common, so that the vagina and vulva become markedly edematous and tender. The vulva may be covered with a tenacious, gray-white frosting (Fig. 2–14) or there may be marked edema due to recurrent scratching. The most common symptoms of monilia are intense itching, burning and swelling. Itching is likely to persist or reappear unless the fungus is completely eliminated by treatment. A whitish, curdlike vaginal discharge, often with a yeasty or disagreeable odor, may develop as the infection becomes more severe. If chafing occurs, a secondary inflammation or dermatitis of the thighs may

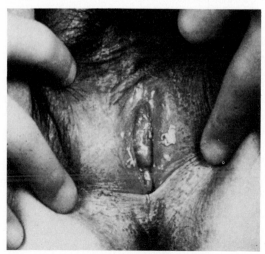

Fig. 2–14.—Moniliasis of vulva.

also be present. Sexual intercourse may be painful or impossible because of the swelling, abrasion and inflammation. Walking may be uncomfortable because of chafing.

In some patients, these characteristic features of monilia infection are so obvious that diagnosis may be by inspection alone. In others, e.g., in older patients, in very early stages of infection, and when secondary bacterial infections are present, diagnosis is more difficult.

Diagnosis, as with tinea cruris, may be made by wet smear, gram stain or culture. Nickerson's medium has simplified culturing, since it is available in small vials which may be inoculated and kept in the office at room temperature. A dark brown or black growth occurs on the medium in about 48 hours if monilia is present. Specific treatment is available in the form of nystatin (Mycostatin) vaginal tablets (100,000 units per tablet) and ointment (100,000 units nystatin/Gm.) or trichloromethyl thiohydantoin with benzalkonium (Sporostacin) cream. In severe cases, especially those complicated by gastrointestinal moniliasis, treatment should include the oral administration of nystatin (500,000 units per tablet). Alternative therapeutic agents are 2 per cent aqueous gentian violet (or Gentia-Jel suppositories) which may be instilled in the vagina and painted over the vulva or Propion Gel, a propionate compound jelly, which is used similarly. Pregnancy is no contraindication to the use of these preparations intravaginally. In unregulated diabetes, rapid improvement is noted after metabolic imbalance is corrected.

Monilia vaginitis has been noted to occur more frequently in users of oral contraceptives, particularly of the combined estrogen-progestin type. The effect may thus simulate the hormonal milieu of pregnancy. If the process is recurrent, diabetes or the pre-diabetic state should be excluded by appropriate laboratory tests. Certain patients are less likely to develop monilia while using sequential oral contraceptives and therefore these may be substituted for the combined agents. A few oral contraceptives contain a progestin which has a pronounced anti-estrogenic effect on the vaginal epithelium. In these patients relief may be obtained by the use of a topical cream containing estrogen. In certain patients I have been able to obtain relief by the suppression of endogenous estrogen and progesterone by the administration of Depo-Provera for six to nine months. Since the Depo-Provera is effective as a contraceptive agent, oral preparations need not be taken. The vaginal mucosa becomes atrophic, similar to that seen in postmenopausal women, and thus the hormonal milieu necessary for the growth of monilia is eliminated. For this rather drastic measure I have given Depo-Provera in a dose of 100 mg. every two weeks for 4 doses followed by 200 mg. each month for six months. It should be noted, however, that Depo-Provera is long acting and subsequent ovulation may be delayed for months. (See chapter on steroid therapy.).

Nonspecific Bacterial Vulvitis.—This may be interpreted to mean a vulvitis unassociated with trichomonas or monilia but in which bacterial studies show mixtures of streptococci, staphylococci, Esch. coli and diphtheroids. It includes intertrigo (a diffuse redness involving labiofemoral and inguinal creases usually seen in obese women with excessive perspiration), follicular vulvitis (a Staph, albus infection of the hair follicles), erysipelas and simple acute ulcer. The last is a rare condition characterized by multiple shallow, round or oval ulcers which produce itching, burning and perineal discomfort. The causative factor is believed to be Bacillus crassus, a normal inhabitant of the vagina. Treatment depends on the results of culture and sensitivity tests of the various organisms with specific antibiotics. Trichlorbisonium suppositories (Tribs) and Sultrin or AVC vaginal creams are particularly effective in most gram-negative infections. In most pyogenic infections neomycin ointment or lotion has proved effective. Chronic, recurring hidradenitis suppurativa is an indolent, low-grade infection of the apocrine glands characterized by tender, swollen nodules which perforate the skin over the mons pubis, leaving sinus tracts and scarring. The hair over the pubis should be shaved and cultures obtained. Daily washing with pHisoHex solution, dry heat and specific antibiotics will usually result in rapid improvement.

Senile Vulvitis.—This is usually coexistent with a vaginitis of similar nature. Symptoms include vulvar burning, itching and dyspareunia. Bleeding may occur from ulceration or telangiectasia. This physiologic, atrophic skin change usually starts at the climacteric or after artificial menopause and the generally accepted cause is estrogen deficiency. The entire process is too complex, however, to be explained on this factor alone. Exogeneous estrogen therapy will not reverse or prevent this ultimate change in most individuals. Other hormones and related factors presumably contribute to the general aging phenomenon. The mons pubis becomes less prominent and the labia majora shrink and flatten as the result of loss of subcutaneous fat. The adjacent skin becomes thin and shiny, the hair sparse and tissue elasticity diminished. As a result, the vaginal orifice becomes narrowed or even stenotic, with resultant dyspareunia. A thin watery discharge may be present. Diagnosis is evident by noting the degree of cornification of vaginal cells in a hanging-drop preparation or Papanicolaou smear. For the vaginal component of the disease, local applications of estrogenic creams or small oral doses of estrogens for short periods are quite effective. Combinations of estrogens with androgens will occasionally give superior results, especially when libido has been diminished. Emollient creams, starch baths, sedatives and antipruritic lotions should afford relief in most cases.

Contact Vulvitis.—This common form of vulvitis usually appears in the form of an eczematous dermatitis with erythema, edema, vesicles, oozing and crusting. In the chronic stage the skin may be lichenified with scaling and a typical "shark-skin" appearance. Etiology is variable; the cause may be irritants contained in clothing, toilet tissue, condoms, douches, contraceptives, nail polish, perfumes, deodorants or sanitary napkins. A careful review of the history will usually disclose the cause, and cure follows removal of the offending agent. During the acute phase cool compresses of boric acid or saturated solution of aluminum acetate may be used, together with oral antihistamine therapy. In severe cases hydrocortisone ointment or parenteral administration of cortisone or adrenocorticotropin may be indicated. An increased effectiveness of topical hydrocortisone therapy has been noted if combined with 2 per cent pantothenylol.

The Kraurosis-Leukoplakia Complex.—Medicine has been plagued for decades with confusing terminology due, in large part, to perpetuation of error and the tenacity of the clinician to cling to terminology because of long association. Such is the case with certain so-called precancerous dermatoses of the vulva, occasionally labeled the "leukokraurosis complex." Confusion of terminology in this group of vulvar diseases dates from 1885 when the first cases of leukoplakic vulvitis were associated with marked sclerosis and narrowing of the vaginal outlet. The constriction was thought to be an essential feature of the disease, so that the term "kraurosis" (to shrivel up) was applied. This was most unfortunate since kraurosis, like pruritus, is only a symptom, not a disease. Leukoplakia, by prolonged usage of the term, is a disease entity with specific histologic characteristics. Although the term really means "white plaque," its present connotation is much broader since white plaques may be present in several chronic dermatoses or even in kraurosis. As will be seen, microscopic leukoplakia bears a definite relationship to the development of vulvar carcinoma and it may or may not be associated with a kraurotic vulva. Stated simply, many sclerosing vulvar diseases may be accompanied by kraurosis, but unless true leukoplakia supervenes the malignant potential is small. With the hope of simplification, the following classification has been suggested: (1) simple kraurosis, (2) lichen sclerosus et atrophicus, (3) leukoplakia, (4) carcinoma in situ.

SIMPLE KRAUROSIS.—Simple kraurosis of the vulva is a primary sclerosing atrophy limited to the labia minora, vestibule, urethra and clitoris. It occurs most commonly in postmenopausal women. The labia majora, perineum and perianal regions are not usually involved. In the early stages the skin may be red and glistening with isolated patches of dark red or dull purple (kraurosis rouge). In later stages the skin becomes pale yellow and has a smooth glistening surface, obliterated labial folds, atrophic mons veneris and scanty broken-off pubic hairs (Fig. 2–15). The vaginal orifice is narrowed and barely admits the index finger.

Histologically, there is hyperkeratosis (excess keratin above the epithelium) with flattening of the rete ridges, edema and homogenization of the cutis collagen, separation of the elastic fibers and mild arteriosclerotic changes in the deeper blood vessels (Fig. 2–16). Simple kraurosis bears no known relationship to carcinoma of the vulva.

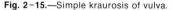

Fig. 2–15.—Simple kraurosis of vulva.

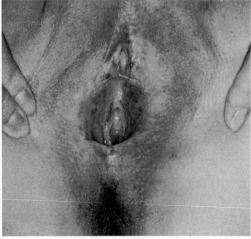

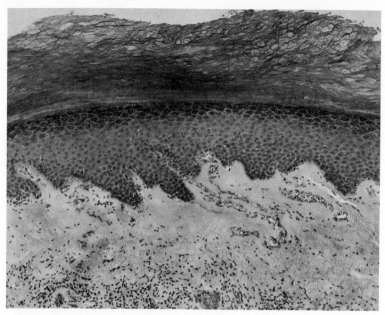

Fig. 2 –16.—Histologic changes in simple kraurosis.

LICHEN SCLEROSUS ET ATROPHICUS.—Like simple kraurosis, this is also a primary sclerosing atrophy of the vulva characterized clinically by typical polygonal, flat-topped, mother-of-pearl papules over the trunk, forearms, neck, axilla and vulva (Fig. 2–17). Occasionally there is a coalescence of papules to form a definite plaque of white, atrophic skin. The labia majora and minora appear atrophic and shrunken and there is stenosis of the vaginal orifice.

Histologically, the appearance is the same as that outlined for kraurosis,

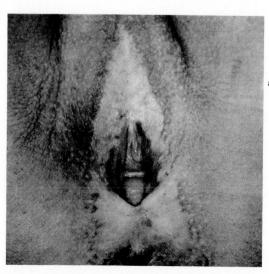

Fig. 2 –17.—Lichen sclerosus et atrophicus of vulva.

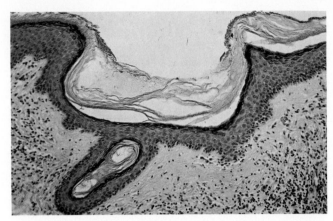

Fig. 2 –18.—Histologic appearance of Lichen sclerosus et atrophicus.

with the possible difference that "follicular plugging" is present in lichen sclerosus (Fig. 2 – 18) and absent in kraurosis. The obliterative blood vessel changes seen in kraurosis are not constant in lichen sclerosus, but most skin pathologists feel that the disease may be considered as the same process and therefore that lichen sclerosus is not causally related to carcinoma.

We would choose to classify both kraurosis and lichen sclerosus as examples of a primary sclerosing atrophy of vulvar structures. It should be remembered, however, that true leukoplakia may occasionally develop in such an area of sclerosing atrophy. Symptoms in lichen sclerosus are variable and in some patients are totally absent in all phases of the disease. In other patients an inflammatory process is prominent, with burning and itching, and in others the complaints may be limited to dysuria, dyspareunia or a simple feeling of vulvar tightness. The diagnosis is made by biopsy.

Treatment is nonspecific and mostly supportive. Spontaneous resolution may occur in several weeks or months or may be delayed for many years. Prolonged bathing should be avoided and the parts should be kept soft with olive oil or a similar preparation. A combination of ichthyol and castor oil is soothing and lubricating. If pruritus is severe, adequate sedation should be given and the patient instructed in the use of colloid baths (2 cups of cornstarch plus ½ cup baking soda in a tub half-filled with warm water). One or 2 tablespoons of liquor carbonis detergens may be added to the bath water. Local cortisone therapy has been tried with encouraging results. In a few patients a mild fungous infection complicates the vulvitis and the use of Mycolog cream is particularly helpful. When used, the preparation should be rubbed in thoroughly every three to four hours. Testosterone propionate in petrolatum has also produced symptomatic and objective improvement. Alcohol nerve block and undercutting procedures afford only temporary relief. The same may be said for vulvar resection and simple total vulvectomy, a recurrence rate of about 65 per cent having been found in patients so treated at the Boston Hospital for Women. Almost all of these patients required repeated surgery in the form of local excision. A categorical statement may be made regarding x-ray therapy in this disease: it should not be used.

LEUKOPLAKIA.—Leukoplakia may be defined as a chronic inflammatory condition, affecting either the entire vulva or a small part thereof, characterized by the formation of whitish plaques of thickened epidermis, with sclerosis of the subjacent connective tissue and absence of elastic fibers, producing a parchment-like consistency of the skin (Fig. 2 – 19). I would add the necessary requisite of epithelial cellular changes including parakeratosis, dyskeratosis and atypism. The plaques may be single or multiple, occasionally bluish areas found usually on the inner surfaces of the labia, about the clitoris and on the perineum. Generally, leukoplakia does not involve the outer surfaces of the labia or anal area. The diagnosis can be made definitely only by microscopic examination and even then failure to appreciate certain histologic details has led to incorrect diagnoses. The commonest errors have been in designating simple kraurosis or lichen sclerosus as a leukoplakic lesion. Because of the precancerous implication of this diagnosis, many unnecessary vulvectomies have, in all probability, been performed. In order to select biopsy sites the vulva should be painted with toluidine blue and then washed with acetic acid. Areas retaining the blue stain should be sampled.

In about 90 per cent of cases of leukoplakic vulvitis there is pronounced itching, whereas in the other 10 per cent only a feeling of burning, chafing or discomfort is present. The exact relationship of vulvar carcinoma to leukoplakia is unknown, although Taussig wrote in 1926 a very pointed opinion: "I believe it [leukoplakia] will inevitably proceed to the development of cancer, but the rate at which this change takes place may be so slow that death supervenes before its accomplishment." He therefore recommended surgical excision of the entire vulva including perineal and

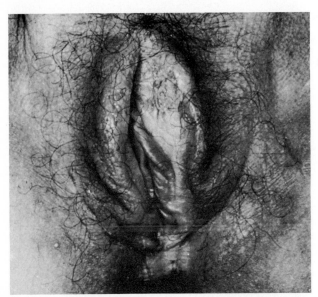

Fig. 2 –19.—Vulvar leukoplakia.

perianal skin for all cases of leukoplakia. That this will not completely prevent vulvar cancer is evident from the cases reported to have developed in recurrent areas of leukoplakia after vulvectomy. True leukoplakia is, by definition, a hypertrophic process. (Previous classifications of an atrophic type were usually lichen sclerosus.) It may develop in the previously mentioned sclerosing atrophy diathesis, in simple senile atrophy or in normal vulvar skin. The process of its development has been described as similar to that of a senile keratosis on mucous membrane—in other words, precancerous.

The important histologic changes are believed to be in the epithelium in the form of hyperkeratosis, acanthosis, dyskeratosis, cellular atypism and absence of polarity. Some surface differentiation may be present. These changes are illustrated in Figure 2 –20. This is at variance with the opinion of Taussig who believed the important changes to be the loss of elastic tissue in the dermis. Changes of increasing degrees of anaplasia, ranging from anaplastic leukoplakia through Bowen-like dyskeratosis to carcinoma in situ and finally to microinvasive carcinoma, explain the pathogenesis of vulvar carcinoma from this entity.

From the literature it has been apparent that the tendency for leukoplakia to develop into carcinoma is great, varying from 23.1 per cent (Miller) to 50 per cent (Taussig). Our own experience at the Boston Hospital

Fig. 2 –20.—Histologic changes in leukoplakia.

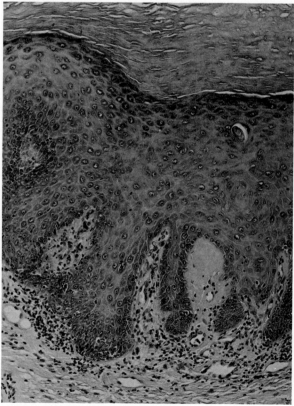

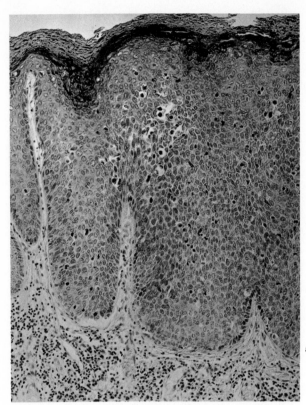

Fig. 2 –21.—Histologic characteristics of carcinoma in situ.

for Women can be cited. An adequate follow-up of three to 25 years was available on 26 patients with what was considered to be definite leukoplakia. Seventeen had some form of surgical excision; in seven of these, there was no improvement or a recurrence developed. Six of the seven were re-operated on. In two of the original 26 patients (7.7 per cent) squamous cell carcinoma developed. A safe conclusion seems to be that many (and perhaps most) squamous cell carcinomas of the vulva arise in true leukoplakia (not lichen sclerosus), but figures are not available to state in what per cent of vulvar leukoplakias (treated or untreated) carcinoma will develop.

Treatment is variable, depending on the extent of the disease and the symptomatology. Simple destruction by electrodesiccation or wide excision will suffice if the lesion is small. If widespread, simple vulvectomy is indicated, but this should be extensive since the recurrence rate is high. The importance of proper diagnosis of a premalignant lesion of the vulva is evident, and follow-up examinations with repeated biopsies of suspicious areas are the only means of prophylaxis against cancer.

CARCINOMA IN SITU.—It is believed that carcinoma in situ is merely an accentuation of the findings noted in leukoplakia. There is no surface differentiation, the abnormal epithelium extending throughout the entire width of the epidermis. Grossly the lesion is not characteristic, since it may look like leukoplakia. Occasionally there may be an elevated, dull red area, sharply demarcated, with ulceration and crusting. The histologic characteristics of carcinoma in situ are seen in Figure 2 –21. The epithelium shows hyperkeratosis with parakeratosis and acanthosis. Rete ridge elongation is striking and the basal layer is intact though not distinct. Numerous atypical, dyskeratotic cells may be seen in the rete malpighii, and there is complete loss of cellular polarity. The individual cell dyskeratosis may be so extreme that "pearls" may be formed in the epidermis. These cells are large and round, with a homogeneous and eosinophilic cytoplasm and a large, irregular, hyperchromatic nucleus. This process of abnormal keratinization has been termed by Lever "individual cell keratinization" or "malignant dyskeratosis." Some of these dyskeratotic cells occasionally demonstrate marked vacuolation and resemble Paget cells. (See Paget's disease.) In carcinoma in situ, however, the intercellular bridges are present, whereas in extramammary Paget's disease involving the vulva these bridges are absent. The treatment of carcinoma in situ is wide surgical excision or extensive simple vulvectomy and careful follow-up.

Systemic Causes of Pruritus

Two important systemic causes of vulvar pruritus, diabetes and uremia, have been discussed in the section on Physiologic Alterations. In addition to these, consideration must be given to drug sensitivities and allergies, chemical irritants, skin diseases and an important but not well-understood entity, neurogenic dermatitis.

Drug Sensitivities and Allergies.—It should be borne in mind that contact dermatitis, dermatitis venenata and eczema are names applied to a dermatitis from an external source to which the patient is sensitized, but that the same reaction may be produced by the same source if it is administered internally. Contact dermatitis may be looked on immunologically in the same light as allergic eczema. Innumerable substances of animal, vegetable and mineral origin may result in an inflammatory, allergic vulvitis. They are varied and may be nonprotein in nature. The following drugs have been described as causing vulvar pruritus: arsenic, aspirin, chlortetracycline, antihistamines, bromides, chloramphenicol, iodides, para-amino-salicylic acid, phenacetin, phenolphthalein, sulfonamides and oxytetracycline. Obviously this is a small and incomplete list. Other causes of allergic vulvitis are food proteins, hair, pollens and bacteria. The importance of nervous tension as a predisposing factor to allergic eczema of the vulva has not received adequate attention, but in the treatment of these conditions its importance must not be minimized. The lesions identified in allergic vulvitis are many: erythema, urticaria, angioneurotic edema, purpura, eczema with vesiculation, acneform dermatitis and ulceration. Treatment should be initiated by eliminating the drug or substance responsible for the vulvitis. If it is a common allergen, desensitization may be tried. Antihistamines, sedatives, cortisone, ACTH and epinephrine are used as indicated. Aluminum subacetate (1 per cent) may be applied to the vulva as cool, wet compresses, followed in a week or so by hydrocortisone ointment or an antihistamine cream. Cornstarch and baking soda baths are helpful, and the patient should soak for an hour twice a day. The affected parts should then be patted dry but not rubbed. All soaps should be avoided.

Chemical Irritants.—These have been discussed in the section on contact vulvitis but they may also cause a generalized, systemic reaction or a widespread dermatitis. Frequently the patient does not realize that such a noxious chemical substance is being utilized and only thorough questioning will elicit this information. Nylon panties, new soaps, girdles, douche nozzles, douche solutions, condoms and deodorants are common offenders. Treatment is the same as that for allergic vulvitis.

Skin Diseases

Since the labia majora may be classified as skin, any disease found elsewhere on the skin may similarly affect the vulva. These diseases will be considered under animal parasites and the exudative and scaly dermatoses.

Animal Parasites.—SCABIES.—Scabies is caused by the female itch mite, Sarcoptes or Acarus scabiei. Examination will reveal similar lesions in the sides and webs of the fingers, the palms, axillae, wrist flexures and over the nipples. Pruritus may be intense but is usually nocturnal. The face is almost always uninvolved. Diagnosis is made by obtaining the acarus from a skin burrow with a needle and examining it under the microscope. Either Kwell ointment, Topocide (benzylchlorophenothane ethyl aminobenzoate) or 25 per cent benzyl benzoate in equal parts of tincture of green soap and water may be used to treat the infestation. A severe dermatitis should first be treated with soothing baths and lotions and topical use of an antibiotic if necessary. It is best to have the patient begin treatment with a prolonged soap-and-water bath, then rub the selected scabicide into the skin, bathe again only after 24 hours and change the bed linen and clothing.

PEDICULOSIS PUBIS.—The pubic or crab louse (Phthirus pubis) pierces the skin and secretes a noxious substance which produces severe pubic and vulvar pruritus. The disease is spread by coitus but possibly also by bedding or toilets. The lice may be found attached to the hairs about $\frac{1}{2}$ in. above the skin or at the skin-hair junction. Diagnosis is made by removing the hair and examining it under the microscope. Topocide, Kwell ointment or Bornate are equally effective therapeutically.

OXYURIASIS.—The vulva of children may be affected by an intestinal focus of Oxyuris vermicularis (pinworms). Treatment includes application of chlorcyclizine hydrochloride cream (1 per cent Perazil) to the perianal and vulvar area and oral administration of either piperazine citrate (Antepar) or phosphate (Piperazate). Pyrvinium chloride (Vanquin) or dithiazanine (Delvex) are also highly effective against the pinworm.

Gentian violet in enteric-coated tablets is an effective, inexpensive agent for the treatment of enterobiasis. Therapy for 10 consecutive days is effective and relatively well tolerated, although nausea, vomiting and abdominal pain are not uncommon.

Exudative Dermatoses.—HERPES PROGENITALIS.—This lesion is caused by a virus and is similar in many respects to herpes simplex, the common fever blister of the perioral area. In many cases its occurrence coincides with the onset of menstruation, and it usually lasts about a week. Characteristically, there are clusters of pinhead-sized vesicles which contain a clear then a seropurulent exudate. After these rupture, a crust is formed over the coalescent lesion which heals without scarring. Treatment consists of wet dressings of Burow's solution diluted 1:10 (saturated solution of aluminum acetate) in the acute stage, and later neomycin ointment to prevent secondary infection. There is some evidence that desensitization by vaccination with vaccinia virus every week for six or eight weeks is effective in preventing recurrence. In patients who had recurrent herpes progenitalis with menstruation we have successfully prevented it by inhibiting ovulation for three or four consecutive months. The anovulatory bleeding episode is not attended by the herpetic rash.

HERPES ZOSTER.—Fortunately this is a rare condition but it may involve the vulva and even the vagina in old and debilitated women. It is virus-caused and is limited to the nerve distribution from one or more posterior ganglia. Onset may be heralded by fever and neuralgic pain. This is followed by a vesicular eruption, usually unilateral, which causes itching, tenderness and severe pain. After the clear vesicular fluid becomes turbid, the vesicles rupture and crusting follows. Some lesions may become hemorrhagic and these are followed by deep scars. Because of the severity of the pain analgesic drugs are necessary during the acute phase, although ACTH and cortisone have been noted to possess analgesic properties and perhaps augment healing. Local treatment is best carried out using an occlusive dressing of collodion containing 10 per cent ichthyol for a week or so; following this, chlortetracycline or tetracycline ointment should be applied. Postherpetic pain may necessitate pudendal nerve block. An aerosol spray of balsam of Peru is occasionally effective.

PEMPHIGUS VULGARIS (TRUE PEMPHIGUS).—The genitalia, face, mouth or neck of older and debilitated women may be affected. Although the exact etiology is unknown, a virus is strongly suspected as the causative organism. The clinical picture is variable but in the usual situation crops of bullae appear, then rupture and form ulcers with subsequent oozing and bleeding. Pemphigus involving the genital tract does not, as a rule, result fatally as is often the case when it involves the mouth or throat. Treatment should be immediate and complete. ACTH (25 mg. in 500 cc. of 5 per cent glucose in water) should be given intravenously slowly over eight hours. This dose may then be increased to 50 or 100 mg. in 500 cc. of 5 per cent glucose in water. Cortisone (500–750 mg. daily) should also be administered orally until recession of bullae occurs. After this a gradual diminution in dosage may be tried.

Dry Scaly Dermatoses.—LICHEN PLANUS.—This inflammatory dermatosis of unknown origin is characterized by multiple, small, flat-topped, polygonal papules that have a peculiar violaceous color and are covered with an often umbilicated horny film usually associated with lesions elsewhere on the body (wrists, ankles, inner thighs). It may be confused with leukoplakia, kraurosis or neurodermatitis. Diagnosis is made by biopsy, which shows acanthosis, hyperkeratosis, absence of parakeratosis, saw-toothed rete ridges and a bandlike infiltration of chronic inflammatory cells in the upper cutis (Fig. 2–22). Treatment includes general measures such as sedatives, rest, avoidance of sweating and the use of tranquilizers of the meprobamate group. Locally, colloid baths, aluminum acetate solution and an ointment such as:

phenol	1.20
salicylic acid	1.80
liq. carbonis detergens	3.00
ungt. zinc oxide	60.00

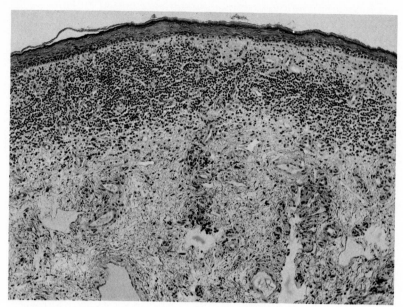

Fig. 2–22.—Lichen planus.

may be tried. Corticosteroid creams are by themselves of little help but their effect may be enhanced by an occlusive dressing of plastic material and cellophane tape. In hypertrophic lesions, injection of small amounts of triamcinolone acetate suspension may be efficacious.

PSORIASIS.—This is an inflammatory dermatosis of unknown origin characterized by dry, scaling patches of various sizes covered by silvery white or grayish white scales. It may involve the vulva, although the sites of predilection are the scalp, nails, the extensor surfaces of the limbs and the sacral area. If vulvar lesions are present, usually there are lesions on these other areas. The disease commonly has periods of exacerbation and remission which may or may not be associated with subjective symptoms. The diagnosis may be obvious, but biopsy frequently is necessary. Microscopically there are a uniform parakeratosis, thin suprabasal epidermal plates, uniform rete ridge elongation with clubbing and microabscesses in the stratum corneum. During periods of exacerbation, improvement may be noted with sunbaths, ultraviolet light or the application of crude tar (2–5 per cent) or salicylic acid (2–10 per cent) ointments. Arsenic in the form of Fowler's solution (3 drops twice daily for six weeks) is effective but should only be used in patients over age 60 since its recurrent use over long periods may be carcinogenic. A low-fat diet should be prescribed, use of alcoholic beverages kept at a minimum and adequate sedation administered. Other medications which have benefited some patients are Granulestin (a phospholipid concentrate), vitamin B12, autohemotherapy, ACTH and cortisone.

Neurodermatitis.—This is a relatively common vulvar disease occurring predominantly in overactive, oversensitive persons, particularly those who also suffer from allergic disorders. Many of this same group have also been found to have psychoneuroses. The disorder may be present in any age group but is more prevalent during the childbearing period. Symptoms include severe itching, usually of long duration and often localized to a small area. Primary infection, discharge or other local cause is usually absent since the patient may have tried many medications or will have seen a number of other physicians. Psychogenic disturbances such as marital friction, frigidity, masturbation, dyspareunia or fear of pregnancy may be elicited by close questioning. The response to all forms of therapy is commonly short-lived.

The lesions are usually on the labia majora or periclitoral area and often scratch marks may be seen. The diagnosis may be made by this characteristic appearance and by the presence of psychoneurotic personality traits

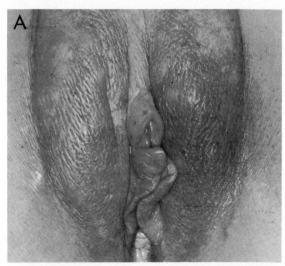

Fig. 2–23.—Vulvar neurodermatitis. **A**, edema and lichenification of early stage. **B**, extensive hyperkeratosis in late stage.

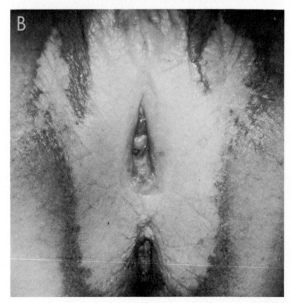

and chronicity of the lesion. Figure 2–23 illustrates the early and late stages of this process. Biopsy reveals the picture of a typical chronic dermatitis: irregular acanthosis, hyperkeratosis, parakeratosis, elongation of rete ridges, thinning of suprabasal epidermal plates and mild inflammatory infiltration in the upper dermis (see Fig. 2–13). Local measures of treatment include (1) avoidance of soap; (2) potassium permanganate wet dressings (1:8,000) and calamine liniment for lesions with pronounced exudation; (3) relief of excess dryness with a bland ointment such as Aquaphor; (4) as the lesions become subacute, 3 per cent ichthyol in 30 per cent zinc oxide ointment; (5) hydrocortisone, if used regularly and in adequate amounts; e.g., Synalar cream (0.025 per cent) applied four to six times daily and rubbed into the skin. Application of testosterone propionate in petrolatum (50 mg. per cc.) has been reported to produce symptomatic and objective improvement. General measures for functional disease and prolonged psychotherapy are the basis for permanent cure. The judicious use of the meprobamate compounds has proved of temporary value.

Benign Neoplasms

The most common benign neoplasms of the vulva are papillomas, lipomas, fibromas and hidradenomas. Less common are neurofibromas, lymphangiomas, hemangiomas and myxomas.

Papilloma.—The dermal papilloma may occur on the vulva as a benign skin tumor of verrucous type, having a brown color. It may be single or multiple, and histologically it shows striking hyperkeratosis with acanthosis and elongation of the rete ridges. Although the proper name for this lesion is nevus verrucosus, nevus cells are not present in the usual case. It is cured by simple excision.

A much commoner type of papilloma is that known as condyloma acuminatum (venereal wart). These lesions should not be confused with condyloma latum, the secondary lesion of syphilis. They are frequently associated with chronic vaginal discharge such as that of trichomoniasis or moniliasis

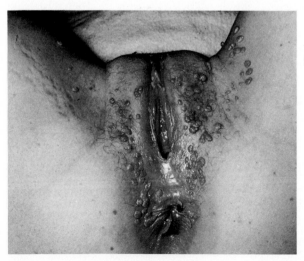

Fig. 2–24.—Condylomata acuminata.

and are benign epithelial growths of viral origin. Their size varies from 0.5 mm. to 1–2 cm., and they tend to be grouped in clusters. Figure 2–24 illustrates a typical pattern of growth with involvement of the inner thighs. If extensive, a cauliflower-like appearance is evident. During pregnancy they enlarge rapidly and may occasionally completely fill the vagina and cover the labia, whereas during the puerperium regression occurs. The histologic appearance is rather characteristic although, on occasion, a close similarity to a papillary squamous cell carcinoma is present. There is slight thickening of the stratum corneum with extensive parakeratosis, marked acanthosis and papillomatosis with thickening and elongation of the rete ridges (Fig. 2–25). This gives an arborescent pattern on low power. Cells of the rete malpighii demonstrate intracellular edema with a fairly large number of mitoses. However, the cellular pattern is orderly, polarity is retained and the junction of the epidermis and corium is sharp—all of which differentiate this lesion from carcinoma (Fig. 2–31). The corium contains many dilated blood vessels and a dense infiltration of lymphocytes and plasma cells.

Diagnosis is usually evident on gross inspection but biopsy should be done in atypical cases or if the lesion does not respond to treatment. If the lesions are small or scanty, the local application of 25 per cent podophyllin in mineral oil or sandarac varnish will result in rapid disappearance. If the lesions are extensive, electrocoagulation is preferable to simple excision since the base may be lightly touched with the cautery as the lesion is removed. Although condylomata acuminata are generally believed to be benign, several recent reports have noted the development of vulvar carcinoma in such lesions.

Lipoma.—This benign tumor arises from the fatty tissue of the labia majora or mons veneris and usually grows slowly and causes no symptoms except when its size is excessive. When this occurs the mass acquires a

Fig. 2–25.—Photomicrograph of vulvar papilloma.

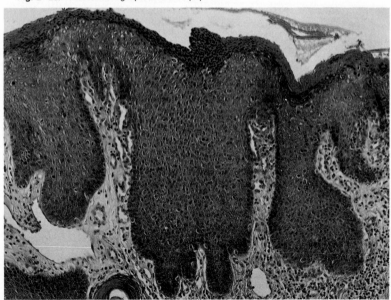

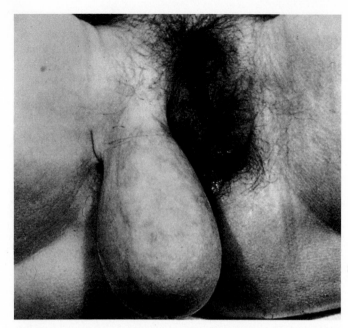

Fig. 2-26.—Lipoma of vulva.

pedicle and hangs from the groin or vulva as a pendulum. If the pedicle is wide it may resemble a hernia (Fig. 2-26). Some lipomas have attained gigantic size but the usual one is not larger than 10-12 cm. The histologic appearance is that of normal fat cells with a connective tissue framework and capsule. The incidence of liposarcoma is extremely rare. Nevertheless, the lesion should be excised since difficulty in walking or in coitus will eventually occur.

Fibroma.—This lesion usually develops as a firm nodule on the labia

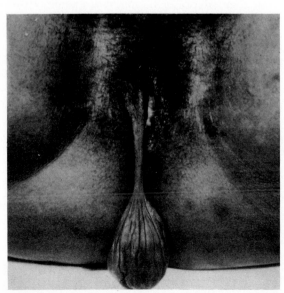

Fig. 2-27.—Fibroma of vulva.

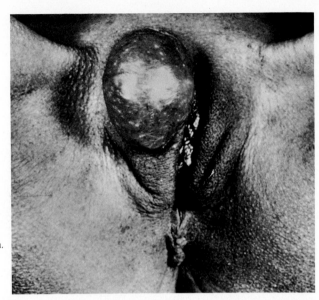

Fig. 2-28.—Vulvar hidradenoma.

majora which then enlarges, develops a pedicle and may hang down for several inches (or feet) so that ulceration and necrosis of the distal portion may occur (Fig. 2–27). The histologic picture is that of any dermatofi-broma, with a well-circumscribed lesion made up of intertwined collagen bundles and fibroblasts. In rare cases the number of nuclei is excessive so that a suspicion of fibrosarcoma is raised. The circumscription of the lesion and absence of mitotic figures and giant cells is usually sufficient to indicate benignancy. These lesions should be surgically removed both for cosmetic effect and for their malignant potential even though it be small.

Hidradenoma.—This is a benign, slow-growing, sweat gland tumor, whose histology simulates that of an adenocarcinoma. It is usually about 1–2 cm. in diameter with a slightly raised, brown surface which may be umbilicated. As seen in Figure 2–28, the lesion may become quite large and cystic change may occur. Histologically this is an adenoma of the vulvar apocrine glands. It is not connected with the epidermis and is usually well encapsulated. The basic pattern is that of a cystlike space in which numerous interlacing villous structures project (Fig. 2–29). These structures, as well as the wall of the cyst, are lined by a single layer of high cylindrical cells with eosinophilic cytoplasm and a large, oval, pale-staining nucleus. The cells are regular and no anaplasia or atypism is evident. A characteristic finding is the layer of myoepithelial cells under the secretory cylindrical cells—a finding similar to that of apocrine tumors in the mammary gland. The lesion is almost always benign, but since a few hidradeno-carcinomas have been reported, all should be excised and submitted to pathologic examination.

Malignant Neoplasms

This broad terminology includes a variety of lesions of separate structure, the most common and most important of which are the squamous

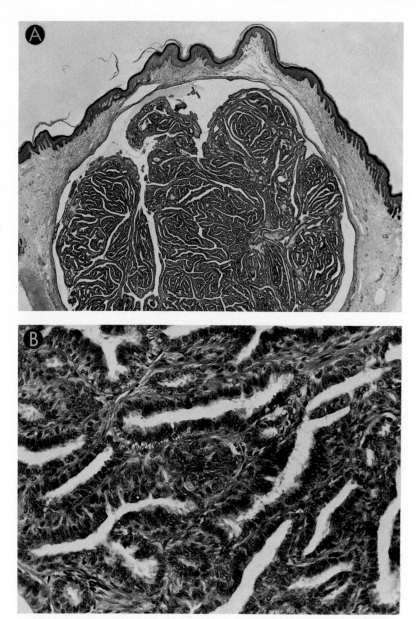

Fig. 2–29.—Hidradenoma. **A,** low power; **B,** high power, showing myoepithelial cells under the secretory cylindrical cells.

cell carcinomas of the labia majora, labia minora and vestibule. Other lesions, fortunately rare, are carcinoma of the clitoris, adenocarcinoma of Bartholin's gland, adenocarcinoma of sweat glands, sarcomas, melanosarcomas, teratomas and Paget's disease. The entire group is said to account for about 1 per cent of all cancers in the female (1.4 per cent of all primary malignant tumors at the Boston Hospital for Women) and for 5–10 per cent of all cancer involving the female genitalia.

CARCINOMA

Vulvar cancer usually occurs in postmenopausal women, about 70 per cent of our patients being between 51 and 70, with an average age of 61.6 years. Youth does not afford complete protection, however, since Way has reported 18 patients between 21 and 40 years. Although postmenopausal bleeding will frequently bring the patient to the physician for examination, abnormalities of the vulva go unnoticed or, if discovered, are self-treated for long periods. A dangerous modesty seems to prevail which accounts for serious patient delay. Added to this is the unexplained hesitancy of many physicians to biopsy vulvar lesions when they are first seen and when opportunity for cure is best. Many months are lost, during which time ointments, salves, lotions and other medications are unsuccessfully tried.

It has become apparent that vulvar carcinoma is not only a disease of the aged but that, as age advances, the incidence of the disease rapidly increases. As the proportion of "old-age" individuals increases in our population, an ever-growing number of vulvar carcinomas will be seen. Thus the importance of diminishing patient delay is obvious if increased salvage is to be realized.

The correlation of leukoplakia, carcinoma in situ and invasive carcinoma has been discussed. It should be reiterated that intelligent observation and treatment of leukoplakia should materially aid in lowering the incidence and mortality rate of vulvar cancer. In most series in which this correlation has been determined, leukoplakia preceded carcinoma in from 12 to 40 per cent of cases. However, Hunt followed 95 patients with leukoplakia and found that carcinoma developed in only five, and in our series at the Boston Hospital for Women, follow-up of 35 patients with definite leukoplakia revealed that only three subsequently had invasive cancer. Other vulvar diseases such as the granulomas and virus-induced condylomas have also been found to predispose to the development of malignancy. Factors such as family history, parity, marital history and race do not predispose to the development of malignancy. In a study of chronic dermatoses both with and without sclerosis, McAdams and Kistner were not able to indict any of these lesions as being precancerous. It is of interest, however, to note that 6–7 per cent of all vulvar carcinomas occur in patients who have another primary carcinoma, usually in the breast, cervix or urethra.

The symptoms complained of most commonly are a localized mass or lump, painful ulcer, discharge, vulvar irritation, dysuria or bleeding. The duration of symptoms in some series has been as long as three or four years but in the cases analyzed at the Boston Hospital for Women it was 13.8 months. Physical examination reveals the lesion to be extremely variable in appearance since in its early form it may merely be an elevated papule or small ulcer. An ulcerative type of vulvar carcinoma is shown in Figure 2–30. The lesion may be a typical everting, ulcerating mass or it may be hypertrophic and resemble a papilloma. Another variety is the non-ulcerating, superficial type which produces severe edema and a peau d'orange effect. About two-thirds of the lesions are found on the labia majora and the remainder on the labia minora, clitoris and posterior commissure. The majority of carcinomas are confined to the anterior half of

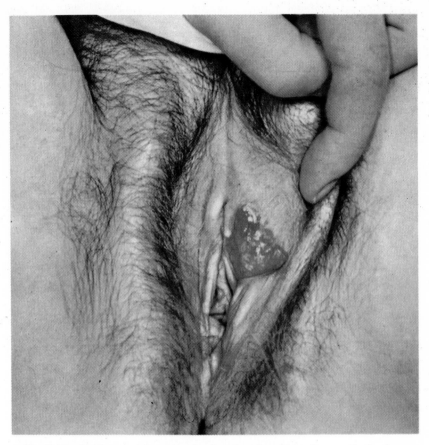

Fig. 2-30.—Carcinoma of the vulva showing ulceration. (From Benson, R.: Carcinoma of the vulva, CA—A Cancer Journal for Clinicians 18: 5, 1968.)

the vulva including the clitoris, and in most cases the external skin surfaces are far more commonly involved than are the medial surfaces of the labia.

Diagnosis is usually obvious except in very early and nonulcerated lesions. Condylomata acuminata, papillomas, ulcerated chancroid, gummas and tuberculous ulcers may be confusing, but biopsy, gram stain and serologic tests will aid in the final diagnosis. The histology is usually that of a moderately well-differentiated, grade I or grade II squamous cell carcinoma. Way, however, found a rather large number of his cases to be of the anaplastic type and stated that these lesions are rapidly growing and rapidly metastasizing. In early lesions the microscopic pattern is that of irregular masses of epidermal cells invading the corium (Fig. 2-31). These masses are composed of differentiated squamous and horn cells and dedifferentiated (atypical or anaplastic) squamous cells. Such anaplasia is expressed by variation in size and shape of the cells, hyperplasia and hyperchromasia of nuclei, loss of polarity, absence of prickles, keratinization of certain cells, presence of mitotic figures and particularly atypical and bizarre mitoses. Differentiation is evident as an increased tendency toward keratinization with the formation of "pearls." These are composed of concentric layers of squamous cells with increased cornification toward the center. Extensive "pearl" formation is seen in Figure 2–32. In the Boston Hospital for Women series, 15 per cent were classified as grade I tumors, 68 per cent as grade II and 11 per cent as grade III.

Clinical staging of carcinoma of the vulva is important, since it refers to the degree of extension of the disease as determined by physical or x-ray examination. It is obvious that survival should be directly correlated with this staging, and this is true not only of carcinoma of the vulva but also of the cervix, breast and endometrium. A workable clinical staging has been proposed by McKelvey:

Stage I   Tumor is 10 sq. cm. or less
Stage II   Tumor is more than 10 sq. cm.
Stage III   Tumor of any size which also involves surrounding structures, such as urethra, vagina, anus or rectum
Stage IV   Tumor of any size with clinically demonstrable intra-abdominal or other distant metastases

Dissemination of vulvar carcinoma is usually by way of lymphatic metastases, probably by tumor emboli rather than by direct permeation (Fig. 2–33). The commonest route of spread is via the superficial inguinal

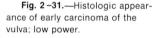

Fig. 2 –31.—Histologic appearance of early carcinoma of the vulva; low power.

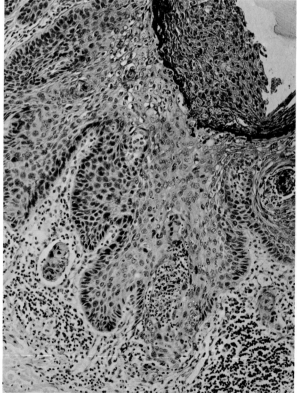

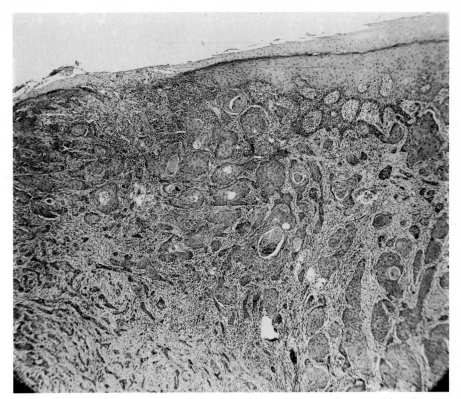

Fig. 2–32.—High-power photomicrograph of carcinoma of the vulva. (Courtesy of Armed Forces Institute of Pathology; no. 70121.)

nodes to the node of Cloquet (the most superior deep femoral node which lies in the upper portion of the femoral canal under the inguinal ligament) and thence to the external iliac nodes. Lesions of the clitoris drain directly to Cloquet's node and lesions which involve the posterior vulva and lower vagina may also bypass the superficial and deep inguinal nodes and drain directly to the external iliac nodes. It is important to realize that contralateral and bilateral spread may occur with a unilateral lesion, so that a bilateral node dissection should be done if surgery is performed. Furthermore, negative findings in superficial nodes do not necessarily mean that the deep nodes are not involved. This situation is more common with lesions involving the posterior labia, posterior vestibule and clitoris. A summation of many reported series shows that involved lymph nodes are found in 55 – 60 per cent of all cases.

The natural history of vulvar cancer is, in general, that of a slowly growing lesion with spread to groin and pelvic nodes and localization in these areas for long periods. Remote metastases are not common until late in the disease when blood-borne spread may occur. If untreated, there is a subsequent fungating, ulcerative process which destroys the vulva, urethra and anus, resulting in painful fistulas. Death may occur from ulceration of large blood vessels, from sepsis or from widespread metastases.

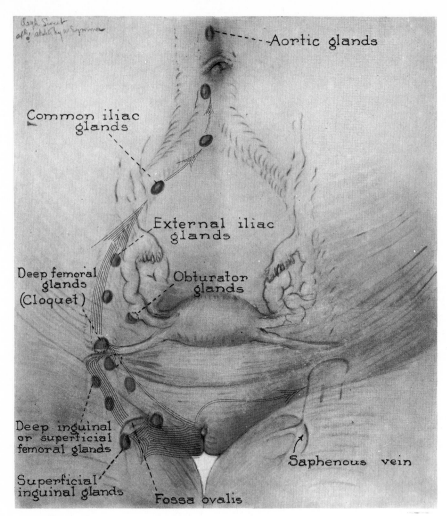

Fig. 2–33.—Lymphatic spread of carcinoma of the vulva. Note: Possible contralateral spread of cancer, especially from anterior vulva and clitoris with possible direct metastasis to a Cloquet node rather than initial involvement of inguinal node. (From Benson, R.: Carcinoma of the vulva, CA—A Cancer Journal for Clinicians 18: 4, 1968.)

Ideals of treatment must emphasize prophylaxis, early diagnosis and early, complete therapy. Although isolated reports have suggested certain dyes, fibers, 3-methylcholanthrene and smegma as carcinogens, no definite evidence exists to support this. The role of scratching, or other trauma, is uncertain since carcinoma is not a sequela of the chronic dermatoses in which pruritus is present. The importance of leukoplakia has been emphasized, and it should be treated as a premalignant state. Chronic discharges, granulomas, syphilis or condylomas should receive prompt and thorough attention. The important point is that any vulvar lesion should be biopsied, watched carefully and rebiopsied whenever necessary.

Definitive therapy in most cases is surgical, and despite the age of the patients, a single-stage radical vulvectomy and bilateral groin resection is almost always possible. The operability rate varies from 50 to 90 per cent and depends on the stage of the lesion and the courage of the surgeon. (It has been 83 per cent at the Boston Hospital For Women). The operation is extensive, although superficial, and to be complete, resection should include the mons, groins and inner thigh down to the muscle and fascia, together with the inguinal, femoral and external iliac nodes and the upper 5–7 cm. of the greater saphenous veins. No attempt is made to preserve the inguinal ligaments or the deep epigastric vessels in the adequate exposure of the deep nodes which are situated anterior and medial to the external iliac vein. The skin flaps may usually be pulled together under moderate tension, but Way insists that if this is possible an adequate amount of tissue has not been removed. Necrosis over the symphysis almost always occurs and may require secondary grafting if the defect is extensive.

Five-year survival depends on the stage of the disease and, therefore, on the incidence of node involvement. In the series at the Boston Hospital for Women only 7 per cent of patients who had nodal metastases survived five years, whereas without metastases the survival rate was 90 per cent. McKelvey reported an 86 per cent operability rate, an absolute five-year cure rate of 44.4 per cent with an 8 per cent operative mortality rate. Way has reported an 87 per cent operability rate, with an operative mortality of 14.6 per cent. The five-year survival rate in patients surviving the operation was 90 per cent. The average five-year survival of 286 patients who had radical vulvectomy and lymphadenectomy (reported by 5 authors) was 65.2 per cent. In those patients in whom the lymph nodes were negative the five-year survival was 83 per cent. Extension of the disease to the vagina, urethra or rectum indicates a grave prognosis, although ultraradical surgery to include partial or total exenteration may increase the survival rate in this group.

X-ray and radium are not used as primary therapy unless the disease is so extensive that surgery is not technically feasible. In such patients judicious use of radium may be of great palliative value. Diathermy coagulation may be used as palliation in large, bulky tumors which distort the vulva and adjacent orifices.

OTHER VULVAR MALIGNANCIES

Carcinoma of Bartholin's gland is a rare finding, and its treatment is that suggested for other carcinomas. It may be mistaken for a benign tumor or a chronic bartholinitis because of its location. A high degree of malignancy exists because of the rich drainage of the gland lymphatics into the deep as well as the superficial lymphatics. Only 109 cases of this entity have been reported, with only nine patients living without disease at the end of five years. About one half of the tumors were adenocarcinoma, one-third were squamous and the rest were mixed or undifferentiated.

Basal cell carcinoma of the vulva is also rather rare, about 75 cases having been reported. It tends to recur locally rather than to spread by lymphatic and blood channels but, unlike basal cell carcinomas elsewhere on the skin, the prognosis is poor. There is some evidence that these tumors do not arise from the basal cells of the epidermis but from hair sheaths or distorted primordia of dermal adnexae. Lever believes them to be nevoid tumors (hemartomas) derived from arrested, embryonal, primary epithelial germ cells. No relationship between leukoplakia and basal cell carcinoma has been demonstrated. Treatment should include a wide and deep local excision, best performed as a unilateral vulvectomy.

Only about 30 cases of *sarcoma* of the vulva have been reported. This tumor may arise from the connective tissue of the vulva or from a fibroma. Several cases of reticulum cell sarcoma and lymphosarcoma have recently been added to the literature. The prognosis is poor despite radical surgery. *Melanomas* are malignant tumors arising from a lentigo or pigmented nevus, characterized by a gradually enlarging, deeply pigmented nodule which is usually surrounded by an erythematous area. Later on the lesion ulcerates and satellites may appear. Metastases occur first through lymphatics with involvement of adjacent nodes. Invasion of the blood stream is a late event but when it occurs widespread metastases appear. Treatment should be radical vulvectomy and bilateral groin dissection unless distant metastases have been demonstrated.

Paget's disease of the vulva merits mention as a possible precancerous or early malignant lesion. As a disorder of the mammary gland, it is a well-known entity, having been described by James Paget in 1874. It is accepted that mammary Paget's disease is a primary duct cancer which has extended to the epidermis where it causes a cutaneous lesion. Woodruff, however, feels that Paget's disease of the vulva is an intraepithelial lesion and that Paget cells arise *de novo* in the epithelium or in its appendages. It is entirely possible that this lesion may progress to invasive carcinoma in much the same fashion as Bowen's disease if one accepts the histogenesis as being autochthonous, as suggested by Woodruff. Huber, in describing three new cases of vulvar Paget's disease, found a definite adenocarcinoma of the underlying apocrine sweat glands in one. The fact remains that, even if a subjacent or adjacent apocrine carcinoma is not discovered, this by no means rules out the possibility that Paget cells may have arisen therein.

In the vulva, the lesion occurs in women in the later decades of life whose presenting complaint is usually pruritus. Grossly it is sharply demarcated, florid, red and moist, with occasional crusting. Little islands of whitened skin appear between the reddened areas (Fig. 2–34). The entire vulva may be involved, with spread to the perineum, mons and thighs. The histologic appearance is characteristic (Fig. 2–35). There is acanthosis with elongation and widening of the rete ridges. Paget cells may be scattered or grouped in clusters, usually in the basalis. They are large cells, lacking prickles, and are surrounded by clear spaces. The cytoplasm is very light and the nuclei are large, round and pale. Paget cells do not invade the corium, a fact which militates somewhat against their intraepithelial origin. Treatment should be that of wide and deep excision with careful follow-up, despite the long interval that usually elapses before definitive treatment is employed. Bilateral pelvic lymphadenectomy is not usually employed as adjunctive therapy for Paget's disease of the vulva. Because local recurrences are common, repeated observations and biopsy of suspicious areas are suggested.

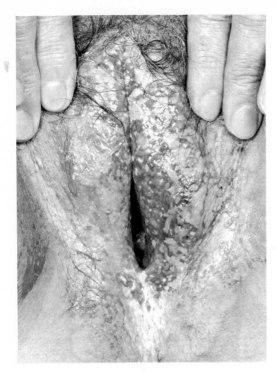

Fig. 2–34.—Gross appearance of Paget's disease of the vulva. The dark areas are velvety red and the white areas are as seen. (From Woodruff, J. D., and Williams, T. F.: The dopa reaction in Paget's disease of the vulva, Obst. & Gynec. 14: 86, 1959.)

Fig. 2–35.—Paget's disease of the vulva, showing marked hyperkeratosis and parakeratosis. Large, irregular cells are seen in the basal layer of the epidermis and infiltrating the upper layers as well. The Paget cells contain clear vacuolated cytoplasm and vesicular nuclei which vary in size, shape and staining quality.

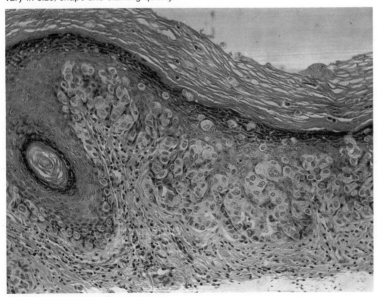

BIBLIOGRAPHY

Anatomy

Anson, B. J.: *An Atlas of Human Anatomy* (Philadelphia: W. B. Saunders Company, 1950).
Lever, W. F.: *Histopathology of Skin* (2d ed.; Philadelphia: J. B. Lippincott Company, 1954).

Embryology

Koff, A. K.: Embryology of the Female Generative Tract, in Curtis, A. H. (ed.): *Obstetrics and Gynecology* (Philadelphia: W. B. Saunders Company, 1933).
Patten, B. M.: *Human Embryology* (2d ed.; New York: McGraw-Hill Book Company, 1953).
Young, H. H.: *Genital Abnormalities, Hermaphroditism and Related Adrenal Diseases* (Baltimore: Williams & Wilkins Company, 1937).

Infections

Beerman, H.: Syphilis, in *Current Diagnosis* (Philadelphia: W. B. Saunders Company, 1966, p. 77).
Charlewood, G. P., and Shippel, S.: Vulval condylomata acuminata as a premalignant lesion in the Bantu, South African M. J. 27: 149, 1953.
Davis, M. E.: Differential diagnosis and treatment of vulvar lesions, S. Clin. North America 30: 267, 1950.
Deacon, W. E., et al.: Identification of Neisseria gonorrhoeae by means of fluorescent antibodies, Proc. Soc. Exper. Biol. & Med. 101: 322, 1959.
Fiumara, N. J.: Gonorrhea, in *Current Diagnosis* (Philadelphia: W. B. Saunders Company, 1966, p. 49).
Gallanis, T. C., Dawson, F. and Harding, H. B.: Laboratory diagnosis of gonorrhea in premenarchal females and in adults, Obst. & Gynec. 29: 401, 1967.
Gray, L. A., and Barnes, M. L.: Lymphogranuloma venereum in the female, Am. J. Surg. 38: 277, 1940.
———, and Kotcher, E.: Vulvovaginitis in childhood, Clin. Obst. & Gynec. 3: 165, 1960.
Greenblatt, R. B.; Baldwin, K. R., and Dienst, R. B.: Minor venereal diseases, Clin. Obst. & Gynec. 2: 549, 1959.
Hester, L. J.: Granuloma venereum of the cervix and vulva, Am. J. Obst. & Gynec. 62: 312, 1951.
Huffman, J. W.: Vulvar disorders in premenarchal children, Clin. Obst. & Gynec. 3: 154, 1960.
Hunt, E.: *Diseases Affecting the Vulva* (4th ed.; St. Louis: C. V. Mosby Company, 1954).
Lang, W. R.: Genital infections in female children, Clin. Obst. & Gynec. 2: 428, 1959.
Schauffler, G. C.: *Pediatric Gynecology* (4th ed.; Chicago: Year Book Publishers, Inc., 1958).

Chronic Vulvitis

Clark, W. H., Jr.: A histological study of kraurosis vulvae, lichen sclerosus et atrophicus and leukoplakia of the vulva; a preliminary report, Bull. Tulane M. Fac. 16: 123, 1957.
Cockerell, E. G.; Knox, J. M., and Rogers, S. F.: Lichen sclerosus et atrophicus, Obst. & Gynec. 15: 554, 1960.
Collins, C. G., et al.: Vulvectomy for benign disease, Am. J. Obst. & Gynec. 76: 363, 1958.
Hyman, A. B., and Falk, H. C.: White lesions of the vulva, Obst. & Gynec. 12: 407, 1958.
Lynch, F. W.: Pruritus vulvae as seen in dermatological practice, J.A.M.A. 150: 14, 1952.
Mering, J. H.: A surgical approach to intractable pruritus vulvae, Am. J. Obst. & Gynec. 64:619, 1952.

Benign Tumors

Anderson, N. P.: Hidradenoma of vulva, Arch. Dermat. & Syph. 62: 873, 1950.
Chung, J. T., and Greene, R. R.: Hidradenoma of vulva, Am. J. Obst. & Gynec. 75: 310, 1958.
de Sousa, L. M., and Lash, A. F.: Hemangiopericytoma of the vulva, Am. J. Obst. & Gynec. 78: 295, 1959.
Duson, C. K., and Zelenik, J. S.: Vulvar endometriosis, apparently produced by menstrual blood, Obst. & Gynec. 3: 76, 1954.
Lacy, G. R.: Hidradenoma and hidradenoid carcinoma of the vulva, Am. J. Obst. & Gynec. 51: 268, 1945.

Leukoplakia and Carcinoma in Situ

Berkeley, C., and Bonney, V.: Leukoplakia vulvitis and its relation to kraurosis vulvae and carcinoma vulvae, Proc. Roy. Soc. Med. 3: 29, 1910.
Collins, C. G., et al.: Non-invasive malignancy of the vulva, Obst. & Gynec. 6: 339, 1955.
Gardiner, S. H., et al.: Intraepithelial carcinoma of vulva, Am. J. Obst. & Gynec. 65: 539, 1953.
Goldberg, L. C.: Bowen's precancerosis with carcinoma: Report of case of organized syphilitic vulvar papules, leukoplakia, Bowen's precancerosis and basal cell carcinoma, Arch. Dermat. & Syph. 36: 47, 1937.
Jayle, F.: Le kraurosis vulvae, Rev. gynec. et chir. abd. 10: 633, 1906.
Jeffcoate, T. N. A.; Davie, T. B., and Harrison, C. V.: Intra-epidermal carcinoma (Bowen's disease) of vulva: Report on 2 cases, J. Obst. & Gynaec. Brit. Emp. 51: 377, 1944.
Ketron, L. W., and Ellis, F. A.: Kraurosis vulvae (leukoplakia) and scleroderma circumscripta: Comparative histological study, Surg. Gynec. & Obst. 61: 635, 1935.

Kindler, T.: Lichen sclerosus et atrophicus in young subjects, Brit. J. Dermat. 65:269, 1953.

Langley, I. I.; Hertig, A. T., and Smith, G. V.: Relation of leukoplakic vulvitis to squamous carcinoma of vulva, Am. J. Obst. & Gynec. 62:167, 1951.

McAdams, A. J., Jr., and Kistner, R. W.: The relationship of chronic vulvar disease, leukoplakia and carcinoma in situ to carcinoma of the vulva, Cancer 11: 740, 1958.

Miller, N. F.; Riley, G. M., and Stanley, M.: Leukoplakia of vulva: II, Am. J. Obst. & Gynec. 64: 768, 1952.

Montgomery, H.: Precancerous dermatosis and epithelioma in situ, Arch. Dermat. & Syph. 39: 387, 1939.

———; Counseller, V. S., and Craig, W. M.: Kraurosis, leukoplakia and pruritus vulvae: Correlation of clinical and pathologic observations, with further studies regarding resection of sensory nerves of perineum, Arch. Dermat. & Syph. 30: 80, 1934.

———, and Hill, W. R.: Lichen sclerosus et atrophicus, Arch. Dermat. & Syph. 42: 755, 1940.

Taussig, F. J.: Leukoplakia vulvitis and cancer of the vulva, Am. J. Obst. & Gynec. 18: 472, 1929.

Woodruff, J. D., and Hildebrandt, E. E.: Carcinoma in situ of the vulva, Obst. & Gynec. 12: 414, 1958.

———, and Novak, E. R.: Premalignant lesions of the vulva: A pathological and clinical survey, Clin. Obst. & Gynec. 5: 1102, 1962.

Carcinoma

Anderson, N. P.: Bowen's precancerous dermatosis and multiple benign superficial epithelioma: Evidence of arsenic as etiologic agent, Arch. Dermat. & Syph. 26: 1052, 1932.

Berlin, H., and Winters, H. S.: Malignant melanoma of the vulva with pregnancy, Obst. & Gynec. 15: 302, 1960.

Berman, W.: Basal cell carcinoma of the vulva, Am. J. Obst. & Gynec. 42: 1070, 1941.

Berven, E. G. E.: Carcinoma of vulva: I. Treatment of cancer of vulva (symposium), Brit. J. Radiol. 22: 498, 1949.

Bonney, V.: Connective tissue in carcinoma and in certain inflammatory states that precede its onset (Hunterian lecture), Lancet 1: 1465, 1953.

Boughton, T. G.: Carcinoma of Bartholin's gland, Am. J. Surg. 59: 585, 1943.

Brack, C. B., and Farber, G. J.: Carcinoma of the female urethra, J. Urol. 64: 710, 1950.

Brunschwig, A. and Brockunier, A.: Surgical treatment of squamous cell carcinoma of the vulva, Obst. & Gynec. 29: 362, 1967.

Buckingham, J. C., and McClure, J. H.: Reticulum cell sarcoma of vulva, Obst. & Gynec. 6: 121, 1955.

Diehl, W. K.; Baggett, J. W., and Shell, J. H.: Vulvar cancer: Critical review, Am. J. Obst. & Gynec. 62: 1209, 1951.

Ellis, F.: Carcinoma of vulva: III. Cancer of vulva treated by radiation; analysis of 127 cases, Brit. J. Radiol. 22: 513, 1949.

Fagan, G. E., and Hertig, A. T.: Carcinoma of the female urethra, Obst. & Gynec. 6: 1, 1955.

Green, T. H.; Ulfelder, H., and Meigs, J. V.: Epidermoid carcinoma of the vulva, Am. J. Obst. & Gynec. 75: 834, 1958.

Hertig, A. T., and Gore, H.: *Tumors of the Female Sex Organs: Part 2. Tumors of the Vulva, Vagina and Uterus* (Washington, D.C.: Armed Forces Institute of Pathology, 1960).

Huber, C. P.; Gardiner, S. H., and Michael, A.: Paget's disease of the vulva, Am. J. Obst. & Gynec. 62: 778, 1951.

Kottmeier, H. L.: *Carcinoma of the Female Genitalia.* The Abraham Flexner Lecture Series, no. 11 (Baltimore: Williams & Wilkins Company, 1953).

McKelvey, J. L.: Carcinoma of the vulva, Obst. & Gynec. 5: 452, 1955.

Newell, J. W., and McKay, D. G.: Clinical review of carcinoma of vulva, West. J. Surg. 60: 388, 1952.

Palmer, J. P.; Sadugor, M. G., and Reinhard, M. C.: Carcinoma of the vulva: Report of 313 cases, Surg. Gynec. & Obst. 88: 435, 1949.

Pund, E. R., and Cole, W. C.: Carcinoma of Bartholin's gland, Am. J. Obst. & Gynec. 43: 887, 1942.

Rubin, A. R.: Granular-cell myoblastoma of the vulva, Am. J. Obst. & Gynec. 77: 292, 1959.

Rutledge, F. N.: Cancer of the vulva and vagina, Clin. Obst. & Gynec. 8: 1051, 1965.

Sadler, W. P., and Dockerty, M. D.: Malignant myoblastoma vulvae, Am. J. Obst. & Gynec. 61: 1047, 1951.

Taussig, F. J.: Leukoplakia and cancer of vulva, Arch. Dermat. & Syph. 21: 431, 1930.

Ulfelder, H.: Radical vulvectomy with bilateral inguinal, femoral and iliac node dissection, Am. J. Obst. & Gynec. 78: 1074, 1959.

Way, S. C.: Carcinoma of the vulva, Am. J. Obst. & Gynec. 79: 692, 1960.

Way, S.: Results of a planned attack on carcinoma of the vulva, Brit. M. J. 2: 780, 1954.

Way, S. and Hennigan, M.: Late results of extended radical vulvectomy for carcinoma of the vulva, J. Obst. & Gynaec. Brit. Commonwealth 73: 594, 1966.

Woodruff, J. D.: Paget's disease of the vulva, Obst. & Gynec. 5: 175, 1955.

———, and Brack, C. B.: Unusual malignancies of vulvourethral region, Obst. & Gynec. 12: 677, 1958.

Woodruff, J. D. and Williams, T. F.: The dopa reaction in Paget's disease of the vulva, Obst. & Gynec. 14: 86, 1959.

CHAPTER 3

The Vagina

THE VAGINA (L., sheath) is a tubular, fibromuscular structure, lined by strat-ified squamous epithelium, which extends from the vestibule to the uterus. Its function is to receive the penis during coitus and in so doing affords the seminal fluid protective entrance through the external os of the cervix. The reproductive function of the vagina is fulfilled during parturition since it represents the lowermost part of the birth canal. A third function is that of an excretory duct for menstrual discharge. From the viewpoint of the clini-cian, a fourth function is the opportunity it provides for the examination of the internal genitalia.

Embryology

Embryologically the vagina may be looked on as having a double origin, that is, from the urogenital sinus and from the müllerian ducts. As men-tioned in Chapter 2, the terminal ends of the müllerian ducts impinge on the urogenital sinus at the termination of their caudad growth, thus form-ing the müllerian tubercle (Fig. 3–1). Later this tubercle disappears as two mesenchymal outgrowths appear on the dorsal surface of the posterior wall of the urogenital sinus. These are the sinovaginal bulbs from which the lower vagina develops. The epithelium of the caudal portion of the uterovaginal canal later proliferates and completely occludes the canal. Thus a solid cord of epithelium is formed, derived from the uterovaginal canal above and the sinovaginal bulbs below. When the embryo is about 150 mm. in length the central cells of this cord degenerate and a hollow tube is formed. Eventually penetration and invasion of this müllerian tube by urogenital sinus epithelium occurs and, when complete, the vagina is lined by stratified cuboidal epithelium derived from the urogenital sinus. The latter then differentiates into stratified squamous cells. A vaginal occlusion is thus the result of a failure of urogenital cells to invade the mül-lerian tube. Normally the replacement of müllerian with squamous epithe-lium ends at the external os of the cervix, but occasionally it ends distal to the os, leaving an area of columnar epithelium, the so-called "congenital erosion" or eversion. In other cases the squamous epithelium invades the endocervix for varying lengths and may remain there permanently. This process has been termed "epidermization." By contrast, "squamous meta-plasia" may occur in the endocervix and produce the same histologic effect, but here the columnar epithelium (müllerian) undergoes a change

Fig. 3-1.—Formation of the lower vagina. The müllerian tubercle is formed by impingement of the terminal ends of the müllerian ducts against the urogenital sinus. The vagina has a double origin, therefore, from the müllerian tubercle and from outgrowths of the urogenital sinus.

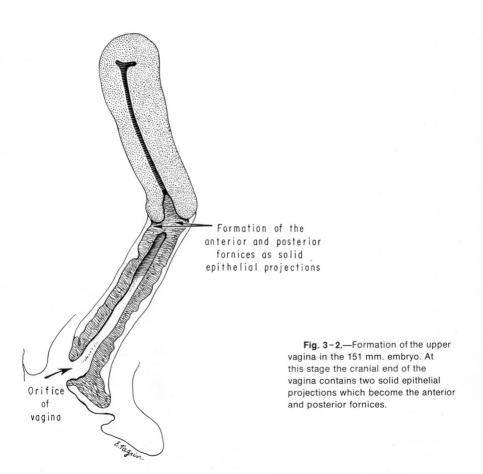

R. Wolffian duct

L. Wolffian duct

Müllerian duct

Primordium of vaginal cord

Müllerian tubercle

Urogenital sinus

Formation of the anterior and posterior fornices as solid epithelial projections

Orifice of vagina

Fig. 3-2.—Formation of the upper vagina in the 151 mm. embryo. At this stage the cranial end of the vagina contains two solid epithelial projections which become the anterior and posterior fornices.

to a squamous type and is not actually replaced. To summarize the conclusions of Koff in relation to the development of the vagina, the following points are of importance:

1. The müllerian ducts appear in the 11 mm. embryo as invaginations of the coelomic epithelium lateral to the cranial extremity of the mesonephros and lateral to the wolffian duct.

2. The solid tips of the müllerian ducts tunnel caudally through the mesenchyme, cross the wolffian ducts anteriorly at the level of the lower end of the mesonephros, approach each other in the midline, fuse and reach the posterior wall of the urogenital sinus and push it forward to form the müllerian tubercle in the 30 mm. embryo.

3. The fusion of the müllerian ducts is complete in the 56 mm. embryo to form the uterovaginal canal.

4. In the 63 mm. embryo the sinovaginal bulbs are formed by bilateral posterior evaginations of the urogenital sinus. Owing to the formation of these structures, the müllerian tubercle is obliterated. At the same period, there is a stratification of the cells lining this portion of the urogenital sinus, and the solid cells composing the tip of the uterovaginal canal show involutional changes due to compression by the paired sinovaginal bulbs.

5. The wolffian ducts show involutional changes throughout. When they do persist, their caudal ends migrate cranially with the growth of the sinovaginal bulbs.

6. The sinovaginal bulbs become solidified by proliferation of lining epithelium and fuse with the tip of the müllerian ducts, which later solidify by the same process and form the solid vaginal plate.

7. The solid primitive vaginal plate grows in all dimensions by the formation and fusion of trabeculae.

8. The central cells of the now solid vagina break down to form the cavity of the vagina.

9. The cranial end of the vagina is demarcated in the 151 mm. embryo by the formation of the anterior and posterior fornices as solid epithelial projections (Fig. 3–2). The caudal end expands, pushes in the posterior wall of the urogenital sinus and extends along the posterior wall to form the caudal segment of the hymen; the anterior paired segment is formed where the evaginations of the urogenital sinus occur to form the sinovaginal bulbs.

Anatomy and Histology

The anterior vaginal wall is in contact with the membranous urethra and bladder and is separated only by a thin layer of endopelvic fascia, the pubovesicovaginal fascia. The most cephalad portion of the anterior vaginal wall ends in a blind pouch, or fornix, and its epithelium is continuous with that of the anterior lip of the cervix which projects forward into the upper vagina. The posterior vaginal wall is in contact with the structures of the perineal body and rectovaginal fascia but its upper extension, the posterior fornix, is more cephalad than its anterior counterpart and attaches to the cervix just below the uterorectal fold of peritoneum. The latter is known as the posterior cul-de-sac of Douglas and is of clinical importance since the peritoneal cavity may be easily entered through the posterior vagina without damage to adjacent organs or structures. The epithelium of the posterior fornix is also continuous with that of the posterior cervix. That portion of the cervix which juts forward into the vagina and is covered with stratified squamous epithelium is called the portio vaginalis (Fig. 3–3).

The vagina is a potential cavity, but in the normal state the walls are in apposition. In multiparous women the potential space becomes an actual

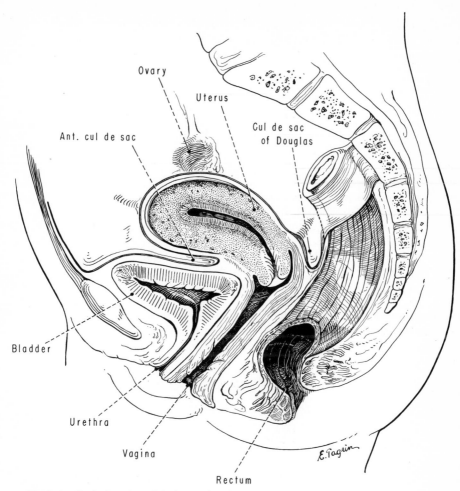

Ovary

Uterus

Cul de sac
of Douglas

Ant. cul de sac

Bladder

Urethra

Vagina

Rectum

E. Tagrin

Fig. 3–3.—Sagittal section of the human female pelvis showing the anatomic relations of the vagina.

one due to the stretching and tearing of the vaginal supports. If the vagina is transected in its medial portion, it presents an H-shaped appearance, the lateral limits being moderately convex toward the midline. The vaginal length is variable but the posterior wall approximates 8–9 cm. and the anterior wall 6–8 cm. The bore follows the usual pattern of constriction at the outlet, distensibility in the midportion and narrowing at the fornices. This is exemplified at the time of delivery when the vaginal outlet must be incised to allow passage of the fetal head. The lateral aspects of the most cephalad portion of the vagina are known as the lateral fornices or vaults.

A longitudinal ridge is usually visible running along the anterior and posterior vaginal walls. These ridges are termed the vaginal columns and represent the line of fusion of the two müllerian ducts. Extending laterally from these columns are numerous elevations, the rugae, and between the rugae are intervening furrows. Seen in microscopic section these appear as simple elevations of the surface epithelium over the dermis. The rugae are formed by the ingrowth of numerous solid epithelial projections into the subjacent mesenchyme when the vaginal lumen is not completely filled with epithelium. The rugated appearance of the vagina is prominent in young adolescents and adults but disappears with multiparity and senescence. Postmenopausally the vaginal mucosa is smooth and shiny.

The wall of the vagina is made up of three layers: (1) mucous membrane, (2) muscularis and (3) adventitial connective tissue.

The mucous membrane consists of a lamina propria of dense connective tissue and a surface epithelium (Fig. 3–4). The latter is made up of six to 10 layers of stratified squamous cells which do not show cornification although keratohyalin granules may be present. The cells, even when desquamated, contain glycogen if adequate estrogen stimulation is present. In vaginal prolapse this is altered, and marked hyperkeratosis may be present. Under ordinary circumstances the glycogenated vaginal cells stain a deep brown with iodine (Schiller's) solution, whereas if hyperkeratosis has occurred this staining property is lost. Dermal papillae are rather prominent in the posterior wall together with irregular rete ridges, whereas in the anterior wall the epidermis is more regular. Beneath the epithelium an interlacing network of elastic fibers is evident in the connective tissue. Interspersed are foci of lymphocytes and numerous blood vessels. There are no glands in the vagina under normal conditions, but occasionally misplaced endocervical glands, wolffian duct remnants or epidermal inclusion cysts are found. The vagina is lubricated by secretions from the

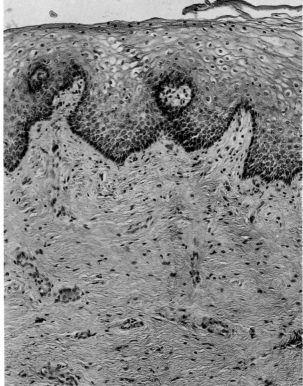

Fig. 3–4.—Photomicrograph of the adult vaginal epithelium and stroma.

cervix and Bartholin's glands, although during sexual stimulation fluid has been described as originating from the vaginal epithelium.

The muscularis is made up of external longitudinal and internal circular layers. The latter are interspersed liberally into the fibroelastic tissue of the lamina propria.

The adventitial coat is an outer layer of dense connective tissue in which are numerous blood vessels and nerves. It blends imperceptibly with the perivaginal (rectovaginal and vesicovaginal) fascia and is in itself supportive.

Malformations

During the first three months of embryonic development there is a close association and correlation of development of the vagina, urinary system, urogenital sinus, cloaca and rectum, so that abnormalities of one are commonly integrated with abnormalities in any or all of the others. It has been pointed out previously that the müllerian ducts normally fuse to form the uterus and vagina, but this process may be arrested at any point. Of particular importance is the process of differentiation of the müllerian tubercle. This structure opens into the urogenital sinus, as does the urinary tract. The process of separation of the two systems is brought about by the descent of this tubercle, creating a septum between the openings of the urethra and vagina in their normal position in the vestibule. The descent of the müllerian tubercle is believed to be a function of estrogenic stimulation so that if relative excesses of androgens are present (as in adrenal hyperplasia) the ultimate position of the vaginal orifice is altered. Thus the vagina may then connect with the urogenital sinus so that a common exit is present at birth. Another variant is due to incomplete fusion of the müllerian ducts, resulting in the formation of a double uterus (uterus didelphys), double cervix and double vagina (Fig. 3–5). In rare cases canalization of the solid müllerian tube does not occur and total absence of the vagina results.

Congenital absence of the vagina seems to be a more common developmental defect in Finland than in other European countries. Turunen has seen more than 200 such cases and has operated on 145 of them. Affected patients show normal constitutional development, though they are frequently of small stature. The secondary sex characteristics, breasts and hair distribution are normal, as are the external genitalia in most cases. The uterus is usually of the rudimentary, bicornis separatus type but occasionally it is normal. In 5 patients Turunen was able to establish continuity between such a uterus and an artificial vagina with subsequent menstruation. Three of these patients became pregnant. This series also showed a large number of abnormalities of the thoracic spine, chiefly wedge vertebrae, fusions, rudimentary and supernumerary vertebrae.

If the cells of the urogenital sinus do not penetrate the müllerian tube, there may be a total occlusion of the vagina. Occasionally both the vagina and rectum open into the urogenital sinus or into the urethra.

The first-mentioned abnormality, urovaginal connection, is seen frequently in patients with female hermaphroditism associated with adrenal hyperplasia. The findings include (1) a persistent urogenital sinus into which the vagina opens, (2) an enlarged clitoris, (3) hypoplastic or infantile

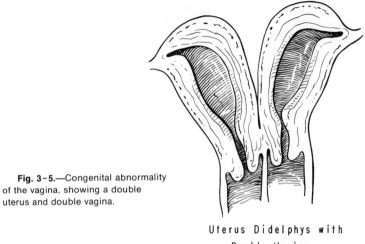

Fig. 3-5.—Congenital abnormality of the vagina, showing a double uterus and double vagina.

Uterus Didelphys with
Double Vagina

uterus and ovaries and (4) greatly enlarged adrenals with hyperplasia of the androgenic zone. Correction of these defects is possible by vaginal plastic surgery in combination with the administration of cortisone. Pregnancies subsequent to this therapy have been reported in such individuals. In those cases caused by adrenal neoplasm surgery will be required, whereas in those due to hyperplasia or hyperfunction cortisone therapy alone may be effective. If the abnormality is that of a double vagina alone, this may be corrected by excision of the septum. If there is associated duplication of the uterus, serious difficulties may be encountered in the form of infertility, abortion or dystocia. The construction of an artificial vagina in patients in whom it is completely lacking has become rather commonplace, and many recent reports indicate excellent results utilizing skin grafts and obturators of various types. Unfortunately the uterus in most of these patients is not sufficiently well developed to allow menstrual function or conception. Although the uterus is frequently said to be absent, more often than not it may be found at laparotomy as a small rudimentary nubbin of tissue in the midline or along the lateral pelvic wall. For a complete description of these abnormalities and their treatment the reader is referred to the works of Wilkins *et al.*, Jones and Young. (See also Chapter 16, Cytogenetics.)

Physiologic Alterations

Before the various forms of vaginitis are considered, it is appropriate to review certain fundamentals of vaginal physiology which deal specifically with the subjects of acidity and bacterial flora. It has been known since 1877 that the vaginal discharge is acid and since 1892 that this acidity is due to the presence of gram-positive organisms, the Döderlein bacilli. The acidity is directly correlated with the amount of lactic acid present, although it has been suggested that perhaps other acids may be effective in certain cases. The exact origin of vaginal lactic acid is unknown but most evidence suggests that it represents a breakdown product of glycogen.

Glycogen is deposited in the cells of the vaginal epithelium under the influence of estrogen although the administration of progesterone in castrates will accomplish the same effect. This is probably due to conversion of progesterone to estrogen. Diminution in the amount of estrogen results in the disappearance of cellular glycogen. Conversely, when estrogen levels are high, vaginal glycogen is abundant. Cellular glycogen may be converted directly to lactic acid by the action of Döderlein's bacilli or it may be fermented to simpler carbohydrates by vaginal enzymes and then reduced by bacteria to lactic acid. Other possibilities are that glycogen is converted to lactic acid by enzymes alone or that bacteria other then Döderlein's are capable of fermenting carbohydrates. Döderlein's bacillus is probably identical with Lactobacillus acidophilus, a facultative anaerobic, nonmotile, gram-positive rod.

The pH of the human vagina has been extensively studied with glass electrodes and various indicator dyes. The vagina of the newborn has a pH of about 5.7, the elevation presumably being due to the presence of alkaline amniotic fluid. Döderlein's bacilli appear about the fourth day and the pH falls to about 4.8. There is then a rise beginning on the eighth day to neutrality, and neutral values persist until the onset of puberty. Following onset of the menarche the pH varies between 4.0 and 5.0, depending on the stage of the menstrual cycle. Lowest values have been found at ovulation and premenstrually. This parallels the curves of estrogen excretion for the normal cycle. There is also a pH gradient, depending on the area of the vagina sampled. Thus, the lowest values are found near the anterior fornix, intermediate ones in the midvagina and highest ones near the vestibule. A pH of 4.0 or less is found during pregnancy, whereas in the postmenopausal women neutral or alkaline values may be seen. The clinical importance of this maintained acidity is emphasized by the fact that most pathogenic bacteria disappear when the pH is kept between 4.1 and 4.9.

During pregnancy the vaginal epithelium reaches a maximum thickness, with concomitant increased glycogen content. Accordingly, the amount of lactic acid production is increased and the pH varies between 3.8 and 4.4. In the newborn infant the vagina is of adult histologic type as a result of maternal estrogen. After a few weeks, however, the epithelium diminishes in thickness and after a few months it is quite thin. This condition is maintained until puberty, with the result that the natural barriers to disease during this time are minimal and gonorrheal and nonspecific vaginitis are common. At puberty the epithelium thickens, glycogen is deposited and the pH is lowered to about 4.0. A vaginal discharge may be noted at this time similar to that occasionally seen in the newborn infant. Microscopically it is made up of precornified and cornified vaginal epithelial cells, leukocytes and many Döderlein's bacilli. Menopause brings about changes in the vaginal epithelium similar to those found before puberty. The epithelial thickness is then greatly reduced and the surface appears smooth and shiny. The individual cells contain little glycogen and Döderlein's bacilli are scarce, so that a pH of 6.0 is common. Vaginal smears show mostly basal cells and leukocytes. The vagina during this stage is quite susceptible to infection and trauma. Interesting observations have been made on artificial vaginas constructed of homologous donor skin. In most cases the glycogen content, acidity, bacterial flora and cytology closely resemble those of the normal vagina.

Cytology

The desquamated epithelial cells of the human vagina lend themselves to easy collection and have thus been extensively studied. This is a fortunate circumstance since much may be learned by microscopic examination of either nonstained or stained material. From such observations one may determine the functional state of the ovaries as regards the secretion of hormones, the presence of infection or carcinoma, the therapeutic responses to hormones, drugs or radium or even whether or not the membranes of a parturient are ruptured.

The cytologic examination of the vaginal secretion is done by aspirating the so-called "vaginal pool" from the posterior fornix with a glass tube to which is attached a rubber bulb. The aspirate is immediately spread in a thin film on a glass slide and immersed in solution made up of equal parts of 95 per cent alcohol and ether. Scrapings from the lateral vaginal wall may also be used. After fixation for 30 minutes the slide is allowed to dry and is stained by the method of Papanicolaou. The usual smear will show a preponderance of vaginal cells but also leukocytes, erythrocytes, fibrin, mucus and a varied bacterial flora. Two major groups of cells are immediately recognizable: cornified cells (containing eleidin, a horny substance which gives the cells birefringence) which stain orange-red, and uncornified cells which stain blue or various shades of blue-green. The cornified cells represent the maximum differentiation of the vaginal epithelium brought about by estrogen. The level of effective estrogen may be estimated by the proportionate number of cornified and precornified cells in stained smears, although vaginal infections will alter the cells and negate the importance of such determinations. Hormonal evaluation of cells is best obtained by scrapings from the lateral vaginal wall.

Typically the cornified pyknotic cell is a large, thin, polygonal cell with smooth edges and a bright red-orange color. The cytoplasm is delicate, transparent and homogeneous. The nucleus is small and pyknotic without definite clumping of the chromatin. These nuclei may have a vacuole beside them or may be surrounded by a clear perinuclear halo. Another characteristic of the cornified cells is the pyknotic nucleus so that this group may be termed "cornified karyopyknotic" cells. The origin of these cells is the superficial and granular layer of the epithelium. Uncornified cells originate from three layers: superficial, intermediate and deep. The karyopyknotic uncornified cells (sometimes called "pre-corns") are similar to the cornified cells except that their cytoplasm has an affinity for basic dyes and stains clear blue or violet. The intermediate cells are polygonal in shape and rather large but have the nuclear pattern of the deep cells. They arise from the stratum spinosum where the presence of intracellular bridges is so marked as to give a spiny or prickle cell appearance. The deep cells are small in comparison with those just described but are larger than leukocytes. They are round or ovoid with well-defined edges. The nucleus is large and centrally placed and the cytoplasm forms a perinuclear zone which lightly stains clear blue or violet.

Three types of smears are evident by examination of the cell types. They are (1) follicular, (2) progestational and (3) atrophic. About the middle of the ovulatory cycle and corresponding with the peak of estrogen, the vaginal smear is characterized by a predominance of cornified cells. The cells are large, smooth and polygonal with pyknotic nuclei, and the cytoplasm is free from folding or wrinkling. Mucus is scant and leukocytes are infrequent. After the corpus luteum is well formed and progesterone is being secreted in adequate amounts, the smear takes on a different appearance. Uncornified cells of the intermediate zone are predominant and they present themselves in groups with doubled-over edges and folded or vacuolated cytoplasm. There is an abundance of mucus, leukocytes and bacteria. Certain unusual cells are evident during the progestational phase because of changes in morphology. The "oyster" or "navicular" cells are due to variations of the cell edges, with doubling over. They are especially common during pregnancy or when progesterone secretion is elevated. If neither estrogen nor progesterone is present in adequate amount, the smear has an atrophic appearance. The deep cells predominate here and there may be complete absence of cornified cells. Considerable mucus, bacteria and leukocytes are present. This smear is found during the prepuberal and menopausal periods and in patients with ovarian insufficiency. That these effects are due to lack of estrogen and progesterone has been shown in castrate females with atrophic smears. The sequential administration of estrogen and progesterone will produce both the follicular and the progestational smears followed by regression to the atrophic type after hormone withdrawal.

Exfoliative vaginal cytology has an important role in present-day obstetrics because it reflects the balance of the female hormones, it is simple to perform in the antenatal clinic, does not inconvenience the patient, and does not add an impossible burden to the work of the pathology department.

A reasonably constant feature in pregnancies threatening to abort, but in fact continuing undisturbedly, is the persistence of a normal or nearly normal pregnancy smear. An increase of the pyknotic index from 15 per cent (the normal level during pregnancy) to a figure around 25 per cent carries a good prognosis. The persistency of cytolysis, the presence of navicular cells in clumps, the basophilic staining reaction and a reasonably low pyknotic index (below 30 per cent) all are favorable signs in a threatened abortion. These cytologic data indicate that the amount of progesterone secreted by the corpus luteum or the placenta is sufficient to maintain the pregnancy. In contrast, the vaginal smear in cases of inevitable abortion shows a more or less uniform picture. The discrete arrangement of the cells, the low incidence of navicular cells, the clean background, the absence of cytolysis and high level of pyknosis are all distinctive features.

Morphologic changes in the vaginal cells have been used as a presumptive diagnostic criterion for ovulation. However, since progesterone may be secreted from the theca interna cells of a luteinized follicle, this is not absolute. The use of vaginal and cervical cytology for the diagnosis and follow-up of cervical cancer is discussed in Chapter 4.

Leukorrhea

About one fourth of all patients who visit the average gynecologic clinic do so because of a vaginal discharge called leukorrhea. The majority of these discharges are due to infections of the vaginal epithelium, and the rest to malignancies of the cervix, uterus or vagina, to cervical ectropions and to senescent changes during menopause. With a decrease in vaginal acidity, bacterial invasion occurs and glycogen and Döderlein's bacilli are reduced. The pathogenic organisms which usually produce vaginitis prefer this elevated pH, so that the vaginal secretion with a pH of 5–6 favors continuation of the disease. These changes occur most frequently during menstruation, menopause and following parturition.

The major causes of leukorrhea are: (1) Trichomonas vaginalis and (2) Candida albicans vaginitis, (3) nonspecific vaginitis, including Hemophilus vaginalis vaginitis, (4) senescent vaginitis and (5) chronic cervicitis.

TRICHOMONIASIS

Trichomoniasis is an extremely common finding and frequently is asymptomatic. In a study of 1,197 pregnant women, examination of routine wet smears revealed trichomonads in 26.8 per cent, and it has been demonstrated that one of every five adult women harbors the organism. In other women, however, it causes an acute vaginitis with a frothy, yellow-green or clear, sometimes watery discharge. Occasionally the discharge is mucopurulent. Usually it is profuse and produces an irritating vulvitis that results in marked pruritus, chafing and dyspareunia. Even digital examination or the passage of a speculum may be painful, and there may be generalized complaints of headache, backache or pelvic pressure. A characteristic fetid odor may be the only complaint noted by the patient. Examination reveals reddening of the labia minora, occasionally with intertrigo of the inner thighs, a typical discharge oozing from the introitus and a vaginal membrane which may be fiery red. The portio vaginalis of the cervix is often involved and bleeds easily when wiped with a cotton swab. The vagina may be covered with multiple round, red papules giving a strawberry-like appearance to the epithelium. It has been definitely established that this vaginal inflammation is due to the protozoan flagellate, Trichomonas vaginalis, since bacteria-free cultures of the organism have produced the inflammation, whereas disappearance of the trichomonads from the vagina is associated with the cessation of symptoms and signs of the disease. The average pH of the vagina in affected patients varies from 5.1 to 5.4, and it has been found that cultures of trichomonads will not grow below pH 5.0 or above pH 7.5. The source of infection has not been definitely solved but various studies have suggested the gastrointestinal tract, the urinary tract, contamination from towels and water, and coitus as possible avenues. Although the male may have negligible symptoms or signs there is little doubt that he may infect and reinfect his sexual partner. In a study of 246 men with nonspecific urethritis the incidence of T. vaginalis was 37 per cent. In another report of 36 men whose wives had trichomoniasis, 58 per cent of semen cultures showed trichomonads. The incidence of trichomonas infestation in the male has been estimated at about 15 per cent. Treatment should, therefore, include the male as well as the female to be most effective. Other recurrences may be due to the presence of the organism in the endocervix, urethra, paraurethral glands, Bartholin's glands or anus.

The diagnosis of trichomoniasis is made by placing a drop of the secretion on an ordinary or hanging-drop slide, adding a few drops of warm saline solution and examining the preparation under high-dry magnification. The slide should be looked at immediately since the flagellate will no longer be motile if the preparation stands for any length of time. To aid in the visualization of the flagellate 1 drop of 1 per cent cresyl blue solution in isotonic sodium chloride may be mixed with 1 drop of the discharge. This will separate the cells, and the vaginal cells will appear violet while only the trichomonads and a few living polymorphonuclear leukocytes will be white. Two precautions are necessary: the examination should not be made in an excessively cold place since cold suppresses trichomonal activity, and isotonic sodium chloride should be used rather than water since water causes the organism to become immobilized and swollen. Giemsa stains and cultures are useful in assessing cure and in detecting extravaginal sources of infection. Trichomonas vaginalis is morphologically similar to T. hominis with two exceptions: the marginal filament along the undulating membrane is not prolonged into a free flagellum and the parabasal body is well defined. The undulating membrane is about one-third to two-thirds the length of the body and there are four anterior flagella and a thin projecting axostyle at the posterior end. The usual preparation will contain many desquamated vaginal cells and leukocytes (Fig. 3–6). By comparison, T. vaginalis is larger than the leukocyte but about one-half the size of a cornified epithelial cell. The average body length is about 15–20 μ and contains an oval nucleus in which are scattered chromatin granules.

TREATMENT.—Temporary relief from symptoms is usually accomplished easily but permanent cure is difficult and at times seems almost impossible. A combination of restoration of vaginal acidity and destruction of the parasite is desirable. This may be accomplished by mild acid douches (2 tablespoons of white vinegar or 2 teaspoons lactic acid per quart of warm water) and the concomitant use of a trichomonacide.

An oral preparation, Flagyl (metronidazole), has given excellent results when administered to both husband and wife for a 10-day period. It has been most effective in resistant cases.

Clinical and experimental studies have shown Flagyl to be highly trichomonacidal in low concentration. It is readily absorbed from the intestinal tract. Flagyl has been proved effective in the treatment of trichomonal

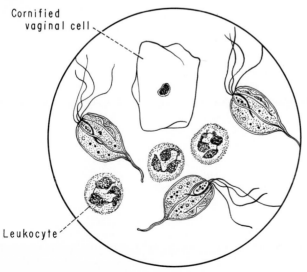

Cornified
vaginal cell

Leukocyte

Fig. 3–6.—Trichomonads as seen in the wet smear. They are about one-half the size of a cornified vaginal cell but larger than leukocytes.

vaginitis, cervicitis, urethritis and prostatitis. Flagyl is indicated in the treatment of trichomoniasis in both male and female patients when the presence of the trichomonad has been demonstrated by wet smear or culture, and for the sexual partners of those patients who have a recurrence of the infection provided trichomonal infection is demonstrated in the urogenital tract of the sexual partner. There is no evidence that the drug is effective against organisms other than trichomonas vaginalis and it should not be employed for the treatment of other conditions for which specific agents should be used.

Although Flagyl has had no significant effect on the blood or blood-forming elements in the patients studied to date, it should not be given to patients with evidence of or a history of blood dyscrasia because of its chemical structure. Also, it is recommended that Flagyl be withheld from patients with active disease of the central nervous system. At the present time, the use of Flagyl during pregnancy is contraindicated, since the preliminary studies have indicated that the drug passes the placental barrier and enters the fetal circulation rapidly.

For women the recommended dosage is one tablet of 250 mg. orally three times a day for ten days, or in stubborn cases two tablets orally and one vaginal insert of 500 mg. daily for the same ten days. Vaginal inserts are not recommended as the sole treatment. In the male Flagyl should be prescribed only when trichomonads are demonstrated in the urogenital tract. One 250-mg. tablet two times daily for ten days is recommended as a course of treatment. When Flagyl is prescribed for the male in conjunction with the treatment of his female partner, the medication should be taken by both partners over the same ten-day period. When repeat courses of the drug are required it is recommended that an interval of four to six weeks elapse between courses and that leukocyte counts be made before, during and after treatment.

It is equally important that instructions in personal hygiene be given. The patient is instructed (1) always to sweep toilet tissue in a posterior arc away from, rather than toward, the vagina, (2) to avoid use of enema tips for douching, (3) to use vaginal tampons rather than sanitary napkins during the menses, (4) to cleanse the vulva and perianal skin daily with Dial soap, then wash away all soap and dry. If the skin is excoriated, a bland ointment should be applied during therapy.

The treatment outlined seems to alleviate the vaginitis in about 90 per cent of patients, and smears give negative results in the majority of individuals. In the other 10 per cent, owing either to resistance of the parasite or to incompleteness of treatment, smears continue to show trichomonads and the patient is unimproved. About one fourth of all patients who are relieved of symptoms by initial therapy have recurrences. It is in these two groups that treatment must be varied and all possible efforts made to isolate the source of the infection. The following scheme has proved of value in the management of such cases. (1) The husband is referred to a urologist for a diagnostic survey and for treatment if he harbors the flagellate. (2) All possible foci (endocervix, periurethral glands, vulvovaginal glands, bladder, anus) are investigated and treated accordingly if trichomonads are found. Particular attention should be paid to the possibility of an intravesical infection, and the urine should be carefully examined and cultures made to exclude infection in this organ. (3) Coitus is prohibited for several weeks and then is permitted only with the use of a condom. (4) Simultaneous treatment of the consort and patient is started with metronidazole, 1 tablet orally three times daily for 10 days. (5) The possibility of a mixed infection must be entertained, proper diagnosis undertaken and systematic treatment instituted. Streptococci, staphylococci, diphtheroids or even Candida albicans may be involved. In postmenopausal or surgically castrated patients an atrophic vaginitis may be present. Preliminary treatment with an estrogenic vaginal cream should precede the active treatment of trichomoniasis. (6) There is recent evidence that recurrent vaginitis due to T. vaginalis may be correlated with emotional stress and is common in women who have symptoms of nervousness or fatigue, sleep disturbances, digestive upsets, headaches, menstrual irregularities and painful breasts. An immature, dependent personality is often concealed by strong dominant drives and outward aggression. Treatment of such patients should include reassurance, explanation and establishment of insight into the patient's problem. Sedation, diminished physical activity, daily rest periods, abstinence from coitus and psychotherapeutic measures should be suggested.

The status of the term "cure" in trichomoniasis has not been adequately defined. Most clinicians, however, are agreed that if examination for three consecutive months is negative for flagellates and the patient is asymptomatic, the patient may be said to be cured.

It has been recognized that the presence of T. vaginalis will produce morphologic changes in vaginal cells of sufficient degree to produce a class III or suspicious Papanicolaou smear. These abnormal cells disappear subsequent to adequate therapy. The clinician should not rush such a patient to the operating room for a conization of the cervix nor should he biopsy the cervix during the process of inflammation. After 10 days of Flagyl therapy the smear should be repeated, the cervix stained with Schiller's solution and then, if Schiller non-staining areas are present, biopsies should be done.

A recent report by Szell et al indicated a correlation of trichomonal vaginitis and the development of permanent atypical epithelium. In a study of 1,500 women, ages 15 to 82, carcinoma of the cervix was found in 3.3 per cent of patients with chronic infection as against 0.6 per cent of non-infected ones.

MONILIASIS

Moniliasis is the second most common cause of vaginal discharge. The vaginal mucosa is grayish or dull red, and there is a thick, caseous, yellow-white discharge that strongly resembles cream cheese. Moniliasis is caused by a yeastlike organism, Candida albicans. Frequently the amount of discharge is small but the patient complains bitterly of vulvar and vaginal pruritus and burning. These complaints may be severe enough to interfere with ordinary activities and sleep. Intercourse causes severe pain. If the patient is obese or if the discharge runs down over the thighs a marked intertriginous rash may develop. Diabetes and pregnancy are predisposing factors. It has been estimated that in about 25 per cent of all pregnant women fungi of some variety are present in the vagina, and this has been

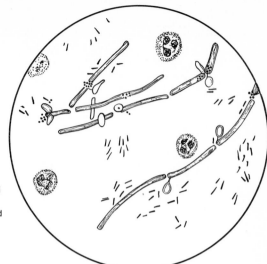

Fig. 3-7.—Fiber-like mycelia and spores of Candida albicans seen in a wet smear. Several leukocytes and Döderlein's bacilli are also shown.

correlated with the increased vaginal glycogen during the pregnant state. The exact relationship between diabetes and moniliasis has not been established. Thrush in the newborn may be etiologically related to vaginal candidiasis, the infant being infected at the time of delivery.

Another causative factor in the development of monilia vaginitis has been the extensive use of systemic antibiotics, particularly the tetracyclines. Their administration results in a reduction of the normal acid-forming vaginal bacilli, permitting fungi of the normal vagina to grow in abundance. A state similar to pregnancy may be produced by the use of oral contraceptives. It is important therefore in taking the history of a patient with pruritus vulvae to ascertain whether she (1) is pregnant, (2) is a diabetic (3) has recently taken a wide-spectrum antibiotic or (4) has been using oral contraceptives.

Examination reveals a hyperemic, edematous vulva which may be covered with a gray-white frosting (see Fig. 2-14, p. 41) and which frequently bears evidence of marked scratching. When a speculum is introduced into the vagina, the typical, cheesy or curdlike, adherent discharge is evident. It may be difficult to tease the discharge from the underlying membrane, which may be red or violaceous. The vagina is usually edematous and tender. Its pH is acid and the vaginal smear characteristically shows mature, well-cornified epithelial cells without trichomonads.

The diagnosis is suggested by the history and examination but is corroborated by microscopic hanging-drop study of the caseous material. A small amount of the discharge is taken from the vagina and a drop of potassium hydroxide is added to thin out the preparation. It may be examined as a hanging drop or it may be stained with Gram's iodine. Characteristically, Candida albicans is a thin-walled, yeastlike structure measuring 2-4 μ. Budding cells (conidia) are usually seen attached to fiber-like structures resembling bamboo shoots (mycelia). Frequently there is a tangled network of fine mycelia with clusters of spores (Fig. 3-7). The organism may be cultured on corn-meal agar or dextrose agar, mycelial development being best seen in colonies grown on the former. Individual culture tubes of Nickerson's medium are available for office use and do not need incubation. A small amount of discharge is placed on this medium, the cover replaced and in about 48 hours, if Candida albicans is present, multiple 1-2 mm. black colonies will be evident. It should be remembered that seven varieties of Candida have been described in cultures from man, but exacting cultural methods are necessary for this differentiation. Moniliasis may also involve the nails, feet, webs of the fingers, oral mucosa, gastrointestinal tract, anus and lungs. A generalized cutaneous form with meningeal involvement and death has been reported, although this is rare.

TREATMENT.—Treatment of monilia vaginitis is effective in producing a high percentage of cures except during pregnancy when mere palliation is achieved. If the patient is diabetic, excess glycosuria should be corrected and the general metabolic disorder controlled. If there has been excessive scratching with resultant vulvar edema, cool tap water or witch hazel compresses (or an ice cap) are applied locally and an antihistamine given orally. Occasionally codeine or codeine plus a barbiturate should be given for several nights so that the patient does not scratch the vulva during sleep. If tap water compresses alone do not bring about sufficient relief, the following prescription is applied to the vulva after the compresses.

starch	6.0
water	30.0
polysorb	ad 60.00

Specific treatment of the vaginitis is best carried out with the use of Mycostatin vaginal suppositories, each containing 100,000 units of nystatin. The usual method is to insert 1 or 2 tablets high into the vagina every night before retiring, for 10-14 days. If the infection is extensive or if there is reason to believe there is gastrointestinal involvement, the oral administration of Mycostatin tablets (500,000 units per tablet) three times daily is suggested. During pregnancy this treatment may have to be repeated several times and there is no contraindication to the continuation of treatment until the onset of labor if the membranes have not ruptured. Other local therapy such as cleansing or douches is not necessary since relief is usually achieved within 48 hours. Occasionally a patient will not be helped by Mycostatin, and in this group the use of 2 per cent aqueous gentian violet is effective. This solution is painted over the entire vaginal mucous membrane including the portio vaginalis of the cervix and over the vulva if this is affected. Since this treatment is rather messy, instructions are given to protect bed linen and lingerie from the medication. The patient is also given a prescription for Gentia-Jel vaginal inserts and instructed to use one each night for six nights. Gentian violet Supprettes are also available for home use. At the end of one week examination is repeated in the office and the vagina is again painted with the solution. Home treatment is repeated for six additional nights, followed by an office visit for a final check. Usually by this time the vaginitis has cleared and smears give negative findings. Re-treatment with gentian violet inserts or Supprettes is suggested for one week after the next three menstrual periods. The excessive use of gentian violet may prove to be locally irritating in some patients; simple withdrawal of the medication will suffice if this occurs.

In recent studies of patients with recurrent infections, the urine has been found to harbor candida in about 45 per cent of cases, whereas the urine of the husbands gave positive cultures in about 30 per cent. In such cases, the husband should be treated with oral Mycostatin and a careful search for a focus of infection in the urinary tract is initiated. The wife is treated simultaneously and coitus prohibited until improvement is noted. Alkaline medications are not recommended in the treatment of vaginal moniliasis, although candida grows easily in the highly acid vagina. The use of estrogens or estrogenic creams is not indicated since the vagina is already well glycogenated. It has been suggested that, during pregnancy, the relative deficiencies of vitamins B and C predispose to vaginitis, and thus these substances should be added to the diet.

Several other methods of treatment have been suggested which apparently are just as effective as those just mentioned. They are: (1) Propion Gel. (2) Tricofuron, a specific moniliacide, Micofur (nifuroxime), in combination with a trichomonacide, Furoxone (furazolidone). (3) Sporostacin.

A few patients develop recurrent monilia vaginitis while using oral contraceptives. Some of these are benefited by changing from the combined estrogen-progestin combinations to sequential agents. In other patients it is necessary to have them repeat one of the anti-monilia agents each month usually immediately after the withdrawal flow. Rarely a patient will have to select another type of contraceptive because of the tendency to persistence or recurrence. All such individuals should have a 2-hour postprandial blood sugar determination or a glucose tolerance test to exclude the possibility of diabetes. (See also Monilia in Chapter 2.)

Nonspecific Vaginitis

The discharge accompanying this vaginitis may be described as somewhere between those of trichomonas and monilia infections. It is neither frothy and greenish like that of trichomoniasis nor cream-cheesy like that of moniliasis. The hanging drop reveals neither trichomonads nor mycelia and the gram stain does not reveal gram-negative intracellular diplococci. The organisms usually found are staphylococci, streptococci and Escherichia coli. There is evidence to support the fact that many of these "nonspecific" vaginal infections are due to a recently discovered pathogen, Hemophilus vaginalis. This organism is a gram-negative, nonmotile, pleomorphic rod that may be isolated readily on proteose blood agar and has fulfilled Koch's postulates for pathogenicity. The organism has been cultured from the urethras of the majority of men whose wives harbor the infection. The commonest symptom associated with this entity is itching or burning of the vagina; also present is a moderate, gray-white, frothy discharge.

In other patients, a specific streptococcal infection is evident. The inflammatory process may vary from a mild to a severe reaction and it may be acute or chronic. It is entirely possible for the pathogenic organisms to ascend through the uterus into the tubes and peritoneal cavity. Streptococcal infections produce generalized reddening of the vaginal walls with irregular patches of marked erythema and a thin discharge. The discharge associated with staphylococcal infections is usually sticky and purulent and the labia may be involved and matted together. Escherichia coli produces a greenish yellow, purulent exudate.

The diagnosis is usually not evident by hanging drop or gram stain, and culture must be carried out. In many cases there is a mixed infection and anywhere from 3 to 12 organisms may be isolated in a given case. A good bacteriologic laboratory is necessary for adequate diagnosis in this group of vaginal infections, since sensitivity studies of various antibiotics will greatly aid rapid and complete treatment.

TREATMENT.—Specific therapy is determined by the type of offending organism and by its sensitivity to the available antibiotics and sulfonamides. Since alteration of the vaginal pH to alkalinity may predispose the mucosa to infection, this should be remedied by lactic acid douches or buffered vaginal creams. Occasionally this type of vaginitis follows use of a douching agent that has traumatized the vaginal mucosa. Removal of the offending agent plus cool tap-water douches produce rapid relief from symptoms. An impacted pessary or foreign body may be the inciting cause and cure results promptly after removal.

In most streptococcal, diphtheroid and colon bacilli infections treatment is best accomplished with vaginal jellies or creams such as Sultrin, AVC or Betadine. Staphylococcal infections have responded to the combined oral and local use of erythromycin. Sterisil vaginal cream is effective against Hemophilus vaginalis and should be applied every other night for a total of six applications. Treatment should be continued through the next menstrual period. Sterisil is also effective against monilia and trichomonas. Systemic administration of ampicillin also has been reported as effective therapy in the treatment of hemophilus infections.

SENESCENT VAGINITIS

This is usually not a primary infection but consists of an inflammatory reaction together with ulceration and telangiectasia in a mucous membrane thinned by inadequate estrogenic stimulation. Occasionally, secondary infection by T. vaginalis, monilia or streptococci may supervene. Since the discharge is frequently blood tinged or mucoid, the possibility of cervical or endometrial cancer must be considered and diagnostic procedures accomplished. A thorough uterine curettage under anesthesia is mandatory in all patients who have postmenopausal bleeding or a bloody mucoid or watery pink discharge.

The usual symptoms are discharge, burning, itching or perineal soreness. Frequently the only complaint is that of dyspareunia. Examination reveals the vagina to be smooth, shiny and tender with the normal rugae lacking. The posterior commissure may be reddened or even ulcerated. The mucous membrane is pale with numerous red petechiae, ecchymoses, telangiectasia or actual ulceration. Diagnosis is made by inspection and by a hanging drop of the secretion which shows a typical "atrophic" smear with basal cells, leukocytes and bacteria.

If cancer is not present, treatment should be twofold: the vaginal acidity should be restored with lactic acid douches or creams, and local estrogen should be given in the form of suppositories or creams. We have used Dienestrol or Premarin vaginal cream successfully in such cases. The cream should be used every night for one week and then at regular intervals every six weeks. It should not be administered continuously for long periods since absorption of the estrogenic substance may lead to endometrial proliferation and irregular uterine bleeding. If the uterus is surgically absent, estrogens may be given orally (e.g., ethinyl estradiol, 0.05 mg. daily), until a desired result is obtained.

CHRONIC CERVICITIS

The discharge associated with a cervical erosion or ectropion is usually white or clear with an abundance of mucus. If infection is present, the discharge may be purulent. Although this entity is a common cause of leukorrhea, it will be discussed in detail in the chapter on the cervix.

GONORRHEAL VAGINITIS

Although the glandular epithelium of the periurethral glands and endocervix is the initial focus of growth in gonorrheal infection, the mucous membrane of the vagina may become secondarily involved, with resultant edema and inflammation. In immature females the commonest cause of vaginitis is the gonococcus. The thinness of the mucous membrane in this age group makes it particularly susceptible to this organism.

Although gonorrheal vaginitis is usually spread by sexual contact, in children it may be disseminated by direct contact with towels, toilet seats, fingers, etc. In institutions for young children it may become widespread before being detected and adequate therapy instituted. The symptoms include a profuse, yellow or yellow-white discharge, vaginal itching, burning and dysuria. In children the discharge may be slight and the symptoms minimal so that attention to the disorder is not immediate. In adults there is often involvement of Bartholin's glands, with an actual abscess occasionally found. Concomitant urethritis and skenitis may be present and should be looked for by gently exerting pressure under the terminal urethra and the openings of Skene's ducts. Pus, if present, can generally be expressed and smears and cultures obtained. The glands of the endocervix and the oviducts may be involved as part of either an acute or a chronic process. When the gonococcus reaches the internal genitalia signs of pelvic peritonitis are frequently demonstrable.

The diagnosis of gonorrhea is made by placing a drop of secretion on a slide and examining it by Gram's method. A typical, coffee-bean, gram-negative, intracellular diplococcus is usually seen. Treatment should not be administered on the basis of the smear alone since many other organisms may simulate the gonococcus. A culture should be taken at the time the smear is made and positive diagnosis should await this report. A complement fixation test is available to settle the diagnosis in borderline cases. A fluorescent antibody technic has been introduced by L. H. Shapiro to aid in diagnosis. This involves the visualization of a specific antigen (e.g., Neisseria gonorrhoeae) under ultraviolet illumination. The specific antibody is "tagged" with a fluorescent dye. Thus, when antigen-antibody reaction occurs, the pathogen (N. gonorrhoeae) may be easily identified.

Most of the strains of gonococci now encountered are sensitive to adequate dosage of any of the following antibiotics: penicillin, streptomycin, chlortetracycline, oxytetracycline, chloramphenicol and carbomycin. In the mature female (after positive findings on smear and culture) treatment now consists of an injection of 4.8 million units of penicillin G preceded by an injection of probenecid one hour previously to delay excretion. If the patient gives a history of penicillin sensitivity, tetracycline in a dose of 250 mg. four times daily for four days is administered. All local therapy is avoided, and showers rather than tub baths are suggested during the first day or so of treatment. The patient is then asked to return at weekly intervals for follow-up smears and cultures. In the immature female, oral penicillin in a total daily dose of 400,000 units given for four days is usually adequate for cure. In most cases it has not been necessary to add estrogenic substances to this therapy, although the use of vaginal suppositories containing 100,000 units of estrogen for three to four weeks following antibiotic treatment is of value in certain patients. The oral or parenteral use of estrogen is not advised because of the possible side effects, namely, breast hypertrophy, uterine bleeding, and epiphyseal closure. (See also Gonorrhea in Chapter 2.)

Vaginal Relaxation

The most common abnormalities of the vagina are due to relaxations of the endopelvic and associated fascia, resulting in cystocele, urethrocele, rectocele, enterocele or colpocele (Fig. 3–8). Occasionally an obturator hernia or pelvic lipoma will protrude into the vaginal canal, but these are uncommon.

Cystocele.—A cystocele results from a herniation of the bladder base into the vaginal canal and is best demonstrated by asking the patient to strain slightly. It is usually due to a laceration and retraction of the urogenital diaphragm and adjacent portions of the pubococcygeus muscle in association with relaxation of the musculofascial coverings of the bladder and anterior vaginal wall. The major etiologic factor is childbirth but large cystoceles are occasionally seen even in nulliparous women. Complaints referable to a cystocele vary. Most women complain of a bulge, a lump or a dropping in the region of the introitus. Some note only a sense of heaviness or pressure in the pelvis after being on their feet for long periods, whereas others note symptoms of urinary frequency or dysuria. The latter symptoms are due to an increased amount of residual urine after voiding, with stasis and subsequent infection of the bladder trigone. Occasionally the symptoms are severe yet only minimal displacement of the bladder is found at examination. It is important to examine these patients in the standing position, for only then will the cystocele be evident. The bladder should also be catheterized after voiding to determine if a large quantity (40 cc. or over) of residual urine is present.

Urethrocele.—This is a protrusion of the inferior aspect of the urethra in an arc away from the pubis toward the vagina. It is frequently associated with a cystocele and is due to lacerations of the urogenital diaphragm with tearing of the pubococcygeal fibers and connective tissue which attach the urethra to the symphysis pubis. There is an associated flattening out and enlargement of the urethral bore as its musculofascial sheaths separate. The anatomic changes thus incurred bring about a change in the urethrovesical angle so that urinary continence is impaired. Such incontinence is most marked when the patient strains, coughs, sneezes or runs and is therefore known as "stress" incontinence. This should be differentiated from "urge" incontinence which is characterized by preliminary loss of urine when the patient has a strong urge to void. The latter is associated with a chronic cystotrigonitis and may be due to a cystocele with a large

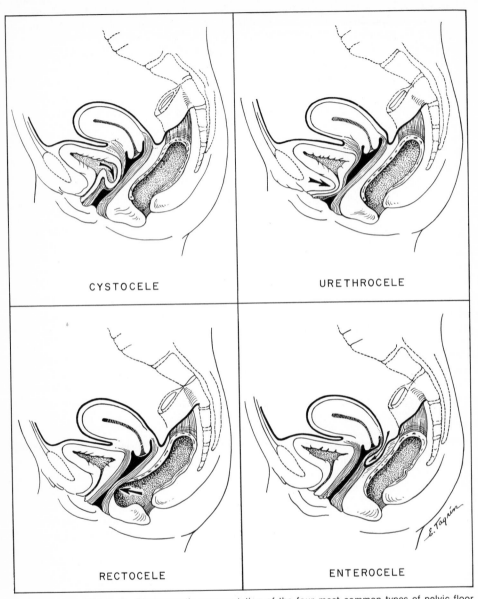

CYSTOCELE

URETHROCELE

RECTOCELE

ENTEROCELE

Fig. 3-8.—Diagrammatic representation of the four most common types of pelvic floor relaxation: cystocele, urethrocele, rectocele and enterocele. Arrows depict sites of maximum protrusion.

amount of residual urine and long-standing bladder infection. In all urinary tract difficulties in the female, especially incontinence, the clinician must not be misled by obvious anatomic deformities, since the symptoms may be due to neurologic causes such as cord lesions, tabes dorsalis or spina bifida. Therefore a thorough neurologic examination should be done in all patients with symptomatic cystourethrocele and cystometric studies done when indicated.

Rectocele.—A rectocele is a hernia of the lower rectum through its surrounding fascial envelopes into the vagina. Injury sustained at the time of pelvic delivery is the predominant etiologic factor, although an innate developmental weakness combined with increased intra-abdominal pressure from hard physical work may bring about the same situation. The anatomic defect is due to stretching, tearing and separation of the musculofascial sheaths of the rectum and vagina, the urogenital diaphragm, the levator ani and frequently portions of the sphincter ani muscle. The perineal body may or may not show evidence of laceration. Frequently an episiotomy has been performed at delivery and the perineum and introitus appear normal, but if the patient is asked to strain or cough the posterior vaginal wall bulges out beyond the introitus. A high rectocele may not be evident unless the patient is examined in the erect position. A rectocele is frequently asymptomatic and, even when large, may cause no particular distress. In other cases there are symptoms of backache, protrusion, pelvic pressure or discomfort, heaviness or perineal burning. These are aggravated by long hours in the standing position or by frequent constipation. Occasionally feces collect in the dilated lower rectum and become inspissated or impacted. It may sometimes be necessary for the patient to aid evacuation by digital pressure through the vagina. The diagnosis is obvious by inspection although a combined rectovaginal examination is often useful to delineate the extent of the rectocele. A high rectocele may be differentiated from an enterocele by placing a Sims speculum in the vagina with the blade held tightly in the posterior cul-de-sac, gently lifting the cervix. A finger in the rectum outlines the upper limits of the rectocele. If an enterocele is present, it will be seen to roll down from the apex of the vagina over the rectocele as the patient strains.

Enterocele.—An enterocele is a herniation of the peritoneum lining the posterior cul-de-sac into the posterior vaginal fornix behind the cervix. Small bowel may be present in an enterocele but almost never becomes incarcerated therein. The condition is frequently associated with a congenitally deep or wide cul-de-sac with separation and attenuation of the uterosacral ligaments. In a primary enterocele the thin-walled peritoneal sac forms behind the cervix and lies between the posterior vaginal wall and the anterior rectal wall in the rectovaginal septum. A secondary enterocele is a herniation through the floor of the pelvis after total abdominal or vaginal hysterectomy. A small enterocele is usually asymptomatic, but after it gains sufficient size it may protrude beyond the introitus so that the chief complaint is one of prolapse. This is especially disconcerting if it occurs after a vaginal hysterectomy and vaginal plastic repair since the patient cannot differentiate it from a cystocele or rectocele, the condition for which the original surgery was performed.

Colpocele.—This is a herniation of the vaginal wall beyond the introitus in association with a complete uterine prolapse. The symptoms are those of protrusion, although ulceration and infection of the vaginal mucosa may occur from long-standing eversion.

Perineal Lacerations.—Frequently these lacerations are seen in association with a rectocele since the etiologic factor is usually difficult delivery. During the time the fetal vertex impinges against the pelvic floor, producing "bulging" and "crowning," there is a combined stretching and tearing of the fibromuscular support of the perineal body. If this stage of labor is prolonged or if episiotomy is not utilized to minimize the trauma, separation or avulsion of the superficial perineal muscles, both layers of the superficial fascia and usually the deep perineal fascia occurs. When delivery is extremely difficult, there may actually be avulsion of the external anal sphincter, urogenital diaphragm and levator ani muscle. These injuries should be repaired at the time of delivery, with particular attention to realignment of fascial layers without tension. Frequently, however, the obstetrician does not recognize the damage or feels incompetent to repair it. In other cases hematomas or infection supervene and a poor result follows. Simple, incomplete perineal lacerations, if unaccompanied by a rectocele, are usually asymptomatic. There is some gaping of the introitus, so that water enters the vagina rather freely during bathing and the patient may note dribbling for a short time after. In other cases a pinpoint fistulous tract occurs between the rectum and vagina so that gas (but not feces) enters the vagina and the patient complains of recurrent passage of gas per vagina. In complete perineal lacerations (Fig. 3-9) the sphincter ani muscle has been completely divided, a modified cloaca thus being formed. Although fecal incontinence may be noted during episodes of diarrhea, these patients are in general able to control bowel movements rather well. Vaginal contamination with feces is, however, unavoidable.

Treatment.—The management of vaginal relaxations, if symptomatic, is surgical. The possible exception to this is a urethrocele with stress incontinence which, after a series of specific pubococcygeal exercises, will regain sufficient tone to be asymptomatic. In the surgical repair of vaginal relaxation, known as a vaginal "plastic" or colporrhaphy, basic surgical principles of hernia repair are employed. Thus in a cystocele repair (anterior colporrhaphy) the bladder is freed from the vagina and mobilized from the cervix. The investing fascia which has spread laterally is mobilized and approximated in the midline with fine catgut sutures. Any excess vaginal mucosa is trimmed and the edges brought together. A urethrocele repair (urethroplasty) is somewhat more difficult, in that the urethra must be freed from scar tissue and its angle of entrance into the bladder base restored. This is usually accomplished by mobilizing musculofascial tissue and approximating it in a slinglike fashion under the proximal urethra. In recurrent cases this may be done by bringing a band of rectus fascia (obtained through an abdominal incision) retroperitoneally and directing it underneath the urethra, thus producing a supporting sling. Another method, entirely suprapubic, approaches the urethra through the space of Retzius. The urethra is suspended by suturing the periurethral fascia and vagina to the posterior aspect of the symphysis pubis and anterior rectus sheath.

A rectocele repair (posterior colporrhaphy) entails separation of the rectum from the vagina and interposition of the musculofascial layers, including the pubococcygeus and puborectalis, between the two structures. If a lacerated perineum is present, this is usually repaired simultaneously by excision of scar tissue and mobilization of the superficial perineal fascia (perineorrhaphy). In a complete perineal laceration the sphincter ani muscle must be dissected free and its ends approximated before the usual posterior colporrhaphy and perineorrhaphy are done.

An enterocele is corrected by incising the posterior vaginal wall to the level of the enterocele, isolating and mobilizing the peritoneal sac, which is

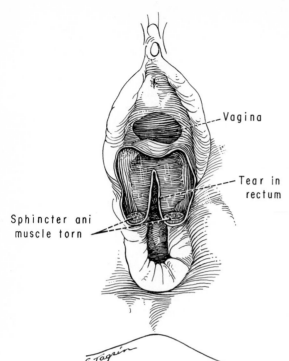

Vagina

Tear in
rectum

Sphincter ani
muscle torn

Fig. 3–9.—Complete laceration of
the perineum, showing division of the
sphincter ani muscle and laceration
of the anterior rectal wall.

excised, and repairing the defect by plication of the uterosacral ligaments
and by mobilization and approximation of sufficient lateral fascia. If adequate structural support cannot be obtained vaginally, the abdomen may
be opened and the posterior cul-de-sac partially obliterated by approximating the uterosacral ligaments. If a deep cul-de-sac is noted at the time of
total abdominal hysterectomy and an incipient enterocele is anticipated,
the posterior cul-de-sac should be obliterated by plication of the uterosacral ligaments. This produces a shelf behind the vagina with just sufficient space for the rectosigmoid to pass through. In a vaginal hysterectomy,
steps should be taken to prevent the development of an enterocele by
incising the posterior vaginal wall to an adequate level so that the important uterosacral ligaments may be brought together in the midline and thus
form the apex of the posterior wall repair.

Benign Neoplasms

The two most common benign neoplasms of the vagina are cystic structures, one derived from remnants of the mesonephros and the other from
surgically implanted fragments of perineal or vaginal epithelium. As
shown in Figure 3–1, the mesonephric remnants course along the supero-
lateral aspect of the vagina, and occasionally some displaced fragments of
tissue are stimulated to grow. In so doing, one or more small, cystlike structures are formed, and these are seen in the anterolateral portion of the
vagina as clear-walled, soft, compressible masses (*Gartner duct cyst*).

Rarely one of these becomes extremely large and pedunculated and may appear to bulge through the introitus (Fig. 3–10), resembling an enterocele.

Microscopically these cysts have a variable lining but usually the cells are tall columnar to cuboidal and are sometimes ciliated. Stratified squamous epithelium has occasionally been described as lining the cysts but this may represent an inclusion of vaginal epithelium as the cyst forms. The cyst wall is made up of fibrous connective tissue which sometimes is hyalinized, and the contents are usually a clear, colorless or amber, serous or mucinous fluid. No malignancies have been reported to have developed in these cysts, but they should be differentiated from epidermal inclusion cysts which usually occur in the distal, posterior vaginal wall and from endometriotic "implants." Treatment of Gartner duct cysts consists of complete surgical excision.

Abnormal configurations of the bladder or urethra such as cystocele, diverticula or urethrocele may usually be diagnosed by passing a catheter or metal probe into the urethra and noting its position. An enterocele may best be demonstrated by holding back the anterior and posterior vaginal walls with a Sims speculum and having the patient exert intra-abdonimal pressure. Other conditions which rarely will present intravaginal masses are: hematocolpos, accessory ureteral cysts and vaginitis emphysematosa.

Vaginitis emphysematosa is characterized by multiple gas filled cysts in the vaginal and cervical mucosa. It is accompanied by a vaginal discharge, which may be the only symptom. It is more common in pregnancy, which may favor infection with Trichomonas vaginalis or Hemophilus vaginalis due to the altered physiology of the vagina. It is seldom diagnosed radiologically and needs to be distinguished from emphysematous cystitis, gangrene of the uterus, vaginal tampon, pelvic abscess or pelvic bowel gas shadows.

Vaginal *inclusion cysts* are quite common but are of little significance unless large. They are formed by bits of stratified squamous epithelium which are buried under the vaginal mucosa at the time of an episiotomy

Fig. 3–10.—Prolapse of a Gartner duct cyst through the introitus, simulating a large prolapsed enterocele.

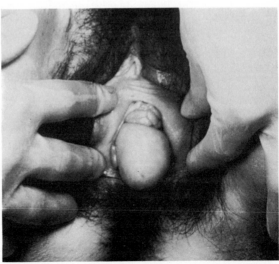

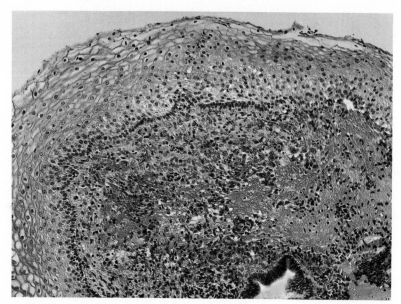

Fig. 3-11.—Photomicrograph showing "menstrual" endometriosis under the vaginal epithelium. Biopsy was obtained from a typical "blueberry" nodule in the vaginal apex during the time of menstruation. (From Kistner, R. W.: Fertil. & Steril. 10:547, 1959.)

repair or posterior colporrhaphy. The epithelium so displaced continues to desquamate cells and keratin which undergo degeneration to form a yellow or yellow-white cheesy material. This becomes encased in a thin-walled structure which is usually firm to palpation and is located in the lower third of the vagina on the posterior or posterolateral wall. The cysts are frequently discovered by the patient but are otherwise asymptomatic unless they are so positioned as to cause dyspareunia. In general, no treatment is necessary but they are usually easily removed at the time of a subsequent episiotomy or vaginal repair.

Endometriotic cysts of the vagina may cause considerable pain and dyspareunia, especially if they contain functioning endometrial tissue. They are usually found behind the cervix in the posterior vaginal fornix and have a typical bluish color. During the premenstrual and menstrual phase of the cycle they may be acutely tender. Microscopically, the typical picture of endometriosis is found, although glands may be infrequent (Fig. 3-11). The endometrial stroma shows varying amounts of hemosiderin-laden macrophages, lymphocytes and old blood. In some areas considerable fibrosis occurs. Such lesions may be treated hormonally or by surgical excision. Following menopause or oophorectomy, vaginal endometriosis regresses. (See treatment of Endometriosis in Chapter 8.)

Premalignant Neoplasms
CARCINOMA IN SITU

Carcinoma in situ of the vagina is seldom diagnosed, except as a direct extension from carcinoma of the cervix. The epithelial changes adjacent to invasive carcinoma of the cervix are generally accepted and involvement of the vagina is being reported with increasing frequency. The direct continuity of in situ lesions of the cervix involving the vagina is a more recent observation but, at the Boston Hospital for Women, diagnostic procedures to determine the presence of vaginal involvement has been routine prior to all hysterectomies for carcinoma in situ of the cervix. A Schiller test of the vagina is performed prior to surgery and all nonstaining areas are biopsied (see Chapter 4).

Intra-epithelial carcinoma confined to the vagina without relation to cervical carcinoma is an apparent rarity. Fourteen patients who fulfilled this criterion have been observed at the Boston Hospital for Women. All but one case were detected by routine cytologic examination. The gross appearance of the lesions was not striking, having been described as "whitish" or "telangiectatic." The classic "blush" or "sugar coating" of cervical carcinoma in situ was not evident. The majority of patients were treated by local surgical excision, some requiring simultaneous hysterectomy. Radium was utilized as adjuvant therapy in 1, and was the primary treatment in 2 patients. Electrical and chemical coagulation was used in 2 others.

A patient with in situ vaginal carcinoma should be as curable as one with in situ cervical carcinoma. Partial vaginectomy is preferable to intravaginal radium in young patients. It is important to follow patients with cytology every three months during the first year after a hysterectomy for cervical carcinoma in situ; cytologic examinations are then performed every six months during the next four years, every 12 months thereafter.

Malignant Neoplasms
CARCINOMA

Primary Carcinoma.—Primary carcinoma of the vagina is almost always a squamous cell type, whereas adenocarcinoma is usually metastatic from another source. As a primary tumor, vaginal carcinoma makes up about 1 per cent of all genital malignancies and its relative incidence to that of cervical cancer is about 1:50. The average age is somewhere between 48 and 55 years, although this malignancy has been reported in the late twenties.

There are no known predisposing factors that seem to affect the development of vaginal carcinoma. Thus the family history, parity, marital history, previous diseases, concomitant diseases or exposure to irritants are of no etiologic significance. A vaginal cancer is found rarely in a patient who has been wearing a pessary for a long time but this is believed to be coincidental.

The usual symptom is abnormal bleeding or a blood-tinged discharge. The bleeding is usually first noticed after intercourse or douching but occasionally may begin as a severe hemorrhage. If the disease is extensive the discharge may be profuse, foul smelling and cause a rather marked vulvitis with pruritus. A normocytic-hypochromic anemia may be found and generalized symptoms such as weakness, dyspnea, dizziness and malaise may be secondary to it. If the tumor has invaded the bladder, symptoms of dysuria, frequency and hematuria may be present, whereas with rectal involvement the patient may complain of tenesmus, diarrhea, melena and pain.

The diagnosis of vaginal carcinoma is usually obvious by speculum examination but should be corroborated by tissue biopsy. Early lesions or carcinoma in situ may be diagnosed by cytologic methods before symptoms develop or before the lesion becomes obvious to the clinician. The value of routine vaginal cytology even in women who have had total hysterectomy has been demonstrated to us on several occasions by the finding of vaginal carcinoma in situ as a completely unexpected lesion. Biopsy of the vagina in cases in which the cytology is suspicious or positive may be aided by painting the entire vagina with Schiller's solution, since atypical epithelium, whether anaplastic, carcinoma in situ or actual carcinoma, will not stain with this iodine solution. In differential diagnosis consideration must be given to cervical cancer, sarcoma botryoides, endometriosis and the granulomas. Biopsy is necessary for definitive diagnosis.

The carcinoma may appear in several forms. It may be a large, fungating, cauliflower-like mass which fills the entire upper vagina or it may be flat, superficial and locally infiltrative (Fig. 3–12). A third type presents as a deep, ulcerating, locally destructive lesion. The tumor is most often found on the posterior wall in the upper third of the vagina. When the carcinoma involves the lower third, prognosis is poor. This is probably due to involvement of different lymphatics and quicker vascular dissemination. There is some evidence that the prognosis is better if the lesion is found on the anterior wall but this may be due to a higher incidence of less extensive tumor in that area.

The disease usually spreads upward toward the cervix and is confined for a fairly long time to the superficial portion of the vagina. If there is involvement of the cervix, it is difficult to determine whether the tumor is a primary cervical lesion with spread to the vagina or vice versa. However, if the lesion is most extensive in the vagina and just involves the edges of the cervical portio, it may be properly termed a primary vaginal tumor. The

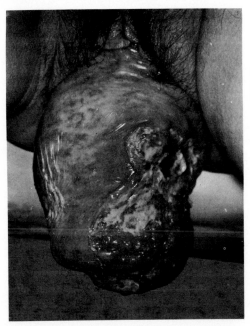

Fig. 3–12.—Extensive primary carcinoma of the vagina in association with procidentia. (From Kistner, R. W.: Obst. & Gynec. 10:483, 1957.)

growth pattern is usually one of rather localized spread, first up and then around the diameter of the vaginal tube before deep extension into the bladder or rectum occurs. In the ulcerative form, however, deep craters

CLINICAL STAGES OF CARCINOMA OF THE VAGINA

Stage I	The carcinoma is limited to the vaginal wall.
Stage II	The carcinoma has involved the subvaginal tissues but has not extended onto the pelvic wall.
Stage III	The carcinoma has extended onto the pelvic wall.
Stage IV	The carcinoma has extended beyond the true pelvis or has involved the mucosa of the bladder or of the rectum; however, bullous edema, as such, does not permit one to classify a case as Stage IV.

NOTE: A carcinoma that has extended to the portio should be classified as carcinoma of the cervix.

into the adjacent viscera may occur. Vesicovaginal and rectovaginal fistulas are usually late findings. The carcinoma spreads by contiguity and also by lymphatics. The upper vagina drains into the same lymphatic chain as the cervix (iliac, ureteral, hypogastric and obturator nodes), whereas the lower vagina duplicates the drainage of the vulva (inguinal, femoral, Cloquet's nodes) (Fig. 3–13). Intermediate lesions may spread to the obturator or to either of the other pathways.

TREATMENT.—In the past it has been stated that vaginal carcinoma is the most difficult of female genital cancers to treat. Taussig is quoted as having said "we acknowledge our total inability to do anything effective for primary carcinoma of the vagina." This statement does not coincide with the recent attitude of most gynecologists who favor a radical surgical approach. Before 1945 only about 25 per cent of patients were deemed suitable for surgery, but in recent years an increasing number are being selected for this approach. In lesions which are apparently confined to the vagina, especially in the upper third, preliminary radium in the form of a plaque or surface mold may be applied to the carcinoma, followed in four to six weeks by a radical hysterectomy, extensive vaginectomy and node dissection. If the lymph nodes are involved or there has been gross extension of the disease at the time of surgery, postoperative x-ray therapy is given. In tumors which involve the anterior vaginal wall extensively and which seem to involve the vesicovaginal septum or fascia, preliminary radium therapy is followed by anterior exenteration. This includes radical hysterectomy, cystectomy, vaginectomy and node dissection. The ureters are best transplanted to an ileal conduit. When the posterior vaginal wall and adjacent fascia and/or rectum are involved, preliminary radium is given, followed by posterior exenteration (radical hysterectomy, node dissection and abdominoperineal resection). In rare cases in which there is extension to bladder and rectum but not lateral fixation to the pelvic wall a total exenteration is sometimes indicated. The ureters are transplanted to an ileal conduit whose stoma is brought out on the right side of the abdomen; a sigmoid colostomy is brought out on the left side. If the lower third of the vagina is involved, an extraperitoneal inguinal and femoral node dissection is also performed. It should be noted that these major surgical procedures are difficult and time-consuming, and usually the operative mortality is 15–25 per cent. They should only be carried out in centers

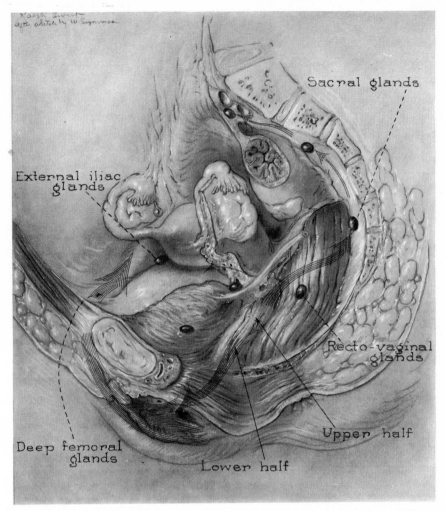

Fig. 3-13.—Lymphatic spread of carcinoma of the vagina. Extension of cancer of upper half of vagina is similar to carcinoma of cervix, while cancer in lower half spreads like vulvar cancer. (From Benson, R.: Carcinoma of the vagina, CA–A Cancer Journal for Clinicians 18: 7, 1968.)

where blood replacement, electrolyte studies and optimum postoperative care are possible. If these criteria cannot be met or if the patient is not a good risk for such operations, treatment should be accomplished with radium and x-ray.

Almost all studies have shown that the prognosis depends on the stage of the disease when it is first treated. Thus, prognosis is good for small lesions which are confined to the upper third of the vagina and which show negative nodes and clear lines of surgical excision. When the lymph nodes are positive or tumor has been transected the results are poor. Radiation therapy alone has been disappointing and a radical surgical approach is the treatment of choice in all operable lesions. An insufficient number of patients have been treated by radical surgery in our clinic to state the exact survival rate, but in other series a survival rate of between 30 and 40 per cent has been reported although not all reports were five years after treatment. Merrill reviewed the treatment of 25 patients followed for five years or longer and noted a survival rate of 28 per cent. All but three of these patients were treated with radiation but most did not have far-advanced disease when first seen. The five-year survival rate was 26.5 per cent and the ten-year survival rate was only 15.3 per cent in the series of patients reported from the Radiumhemmet in Stockholm. Rutledge reported the highest salvage rate in patients treated by radium and x-ray, 44 per cent of 70 patients living and well without evidence of disease after 5 years. As a result of his experience, Rutledge believes that radiation is the preferable initial therapy for vaginal cancer and, if the lesion fails to respond, surgery can be done later.

In my opinion, radium therapy is ideally suited for the widespread, superficial polypoid lesion. The more common ulcerating or papillary growth usually has reached the rectovaginal or vesicovaginal septum by the time it is diagnosed. Thus, if radiation therapy is adequate, a fistula is practically assured.

When the tumor is located in the posterior vaginal wall, I prefer to do a posterior exenteration with total vaginectomy and pelvic lymphadenectomy. If the lesion involves the anterior wall, an anterior exenteration, total vaginectomy and pelvic lymphadenectomy is done. If the lesion involves the lower third of the vagina, a radical vulvectomy with inguinal and femoral node dissection is combined with the procedures noted above.

Death usually occurs from ureteral obstruction or wide dissemination of metastases, although rarely massive hemorrhage from erosion of a large blood vessel may be lethal.

Secondary Carcinoma.—This type is much commoner than primary cancer and is most often associated with metastases from the cervix, the endometrium or the ovary. Cervical cancer may spread by direct contiguity, either along or underneath the epithelium, or possibly also by lymphatics. If it involves the upper vagina, the cervical cancer is then said to be a Stage II-A. The diagnosis must be made by visualization of the cervix, and exact details of the areas biopsied must be known since the microscopic sections of the cervix and vagina may be identical. Frequently in cervical cancer there is spread along the uterosacral ligaments, which aids in making the differential diagnosis.

Endometrial cancer may also involve the vagina although there is considerable speculation as to the exact mode of spread. These metastases are found most commonly in the vaginal vault and under the urethra and have been reported in about 10 per cent of all patients with endometrial cancer. The tumor in the vault may be due to implantation at the time of hysterectomy or it may merely represent later growth of cancer cells which were under the vaginal mucosa in lymphatic or blood vessels at the time of surgery. The metastases under the urethra cannot be looked on as being due to implantation of cancer cells but probably represent growth of tumor emboli which are trapped in the cross-circuit between the uterine and vaginal circulations. This is the area where the uterine blood supply ends and the pudendal begins. This same area is a common site for the metastatic vaginal lesions of hypernephromas, which must reach this area by vascular dissemination.

Ovarian carcinoma may occasionally invade the vagina by direct extension through the posterior cul-de-sac, and we have seen several large fungating masses which seemed to arise from the posterior vaginal wall but proved to be adenocarcinomas of a very anaplastic type. The finding of psammoma bodies in these microscopic sections suggested the ovarian origin of these lesions.

A variety of other metastatic carcinomas may be found in the vagina and will be diagnosed correctly only after biopsy, cystoscopy, proctoscopy, intravenous urograms and x-rays of the colon. The commonest sites of the primary lesions are the rectum, bladder, urethra, breast, cecum, Skene's glands, Bartholin's glands and left kidney. Blood-borne metastases from a hypernephroma of the left kidney may reach the vagina via the left ovarian vein which drains into the left renal vein. The uterovaginal veins are secondarily involved from the ovarian vein. A choriocarcinoma may metastasize to the vagina and presents as a characteristic blue or dark red nodule or cystic mass which may resemble a hemangioma. Biopsy of this mass may be the first indication of the exact nature of the disease process and may lead to diagnosis before pulmonary metastases are seen by x-ray. A malignant melanoma may occur in the vagina but is usually secondary to a melanoma of the skin, eye or vulva. Although about a dozen apparently primary vaginal melanomas have been reported, it is imperative that a detailed search for another possible source be carried out. Teratomas also may involve the vagina but are usually secondary lesions.

Sarcoma

Sarcoma of the vagina is an extremely rare lesion, usually occurring as two major types: in childhood as sarcoma botryoides and in adult life as a dysontogenetic tumor of mixed cell type. Sarcoma botryoides, a grapelike sarcoma, is usually found in infancy or early childhood although a few cases have been reported in later life. It is really a type of mixed mesodermal tumor with a rather loose-textured, but not too anaplastic, sarcomatous pattern mixed with embryonic striated muscle cells or masses of myxomatous tissue. It may arise from the cervix as well as from the vagina and it appears as a simple polypoid mass or a fungating, grape cluster protruding from the vagina. Despite the fairly differentiated cellular pattern the tumor is usually extremely malignant. Radical surgery has not changed the poor prognosis. The incidence of polypoid masses of benign nature in the vaginas of children is so small that the mere presence should make one suspicious of sarcoma botryoides and biopsy should be done without hesitation.

The sarcoma occurring in adults is equally malignant although it may not be so easily discovered. It occurs as a mucosal type which is raised, exophytic and rapidly growing or as a deep or parietal type which permeates the subvaginal mucosa rather extensively before ulcerating the surface. Histologically the tumor is of a mixed mesodermal variety and is thought to arise from displacements of embryonal anlage of the urogenital region. Thus it may contain striated muscle, smooth muscle, lipomatous material, cartilage, bone and nerve tissue. In some cases the predominant cell type is of connective tissue variety, being either spindle cell, round cell or a mixture. Hematogenous metastases usually occur to lungs, pleura or brain and result fatally in almost all instances.

BIBLIOGRAPHY

Anatomy

Anson, B. J.: *An Atlas of Human Anatomy* (Philadelphia: W. B. Saunders Company, 1950), pp. 358–391.

Embryology

Jones, H. W., and Jones, G. E. S.: The gynecological aspects of adrenal hyperplasia and allied disorders, Am. J. Obst. & Gynec. 68:1330, 1954.

Koff, A. K.: Development of the Vagina in the Human Fetus, in *Contributions to Embryology* (Washington, D. C.: Carnegie Institute, 1933), vol. 24.

————: Embryology of the Female Generative Tract, in Curtis, A. H. (ed.): *Obstetrics and Gynecology* (Philadelphia: W. B. Saunders Company, 1933).

Wilkins, L., *et al.*: Further studies on treatment of congenital adrenal hyperplasia with cortisone, J. Clin. Endocrinol. 12:257, 1952.

————: Diagnosis of adrenogenital syndrome and its treatment with cortisone, J. Pediat. 41:860, 1952.

Young, H. H.: *Genital Abnormalities, Hermaphroditism and Related Adrenal Diseases* (Baltimore: Williams & Wilkins Company, 1937), pp. 23–45.

Physiology

DeAllende, I. L. C., and Orias, O.: *Cytology of the Human Vagina* (New York: Paul B. Hoeber, Inc., 1950).

Lang, W. H.: Vaginal acidity and pH: A review, Obst. & Gynec. Surv. 10:546, 1955.

Infections

Buxton, C. L., and Weinman, D.: Vaginal Infections Due to Trichomonas Vaginalis and Candida Albicans, in Meigs, J. V., and Sturgis, S. H. (ed.): *Progress in Gynecology* (New York: Grune & Stratton, Inc., 1957).

Kistner, R. W.: Vaginal Infections, in Conn, H. F. (ed.): *Current Therapy* (Philadelphia: W. B. Saunders Company, 1957).

Trussel, R. E.: *Trichomonas Vaginalis and Trichomoniasis* (Springfield, Ill.: Charles C. Thomas, Publisher, 1947).

Carcinoma

Corcaden, J. A.: *Gynecologic Cancer* (New York: Thomas Nelson & Sons, 1951).

Kistner, R. W.: Cervical carcinoma complicating procidentia, Obst. & Gynec. 10:483, 1957.

Merrill, J. A., and Bender, W. T.: Primary carcinoma of the vagina, Obst. & Gynec. 11:3, 1958.

Prangley, A. G.: Premalignant lesions of the vagina, Clin. Obst. & Gynec. Vol. 5. No. 4 December, 1962, p. 1119. Ed. by Kistner, R. W.

Rutledge, F.: Cancer of the vagina, Am. J. Obst. & Gynec. 97:635, 1967.

Smith, F. R.: Primary carcinoma of the vagina, Am. J. Obst. & Gynec. 69:525, 1955.

Way, S.: *Malignant Disease of the Female Genital Tract* (Philadelphia: Blakiston Company, 1951).

Whelton, J., and Kottmeier, H. L.: Primary carcinoma of the vagina, Acta obst. gynec. scand. 41: 22, 1962.

CHAPTER 4

The Cervix

Revised by C. THOMAS GRIFFITHS, M.D.

Embryology

THE EMBRYONIC DEVELOPMENT of the cervix remains a poorly understood and controversial subject. However, newly acquired knowledge in this area has relevance to the clinician's insight into histologic and anatomic processes which are intimately associated with pathogenesis. Embryonic development of the cervix is merely the beginning in a continuum of change which extends beyond the reproductive years.

As outlined in Chapter 3, fusion between the urogenital sinus and müllerian vaginal tube is followed by an upward growth of squamous epithelium which terminates near the external cervical os. Traditionally, the columnar epithelium of the endocervix has been thought to differentiate directly from mesoderm in the müllerian tubercle. This concept has been challenged by Fluhmann who postulates continued upward growth into the cervical canal of urogenital squamous epithelium with subsequent transformation into columnar epithelium. Thus, the endocervical lining, like that of the vagina, would have an entodermal origin. Song, on the other hand, presents evidence that the endocervical columnar epithelium is a product of endocervical stromal cells which in turn have been transformed from endometrial stromal cells at about the 25th week of gestation. In addition to the surface columnar cells, differentiation of deeper stromal cells results in the formation of tubular glandlike structures lined by mucus-secreting columnar epithelium which open onto the surface. From the 28th week until birth an accelerated linear growth of endocervical mucosa occurs resulting in deep infolding of surface epithelium to form clefts within the stroma. The largest of these clefts, visible grossly, are known as the plicae palmatae.

Traditionally, the endocervical glands have been described as racemose in type, that is, made up of numerous branching ducts terminating in acini. Fluhmann, however, by meticulous three dimensional plastic reconstructions, has shown that these glands consist only of deep clefts in the stroma from which multiple blind tunnels branch forth in all directions. Cross-sections of these tunnels in histologic preparations appear to be acini. It may be that the tunnels described by Fluhmann are the early tubular "glands" which have been carried downward with the formation of the clefts and whose ostia henceforth open into the clefts.

The excessive proliferation of endocervical mucosa occurring after the 28th week produces the so-called congenital erosion found in about 50 per cent of female neonates. This term incorrectly implies epithelial denudation. The extension of endocervical mucosa onto the portio vaginalis is more properly termed an eversion or ectropion. The squamocolumnar junction in this condition lies distal to the external os and is clearly visible as a peripheral, circumferential line of demarcation on the portio. In some neonates, the entire portio may be covered by columnar epithelium with the squamocolumnar junction lying in the vaginal fornices. Although previously considered an anomaly attributed to the failure of ascending squamous epithelium to reach the external os, it is now apparent that congenital eversions are secondary to extension of rapidly proliferating endocervical mucosa.

Abnormalities in the development or fusion of one or both müllerian ducts may result in a malformation of the cervix. This may be a double cervix with a septate uterus and double vagina, a double cervix with bicornuate uterus and single vagina, a double cervix with didelphys uterus or, occasionally, a complete atresia of the cervix. (See Fig. 5–8.)

In a consideration of the embryology of the cervix, mention should be made of the importance of mesonephric remnants in this structure. Huffman has confirmed the earlier work of Robert Meyer by examining serial sections of about 1,200 cervices and finding remnants of the fetal mesonephros in about 1 per cent. Meyer had previously reported an incidence of about 20 per cent. These structures characteristically are found as minute tubules or canaliculi in the lateral cervical wall. They are lined by non-secretory, ciliated low columnar or cuboidal cells with translucent cytoplasm and large, round, clearly staining nuclei. Bizarre tumors of both benign and malignant varieties may arise from these remnants and may prove to be histogenetically confusing if their origin is not appreciated. Huffman described one cyst from adenomatous proliferation and one adenocarcinoma which were architecturally and topographically of mesonephric origin.

Anatomy

The cervix (L., neck) is the narrowed, most caudad portion of the uterus. It is somewhat conical in shape, with a truncated apex directed downward and backward. It is about 1 in. long and is continuous above with the inferior aspect of the uterine corpus, the point of the juncture being known as the isthmus—an area of slight constriction. The vagina is attached obliquely around the center of the cervical periphery, thus dividing the cervix into two segments, an upper or supravaginal portion and a lower or vaginal portion. The cervix enters the vagina at an angle through the anterior vaginal wall and, in the normal situation, its vaginal portion is in contact with the posterior vaginal wall. The supravaginal part of the cervix is separated anteriorly from the bladder by a layer of endopelvic fascia, the pubovesicocervical fascia. Laterally this same level of the cervix is in continuity with the paracervical ligaments (cardinal ligaments of Mackenrodt) and the uterine vessels which they contain. Posteriorly, the supravaginal cervix is covered by peritoneum as it reflects off

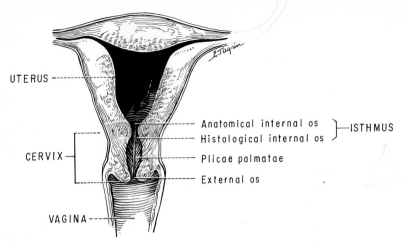

UTERUS

Anatomical internal os ⎫
Histological internal os ⎬ ISTHMUS
                        ⎭

CERVIX

Plicae palmatae

External os

VAGINA

Fig. 4-1.—Frontal section of uterine cervix and corpus.

the uterosacral ligaments downward toward the apex of the vagina.

The vaginal portion of the cervix (portio vaginalis, anatomic portio, exocervix, ectocervix) projects into the upper vagina between the anterior and posterior fornices as a convex prominence of rather elliptical shape. A small aperture, usually round or slit-like in the nullipara, is in the center of the projection—the anatomic external cervical os. This orifice connects the uterine cavity with the vagina. The external os is surrounded by the anterior and posterior lips, both being covered with stratified squamous epithelium in the normal state.

The cervical canal extends from the anatomic external os to the internal os, where it joins the uterine cavity (Fig. 4-1). It is somewhat fusiform or spindle shaped, flattened from before backward and wider at the middle than at either extremity. Anterior and posterior longitudinal ridges are evident on the walls of the canal. They represent the lines of fusion of the müllerian ducts. Fanning out laterally from these ridges is a series of folds (plicae palmatae) which look much like branches off a tree stem. When these are hypertrophied, the insertion of a uterine sound or dilator is hindered since the ridges simulate false passages in the canal. In some patients anesthesia may be necessary to get beyond these folds.

The *isthmus* of the uterus is of importance in the process of labor. It is defined as that area of the uterus between the anatomic internal os above and the histologic internal os below. The latter is an area where there is a transition from endometrial to endocervical glands. The isthmic musculature is thinner than that of the corpus since it is the area in which effacement and dilation occur during early labor. During pregnancy and labor the isthmus is referred to as the lower uterine segment.

Histology

An oversimplified consideration of the normal histology of the cervix consists only of descriptions of the squamous and columnar epithelium and their subjacent stroma. Of particular significance in the pathogenesis of cervical neoplasia, however, is the area of transition between the two epithelial types. Thus, according to Johnson, it is appropriate to discuss cervi-

HISTOLOGIC ZONES

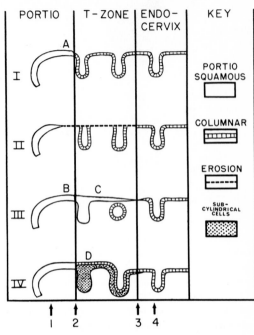

Fig. 4-2.—Schematic relationship of the histologic zones to anatomic areas as determined by the location of the anatomic external os. The histologic zones are the portio, transitional zone, and endocervix. The anatomic areas are the portio (to the left of any given arrow) and the endocervix (to the right of any given arrow). The four types of squamocolumnar junction are: I normal; II pathologic erosion; III erosion healing by squamous epithelization; IV reserve (sub-cylindrical) cell metaplasia which becomes squamous metaplasia after sloughing of the overlying columnar cells. Possible sites of origin of carcinoma in situ are: (A) basal cells of the portio epithelium; (B) basal cells of the portio epithelium at the margin of an old pathologic erosion; (C) basal cells of squamous epithelization; (D) reserve cells within the transitional zone. (From Johnson, L. D., *et al.:* Cancer 17:213, 1964.)

cal histology and histopathology in terms of three histologic zones: the histologic portio, the transitional zone, and the histologic endocervix.

The histologic portio is defined as cervical stroma without glands covered with stratified squamous epithelium (Fig. 4-2). The portio epithelium is 15 to 20 cells in thickness and demonstrates a progressive and orderly maturation from the lowermost basal layer through the prickle cell layer to the superficial zone where the cells cornify under the stimulus of estrogen (Fig. 4-3). The basal layer (stratum germinativum) consists of a single row of small cylindrical cells with large nuclei and scanty cytoplasm. A few mitotic figures are normally seen. Above the basal cells is a layer of larger polyhedral cells, 4 to 10 cells in thickness, arranged in an irregular mosaic pattern and connected by characteristic intercellular bridges. These cells are known as prickle, parabasal or spinal cells. The cytoplasmic basophilia of the basal and prickle cells is attributable to their ribonucleic acid content. Above the prickle cells is a layer of larger, oval or navicular shaped

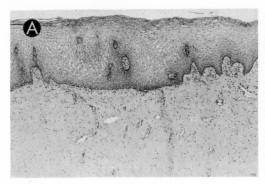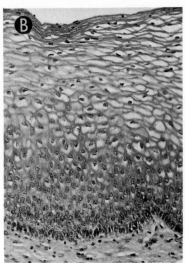

Fig. 4-3.—A, normal exocervix; ×50. **B,** high-power magnification to show process of stratification and cornification; ×150.

cells with relatively small nuclei. Their cytoplasm is rich in glycogen but appears clear in histologic sections since the glycogen is washed out during fixation. This layer has been called the intermediate, clear cell, or navicular zone. The superficial layer or stratum corneum consists of flattened elongated cells with small pyknotic nuclei. These are the cornified cells or squames seen in cytologic preparations. Glycogen is present normally in the superficial and intermediate cells and may be demonstrated by histochemical staining or by the application of iodine.

The basal layer of epithelium of the cervix is usually quite regular and does not show the rete ridge formation seen in the vulva and vagina. Traditionally, the squamous epithelium of the cervix rests on a basement membrane of ground substance. It now appears that this structure, inconsistently seen under the light microscope, actually consists of a condensation of stromal collagen. A "true" basement membrane has been identified under the electron microscope.

The *transitional zone,* found in 99 per cent of uncauterized cervices during the childbearing years, lies between the histologic portio and the endocervical mucosa and consists of endocervical stroma and glands covered by squamous epithelium (Fig. 4-2, III). Squamous epithelium comes to lie on the surface of the endocervical stroma by several physiologic or pathologic processes to be described later. Although these processes result in an upward or proximal displacement of the squamocolumnar junction, the junction between the histologic portio and transitional zone can be termed the original squamocolumnar junction. As can be seen by the location of the numbered arrows in Figure 4-2, the transitional zone may lie above or below the anatomic external os. The latter situation almost always prevails in the childbearing age (Arrows 3 and 4).

The *histologic endocervix* (Figs. 4-2 and 4-4) is lined by tall columnar epithelium characterized by dense basal nuclei and cytoplasm which stains a pale pink with hematoxylin—eosin preparation. The slight variation in height of the cells gives the appearance of a picket fence in sagittal section. Two types of cells are found in the endocervix, a mucus-secreting

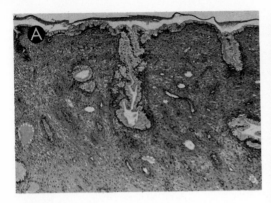
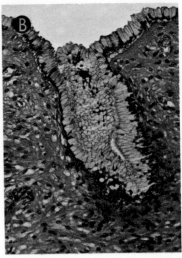

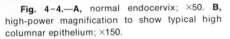

Fig. 4–4.—A, normal endocervix; ×50. B, high-power magnification to show typical high columnar epithelium; ×150.

cell and a ciliated cell located in patches in the cervical canal and in gland orifices. The development of the endocervical glands has been discussed in light of Fluhmann's widely accepted concept of clefts and tunnels. Although this concept renders the term "gland" a misnomer, common usage most likely will dictate continual reference to endocervical glands. The cleft arrangement increases the surface area of endocervical mucosa and permits increased mucus production. The secretion of endocervical mucus is dependent upon estrogen. Maximum production and secretion occur prior to ovulation and, in certain patients, a true mucorrhea exists.

The stroma of the cervix is composed of connective tissue, with unstriated muscle fibers and elastic tissue. The elastic tissue is found chiefly around the walls of the larger blood vessels. An area of transition separates the connective tissue of the cervix from the muscle of the lower uterine segment. This zone is usually about 10 mm. in length but occasionally it is absent and the cervical-uterine junction is abrupt.

For some years controversy has arisen between clinicians and pathologists in regard to the location of cervical lesions, particularly those of a neoplastic nature. This is a consequence of the erroneous assumption that an anatomic area is synonomous with a histologic zone of the same or similar designation. For example, the clinician defines a lesion of the portio as one existing on that portion of the cervix which can be visualized with a speculum. The pathologist, on the other hand, defines a lesion of the portio as one arising in the squamous epithelium of the histologic portio. A lesion arising in the transitional zone (overlying endocervical glands) or in the columnar epithelium, is classified pathologically as endocervical even though it is located on the anatomic portio. Obviously, the anatomic location of a lesion must be clearly distinguished from its histologic location.

The relationship between *histologic zones* and *anatomic areas* depends upon the position of the external os with reference to the histologic zones as illustrated in Figure 4–2. If the external os lies at arrow 2, the anatomic portio and histologic portio are the same in all 4 variations of the squamocolumnar junction. But if the external os lies at arrow 3, the anatomic portio will consist of histologic portio and either histologic endocervix

(Fig. 4–2, I) or transitional zone (Fig. 4–2, III, IV). With the external os at arrow 4 all three histologic zones will be present on the anatomic portio.

It is important that clinicians be aware of the fact that the majority of early neoplastic lesions in women of the child-bearing age, and particularly pregnant women, occur on the anatomic portio. Thus they are readily available for biopsy. It should be emphasized that reports from histopathologists which indicate that the majority of these lesions occur in the endocervix refer only to their histologic position.

From the anatomic and histologic characteristics described, it is obvious that the cervix differs from the uterine corpus in many important ways.

1. The cervix has only a small surface covered by peritoneum.

2. About 85 per cent of the cervix is made up of fibrous connective tissue.

3. There are no cervical venous sinuses.

4. The mucous membrane of the cervix presents numerous folds, and the glands secrete a clear, viscid, tenacious mucus.

5. The cervical mucosa does not undergo marked menstrual change as does the endometrium. There are some cyclic changes dependent on estrogen and progesterone.

6. The vaginal cervix is covered by stratified squamous epithelium.

Physiology

The cervix functions passively as a segment of the birth canal and as a channel for the exitus of the menstrual discharge. Its primary physiologic function, however, is the secretion of mucus which facilitates the transport of spermatozoa and subsequently acts as a plug to seal off the impregnated uterine cavity from the external environment.

Changes in physical properties and in pH of the cervical mucus are of importance in infertility since it has been shown that the mucus becomes thinner and permits penetration by spermatozoa at the time of ovulation. Studies of flow elasticity and elastic recoil have proved to be a very practical objective method for determining viscosity of the mucus. The German term *spinnbarkeit* has been applied to this unusual characteristic.

Cyclic variations in certain characteristics of cervical mucus have been extensively studied and may be of considerable assistance in clinical diagnosis. In the immediate postmenstrual phase the cervical mucus is sparse, viscid, and sticky and if allowed to dry on a slide reveals abundant vaginal and cervical cells, leukocytes and particles of mucus. From the eighth day until the time of ovulation the amount of mucus increases, its viscosity decreases, and it becomes permeable to spermatozoa. Just before ovulation the mucus is glassy, transparent and highly elastic. If allowed to dry on a slide, only a few cells are seen; however it assumes the form of fern or palm leaves (Fig. 4–5) and thus the term "fern test" has been applied to this finding. After ovulation the mucus remains transparent and elastic until about the twenty-second day of a 28 day cycle. Drying reveals a failure of arborization, with mucous threads and the usual cells and leukocytes.

FERN TEST TECHNIQUE.—The specimen of mucus should be aspirated from the external os after initial dry cleansing. Usually two aspirates are obtained and placed on separate slides, since the response may be positive on the second but negative on the first. The mucus is permitted to air dry for 20 minutes and is then examined under magnification of about 100×. False interpretations are possible if (1) the aspirating

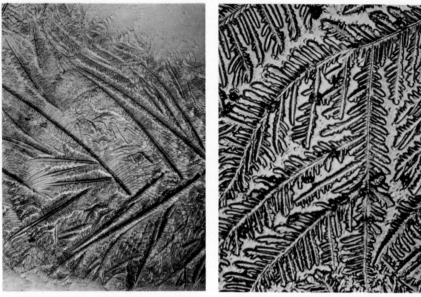

Fig. 4-5.—Fern phenomenon in cervical mucus during the normal menstrual cycle between days 12 and 16. *Left,* low power; *right,* high power. (Courtesy of Dr. Maxwell Roland.)

tube is wet; (2) salt solution has been used in cleaning or sterilizing the tube—always sterilize in distilled water; (3) excessive blood is mixed with the mucus.

Zondek has shown that mucous secretions and most body fluids show the phenomenon of ferning or arborization in a dried state, and Rydberg found that this arborization represents a special form of crystallization of sodium chloride in the medium of drying cervical mucus. Although arborization per se is a nonspecific process, its occurrence in cervical mucus is dependent on adequate estrogenic stimulation.

From a clinical viewpoint, the examination of cervical mucus is a simple test of ovarian function. Thus in the human castrate small amounts of exogenous estrogen will cause arborization of salt-containing mucus, whereas progesterone modifies the action of estrogen. Thus in amenorrhea a persistently negative fern test suggests insufficient estrogenic stimulation. In functional amenorrhea this may be reversed by the administration of estrogens, but in the amenorrhea of pregnancy exogenous estrogens will not produce the fern phenomenon. As a matter of fact, if the mucus shows strong arborization, pregnancy can be ruled out. Although the logical conclusion as to the mechanism involved in pregnancy is that high progesterone levels negate the estrogen effect, recent investigation has shown that the cervical cells during pregnancy do not permit permeation of electrolytes. It may be that the *effect* of progesterone is to prevent imbibition of sodium chloride by the endocervical cells.

Physiologic Alterations

The unique position held by the uterine cervix as a focal point for the histologic and colposcopic study of oncogenesis has also shed considerable light on its response to several physiologic processes. Thus, many of the gross and microscopic variations previously considered abnormal or even pathologic are now regarded as normal physiologic alterations. Prominent among these is prolapse of endocervical mucosa onto the anatomic portio. It now appears that this cervical *eversion* is related to age, the first pregnancy and estrogen stimulation. One of the most significant contributions to an understanding of cervical eversions as well as to dissolution of confusion between anatomic areas and histologic zones was made by Schneppenheim and associates. These workers meticulously examined 853 unselected uteri and showed that the length of the *gland-bearing* endocervical mucosa is relatively constant throughout life. However, the location of endocervical mucosa in relation to the anatomic cervical canal varies with age. During the childbearing years endocervical glands are found just below the internal os and extend below the external os, i.e., on to the ana-

Fig. 4–6.—Postpartum cervical eversion associated with a transverse laceration of the external os. The application of Schiller's solution stains the normal squamous epithelium dark brown. The endocervical epithelium does not stain.

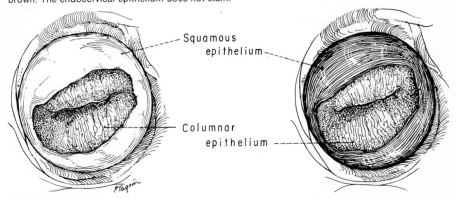

Squamous
epithelium

Columnar
epithelium

Schiller Test

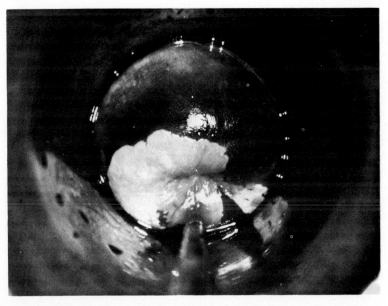

tomic portio (Fig. 4-2, arrows 3 and 4). After age forty, due to waning ovarian activity, the endocervical mucosa ascends the canal so that during postmenopause the lowest glands, the original squamo-columnar junction, and the transitional zone lie at or above the anatomic external os (Fig. 4-2, arrows 1 and 2). Schneppenheim *et al.* attribute the downward shift and eversion of the endocervix to an increase in volume of the mucosa during the years of maximal estrogen stimulation. This concept is in agreement with those of Coppleson and Reid, and Song and explains the increase in eversions noted after the first pregnancy (Fig. 4-6).

That growth and development of the cervix parallels stimulation by estrogen has also been demonstrated by Rosenthal and Hellman who studied the cervices of 80 premature or mature infants who were either stillborn or died neonatally and later by Hellman and co-workers who studied the effects of estrogen on the cervices of postmenopausal women. The bulbous cervix of the newborn comprises about five-sixths of the entire uterus and the changes in the epithelial structures of the endocervix show a high degree of development, with glandular and epithelial hyperplasia and hypersecretion. The endometrium by contrast is incompletely developed, usually inactive, and presents only a few tubular glands. It is assumed that these changes in the fetal endocervix are brought about by maternal estrogen since the same morphologic findings may be produced in postmenopausal women by exogenous estrogens. The squamous cells of the ectocervix of the newborn infant also demonstrate the effect of maternal estrogen since they are well stratified and contain abundant glycogen. In some instances hyperplasia of the basal cells has been noted in a degree which simulates that of the adult. At puberty, under the stimulation of estrogen from growing ovarian follicles the above changes presumably occur again although adequate morphologic studies in this age group preclude definitive description.

The transitional zone itself, now recognized as a usual finding, has in the past been considered an abnormal squamous cell proliferation. The histogenesis of the transitional zone involves the replacement of surface and glandular columnar cells by one of two mechanisms: (A) squamous metaplasia, (B) squamous epithelization.

SQUAMOUS METAPLASIA

It is now generally accepted that this type of epithelium is the end result of a process known as reserve cell metaplasia (subcolumnar or subcylindrical cell metaplasia, squamous prosoplasia). Reserve cells are undifferentiated spherical or polygonal cells with plump, centrally placed, dark nuclei and scanty cytoplasm. Their origin is controversial. It has been proposed that they are derived from (1) embryonal rests of urogenital sinus epithelium, (2) direct or indirect metaplasia from columnar cells, (3) basal cells of the portio, (4) stromal cells. There is accumulating evidence favoring the latter (Coppleson and Reid, Song). Although Hellman and associates demonstrated a striking increase in reserve cell hyperplasia and metaplasia with the administration of large doses of estrogen to postmenopausal women, DeAlvarez was able to relate the process only to age, i.e., the childbearing years, and the presence of cervical eversion. Coppleson and Reid present evidence that the metaplastic process is initiated by the

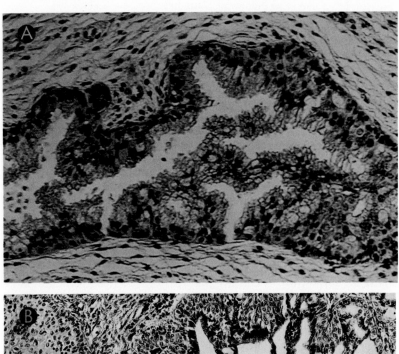

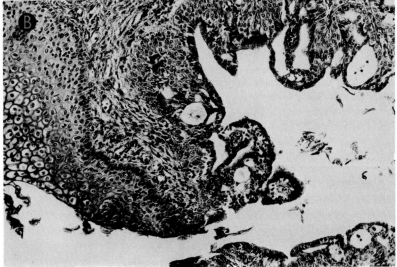

Fig. 4–7.—A, hyperplasia of the reserve cells in the endocervix. **B,** squamous metaplasia from reserve cells of the endocervix occurring at the histologic external os. Normal stratified squamous epithelium is seen at left. (Courtesy of Drs. Louis M. Hellman and Alexander Rosenthal.)

exposure of the endocervical mucosa to the lower pH of the vagina and suggest that estrogen plays a secondary role by promoting endocervical hyperplasia and prolapse and in lowering the pH of the vaginal environment.

The probable sequence of events in the metaplastic process may be outlined as follows:

1. Endocervical eversion
2. Reserve cell hyperplasia (Fig. 4–7, *A*)
3. Reserve cell metaplasia (squamous-like epithelium) (Fig. 4–7, *B*)

4. Sloughing off of overlying columnar epithelium

5. Differentiation into a multi-layered immature squamous epithelium

Although squamous metaplasia may rarely differentiate into a mature cornified form, it tends to remain immature and is sharply demarcated from the normal portio epithelium. Particularly active squamous metaplasia filling multiple glands has been confused with carcinoma in situ. However, examination of these cells under a high power microscope will reveal distinct morphologic characteristics. There are no clearly visible basal or prickle cell layers and the individual cells are of uniform size without intercellular ridges. Hyperchromatism, nuclear pleomorphism and abnormal mitotic activity are not seen in reserve cell hyperplasia or squamous metaplasia.

SQUAMOUS EPITHELIZATION

The second mechanism by which squamous epithelium overlies endocervical stroma has been called epidermization, epidermidization, or epidermalization. Since the analogy to skin is somewhat remote, Johnson's preference for the term squamous epithelization is more appropriate. This squamous epithelium is continuous with that of the histologic portio from which it is indistinguishable in its mature form. The most likely initiating event is a true pathologic erosion of the distal endocervix, a fairly common occurrence (Fig. 4–2, II), followed by an ingrowth or overglide of portio squamous cells. In the early stages of erosion healing, the squamous epithelium may be seen as a tenuous strand of immature squamous cells gradually decreasing in height as it is stretched over an otherwise denuded and inflamed stroma (Fig. 4–2, III). As with many regenerative processes, there may be considerable mitotic activity or a hyperplasia of basal or prickle cells. However, the nuclear changes characteristic of malignancy are absent. Whether these squamous cells are capable of actually displacing intact columnar epithelium is a subject of controversy. This property can be attributed only to metaplastic squamous cells. However, in its upward extension over denuded stroma the new epithelium does cover the mouths of the short glands of the distal endocervix. These occluded glands become mucous retention cysts (Nabothian) seen after childbirth and incomplete cervical cauterization. They are grossly visible on the portio as spherical elevations or as vesicular clear cysts 2 to 4 mm. in diameter. Microscopically the cystic space is seen to be lined by low cuboidal or flattened endocervical cells. Since the malignant potential of these cysts is practically nil, they may be treated by electrocauterization without biopsy. The small nasal tip is introduced directly into the cyst, rupturing it and allowing the thick glairy mucus to escape. This may be removed with a long forceps and the entire cavity thoroughly cauterized. Since these cysts have a tendency to recur, repeated cauterizations may be necessary to effect cure.

Pathologic Alterations

INFLAMMATION

From the time of the earliest clinical and microscopic descriptions of cervical disease, inflammation or more specifically "chronic cervicitis" has been an ubiquitous finding. Either alone or coexisting with other diseases it has been implicated in the pathogenesis of cervical eversion, squamous metaplasia, epithelization, basal cell hyperplasia, leukoplakia, endocervical polyps, and cancer. The histologic diagnosis of inflammation is based on the presence of two of the five cardinal signs of inflammation, redness and leukocytic infiltration. Although the former sign may be the result of increased stromal vascularity, it is just as likely the result of the thinness of transitional zone epithelium overlying its subjacent capillary bed. The leukocytic infiltrate consists primarily of lymphocytes with a few plasma cells and occasionally polymorphonuclear leukocytes. Leukocytic infiltration was found in 98 per cent of 400 cervices examined by Howard and associates and is described in nearly every specimen of cervical tissue examined at the Boston Hospital for Women. It has also been described in the cervices of the newborn and children. Extensive bacteriologic studies in all age groups rarely reveal pathogenic organisms. Thus, there is now general agreement with Song's opinion that in most instances cellular infiltration of the stroma is a unique physiologic phenomenon without clinical significance.

Although an attempt has been made to place the term "chronic cervicitis" in proper perspective, it cannot be denied that specific types of acute and chronic cervicitis do exist.

ACUTE CERVICITIS

The commonest cause of acute cervicitis is an infection brought about by the gonococcus. It involves chiefly the endocervical glands but may spread to the squamous epithelium and subjacent stroma by contiguity. Other organisms may also affect the cervix. These include streptococci, staphylococci, enterococci and Hemophilus vaginalis. An acute streptococcal cervicitis may be seen as part of a generalized pelvic cellulitis secondary to a criminal abortion, or it may follow instrumentation such as biopsy or insertion of a stem pessary. Usually such an infection is not confined to the cervix but spreads into the uterus and laterally into the lymphatics of the broad ligament. Symptoms of acute cervicitis are: (1) a tenacious, jelly-like but yellow or turbid discharge—in gonorrhea the admixture of pus is characteristic, and (2) a sensation of pelvic pressure or discomfort. If the inflammatory process is confined to the cervix, generalized symptoms are not evident.

Diagnosis is made by inspection of the cervix and examination of the discharge by stains and culture. There may be hyperemia and edema of the entire cervix together with an acute vaginitis from the infected discharge. Motion of the cervix at the time of pelvic examination may cause pain. Biopsy of the cervix should not be performed if an acute cervicitis is suspected. Cauterization is also contraindicated, since a fulminating pelvic cellulitis may be initiated by this procedure.

Treatment consists of: (1) avoiding instrumentation, and interdicting coitus; (2) limitation of activity; (3) lactic acid douches; (4) specific sulfonamide or antibiotic therapy, depending on the type and sensitivity of the responsible organism; (5) chemical debridement using a fibrinolytic agent, such as a combination of fibrinolysin and desoxyribonuclease in petrolatum and polyethylene (Elase).

Chronic Cervicitis

Although some authors would eliminate this term, its retention in a restricted sense seems appropriate. It is otherwise difficult to explain the everted cervix with beefy, friable, papillary appearing endocervical mucosa that bleeds profusely on contact. There is an associated thick yellow mucopurulent discharge, which on culture yields such misplaced organisms as *Escherichia coli, Streptococcus viridans,* or *Aerobacter aerogenes.* Histologically, there may be a true erosion or denudation of endocervical mucosa (Fig. 4–2, II) with beginning epithelization or squamous metaplasia. Granulation tissue is usually present and this plus epithelial necrosis and neutrophilic infiltration are Song's criteria for a diagnosis of true chronic cervicitis as opposed to the physiologic variety.

The symptoms of chronic cervicitis are vaginal discharge, usually yellow-white, thick and tenacious, and postcoital or post-douche spotting or bleeding. Complaints of pelvic pressure or heaviness with or without urinary symptoms suggest an associated "pelvic congestion syndrome" which is described in Chapter 5. In some cases the alteration of cervical mucus may contribute to a complaint of infertility.

A tentative diagnosis can be made on inspection of the cervix but biopsy and tissue diagnosis are mandatory. Chronic cervicitis as defined here is grossly indistinguishable from carcinoma in situ or early invasive cancer. In too many instances expectant management or ill-advised cautery has permitted cancer to progress to incurable stages. The inflammation and bleeding associated with chronic cervicitis render Papanicolaou smears unreliable in excluding carcinoma. Biopsies are obtained from the squamocolumnar junction and should include any transitional zone epithelium which fails to stain with the application of Gram's iodine solution (Schiller test).

Treatment of chronic cervicitis should be undertaken only after necessary tests have excluded cancer, cancer in situ or areas of dysplasia. The optimum treatment for this condition is electrocauterization. Following such treatment an enlarged, boggy cervix will usually be converted into one which closely resembles that of a nulliparous woman. Occasionally repeat cauterization is necessary. Failure to heal should raise the suspicion of malignancy. Cauterization of the cervix in the postpartum state is advisable if it appears abnormal but it should be deferred until cytologic study has been performed. If the cervix appears acutely inflamed at the six weeks postpartum visit, treatment with local antibacterial agents should be instituted and cauterization postponed until the eighth or twelfth week.

Keratinization

Since keratinization is not a physiologic property of cervical squamous epithelium, any tendency in this direction must be considered abnormal. However, some degree of focal keratinization is frequently observed in the absence of other abnormalities and its significance has been questioned. Since the keratin layer does not contain glycogen, focal lesions give a Schiller-positive staining reaction and should be studied by biopsy. The commonest abnormality in this group has been termed *leukoparakeratosis* and is characterized microscopically by an abrupt change in the staining quality of the cells with a sharp (usually oblique) line of demarcation between the normal glycogen-containing cells of the portio and the more densely staining, immature, nonglycogenated cells. (See Fig. 4–15,B.) Grossly the area of leukoparakeratosis may appear perfectly normal except for a faint ground-glass appearance. It is benign squamous epithelium and is responsible for most positive Schiller test results. After the solution is applied, the lesion appears as a flame-shaped area, radiating peripherally from the squamocolumnar junction, though not infrequently it is distal to this junction. Occasionally it involves most or all of the cervix and, may even extend onto the vaginal walls in any direction or may involve the entire cervix and the upper third of the vagina.

Leukoplakia of the cervix refers to a white, raised, smooth or sometimes roughened area which is usually grossly visible on the portio. The microscopic features are: (1) hyperkeratosis, (2) epithelial thickening with occasional rete ridge hyperplasia, (3) basal layer pleomorphism and a moderate degree of cellular differentiation and anaplasia. Unlike other squamous epithelial surfaces in the body, the relationship of leukoplakia to carcinoma is vague at best. Younge, however, has observed that if the leukoplakic area is in or adjacent to an eversion (transitional-zone) it may be malignant. When the leukoplakic area is distal to and not in continuity with the squamocolumnar junction it is usually benign. Because of the marked hyperkeratosis, leukoplakia does not stain with iodine. The diagnosis can be made only by biopsy and the treatment is local excision or extensive cauterization.

Hyperkeratosis is not a common finding in the cervix except in extensive prolapse when the epithelium actually is transformed into a skinlike covering. In this condition a homogeneous surface layer of keratin is produced by the squamous cells. There are usually dark-staining granules in the keratoeleidin layer but the surface cells are not nucleated. As previously noted, hyperkeratosis is one of the pathologic features of leukoplakia. *Parakeratosis* refers to a process of excessive surface keratin formation but in which the nuclei are retained. It probably represents a stage in the development of acellular hyperkeratosis.

Diagnostic and Minor Surgical Procedures

Biopsy of the Cervix

Cervical biopsy is the minor surgical procedure most often performed by the gynecologist. Its increasing use is partly responsible for the large numbers of early carcinomas of the cervix diagnosed during recent years. The procedure is simple, relatively painless and may be performed as part of a routine office examination. Indications for biopsy include any departure from the normal as determined by gross inspection. Thus erosions, eversions, ectropions, leukoplakia, ulcerations and polyps should be routinely sampled. The exact site to be biopsied is sometimes difficult to determine, especially if the cervix is hypertrophied and an extensive erosion is present. The use of Schiller's solution will facilitate the selection of biopsy sites since it will stain the normal glycogenated squamous epithelium a deep brown but will leave areas of columnar epithelium or abnormal (keratinized or neoplastic) epithelium unstained.

Only a few contraindications to cervical biopsy exist. These include acute or subacute pelvic inflammatory disease and acute purulent cervicitis. However, following treatment of the primary disorder biopsy should be carried out whenever indicated.

Numerous reports have indicated that early invasive cancer (microcarcinoma) and carcinoma in situ of the cervix may often be asymptomatic and that gross inspection is inadequate for diagnosis. The combination of cytologic examination and biopsy will secure more positive diagnoses than either method alone. Frequently, symptoms of postcoital or postdouche spotting will be the presenting complaint. In these patients biopsy of the normal-appearing cervix plus endocervical curettage is indicated. If blood is noted on wiping the portio epithelium, biopsy should always be carried out. Similarly any white or gray area, depressed crater, heaped-up tissue or polyp should be adequately sampled. Pregnancy is no contraindication to biopsy, and since it has been shown that carcinoma of the cervix in the first two trimesters carries with it the same prognosis as in the nonpregnant patient, early biopsy should not be deferred. Several studies have shown no increase in the abortion rate if biopsy is carried out during the first trimester.

TECHNIQUE.—The cervix is visualized by a Graves speculum and adequate illumination is provided. Wiping the eversion with a dry gauze pledget frequently causes bleeding, so we routinely cleanse the cervix with a cotton ball soaked in Alkalol (an alkaline astringent solution) or aqueous zephiran. After it has been thoroughly dried, Schiller's test is done. A fresh solution of iodine, potassium iodide and water in a 1:2:300 dilution is applied liberally to the cervix and upper vagina with a cotton-

Fig. 4–8.—**A,** Younge cervical biopsy forceps. Over-all length is 10 in., and the narrow jaws facilitate insertion into the cervical canal. The front of the lower jaw is elevated and has fine teeth to anchor the bite on the precise area to be biopsied. Serrations on the side of each jaw prevent slippage. A jaw opening of almost 90 degrees and sharp cutting edges insure adequate specimen size. **B,** Kevorkian biopsy curet, for detection of early endocervical lesions and for follow-up investigations. The narrow tip can be inserted without dilatation of the cervix, and the curet can be used without anesthesia. The rectangular cutting blade is slightly curved and obtains specimens that are easily oriented. Endometrial biopsies several centimeters in length may be obtained. **C,** typical biopsy site by Younge's method. (Courtesy of Dr. Paul A. Younge.)

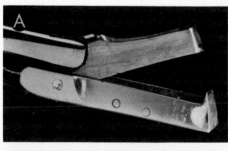
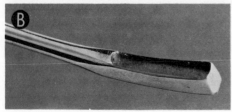
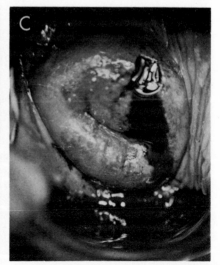

tipped applicator. Results are not conclusive if the patient is postmenopausal, excessive mucus is present or Schiller's solution is not fresh.

Areas of columnar epithelium which appear on the portio (eversion, ectropion) are grossly visible by their fine, pebbly, orange-red appearance and such areas, containing no glycogen, do not stain brown with Schiller's solution. All adjacent areas of squamous epithelium should stain homogeneously, and are designated as Schiller-positive areas if they do not. Biopsies are made of these areas. Care is taken to include a portion of the stained area with the nonstained to provide the pathologist with a comparison of normal and abnormal tissue. The ectropion or eversion is also biopsied to provide a portion of squamous epithelium in the fragment.

Proper diagnosis depends on a combination of careful selection of the site, skillful procurement of the specimen, and prompt fixation and intelligent imbedding of the biopsy specimen in paraffin. In order to provide the pathology technician with a recognizable fragment so that the tissue may be oriented for maximum study, Dr. Paul Younge has modified the Yeoman biopsy punch (Fig. 4–8, *A*). Use of this instrument facilitates biopsy in deep vaginas and enables one to get an adequate rectangular fragment which provides a maximum length of epithelium without excess stroma. Postbiopsy bleeding is also minimized. A typical biopsy site is shown in Figure 4–8, *C*.

The tissue is placed immediately in Bouin's solution, and appropriate designation is made as to where each fragment was located on the cervix. This facilitates further studies should one of multiple biopsies show anaplasia or carcinoma in situ.

A small vaginal tampon is placed against the cervix and the patient is instructed not to douche or to have intercourse for two weeks. If the biopsy tissue proves to be benign, cauterization of abnormal areas is performed at the end of that time. Cauterization is *never performed at the time of biopsy* or without previous biopsies except at the six-weeks postpartum examination and then only if cytology has been normal. If oozing is bothersome, Oxycel or Gelfoam may be placed against the bleeding point and the vagina packed. Occasionally a figure-of-eight catgut suture is necessary for hemostasis.

Cauterization of the Cervix

This procedure may be performed in the office or operating room. Although it is relatively painless, some patients are cognizant of the heat transmitted to the speculum and others may complain of uterine cramps. In young, nulliparous females who have discharge from large cervical ectropions or in extremely apprehensive patients a more thorough cauterization may be performed under light Pentothal anesthesia. Excellent results have been reported utilizing cold cauterization with liquid nitrogen as the refrigerant delivered through a special cervical probe. Several reports have indicated that this method of cryosurgery may offer several advantages when compared to more conventional electrocauterization.

The usual indications include chronic cervicitis with eversion or ectropion, nabothian cysts, polyps and postpartum eversion. Cauterization is done less commonly for leukoplakia, leukoparakeratosis, endometriosis and papillomas, although it is equally effective in securing good results in these entities. Cervical disease associated with infertility may benefit from judicious cauterization.

Electrocauterization should not be done in the presence of an acute cervicitis, such as that brought about by gonorrhea. Adequate cytologic and biopsy studies should have ruled out carcinoma, carcinoma in situ and cellular atypias such as dysplasia and basal cell hyperplasia, since other definitive therapy or follow-up would be indicated. Acute or even subacute pelvic inflammatory disease is a definite contraindication and, in general, it is better not to perform cauterization during the menstrual period. An ideal time is five to seven days after the cessation of menstrual flow. Although cauterization of the postpartum cervix is usually performed at the six-weeks checkup, occasionally it is desirable to wait eight to 12 weeks for further involution.

TECHNIQUE.—A nasal-tip cautery (Fig. 4–9) is adequate and several cautery transformers are available. The tips vary in size so that the endocervix may always be treated. A bivalve speculum is inserted into the vagina and the cervix completely exposed in good light. The cervix is then cleansed of mucus with Alkalol and dried

Fig. 4–9.—Cauterization of the cervix using the electric cautery. If visualization is good, use of the tenaculum is unnecessary. The cautery should not be introduced too far up the endocervical canal to avoid destruction of all endocervical glands.

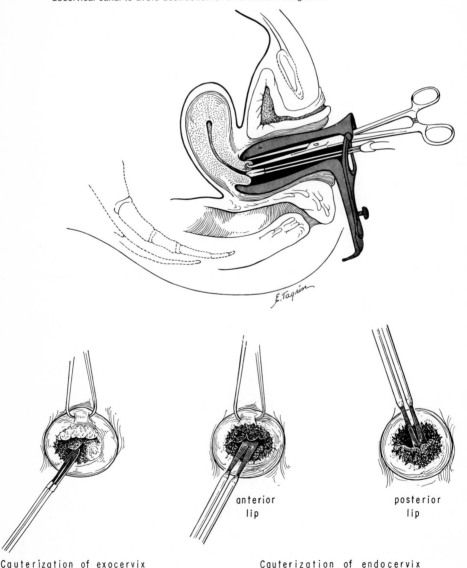

anterior lip

posterior lip

Cauterization of exocervix   Cauterization of endocervix

with cotton pledgets. The cautery is brought to a dull red before insertion into the vagina, and care must be taken not to touch the vaginal walls during insertion. The erosion or eversion is deeply cauterized throughout its entirety, thus removing all of the infected or abnormal tissue. The author no longer limits this procedure to linear streaking because of the possibility of inadequate treatment, unless of course the lesion or cyst is small. The endocervix is also thoroughly cauterized by laying the cautery flat against the anterior and then the posterior lip with the tip inserted about 1 cm. into the canal. It is felt that only by this maneuver will the diseased endocervix be sufficiently treated. Stenosis is prevented by passing a uterine sound or small dilators on subsequent visits at six weeks, three months and six months after cauterization. Occasionally visits will have to be scheduled more often.

The patient should be told that a vaginal discharge will be noted in a few days, which after a week or so will be purulent and foul smelling. Bleeding, occasionally profuse, may occur after about two weeks and packing is occasionally needed to control this. The discharge and odor may be minimized by use of an antibiotic or sulfonamide cream for two weeks following cauterization. Coitus and douching are interdicted during this time. At the end of six weeks, the portio is usually well epithelized but may appear pink and bleed easily. A Schiller test at this time is not always conclusive since the cells are not well glycogenated. Repeat cauterization is rarely needed except in extremely large lesions. Nonhealing after cauterization should make the physician suspicious of carcinoma.

Benign Neoplasms
CERVICAL POLYPS

These are usually derived from the endocervix as a result of a chronic papillary endocervicitis and present as soft, spherical, usually glistening red masses of about ⅛ to ¼ in. in diameter (Fig. 4-10). They may bleed readily when touched and are almost always benign. Occasionally dys-

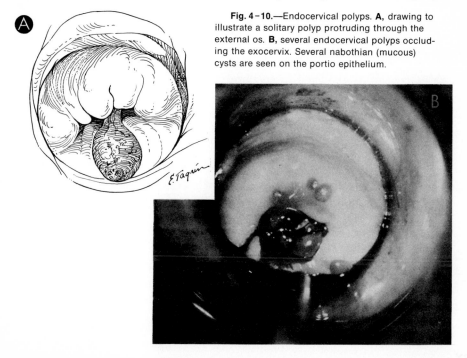

Fig. 4-10.—Endocervical polyps. **A,** drawing to illustrate a solitary polyp protruding through the external os. **B,** several endocervical polyps occluding the exocervix. Several nabothian (mucous) cysts are seen on the portio epithelium.

plasia or carcinoma in situ may be found in a solitary polyp. The base of the polyp may be readily visible at the squamocolumnar junction or it may be higher in the endocervix. Most cervical polyps can be grasped with a clamp and twisted free, and the base cauterized for hemostasis. All should be submitted for pathologic examination even though the malignant potential is small. If the polyp is large or the base cannot be readily identified, its origin from the endometrium must be considered. An adenomyoma pedunculated through the cervix may assume a polypoid shape although it is usually larger and firmer than a true polyp.

Differential diagnosis includes: (1) polypoid fragments of endocervical carcinoma or carcinosarcoma protruding through the os, (2) retained portions of an abortion, (3) the grapelike swellings of sarcoma botryoides which occasionally originate in the cervix and (4) a polypoidal submucous leiomyoma or endometrial polyp which has prolapsed through the cervical os.

ENDOMETRIOSIS

This lesion presents a characteristic gross picture but usually causes minimal symptoms. It is believed to be somewhat rare but actually is common in women who have had cervical biopsies or repairs. A red, elevated streaking over the surface of the portio is usually evident, together with red or reddish blue vesicular areas. These are most evident premenstrually, and biopsies should be performed at this time for adequate pathologic interpretation. This type of endometriosis suggests implantation as its cause, since it frequently is seen a few months after biopsy and cauterization or trachelorrhaphy in menstruating women. Against this idea, however, is the finding of areas of decidual reaction in the cervices of pregnant women who have not had previous biopsies. This suggests the presence of multipotential cells in the stroma of the cervix which are capable of responding as endometrial cells to the influence of estrogen and progesterone. These deciduomas may also be produced in the nonpregnant woman by prolonged administration of moderately high doses of estrogen and progesterone. Treatment following biopsy confirmation should be extensive deep cauterization.

PAPILLOMAS

These rather uncommon tumors are benign epithelial neoplasms of stratified squamous epithelium with supporting connective tissue and are grossly papillary in nature. Only about 100 cases have been reported, and the reader is referred to the list of references for detailed analyses. The author described 14 cases in 1955, reviewed the literature and classified the lesions into (1) papillomas associated with pregnancy, (2) condylomata acuminata and (3) neoplastic papillomas.

Papillomas associated with pregnancy occur in young individuals, are usually discovered during routine examination during the first trimester, require no treatment and disappear spontaneously during the puerperium. They are warty, gray or gray-red lesions of the endocervix which occasionally grow rapidly and which microscopically may show prickle cell hyperplasia with variations in nuclear size, shape and staining intensity. Close study will show that these changes are localized and that most cells differentiate in an orderly fashion. They are always benign and have been called "cockscomb polyps."

Condylomata acuminata may occur on the cervix as well as in the vagina. They have been called "venereal warts" and are presumed to be of viral origin. An associated vaginal discharge is a common finding. Although this lesion may simulate invasive carcinoma grossly, it is not neoplastic and usually is rather characteristic histologically, with prickle cell hyperplasia and acanthosis, an arborescent pattern of squamous cells without anaplasia and round cell infiltration of the stroma (Fig. 4–11). Treatment consists of elimination of the vaginal discharge, biopsy to rule out carcinoma and electrocauterization.

True (neoplastic) papillomas are the most important lesions of the group because they are potentially or actually malignant and occur postmenopausally. Usually the growth is small (less than 4 mm. in height) and has a wide base attached near the squamocolumnar junction. Even when sufficient biopsy material is obtained, histologic differentiation between papillary carcinoma and an active papilloma is difficult (Fig. 4–12). In these patients careful pathologic examination and continued clinical observation

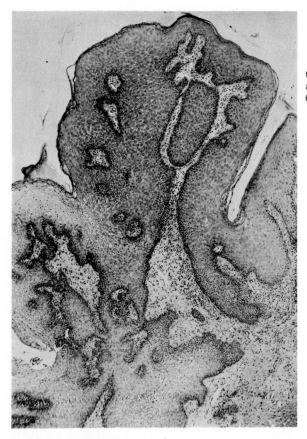

Fig. 4–11.—Condyloma acuminatum of cervix. (From Kistner, R. W., and Hertig, A. T.: Obst. & Gynec. 6:147, 1955.)

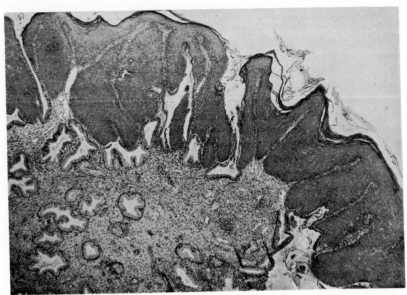

Fig. 4-12.—Papilloma of cervix. (From Kistner, R. W., and Hertig, A. T.:
Obst. & Gynec. 6:147, 1955.)

is mandatory. It should be emphasized that such papillary lesions may
simulate invasive carcinoma grossly and microscopically and conversely—
and perhaps more important—that an occasional low-grade carcinoma
may masquerade under the guise of a benign, papillary acuminate lesion.
Local excision is adequate therapy after cancer has been excluded.

Malignant Neoplasms

SQUAMOUS CELL CARCINOMA

Three decades ago carcinoma of the cervix was the leading cause of
death from malignant disease in American women. However, during the
past 30 years the mortality rate from this disease has declined by more than
50 per cent despite an overall increase in incidence. For the most part the
reduction in mortality is attributable to two factors: (1) the recognition of a
significant preinvasive phase and (2) the means by which the preinvasive
lesion can be detected, namely Papanicolaou smears. The influence of the
detection and treatment of preinvasive cervical cancer on both the death
rate and the incidence of invasive cases is exemplified by the trends in
New York State charted in Figure 4-13.

In 1957 Dr. Paul A. Younge stated that carcinoma of the cervix was a
preventable disease. The results of two long term cytology screening programs support this concept. In Shelby County, Tennessee, where a screening program was inaugurated in 1949, 75 per cent of the white population
over age 20 had had at least one cervico-vaginal smear by 1961. There was
a concurrent 51 per cent reduction in the incidence rate of invasive cancer
and the mortality rate decreased by 59 per cent. A mass screening program
was also initiated in British Columbia in 1949. By 1966, 75 per cent of
women age 20 and over had been screened on at least 1 occasion. Between

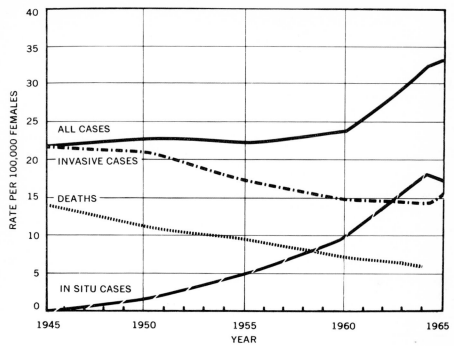

Fig. 4-13.—Graphic presentation of cancer of uterine cervix death rates and incidence rates from New York State (except New York City) 1945-1965. Note: Rate per 100,000 population standardized for age on the 1940 census population of the United States, from the New York State Department of Health. (From Cancer Facts and Figures, 1968, American Cancer Society.)

1955 and 1966 there was a 52 per cent decline in the incidence rate of invasive cancer. The incidence in the screened population in 1966 was 4.8 per 100,000 per year while that in the unscreened group remained at the original level of 29 per 100,000 per year.

The results of a small but carefully controlled cervical cancer demonstration project at the Boston Hospital for Women are tabulated in Table 4-1. There have been no cases of invasive cancer detected after the initial examination and in effect, carcinoma in situ has been eliminated from the study population after the second year repeat examination.

Epidemiology.—Numerous epidemiologic studies reported in the literature have established a positive association between cancer of the cervix and multiple interdependent social factors.

TABLE 4-1.—Pathologic Diagnoses in Boston Hospital for Women Project

Exam	No. Patients	Invasive	Carcinoma in Situ	Dysplasia
Initial	12,077	50	118	221
1 Year	4,205	0	7	35
2 Years	2,278	0	2	11
3 Years	1,522	0	0	3
4 Years	877	0	0	2
5 Years	205	0	1*	0

*Not seen between initial and 5th year examination.

TABLE 4–2.—Association Between Cervical Cancer and Social Factors

1. Socioeconomic
   a) Poverty
   b) Race

2. Marital
   a) Ever married versus never married
   b) Marriage before age 20
   c) Multiple and broken marriages

3. Childbearing
   a) Multiparity
   b) First pregnancy before age 20

4. Sexual exposure
   a) First coitus before age 20
   b) Prostitution
   c) Syphilis

A number of inter-relationships can be seen at first glance and statistical analysis of these data has eliminated several factors. The greater incidence of cervical cancer observed among Negroes is related to their lower socioeconomic status. Multiparity, previously thought to be of etiologic importance, is of no significance independent of age at first marriage and age at first pregnancy. The interdependence of prostitution and syphilis is obvious, and excluding the influence of a marriage license, early first coitus and early marriage are also related factors. Even socioeconomic status is inter-related since an association has long been noted between relative poverty and early marriage and childbearing.

In terms of greatest risk the final common denominator appears to be the onset of regular sexual activity before the age of 20 with continued exposure to multiple sexual partners. The rarity of cervical cancer in nuns, a celibate group, has been observed by 2 investigators and strongly supports this concept. Recently the remark has been made that cancer of the cervix is a venereal disease.

One of the most striking epidemiologic characteristics of cervical cancer is its low incidence in Jewish women, about one sixth that of the general population. This plus absence of penile cancer among Jews has led to the hypothesis that circumcision has a protective effect and that the smegma of uncircumcised males plays a role in carcinogenesis. However, incidence figures comparing Moslems, who also practice ritual circumcision, to otherwise comparable noncircumcised groups have been inconclusive. Difficulties in history taking and variability in the completeness of circumcision have prevented valid comparisons between non-Jewish circumcised and noncircumcised groups in this country.

The epidemiologic evidence strongly suggesting the venereal transmission of a carcinogenic agent coupled with the revival of interest in viral oncogenesis has led to a search for a possible viral etiology of cervical cancer. Type II herpes virus (Herpes progenitalis) has recently been implicated. It is transmitted by coitus and frequently infects noncircumcised males. Naib has reported a 7 per cent prevalence of carcinoma in situ among women with genital herpes as compared to a 0.6 per cent prevalence of this lesion in his control group. Additional evidence has been presented by Rawls and associates who found neutralizing antibodies to type II herpes virus in the sera of a significantly greater number of women with cervical cancer than in the sera of matched controls.

Premalignant Neoplasia

At present there is unanimity of opinion regarding the basic concept of carcinoma in situ of the cervix. A sufficient group of patients, adequately observed, has developed invasive cancer from the in situ stage to warrant the conclusion that such a progression exists. In 1956 Stewart stated that, "every infiltrative cancer must come from an in situ cancer, there being no other thing it can come from, this irrespective of various doubts cast on the relationship." Although it may be conceded that invasive cancer arises from an area of carcinoma in situ, whether the latter originates from a few aberrant cells or at several sites within a larger field of an earlier precursor remains a controversial subject.

Current opinion favors the existence of a precursor to carcinoma in situ which has been termed dysplasia, anaplasia, atypical hyperplasia, and basal cell hyperactivity. Although Hertig's descriptive term, *anaplasia,* has been utilized at the Boston Hospital for Women, *dysplasia* has been accepted and is a preferable term.

Dysplasia.—According to Reagan and Wentz, the term dysplasia designates a group of heteroplastic lesions of the cervical squamous epithelium. These lesions are characterized by a variable increase in the number of immature cells and by evidence of abnormal maturation. There may be active cellular proliferation with an increase in the number of mitoses, normal or abnormal, and there may be associated disorders of keratinization. The lesions are located at the distal end of the transitional zone in juxaposition to the portio epithelium. At the Boston Hospital for Women, criteria for the diagnosis of dysplasia include the cellular abnormalities characteristic of carcinoma in situ. However, the entire epithelial thickness is not uniformly involved and some degree of surface differentiation is observed. In general there is more cytoplasm and less hyperchromatism than with carcinoma in situ. Vesicular nuclei containing coarse clumped chromatin are common as are large bizarre mitotic figures. The dysplasias are categorized into slight, moderate and severe gradations based on the degree of differentiation and maturation. The severe dysplasias are borderline carcinomas in situ and would be diagnosed as such by many pathologists. Evidence supporting the thesis that dysplasia is a precursor of carcinoma in situ may be summarized as follows:

1. Observed progression of dysplasia to carcinoma in situ in from 1.4 to 42.3 per cent of patients. The variation in percentages is the result of differences in criteria used to define each lesion and variable periods of follow up. It has been suggested that diagnostic biopsies remove or alter the dysplastic lesion.

2. The incidence of carcinoma in situ is reportedly higher in a population previously found to have dysplasia than in an otherwise comparable population. (Stern and Neely—64 per 1000 per year versus 0.04 per 1000 per year.)

3. Both histologic studies and colposcopic observations have indicated that carcinoma in situ occurs adjacent to or within areas of dysplasia.

4. The screening and subsequent elimination of women with dysplasia from a study population will greatly reduce the incidence of carcinoma in situ in that population. In the Boston Hospital for Women series, carcinoma in situ was eliminated after the third screening.

5. The average age of patients with dysplasia is consistently 3 to 5 years younger than that of patients with carcinoma in situ.

6. Cells obtained from dysplastic lesions demonstrate chromosomal aneuploidy similar to that found in carcinoma in situ and invasive cancer.

7. Dysplastic cells show abnormal amounts of deoxyribonucleic acid (DNA) by microspectrophotometry and an increased rate of DNA synthesis has been demonstrated in tissue culture.

Despite a significant rate of progression from dysplasia to carcinoma in situ, it is also apparent that a large number of these lesions regress, either spontaneously or as a result of biopsy. Of 129 adequately followed cases reported by McKay *et al.* 20.2 per cent disappeared as evidenced by cytologic smears, biopsies or hysterectomy. In a series of 141 patients reported by Johnson at the Boston Hospital for Women 71.3 per cent regressed during a period of 9 years. However, 21.3 per cent subsequently recurred. The duration of the initial period of dysplasia was less than one year in 81.7 per cent of those demonstrating regression.

McKay and associates' review includes 243 cases of dysplasia diagnosed by cervical biopsies at the Boston Hospital for Women during the years 1945 through 1954 (Fig. 4–14). This was an over-all prevalance of 1.2 per cent of 20,000 cervices examined pathologically during this time. Comparative incidences were 1.3 per cent for in situ carcinoma and 3.4 per cent for invasive carcinoma during the same interval. The average age of the patient with dysplasia was 34.9 years compared with 38 for in situ carcinoma and 48 for invasive carcinoma. Of the 243 patients with dysplasia 129 had adequate study and follow up. About 40 per cent of these had dyplasia coexisting with carcinoma in situ or invasive carcinoma at the time of hysterectomy and a little over 30 per cent had persistent dysplasia at the time the study was completed.

These observations suggest that a spectrum of change exists which may regress in the earlier stages or remain unchanged for long periods of time, possibly for the patient's life span. On the other hand, a biopsy finding of dysplasia should alert the clinician to the possibility of co-existing carcinoma in situ or invasive cancer. A patient having dysplasia of the cervix need not be approached with a sense of urgency. Both ill-conceived and over-zealous treatment may be obviated by following a carefully planned diagnostic regimen.

If repeat cytology and selective biopsies, based on the clinical and/or colposcopic appearance of the cervix and the Schiller test, are compatible with dysplasia, further diagnostic procedures are rarely necessary. At the Boston Hospital for Women dysplastic lesions exhibiting regression are followed cytologically at specific intervals. Persistent dysplastic lesions are treated by high frequency electrocoagulation. Dysplastic lesions bordering on carcinoma in situ in the older age group are an indication for hysterectomy.

Richart and Sciarra have reported the results of cautery in 170 patients with dysplasia. The lesion was eradicated in 89 per cent by the first cauteri-

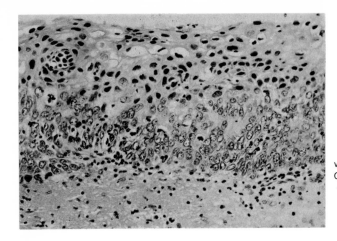

Fig. 4-14.—Dysplasia of cervix. (From McKay, D. G., *et al.*: Obst. & Gynec. 13:2, 1959.)

zation. Repeat cautery was successful in all but two patients who required conization.

Carcinoma In Situ.—Carcinoma in situ is an abnormality of the stratified squamous epithelium of the cervix which resembles carcinoma morphologically but whose extent is confined to the epithelium and epithelial structures. It has been variously termed "intraepithelial carcinoma," "incipient carcinoma," "preinvasive carcinoma" and "Bowen's disease of the cervix." The earliest abnormalities usually begin at the junction of the histologic portio and transitional zone, but it must be remembered that this junction is not always situated in the same area. Thus it may be within the endocervical canal or well out on the portio. Marsh has presented evidence that suggests that squamous cell carcinoma of the cervix often arises from endocervical epithelium located either within the canal or displaced from the canal to the portio as a result of eversion and erosion. This supports the idea of Pund and Auerbach who found 47 cases of carcinoma in situ "located principally or entirely on the gland-bearing portion of the cervical lining near or at the junction of the stratified squamous and columnar epithelia." These authors believed the ultimate source of these cancers to be the endocervical reserve cells. Johnson and associate's meticulous clinicopathologic studies and graphic reconstructions of cervices support the concept of progression from abnormal reserve cell hyperplasia to reserve cell dysplasia to dysplasia and thence to carcinoma in situ. They also propose a more rapid evolution whereby reserve cell dysplasia is converted directly into carcinoma in situ.

At the present time there is no unanimous opinion on the cellular origin of carcinoma in situ. Reagan and Wentz, however, have proposed three types of invasive cancer, whose origins are either the squamous epithelium of the portio, metaplastic epithelium of the transitional zone or subcylindrical cells of the endocervix depending upon which type of tissue is acted upon by the carcinogen.

The characteristic morphologic changes in carcinoma in situ are similar to, but more extensive than, those described in the section on dysplasia. They are: (1) cellular undifferentiation, with absence of normal stratification and maturation; (2) loss of polarity; (3) numerous and atypical mitotic figures throughout the extent of the epithelium; (4) cellular pleomorphism, nuclear hyperchromatism, dyskaryosis (abnormal nuclear changes), and (5) absence of differentiation on the surface (Figs. 4–15 and 4–16). In summary, the cells, both as units and in aggregate, look like cancer. A sharp line of demarcation usually exists between the normal and abnormal cells and this may be detected grossly by the equally sharp line between these areas that is brought into view by Schiller's test. Carcinoma

Fig. 4–15.—A, carcinoma in situ of cervix. (From Hertig, A. T., and Gore, H. M.: *Tumors of the Female Sex Organs,* fasc. 33 of *Atlas of Tumor Pathology* [Washington, D.C.: Armed Forces Institute of Pathology, 1960].) **B,** carcinoma in situ of cervix with gland involvement. An area of leukoparakeratosis is seen at the upper right.

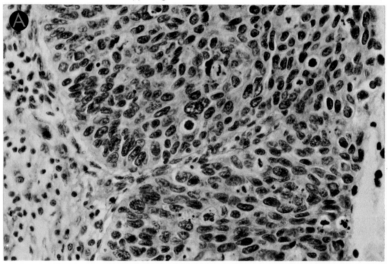

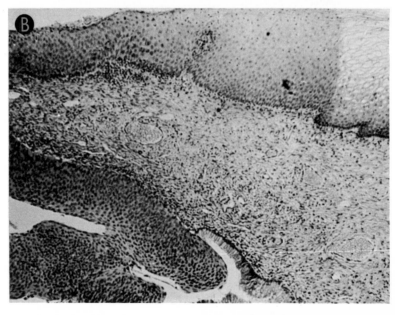

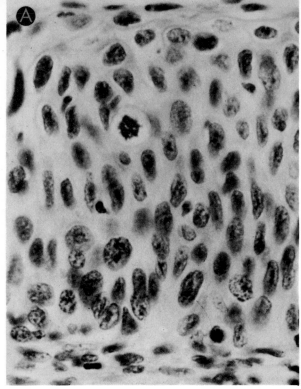

Fig. 4-16.—A, high power of carcinoma in situ of cervix. B, diagrammatic representation of changes in cellular morphology from slight dysplasia to carcinoma in situ. Nuclear-cytoplasmic ratios are shown at the bottom. C, diagrammatic representation of exfoliated cells from the normal cervix compared with variations of exfoliated cells from the neoplastic cervix. (B and C, courtesy of Dr. Paul A. Younge.)

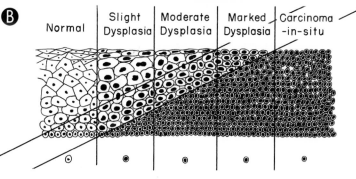

Normal | Slight Dysplasia | Moderate Dysplasia | Marked Dysplasia | Carcinoma-in-situ

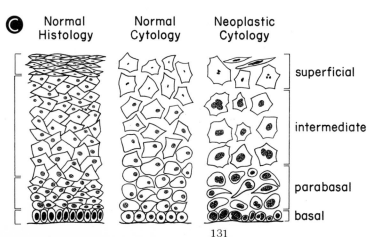

Normal Histology | Normal Cytology | Neoplastic Cytology

superficial

intermediate

parabasal

basal

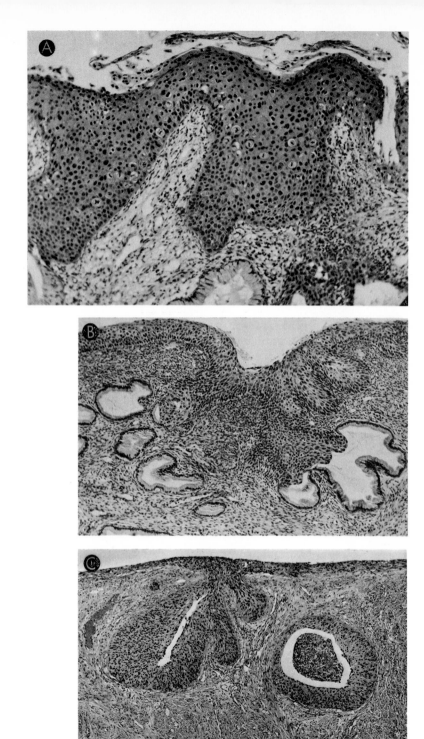

Fig. 4–17.—**A,** carcinoma in situ with surface stratification and differentiation. **B** and **C,** carcinoma in situ with gland involvement. (*A* and *B* from Hertig, A. T., and Gore, H. M.: *Tumors of the Female Sex Organs,* fasc. 33 of *Atlas of Tumor Pathology* [Washington, D.C.: Armed Forces Institute of Pathology, 1960].)

in situ may spread as a surface phenomenon (Fig. 4–17, *A*) before it begins to invade the connective tissue stroma and, as it advances, may replace columnar cells of the endocervix including that of the endocervical glands. This process is looked on as a later phase of the process of intraepithelial spread and has been termed "gland involvement" (Fig. 4–17, *B* and *C*) but is not considered true invasion. It should be noted that squamous metaplastic changes may occur in endocervical glands as a benign undergrowth with displacement of columnar epithelium. The differentiating characteristics from in situ carcinoma have been mentioned.

Whether all invasive cervical carcinomas begin as in situ lesions is unknown but Peterson reported that in one third of 127 untreated patients invasive carcinoma developed *subsequent to* in situ carcinoma at the end of nine years. Masterson found that 28 per cent of 25 untreated patients demonstrated invasive carcinoma at the end of five years.

The prevalence of carcinoma in situ will vary depending on the type of population being screened. At the Boston Hospital for Women the prevalence in ambulatory patients has been stable at 1.2 per cent for 20 years. In contrast, the prevalence of invasive cancer has dropped from over 2 per cent to 0.5 per cent during the same period. As with invasive cancer, epidemiologic evidence from populations with carcinoma in situ has shown that this lesion is associated with low socioeconomic status, early coitus, early marriage and child-bearing, and that it occurs more frequently in Negroes and less frequently among Jews.

The average age of patients with carcinoma in situ at the Boston Hospital for Women was 38, whereas the average age of patients with invasive

Fig. 4-18.—Increasing average age with progression of cancer of the cervix. Note the 10-year age span between patients with carcinoma in situ and those with invasive cancer. (Courtesy of Dr. Paul A. Younge.)

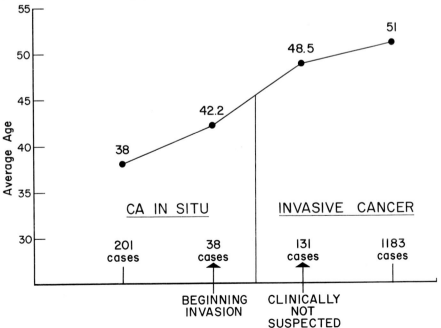

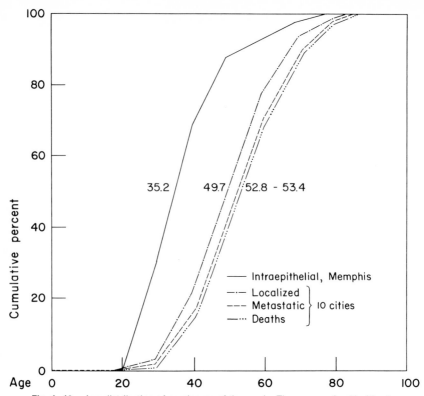

Fig. 4–19.—Age distribution of carcinoma of the cervix. The average for 10 cities is compared with the average of patients having intraepithelial carcinoma in Memphis, Tennessee.

carcinoma was 48 (Figs. 4–18 and 4–19). However, the finding of many cases in the late twenties and early thirties, makes it imperative that each patient be treated individually. Parity, desire for children and the presence or absence of associated pelvic disease are important factors in deciding optimum therapy.

Diagnosis.—The diagnosis of carcinoma in situ must be made by histologic examination of an adequate sample of tissue obtained from the suspect cervix. Subsequent to the extensive use of the Papanicolaou smear for cancer screening, gynecologists and pathologists were faced with the problem of satisfactorily explaining the origin of abnormal cells obtained from grossly benign cervices. Adequate tissue sampling became a necessity and this was expeditiously accomplished by cold-knife conization of the cervix. Diagnostic conization continues to be the keystone of pre-treatment evaluation in most clinics in the United States. However, the necessity for hospitalization and anesthesia has been seriously questioned. Furthermore certain complications, usually hemorrhage and infection, and the end results have led many gynecologists to become disenchanted with this procedure.

For more than 40 years the diagnostic regimen at the Boston Hospital for Women has consisted of multiple biopsies combined with endocervical curettage. These procedures may be performed on ambulatory patients and are extremely accurate. Diagnostic conization has been necessary only rarely. The success of this approach is dependent, however, on the use of a sharp square-jawed biopsy punch (see Fig. 4–8A). This instrument obtains an untraumatized, rectangular specimen which is oriented easily by the histotechnician and sectioned in a plane perpendicular to its epithelial surface. The squamocolumnar junction and the transitional zone must be represented. The sites for biopsy are not chosen randomly but are based on the gross appearance of the cervix and the Schiller test. Endocervical curettage is essential in determining the presence of carcinoma in situ in the endocervical canal as well as excluding invasive cancer in this area. This procedure is performed using the narrow rectangular curette shown in Figure 4–8B. If the specimen is scanty it is combined with clotted blood and is submitted to the pathologist as a "cell block." Carcinoma in situ arising in the canal is evident as strips of anaplastic epithelium whereas invasive cancer is seen as larger fragments of piled-up, malignant squamous epithelium usually showing increased differentiation.

The most serious error encountered in the evaluation of a suspicious cervix is that which leads to inadequate treatment of invasive cancer. The fear of overlooking invasive cancer when biopsies alone are employed is the primary reason for conization. This viewpoint has been supported by several clinical studies. It should be emphasized, however, that in these studies hysterectomy specimens have revealed unsuspected invasive cancer in from 0.8 per cent to 4.0 per cent of patients in whom the preoperative conization specimen disclosed only carcinoma in situ. The diagnostic accuracy of multiple biopsy-endocervical curettage combination from a recent Boston Hospital for Women series is compared with the final diagnosis in Table 4–3. The final diagnosis in each case represents the most advanced lesion discovered on examination of biopsies and surgical specimens (hysterectomy and therapeutic conization). In none of these 513 patients was the lesion grossly visible. The over-all diagnostic accuracy was 94.7 per cent and no patient was under-treated. In a previous series reported from this hospital only one of 125 early invasive cancers was undetected prior to hysterectomy. This is the only instance in which a patient's welfare was jeopardized by this diagnostic approach. If biopsy-diagnosed carcinomas in situ and microinvasive cancers from these two series are combined, the incidence of unsuspected invasive cancer is 1 in 248 patients or only 0.4 per cent.

Diagnosis is frequently confused by lack of criteria for exacting pathologic interpretation. Only a few pathologists have had the experience, or the interest, necessary to differentiate fine nuances of cellular detail. The obvious in situ lesions occasion little difficulty, but the questionable ones

TABLE 4–3.—PREOPERATIVE BIOPSY VERSUS FINAL DIAGNOSIS

BIOPSY DIAGNOSIS	NO. OF PATIENTS	FINAL DIAGNOSIS	NO. OF PATIENTS	% ACCURACY
Ca. in situ	89	Ca. in situ	94	94.7
Severe dysplasia	5			
Ca. in situ	1	Ca. in situ with	9	88.8
Ca. in situ with early stromal invasion	8	early stromal invasion		
Invasive	10	Preclincal invasive	10	100.0
Total	113	Over-all accuracy		94.7

are subject to great differences of opinion. The gynecologist should secure clinical as well as pathologic consultation in such patients before proceeding to therapy.

CONE BIOPSY OF THE CERVIX.—This term implies that a conical segment of cervix including 1.0–1.5 cm. of portio epithelium (the base of the cone) together with all (or as much as possible) of the endocervix is removed as a single piece of tissue. The tissue is then fixed, cut into anywhere from eight to 30 fragments and each block of tissue "step sectioned."

This procedure may be indicated in certain patients in whom the results of cervical smears remain definitely positive for invasive cancer but biopsies have shown only carcinoma in situ. In our clinic, however, this procedure has generally been used therapeutically rather than diagnostically. For example, the young patient desirous of having children, and in whom thorough pathologic studies have shown only in situ carcinoma, may have this procedure as definitive therapy. Of course, should study of the cone reveal invasive cancer, therapy would be given accordingly. If the pathologist is not satisfied that an adequate diagnosis can be made by multiple biopsies, we perform a diagnostic cone biopsy.

TECHNIQUE.—Pentothal anesthesia is adequate. The vagina and cervix are prepared in the usual fashion, and Schiller's test is performed. Cervical dilatation is usually not done, but a wing-tip catheter over a metal introducer is inserted into the uterine cavity and a tenaculum is placed on the anterior lip. This will stabilize the cervix and simplify the procedure. Hemostasis is aided by injecting saline and epinephrine solution into the cervix or by ligating the descending cervical branch of the uterine artery bilaterally. A circular incision is made around the external os, its size depending on the size of the erosion or of Schiller-positive areas. The incision is then carried into the cervical stroma, with angulation toward the canal, and is continued so as to reach the level of the internal os or lower uterine segment. A suture or clip should be placed at 12 or at 6 o'clock for purposes of orientation. If bleeding is excessive, one or two small vessels may have to be sutured. Ordinarily Gelfoam or Oxycel may be placed against the coned area and a vaginal pack inserted for 24 hours. Delayed bleeding (usually at seven to 10 days) may occur at times and necessitate ligation.

Treatment.—The treatment of carcinoma in situ of the cervix has been resolved into two major and somewhat antagonistic groups. Approaches are based on certain premises. (1) Since in situ carcinoma will eventually develop into invasive cancer if left untreated, the only therapy is surgical extirpation, namely total hysterectomy. Further, since some in situ carcinomas have shown invasive carcinoma in the excised specimen, a modified radical hysterectomy should be the optimum method. (2) Since in situ carcinoma does not undergo rapid progression to invasive carcinoma, a period of observation is permissible, especially if conservative procedures for local removal of the in situ lesion are undertaken. At the carcinoma in situ clinic of the Boston Hospital for Women, Dr. Paul Younge has championed the latter approach. The following variations in therapy are used. (1) If the patient is beyond the childbearing age, has completed her childbearing function or has additional pelvic lesions which indicate hysterectomy, surgery is performed. Usually this is a simple total abdominal hysterectomy, although occasionally it is performed vaginally. Just before surgery the entire cervix and vagina are painted with Schiller's solution and the extent of vagina to be removed is delineated. (2) If the lesion is limited to the squamocolumnar junction in an everted cervix and there is proof that the canal is normal, a therapeutic conization or cauterization is recommended. This pertains only if the patient agrees to prolonged follow-up and is anxious to have more children. Of 34 patients so treated by Younge, 12 have had a total of 21 children and seven miscarriages. All are well five or more years after treatment, and in all the results of cytologic and pathologic studies are negative. (3) If the patient does not wish to accept the therapy outlined in 2, or if the lesion is found to extend up into the cervical canal or the disease persists after usual conservative procedures, a simple total hysterectomy is performed. The ovaries are removed only for specific indication in patients under 45.

In summary, each patient with carcinoma in situ presents individual and specific problems, and therefore no broad rules of management can be given. It is just as poor judgment to treat *all* in situ lesions with radical hysterectomy or radiation as it is to treat *all* by conization or cauterization. It should be re-emphasized that adequate evaluation of the cervix by means of six to 14 punch biopsies and endocervical curettage should never miss invasive cancer except in its very earliest stages. Simple total hysterectomy is adequate therapy for the latter. Of the 440 patients treated for in situ carcinoma and followed five years or more in our clinic, *none* has had recurrent cancer despite the fact that nearly 10 per cent had early microscopic invasion at the time of definitive surgery. The clinician, the cytologist and the pathologist should form an investigative team which combines diagnostic procedures, histologic interpretation and specific therapy to the advantage of the patient so that she is neither overexposed to the dangers of cancer nor subjected to excessive irradiation or surgery.

Carcinoma In Situ with Early Stromal Invasion.—A further stage of carcinoma in situ known as carcinoma in situ with early stromal invasion has been recognized as an entity at the Boston Hospital for Women and most likely represents the earliest recognizable transition from carcinoma in situ to invasive cancer. The malignant epithelium remains predominantly intraepithelial but in one or more areas there is minimal breakthrough of the basement membrane by malignant cells. These cells assume the configuration of prongs or tongues several cells in thickness, extending down into the stroma. Typically, they demonstrate increased differentiation with abundant pale cytoplasm, which frequently contains glycogen on PAS staining. The invaded stroma usually responds with a surrounding inflammatory cell infiltrate (Figs. 4–20, *A, B, C*).

This pattern of early invasion was first described and given its name by Fennell who found the lesion in 7 per cent of cases of carcinoma in situ and likened the invasive prongs to lobster claws. Hamperl discovered this pattern of stromal invasion in 12 per cent of cases of carcinoma in situ but is reluctant to accept it as true invasive cancer. After extensive study he concluded that the invasive cells are most often destroyed by the inflammatory reaction in the stroma.

Carcinoma in situ with early stromal invasion must be distinguished from those more advanced lesions termed microcarcinoma (Fig. 4–20, *D*), advanced stromal invasion (Fig. 4–20, *E*) or preclinical carcinoma. Although rare, lymph node metastases have been reported with these lesions. Microcarcinomas have been included among the Stage I cancers at the Boston Hospital for Women.

In reviewing our cases of carcinoma in situ and early invasive cancer

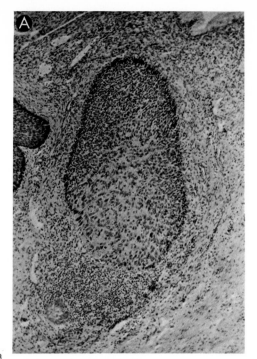

Fig. 4–20.—**A,** earliest phase of stromal invasion from a gland filled with carcinoma in situ. Increased epithelial differentiation and loss of demarcation from the stroma abuts a leukocytic infiltrate. **B,** early stromal invasion with a single tongue of malignant squamous cells from surface carcinoma in situ penetrating the stroma. *(Continued.)*

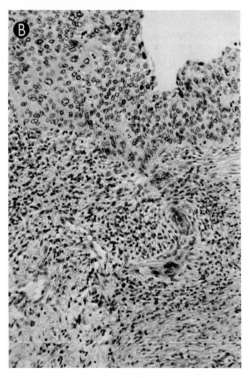

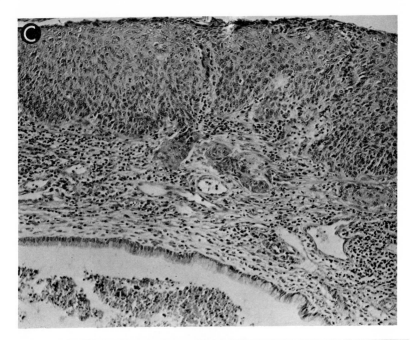

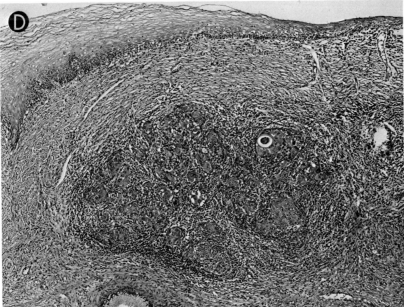

Fig. 4–20 *(cont.)*.—**C,** two invasive buds from surface carcinoma in situ entering a vascular stroma above a normal gland. **D,** microcarcinoma underlying normal portio epithelium. No other area of invasive cancer could be found in this cervix. Carcinoma in situ from which this miniature cancer must have arisen was found in the endocervix. *(Continued.)*

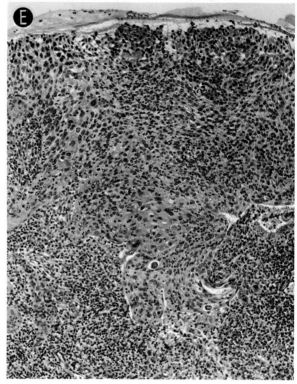

Fig. 4-20 *(cont.).*—**E,** late stromal invasion characterized by a confluence of invasive buds in an inflamed stroma. The surface epithelium is absent on the right but overlying carcinoma in situ is visible on the left.

Griffiths found early stromal invasion in 16 of 163 cases of carcinoma in situ. This incidence of 10 per cent was also found by Friedell in his earlier study of 245 cases from this hospital.

Of the 16 patients, 13 were treated by simple total hysterectomy and three by radical hysterectomy. In seven patients early stromal invasion could not be found in the hysterectomy specimen, the small focus having been removed by the preoperative biopsies. Among the other nine patients there was no extension of tumor beyond the immediate area of stromal penetration. Simple total hysterectomy appears to be adequate treatment since recurrent or metastatic disease has not been seen in any of these patients so treated. Paradoxically, the only death among the 16 patients resulted from late urinary tract complications following radical hysterectomy.

There are several objections to inclusion of patients with carcinoma in situ and early stromal invasion in Stage I. (1) The treatment and results therefrom are identical to those of carcinoma in situ. (2) Lymph node metastases have not been reported with this entity. (3) In the reporting of survival statistics the result in Stage I would be skewed in a favorable direction, erroneously suggesting superior treatment.

The classification proposed by the International Federation of Obstetrics and Gynecology corrects the third objection although there is no provision for separating patients with carcinoma in situ with early stromal invasion from patients with microcarcinoma.

Carcinoma In Situ during Pregnancy.—The occurrence of carcinoma in situ during pregnancy presents several additional problems both in diagnosis and management. Because of changes in both squamous and columnar epithelia brought about by pregnancy, Nesbitt and Hellman have suggested that extreme caution be exercised before a diagnosis of carcinoma in situ is made during the gestational period. Epperson and coworkers reported that five lesions diagnosed as in situ carcinoma during pregnancy disappeared spontaneously at the termination of pregnancy. The implication of these writers is that specific cellular changes are brought about by pregnancy and revert without treatment after delivery. Quite opposite evidence has been reported by Greene and associates, who found in situ carcinoma in 14 pregnant patients and after termination of pregnancy discovered residual in situ foci in 12 of the 14. Marsh followed 20 patients who had a diagnosis of in situ carcinoma during pregnancy and found that four of the 20 biopsies prior to pregnancy revealed the in situ carcinoma. In seven patients the in situ lesion was present in follow-up biopsies taken 13, 19, 21, 26 and 31 months after delivery. Persistence of carcinoma in situ was found in 12 other patients from three weeks to 11 months after delivery. Thus, a total of 19 of 20 patients had in situ cancer both during and after the termination of gestation. Marsh suggests that pregnancy per se does not give rise to a transient morphologic lesion, indistinguishable from true carcinoma in situ, that disappears in the postpartum period.

Both Greene and Marsh have concluded that there are certain changes such as metaplasia, glandular hyperplasia and basal cell hyperactivity which occur frequently during pregnancy but that specific dysplastic or neoplastic changes are not dependent on gestational stimuli. The author agrees with this concept and suggests that a pregnant patient with possible carcinoma in situ should be studied just as completely as the patient who is not pregnant. Multiple biopsies or a cone biopsy may be performed to rule out invasive carcinoma.

Treatment of carcinoma in situ during pregnancy is always conservative. There is no need for hasty or ill-advised surgery if invasive cancer has been adequately excluded. If the patient is young, a primigravida and desirous of more children, the pregnancy should be allowed to continue and the situation re-evaluated by biopsies and cytology six weeks after delivery. Depending on the diagnosis at that time, therapeutic cauterization or conization may be indicated. If the patient is older and has completed childbearing and especially if the disease has been found high in the endocervical canal, subsequent hysterectomy is indicated. If there are other reasons for cesarean section (repeat section, leiomyomas, antepartum hemorrhage), a cesarean hysterectomy with a good vaginal cuff may be performed. Carcinoma in situ of the cervix does not contraindicate pelvic delivery.

Detection of Early Cervical Neoplasms

The importance of mass cervical cytology screening programs in reducing the incidence of cervical cancer has been previously described. Certainly the outstanding contribution of recent decades to the field of gynecology is that of the late George N. Papanicolaou. In studying cells exfoliated from the female genital tract, Dr. Papanicolaou, in the late 1920's, noted characteristic cellular changes associated with cervical cancer. These cellular abnormalities include anomalies of staining reaction, cell gigantism or dwarfing, nuclear irregularity or density changes, clumping and granulation of chromatin, multiple nucleoli, and increased nuclear-cytoplasmic ratio. As with so many important discoveries, fully 20 years elapsed before Papanicolaou's cytologic technique was accepted as a cancer screening measure.

Papanicolaou's classification of the cytologic findings consists of five gradations as follows: I- benign, II- atypical benign, III- suspicious, IV- probably positive and V- positive. Although this classification applies to invasive cancer it soon became apparent that cytology was not only capable of detecting both carcinoma in situ and dysplasia but also revealed cellular abnormalities characteristic of these entities. It has become the practice in many laboratories to equate cytologic findings of carcinoma in situ and dysplasia with the Class IV and Class III designations, respectively. The following classification is currently used at the Boston Hospital for Women:

Class I	Benign
Class II	Atypical benign
Class IIR	Atypical repeat
Class III	Dysplasia
Class IV	Carcinoma in situ
Class V	Invasive carcinoma

In recent years an appreciation of both qualitative and quantitative variations in cell types found in abnormal cytologic smears has enabled cytopathologists to make reasonably accurate diagnostic interpretations. The correlation of specific cytologic characteristics with established histologic criteria for each pathologic entity is mainly a trial and error process. However, the cytologic differentiation between carcinoma in situ and dysplasia was carried to mathematical precision at the Boston Hospital for Women by Okagaki, who performed differential cell counts and found that in cases of proven carcinoma in situ 30 per cent or more of all abnormal cells exfoliated were of the basal cell type. Although time consuming, this technique has shown a predictability of 97.5 per cent.

The diagnostic correlation between the initial cytologic smears and the final diagnosis in 400 recent cases from the Boston Hospital for Women is illustrated in Table 4-4. Although the cytodiagnosis of dysplasia is reasonably accurate, only 37.5 per cent of the carcinoma in situ cases fell into

TABLE 4-4.—CORRELATION OF INITIAL CYTODIAGNOSIS WITH FINAL DIAGNOSIS
AT THE BOSTON HOSPITAL FOR WOMEN (1962-1968)

SMEAR	PRECLINICAL CANCER	CA. IN SITU WITH EARLY STROMAL INVASION	CA. IN SITU	DYSPLASIA
Negative	2	0	16 (23)	60 (96)
Atypical	0	1	3	19
Dysplasia	0	1	40	133
Ca. in situ	3	5	45	12
Invasive	5	2	9	1
Total	10	9	113 (120)	225 (261)

Figures in parentheses include cases detected at the first year repeat examination.

TABLE 4-5.—DISTRIBUTION OF CARCINOMA IN SITU CASES BY
FINAL CYTODIAGNOSIS AT THE BOSTON HOSPITAL FOR WOMEN

Negative	1
Atypical	2
Dysplasia	14
Ca. in situ	93
Invasive	3
Total	113

the corresponding cytologic category. The value of obtaining two or more smears can be observed in Table 4-5 where the 113 patients with carcinoma in situ in whom additional smears were obtained are grouped according to the consensus of all cytologic studies. In this instance there is an 82.3 per cent exact correlation between the cytologic and histologic diagnosis of carcinoma in situ.

Despite the over-all success of exfoliative cytology the awareness of a significant incidence of initially false negative smears has gradually evolved. Although quality control is inherently difficult, false negative reports have occurred in early invasive lesions discovered in concurrent biopsies, subsequent hysterectomy specimens and at the time of interval re-examinations.

The practice of routinely subjecting every abnormal cervix to biopsy was established at the Boston Hospital for Women by Younge in 1936 and has provided a controlled series from which the relative accuracy of cytology could be determined. When the vaginal pool aspiration, initiated in 1947, proved to be negative in nearly 35 per cent of cases of carcinoma in situ, cervical aspiration and scraping were substituted. In considering the cases of carcinoma in situ diagnosed during the years 1962–1968, the cytology was initially negative in 14.2 per cent (Table 4-4). If we can presume that the 7 patients with carcinoma in situ diagnosed at the first year repeat examination had false negative cytology one year previously, the false negative rate increases to 19.2 per cent. Similarly, in a report by Silbar and Woodruff, cytology obtained at the time of biopsy diagnosis of carcinoma in situ was negative in 15.7 per cent of 110 patients. However, the false negative rate taken one to two years prior to diagnosis was 18.2 per cent.

It seems apparent that complete reliance on a negative Papanicolaou smear is not justified and that the adjunctive use of cervical biopsies should be encouraged. Although biopsy of grossly suspicious cervical lesions has always been the rule, cervices involved by carcinoma in situ or microinvasive cancer infrequently arouse suspicion on clinical grounds. On the other hand, these lesions rarely are found in cervices which are completely normal on close inspection. In a 1964 report from the Boston Hospital for Women only 4 of 154 cervices containing carcinoma in situ were considered normal. Even the cervical eversion usually thought of as a normal variant must be viewed with some suspicion since it is found in 85–90 per cent of patients with carcinoma in situ. When the site for biopsy is carefully selected, the initial biopsy will reveal a suspicious or positive lesion in 95 per cent of patients with carcinoma in situ and in 100 per cent of patients with early stromal invasion or preclinical carcinoma.

The infrequent use of routine biopsies in other institutions can in part be attributed to the lack of target areas. However, to quote Younge, "Very little attention has been given to the subtle changes in color, the texture, ability to reflect light, the Schiller test and colposcopic examination." A detailed description of these visible changes and an "atlas" illustrating the application of the Schiller test to a variety of abnormal cervices have been published by Younge.

The Schiller test is positive in at least 83 per cent of cervices harboring carcinoma in situ and, with rare exception, positive biopsies are obtained from Schiller positive areas. In the 1964 Boston Hospital for Women study, two-thirds of the patients with carcinoma in situ and initially negative cervical smears were detected by the Schiller test.

The emergent use of the colposcope in this country 40 years after its introduction in Europe is an indication of the need for an additional detection method and in essence represents an attempt to locate suspicious areas for punch biopsy. Unfortunately it appears that the necessity for training in the use of this instrument will indefinitely curtail its application as a detection method.

TECHNIQUE FOR TAKING VAGINAL AND CERVICAL SMEARS.—The following equipment is needed:

1. Clean glass (microscopic) slides. Those with frosted ends permit easy labeling in pencil with patient's name and also identify "right side" or smeared side of the slide.

2. Rubber suction bulb, 1 or 2 oz. size, with opening that fits snugly over the glass pipet.

3. Glass (Papanicolaou) pipets measuring about 8 in. in length and having a slight curve, with a capillary opening for adequate suction of the cervical secretion.

4. Tongue depressors or spatulas to be used for cervical scrapings to prepare cervical smear.

5. For the fixative, any one of several types of dehydrating agents can be used. Listed in order of preference, these are:

  a) A half-and-half mixture of 95 per cent ethyl alcohol and ether.

  b) Plain 95 per cent ethyl alcohol, or lesser dilutions to 75 per cent.

  c) 75–95 per cent methyl alcohol (wood alcohol) or denatured alcohol.

  d) 75–95 per cent isopropyl alcohol (rubbing alcohol).

  e) Acetone.

The vaginal "secretion" is a mixture of cells shed from the vagina, cervix and endometrial cavity, mixed with leukocytes and mucus. It can be aspirated readily from the cervical os by means of the standard Papanicolaou pipet to which the rubber bulb is attached for suction. Smears are obtained with the patient in the lithotomy position, before digital examination and without lubricants. The latter spoil the staining characteristics of the cells. Douches dilute and wet the cells so that a satisfactory smear cannot be obtained 12–24 hours after douching. The aspirated drop or two of "secretion" is blown out on the slide from the pipet by compressing the aspiration bulb several times quickly and is spread into a film on the slide, with the slide "right" or etched side up. The slide is immersed immediately into a small stoppered bottle containing fixative. Fixation is complete in 15–30 minutes; the slide can be prepared for dry mailing promptly but may stay in fixative indefinitely.

Cervical scrapings may give additional information about suspicious areas on the portio of the cervix. It is possible after the speculum is gently introduced into the vagina to scrape off the superficial layers of epithelium lightly with the tip of a tongue depressor or Ayre's spatula. The scraping is then smeared on a slide. The slide or the requisition form should bear a notation that the specimen is a "cervical scraping". The dried smears may be packed in wooden or cardboard holders, secured with rubber bands and mailed to any competent laboratory.

Invasive Cancer

Carcinoma of the uterine cervix is the fifth leading cause of death from malignant disease among American women, following cancer of the breast, colon, lung and ovary. The estimated number of deaths from cervical cancer for the year 1970 approached 10,000. This disease occurs in about 2 per cent of the female population and will result fatally in approximately 50 per cent of those it affects. This order of incidence and mortality presents a singular challenge to the gynecologist who would attempt to prevent or cure the disease.

PATHOLOGY

Three major types of growth are evident by gross inspection: exophytic or proliferative, endophytic or invasive, and ulcerating or excavating. The vagaries of this gross growth pattern have not been fully interpreted, but in general the exophytic lesion, which may be quite large and may actually completely replace the cervix, has a better prognosis than the endophytic or excavating one. The endophytic lesion is often resistant to radiation therapy and is associated with a high incidence of involved lymph nodes and parametrial spread. The appearance of carcinoma is variable but in extensive lesions is quite characteristic. The cervix cannot be distinguished as such and the vaginal apex is filled with a papillary, necrotic, often bleeding mass which is gray or dark red. Some of the fragments may be removed with the finger or thumb forceps, but if a biopsy is taken the sensation of cutting through unripe fruit is suggested. In less advanced lesions the cervix feels stony hard and there is an area of ulceration near the os. In this case the tumor has advanced under an epithelium which grossly appears normal. With endophytic cancers arising in the endocervix, the cervix may appear grossly normal until the tumor actually protrudes through the cervical os or spreads laterally and produces induration in the broad ligament. The excavating type presents a crater-like depression at the vaginal apex associated with extensive tissue destruction and paracervical fixation.

Most cervical cancers are classified microscopically as being of squamous or "epidermoid" origin. An analysis of approximately 1,200 patients treated at the Boston Hospital for Women revealed the following percentages: squamous carcinoma 90.2, adenocarcinoma 7.1, adenosquamous carcinoma 1.6, double primary, adenocarcinoma and squamous carcinoma 0.8, undifferentiated 0.3.

The microscopic pattern of invasive squamous cell cervical cancer is typical, and in most cases diagnosis is made simply by a glance through a low-power microscope. There is a general disorientation of cells without delineating surface epithelium. Nests and clusters of epithelial cells are seen scattered in an irregular pattern in the stroma and in endocervical glands, and the stroma is usually infiltrated with inflammatory cells of lymphocytic and polymorphonuclear types (Fig. 4–21). It should be emphasized that such a pattern may be simulated by (1) extensive active squamous metaplasia, (2) tangential cut of a poorly mounted biopsy specimen and (3) papillomatosis. Therefore, examination of cellular detail under high power is necessary. The cells of squamous cell carcinoma show the same characteristics described for in situ cancer, namely, undifferentiation

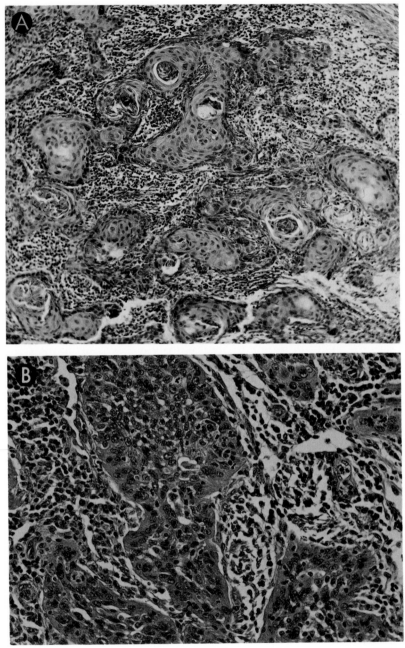

Fig. 4–21.—A, typical grade I squamous cell carcinoma of the cervix. There is extensive keratinization with "pearl" formation and a lymphocytic infiltration of the stroma. (From Hertig, A. T., and Gore, H. M.: *Tumors of the Female Sex Organs,* fasc. 33 of *Atlas of Tumor Pathology* [Washington, D.C.: Armed Forces Institute of Pathology, 1960].) **B,** grade II squamous cell carcinoma of the cervix. Several nests of malignant cells showing pleomorphism, nuclear hyperchromatism and atypical mitotic figures are seen.

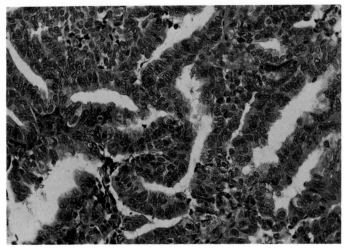

Fig. 4–22.—Adenocarcinoma of the cervix. The malignant cells are arranged in a glandular pattern. The typical cylindrical appearance of the cell has been lost, and numerous cells show atypical mitoses.

with loss of stratification, loss of polarity, presence of numerous and atypical mitotic figures, pleomorphism, nuclear hyperchromatism (Fig. 4–21,*B*) and dyskaryosis. Tumor giant cells may be found, together with areas of necrosis and cellular degeneration.

In adenocarcinoma the microscopic picture is equally typical (Fig. 4–22). The glandular elements are increased greatly in number and show much variation in size and shape. Glandular spaces may be large or filled with papillary fronds of pale-staining epithelium. Much of the stroma may be infiltrated with tumor cells, but an inflammatory response is almost always seen. Under high power the individual cells have lost their characteristic cylindrical appearance and are very anaplastic, with marked enlargement of the nucleus which is often bizarre and hyperchromatic. Mitotic figures are common as are areas of necrosis and degeneration, indicating the rapid growth potential of this tumor.

Histologic Grading of Cervical Cancer.—The degree of differentiation of a cancer cell as viewed under high power determines its histologic GRADE. This should not be confused with the STAGE, or the extent of the disease as determined by physical and radiologic examination. The classification of grading most generally accepted is that of Broders, who in 1920 divided tumors into differentiated and undifferentiated groups and then assigned one of four grades, depending on the relative amount of cellular differentiation. Thus, grade I is the most differentiated and grade IV the least (or most anaplastic). Martzloff subdivided cervical cancers according to the predominance of a certain cell type, e.g., *spinal cell,* similar to the typical superficial or prickle cell; *spindle cell,* similar to the compactly placed basal cells; *transitional cell,* like the intermediate group. The incidence, as given by Martzloff, of the various groups is: transitional 66.8 per cent, spinal cell 15 per cent, and spindle cell 12 per cent (5.4 per cent were adenocarcinomas). Using Broders' classification, about 76 per cent of the cases at the Boston Hospital for Women were placed in grade III, which corresponds to the transitional cell type of Martzloff.

Graham analyzed the problem of grading with particular reference to extent of disease, response to radiation and five-year survival. He reached the following conclusions: **(1)** The histologic grading of cervical cancer is of limited value. **(2)** In the majority of classifications the cure rate for the most anaplastic growths is one-fourth to one-third lower than that for the most differentiated grade when treated radiologically. **(3)** The technique is partially subjective and is limited by the biopsy which may or may not be a good sample of the tumor. **(4)** The degree of anaplasia correlates poorly with the extent of the disease when the patient is first seen but somewhat better with the incidence of metastases in postmortem material.

CLINICAL STAGING OF CERVICAL CANCER

The most important factor in determining the prognosis in cervical cancer is the *clinical* stage of the disease. The five-year survival rate depends on the efficacy of treatment and on the resistance of the patient to the neoplasm, but in the final evaluation it is the stage or *extent* of the disease which allows the clinician to predict a certain percentage of "cures." The histologic *grade* of the cancer influences the survival rate only by its possible effect on the *stage*. Thus a very anaplastic tumor may be associated with a very rapid spread to the pelvic lymph nodes or adjacent viscera. However, in a study of pre- and postirradiation cervical biopsies by Kistner and Hertig, it was not possible to predict the survival rate on the basis of histologic grade. They found, however, a definite relationship between survival and staging.

Staging should be performed under anesthesia so that thorough pelvic and rectal examinations may be performed. In our clinic this is done jointly by the gynecologist and radiotherapist. Proctosigmoidoscopy is carried out before this examination but a barium enema is not done routinely. Excretory urography is an integral part of the preliminary work-up, and the presence of ureteral obstruction may almost always be assumed to be due to extension of cancer. Cystoscopy is usually done at the time of anesthesia examination since the presence of tumor in the mucosa or muscularis may otherwise be missed. The cervix and vagina must be carefully visualized and biopsies taken of any suspicious areas in the vagina. Fractional curettage of the endocervix and endometrium is then done, the specimens being submitted separately. The digital examination is best carried out rectally since the cervix, paracervical areas, uterosacral ligaments and rectovaginal septum may then be thoroughly palpated. The findings are recorded and the final stage decided. This must remain the final staging since it cannot be changed after therapy has been started.

The International Federation of Gynaecology and Obstetrics adopted the following classification in 1962:

CLINICAL STAGES OF CARCINOMA OF THE CERVIX
(International Federation of Gynaecology and Obstetrics)

Stage 0   Preinvasive carcinoma, so-called carcinoma in situ

Stage I   The carcinoma is strictly confined to the cervix (and extension to the corpus is disregarded).

>   Stage I-A Cases with minimal stromal invasion (preclinical invasive carcinoma, i.e., cases which cannot be diagnosed by routine clinical examination)
>   Stage I-B All other cases of Stage I

Stage II   The carcinoma extends beyond the cervix but has not extended onto the pelvic wall. The carcinoma involves the vagina, but not the lower third.

>   Stage II-A The carcinoma has not infiltrated the parametrium.
>   Stage II-B The carcinoma has infiltrated the parametrium.

Stage III   The carcinoma has extended onto the pelvic wall. On rectal examination there is no cancer-free space between the tumor and the pelvic wall. The carcinoma involves the lower third of the vagina.

Stage IV   The carcinoma has extended beyond the true pelvis or has involved the mucosa of the bladder or the rectum. However, the presence of bullous edema is not sufficient evidence to classify a case as Stage IV.

NOTE: It is unavoidable that the personal opinion of the examiner influences his staging of various cases, and this is especially true with those classified as Stage II and Stage III. Therefore, the Cancer Committee recommended that, when reporting results of therapy in carcinoma of the cervix, all cases examined be reported. Also that, in arriving at an opinion of the results achieved at a given institution in Stage II, for instance, the statistics for Stage III be considered simultaneously.

Certain difficulties and misinterpretations are unavoidable in clinical staging. Frequently the examiner interprets pelvic inflammatory processes or scarring from endometriosis as tumor and overstages the disease. Conversely, the lateral pelvis may be soft when palpated but at surgery positive lymph nodes are found. Staging will thus vary somewhat with the experience and tactile prowess of the examiner. Heyman, Kottmeier and Segerdahl independently staged the gross extent of disease in 161 patients and agreed in 89 per cent. The greatest difficulty was encountered in distinguishing between borderline Stage II–Stage III cases. Despite this high correlation among experienced gynecologists, there still exists a discrepancy between staging and actual findings at surgery. Cherry and co-workers compared preoperative staging with postoperative findings and noted that the disease was more extensive than staged in 56 per cent, less extensive in 21 per cent and correctly evaluated in 23 per cent. The two most common causes of error were the inability to detect lymph node metastases and the inability to determine whether thickening in the broad ligament was due to carcinoma or to other causes.

Methods of Spread of Cervical Cancer.—Carcinoma of the cervix spreads principally by direct local invasion and by lymphatics. Hematogenous dissemination is uncommon though occasionally isolated metastases in the lung, pleura, liver, bone, skin and brain do occur when the local process has been eradicated. Tumor growth commonly occurs by *direct contiguity* to the vagina, uterine cavity and laterally through the cardinal and uterosacral ligaments. The lateral spread may occur in the substance of the ligaments or in the areolar tissue adjacent to them. Thus a pathway to the bony pelvis is available for spread, and in this fashion the carcinoma encompasses the ureter as it traverses the paracervical area. The effect of this process, if bilateral, is hydroureter, hydronephrosis, loss of kidney function, uremia and death. Direct extension may also traverse the paravaginal fascia, with extension into the bladder or bowel resulting in vesicovaginal or rectovaginal fistulas.

The spread of cervical cancer via lymphatics has been thoroughly studied as a result of renewed interest in the surgical treatment of this disease. Cherry and co-workers studied the lymphatic drainage in surgical specimens with involved nodes in Stages I and II and found two major routes of spread. One involved the paracervical, external iliac and obturator groups and the other included the hypogastric and sacral groups. The former route was the most common but in 10 patients both avenues contained tumor. They found over 500 lymph nodes with metastatic cancer in 91 patients and only one of these was palpated clinically. Henrikson studied the lymphatic spread in 356 autopsies and concluded that dissemination followed a constant course via the parametrium, primary nodes (paracervical, hypogastric, obturator, external iliac), secondary nodes (sacral, common iliac, aortic, inguinal) and then extension beyond the pelvis. A definite correlation exists between the extent of the disease and the number of involved nodes. Averages of numerous reported series give an incidence of 17 per cent involved nodes in Stage I, 31 per cent in Stage II and 66 per cent in Stage III.

Ureteral compression either in the pelvis or near the kidney, with uremia and/or pyelonephritis, is a major cause of death and is found in about 50 per cent of patients whether treated or untreated. Other causes of death are infection (peritonitis, pelvic abscess, septicemia), uncontrolled hemorrhage and extrapelvic metastases.

In a study of the causes of death in cancer of the cervix, De Alvarez found that 40 per cent were due to urinary tract involvement. Most of these deaths were due to periureteral lymphatic obstruction rather than to occlusion of the ureteral wall by tumor. However, obstruction was also noted secondary to radiation fibrosis producing bilateral, chronic pyelonephritis and subsequently complete renal shutdown. Thirty-one per cent of the deaths were found at autopsy to be due to pulmonary metastases or to extensive pulmonary edema associated with metastases to the perivascular areas in the lung parenchyma. Occasionally this was misdiagnosed as pneumonia clinically. Patients who have completed therapy should have sequential chest x-rays, metastatic series which include the long bones, and intravenous urograms. Routine intravenous urograms should be obtained every six months during the first two years post-treatment, then annually.

Occasionally a patient treated for cardiac failure will have severe pulmonary edema together with edema of the arms and neck. There is usually a plethora of the face and neck. This entity is due to superior vena caval obstruction from metastatic cervical cancer. In 13 per cent of deaths from cancer of the cervix the cause was gastrointestinal tract involvement, usually manifesting itself as large bowel obstruction, particularly of the rectosigmoid. Occasionally perforation of the large or small bowel results in fatal peritonitis. Jaundice may be noted terminally due to extensive hepatic metastases. Diabetic acidosis has been seen as a terminal event in a few patients from extensive pancreatic metastases. If the blood count reveals thrombocytosis and nucleated red cells, splenic metastases should be strongly suspected.

De Alvarez also showed that massive edema of the extremities may be due to a diminution in the serum proteins with alteration and reversal of the albumin-globulin ratio. The alpha-2 globulin has been noted to be specifically elevated. Specific variations in lipid fractions, particularly elevation in the beta lipoprotein and cholesterol, have been described in patients having carcinoma in situ of the cervix as well as in patients with invasive disease.

Left-sided chest pain or cardiac arrhythmias may be due to cardiac metastases, and acute episodes of chest pain may be due to pulmonary emboli from tumor involving the femoral vessels. Although hemorrhage has not been found to be a common cause of death, hypochloremia, hypokalemia and alkalosis have been a rather common cause.

Symptoms and Diagnosis

There are no specific symptoms which characterize cervical cancer, especially in its early stages. Frequently there are no symptoms whatever. Slight intermenstrual, postcoital or postdouche bleeding may be noted or there may be only a pink discharge which is occasionally odorous. Abnormal vaginal bleeding may first be noted as a prolonged menstrual period or as profuse flow at the time of a normal period. As the disease progresses and more blood vessels are eroded, a scant serosanguineous discharge may become grossly hemorrhagic. A common complaint is the daily appearance of a little blood, usually noted just after voiding and seen on the toilet tissue. In advanced cancer a characteristic bloody, malodorous discharge may be present together with pain from either fistula formation or nerve irritation. Pain is a late symptom and is typically of sciatic distribution, with radiation down the back of the buttock, thigh and knee. With endophytic tumors there may be no bleeding or discharge, but the process extends rapidly to the sacral plexus, producing severe pain.

It is obvious that these symptoms, if due to cervical cancer, will originate in lesions of moderate size. The patient should be educated to visit her physician regularly for proper diagnostic procedures at least once a year. Although 35 has been suggested as the minimum age for such examinations, this has been lowered to 20 by many clinicians who have seen advanced cancer in women in the early twenties.

As noted earlier, carcinoma in situ presents no characteristic gross lesion and is detectable only by the judicious use of cervical cytology and adequate biopsies. Similarly, in very early invasive carcinoma, the cervix may appear normal or may present an erosion. If we are to reduce the mortality of this disease, it is necessary that more diagnoses be made and treatment given during the in situ and early invasive phases of cancer. It should not be necessary to emphasize the importance of a digital and speculum examination in women of all age groups. The fact is, unfortunately, that many women are reassured or are advised to take douches for abnormal discharges or bleeding without ever having a pelvic examination. It is this attitude on the part of physicians that keeps the average cure rate in squamous cell carcinoma of the cervix at about 30–35 per cent.

Differential Diagnosis.—The lesions most commonly confused with cervical cancer are eversions, polyps, papillary endocervicitis and papillomas. Tuberculosis, chancres and granuloma inguinale only rarely involve the cervix. It is impossible to differentiate these benign lesions from invasive early cancer by any method except biopsy. In many cases repeat or multiple biopsies are necessary before a final diagnosis is made. This has been particularly true in papillomas of the cervix which are frequently difficult to distinguish from a low-grade, papillary carcinoma.

Secondary carcinoma of the cervix may occur by direct extension from the corpus or vagina. Ovarian, bladder and breast carcinoma have also been reported although the breast cancer may first spread to the ovary and secondarily involve the cervix. Lymphomas, particularly reticulum cell sarcoma, may present as a cervical tumor.

TREATMENT

This aspect of cervical cancer will be discussed under three general divisions: prophylactic, curative and palliative.

The *prophylaxis* of cervical cancer offers great opportunity for the improvement of salvage rates. Epidemiologic studies have re-emphasized the importance of the socioeconomic complex of relative poverty (in early life) with rapid sexual maturation and the desire to begin and terminate early the various phases of reproduction, i.e., marriage, intercourse, pregnancy and the possible sequelae, separation and divorce. Since celibacy and delayed marriage will never attain great popularity as preventive methods, others must be substituted.

Some authors stress the importance of circumcision in the male as being prophylactic, whereas others disagree. Obstetricians should treat abnormalities of the cervix by adequate cauterization or surgical plastic procedures. Congenital eversions should be corrected before marriage and pregnancy. Premalignant lesions must be removed or destroyed as the individual case warrants. All abnormal bleeding or discharge should be investigated thoroughly. Cytology should be a routine practice in examinations of all women over 20. Finally, supracervical hysterectomy should be abandoned except in emergency.

Curative treatment of cervical cancer utilizes two basic modalities, surgery and radiation. Throughout most of the world, radiation therapy is the treatment of choice. In a few medical centers the surgical approach has been renewed and is being evaluated. Bonney in England and Meigs and Lynch in the United States have given the impetus to this resurgence of effort by surgeons to improve upon the results obtained with radium and x-ray. An evaluation of the series treated by surgery reveals that the results compare favorably with those of radiation in early stages of the disease. Unfortunately, the selection of treatment is frequently determined by locale, prejudice or clinical impression. Cade and Lederman summarize this problem succinctly: "Nevertheless, whilst the case for radiotherapy as the method of choice in the treatment of carcinoma of the cervix remains indisputable, it is important not to lose sight of the fact that with a disease such as cancer for which there is no certain method of cure, it is easy to be biased in favor of one or another method of treatment. If a patient is to receive the best treatment it is equally important for her to avoid falling into the hands of a radium enthusiast as into those of a surgical enthusiast. Each employs the method he knows best, and this may not coincide with the best interests of the patient. To safeguard the patient against the risk of misguided enthusiasm she should be seen by both gynecologist and radiotherapist in consultation together, and treatment decided only after such consultation." In the opinion of the author there is a desirable middle ground and the sage advice, "individualize every case" is still applicable. The answer lies in proper selection of patients, some for radiation alone, others for surgery alone and occasionally others for combination therapy.

Radiation Therapy.—This is administered in most clinics in two forms, radium and x-ray, with considerable variation as to types of applicators and sequence of administration. In the past the measurement of radium dosage was expressed in terms of milligram-hours, which was simply a computation of the amount of radium applied (in milligrams) times the number of hours it was in position. Unless, however, this figure is qualified by a statement of distance factors, filtration, arrangement of sources and the volume of tissue irradiated, the term is quite meaningless for clinical therapy. A more logical method of expressing radium dosage is similar to that used in calculating x-ray dosage, that is, in terms of the amount of ionization it produces. This may be expressed in terms of a roentgen, and for radium this is called the gamma roentgen ($r\gamma$). A roentgen may be defined as "that amount of x- or gamma radiation such that the associated corpuscular emission per 0.001293 Gm. (1 cc.) of air produces, in air, ions carrying 1 electrostatic unit of quantity of electricity of either sign." A gamma roentgen has been accurately measured: 1 mg. radium in equilibrium at a point source filtered with 0.5 mm. platinum being accepted as giving 8.25 r per hour at 1 cm. distance.

Numerous radium applicators have been devised and practically every major clinic has made some change in the basic construction. The better known ones are the Stockholm, Fletcher, Paris, Manchester, Ernst and Neary. In addition cervical cancer may be treated by intravaginal cone (x-ray), interstitial needles, interstitial radon seeds, interstitial colloidal gold and radioactive cobalt. All of these methods strive to deliver a cancericidal dose throughout the tumor-bearing area without causing irreversible damage to normal tissues. This can be accomplished only if an understanding of pelvic anatomy and pathology is combined with a knowledge of the essentials of radiation physics and radiobiology (Figs. 4–23, 24, 25).

In order to evaluate and measure the amount of radiation reaching certain areas in the pelvis, the Manchester group suggested specific landmarks. They designated a point 2 cm. above the mucosa of the lateral vaginal fornix and 2 cm. lateral to the uterine canal as Point A and another point 5 cm. from the same landmarks as Point B. Thus the calculated dosage (of both radium and x-ray) will give a fairly good idea of the tumor dosage at the periphery of the cervix (Point A) and in the region of the pelvic lymph nodes (Point B). To control squamous cell carcinoma of the cervix it has been suggested that 7,000–8,000 r be directed to the tumor area. The technique of usage and positioning of the radium is seen to be important, since it is known that the rectovaginal septum will not tolerate more than 6,000 r ± (depending on time-intensity factors, etc.) and the bladder will tolerate only slightly more.

The Stockholm method of treatment with minor modifications by Dr. J. L. Sosman was used at the Boston Hospital for Women from 1954 through 1968. In 1968, Fletcher applicators, as modified by Suit to permit afterloading, were adopted (Fig. 4–26). The use of after-loading technics, in which

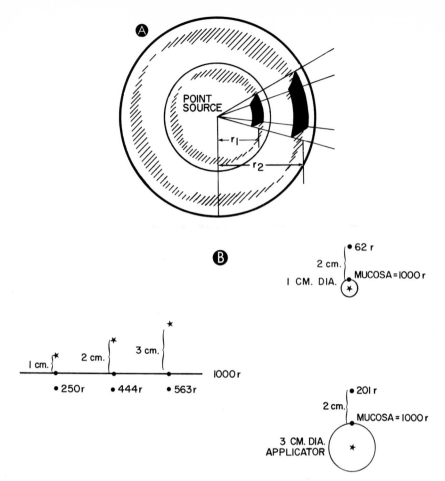

Fig. 4-23.—Inverse square law in brachyradium therapy. **A,** gamma rays travel in a straight line from a point source. The number of rays passing through a given area defined by the rays will be the same regardless of the distance from the source. As the areas increase with the square of the distance from the source, the dose rate from a point source is inversely proportional to the square of the distance from the source; this relationship is known as the inverse square law.

If the dose rate at any distance (r_1) is known, the dose rate at any other distance (r_2) may be found by the following formula:

$$\text{Dose rate at } r_2 = \text{Dose rate at } r_1 \times \frac{r_1^2}{r_2^2}$$

For example, in **A,** the area defined by the rays at distance r_1, is one-fourth the area defined by the same rays at distance r_2, since r_2 is twice the length of r_1. Therefore, the dose rate at r_2 is one-fourth the dose rate at r_1.

B, the depth dose from a point source is increased as the treating distance is increased. In this case, two points are 1 cm. apart and the dose at the near point is limited to 1,000 r. The dose of the far point increases as the distance to the near point increases from 1 to 3 cm.

The principle of the inverse square law is applied to the design of radium applicators. If the dose on the surface of applicators is limited, an applicator of larger diameter will give greater depth dose to surrounding tissues. (Figs. 4-23—4-25 from Fletcher, G. H.; Stovall, M., and Sampiere, V.: *Carcinoma of the Uterine Cervix, Endometrium and Ovary* [Chicago: Year Book Medical Publishers, Inc., 1962], pp. 69-148.)

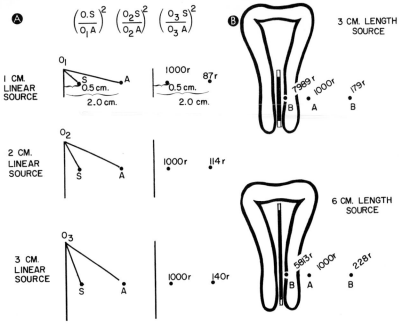

Fig. 4–24.—Length of linear source in brachyradium therapy. The depth dose opposite the center of a linear source of radiation increases as the length of the source increases. In view of this, the linear source used in a uterine tandem should be kept as long as the anatomy will permit **(A).** For example, in **B,** the dose at point *A* is kept constant at 1,000 r. As the length of the source increases, the dose to the mucosa decreases and the dose at point *B* increases.

the unloaded applicators are placed in position in the operating room but the radium sources are not inserted until the patient has been returned to bed, drastically reduces radiation exposure to physicians, operating room personnel, recovery room personnel and x-ray technicians. The operator not being exposed to radiation during the placement period permits a less hurried and more precise application of the radium.

Treatment of carcinoma of the cervix is generally planned to combine external megavoltage radiation and intracavitary radium. Initial therapy is frequently by external proton beam with Cobalt 60 gamma rays or 6 million volt x-rays. Such therapy given over a period of 3 to 4 weeks serves to reduce the local tumor volume. Since the effective dose from radium sources diminishes rapidly with increasing thickness of tissue, preliminary external therapy not only improves placement of the radium sources but also increases the effectiveness of the radium exposure. Two radium insertions, not less than two weeks apart, are usually utilized. Finally, supplemental radiation with external beam is directed to the lateral portions of the pelvis while shielding the central areas.

It should be emphasized that the key to successful radiotherapy is the individualization of each case. No formula for radium or external beam dosage can be outlined in the treatment of carcinoma of the cervix. The gynecologist and radiotherapist must jointly examine and evaluate the patient and the extent of her disease. They must then decide on a plan of

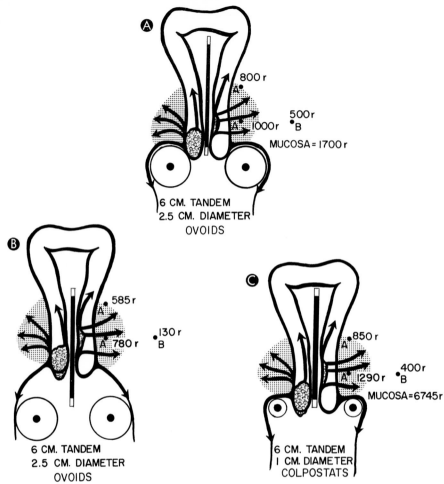

Fig. 4–25.—Variations in dose to the vaginal mucosa, to the paracervical area, and at a point 5 cm. lateral to the internal os with three different radium systems using the same total of 1,000 milligrams hours (mgh). A tumor originating on the portio is illustrated on the right lip of the cervix; on the left side, a tumor originating in the endocervix. The likelihood of involvement of the myometrium of the lower uterine segment is greater with an endocervical lesion. The paracervical area is lateral to the internal os, the endocervix and the lower uterine segment, and is not a point. It is represented by the stippled area, and calculations have been made for two points, A and A_1.

A, 2.5-cm. colpostats are used, and the tandem reaches the top of the fundus. The relationship between the dose to the vaginal mucosa and the dose to the paracervical area is good. The dose at a point B 5 cm. laterally is still favorable.

In **B,** the same two medium ovoids are used, but, because of the cone-shaped vault, have been pushed downward. The tandem is kept in the same position relative to the colpostats as if a one-piece applicator had been used. The vault dose cannot be calculated because the mucous membrane is not stretched over the colpostats. There is a sharp drop in the doses to the paracervical areas, the parametria (point B), and the myometrium.

C, small-diameter colpostats are used. The doses to the paracervical area, and also at point B, are good although the relative proportion is not quite as favorable as in A; however, the dose to the vaginal mucosa is tremendous. If 7,000 or 8,000 mgh are given, or if 7,000 r are delivered at point A, the mucosal dose is in the neighborhood of 35,000 r.

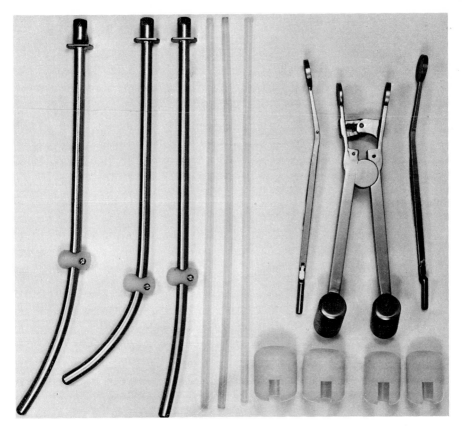

Fig. 4-26.—Fletcher-Suit afterload applicator showing vaginal colpostat and intra-uterine tandems.

treatment evolved on the basis of the nature and extent of the cancer, the anatomic variations of the patient and then, whenever necessary, make departures from a theoretical "standard" regimen.

The use of intravaginal cone x-ray in place of radium has been used with success in some hospitals but seems to offer no appreciable improvement in the five-year apparent cure rate. In Stages II-B or III cancers which extend down the vagina, it facilitates administration of adequate dosage. Interstitial radium needles have been utilized in several clinics in this country and offer the advantage of low-intensity radiation given over a long period. These needles, containing less than 1 mg. of radium element per centimeter of active length, utilize the *radiation* effect to the maximum with a minimum of cauterization effect. This provides a uniform distribution of radium throughout the tumor with the least possible damage to normal structures. Radon seeds are used ideally in small surface tumors, such as recurrent carcinoma in and around the urethra. They seem especially valuable in certain areas that cannot be reached by conventional means and offer the advantage that, once properly placed, they need not be removed.

The prognosis in cancer of the cervix treated by radiation depends on three important variables: (1) the stage of disease, (2) the skill and technique of the radiotherapist and (3) the sensitivity of the tumor to irradiation. These are listed in order of their importance, many radiotherapists feeling that true "radioresistant" tumors are rare. It is apparent, then, that good results will be obtained if *adequate* radiation is administered to early lesions. Nolan and co-workers analyzed reports of several radiation clinics and noted that the percentage of failures in each stage is quite similar to the percentage of patients showing metastatic lymph nodes in surgical and autopsy series, and that there is a tendency to conclude that failure in a given patient is dependent on lymph node involvement rather than on the adequacy of irradiation. In a subsequent study they found that in Stage II lesions (involving Point A) a higher dose of radiation to Point A was reflected in an increased survival rate and that in Stage III lesions (involving points A and B) heavy radiation to points A and B resulted in a statistically significant increase in the survival rate. There does not seem to be any doubt that adequate irradiation will destroy tumor both in the lymph nodes and in the broad ligament. The over-all five-year apparent cure rates obtainable with radiation therapy approximate 60 per cent (Fletcher-61 per cent; Morris-56.8 per cent; Kottmeier-59.7 per cent). Needless to say, a large number of patients in Stages I and II will improve the salvage rate and, if carcinoma in situ is included as Stage I, the results will appear even better.

Radiation therapy is not without a moderate incidence of complications due either to inherent sensitivity or to improper application. The commonest difficulties following radium treatment are cystitis and proctitis. Cystitis is usually delayed a year or more after treatment and is characterized by marked frequency, urgency with occasional incontinence, nocturia, dysuria and occasionally hematuria. Urine specimens and cultures usually give negative findings but the cystoscopic examination is diagnostic. The bladder mucosa is pale and smooth, blood vessels appear constricted and there is a loss of normal elasticity, resulting in diminished bladder capacity. The entire process is due to the late effects of radium, namely a gradual obliteration of capillaries and scarring of supportive tissue. Treatment is frequently unsatisfactory and protracted, but some relief may be obtained with antispasmodics and with bladder irrigations utilizing dilute silver nitrate or analgesic oily solutions.

Proctitis usually occurs shortly after radium administration but is transient in most cases. Symptoms include diarrhea, tenesmus and painful defecation. Relief is obtained with paregoric or deodorized tincture of opium used in conjunction with pectin compounds, such as Kaopectate or Donnagel. Analgesic rectal suppositories are useful if tenesmus persists. In a few patients the radiation reaction may be delayed a year or more and in these there may be constipation, diarrhea and rectal bleeding. Extensive fibrosis may seriously diminish the caliber of the rectosigmoid so that resection or colostomy is occasionally necessary. This condition, however, is due to a combined effect of radium and x-rays.

Vesicovaginal and rectovaginal fistulas are only rarely a result of radium therapy per se. Usually these are due to tumor or the destruction of tumor areas by irradiation. Poor positioning of the radium applicator or overdosage may, however, result in a fistula in the absence of cancer. This is not the fault of the method but of the technique.

Pelvic inflammatory disease is a contraindication to the use of either radium or x-ray since it may be markedly activated or aggravated, with tubo-ovarian abscesses, septicemia and occasionally death resulting. If pyometra is found at the time of uterine curettage, it should be drained and antibiotics given until evidence of infection has subsided. If inflammatory tubo-ovarian masses are present, a preliminary salpingo-oophorectomy should be done before starting radiation therapy. It has been our policy to administer penicillin or one of the tetracyclines during the time that radium is in position and to remove the radium if the temperature exceeds 100 F.

Vaginal stenosis may develop following radium treatment. This may be prevented in younger women by frequent examinations and by breaking up the thin synechiae. Coitus will aid in keeping the vagina of normal size and the use of an estrogen cream locally prevents bleeding from senescent changes that are inevitable. In older women the vagina usually closes off so that the cervix is no longer available for inspection or cytology. Although this causes the patient no difficulty it prevents adequate follow-up by the use of vaginal smears.

The use of x-ray may result in nausea and vomiting (radiation sickness) and in depression of the bone marrow with subsequent mild leukopenia. It is our practice to have a complete blood count performed once weekly during the period of x-ray therapy. Similarly, if severe nausea or vomiting develops during treatment, hospitalization is recommended and pheno-thiazines and intravenous fluids are given. Skin hyperemia is an occasional result of x-ray therapy and in some individuals with fair skin blistering and ulceration may develop. Cessation of treatment for a few days and the use of a soothing ointment will usually permit adequate healing. The skin in these areas remains "tanned" for months, after which there is a gradual whitening with dilatation of capillaries so that extensive telangiectasia may be evident. The use of supervoltage technic has minimized this complication.

Other effects of x-ray and radium therapy include late small bowel obstruction and perforation, loss of libido and menopausal symptoms. Bowel obstruction or perforation may occur as late as 10 years following therapy. More often the patient may note vague lower abdominal crampy pain, irregular bowel habits and blood in the stool. Roentgenograms may give entirely negative findings but exploration will reveal multiple loops of small bowel adherent to each other and to adjacent structures. In the more severe forms, arteriolar occlusion may result in localized areas of necrosis with perforation. It is well to remember this possible complication of radiation therapy in the differential diagnosis of an acute abdomen.

Loss of libido is not common and may be prevented by a frank discussion of the problem with the patient during or at the conclusion of treatment. The use of estrogen creams to keep the vaginal mucosa soft and pliable has been mentioned. In addition, the use of androgenic hormones in subviriliz-ing doses is frequently helpful. Hot flushes and sweats typical of the artificially induced menopause may be troublesome in some patients. Small doses of diethylstilbestrol (0.1 mg.) or estinyl (0.02 mg.) will relieve these symptoms and aid in the maintenance of a more normal extragenital endocrine balance. There is no evidence that such estrogenic therapy will bring about a recurrence of cervical cancer.

Postradiation ureteral obstruction is another serious complication. The old dictum that ureteral obstruction with hydroureter and hydronephrosis is always due to tumor has not been borne out in our clinic. During the past few years we have performed laparotomies on all patients with hydroureter developing after x-ray therapy. Frequently we have found compression due to radiation fibrosis and have relieved this by ureteral transplantation into the bladder or ileal conduit.

Surgical Treatment.—At present the determination of the optimum method of treatment for *operable* cancer is undergoing extensive investigation in numerous surgical centers. It should be restated at the outset that a comparison of results of radiation-treated cases and surgically treated cases is not possible because of the factor of selection. Even in clinics where an attempt is made to perform surgery on every patient, certain cases are found to be inoperable either because of the extent of the disease, complications of the cancer or concomitant disease. The radiologist, however, must treat *all* patients referred to him and usually does so in 96–98 per cent of the cases.

The crux of the problem is reduced to the determination of the radiosensitivity and radioresistance of the cancer together with technical difficulties, such as the adequacy of pelvic lymph node dissection and comparisons of radiation and surgical complications. An important question to be answered if one is to employ a surgical approach is: Is there statistical evidence at present to demonstrate the superiority of surgery over well-planned and carefully executed radiation therapy in the primary treatment of *operable* cases of invasive cervical cancer? To prove this affirmatively, it must be shown that surgery will reduce the 20 per cent mortality obtained by skillful radiotherapists in patients with Stage I lesions and similarly will reduce the 35–40 per cent mortality in patients with Stage II lesions.

In an effort to select patients for surgery on the basis of radiation resistance several screening methods have been developed. The first of these is based on examination of cervical biopsies taken at regular intervals following radium therapy. The response of the *tumor cells* is thus noted at 7, 14 and 21 days after the first dose of radium and again 7 days following the second dose. If the radiation response is good, deep x-ray therapy follows; if the response is poor, surgery is performed. While this method seems logical, it presents certain technical difficulties. In the first place, biopsies may not always be taken in an area where lack of response is present. Secondly, the reaction noted in the cervix may not be representative of the reaction in the parametrium or in the pelvic nodes. Thirdly, the influence of systemic factors on the reaction to radium and x-ray may be more important than the local ones. Lastly, the repeated manipulation of the tumor-bearing area and the trauma of multiple biopsy is believed by some to increase dissemination of tumor cells through lymphatic and blood channels.

The Grahams attempted to select patients with cervical cancer for radiation or surgery on the basis of specific morphologic changes in the normal cells of the vaginal smear, both before and after initiation of radiation therapy. However, this project failed to achieve the salvage rate improvement originally designated and has been abandoned. Gusberg and McKay attempted to gain some degree of selection with a test radiation regimen. In this method biopsies of the cervix are obtained after 10 days of radiation therapy and are studied for "radiation sensitivity." Gusberg and McKay reported an improved salvage rate from 32.5 to 56 per cent if patients with a poor initial radiation response were treated surgically. However, only three-year follow-up statistics are available and the number of patients having poor radiation response is too small to permit significant conclusions. Subsequent observations may prove this method of selection to be of value.

The answer to the problem of selection has yet to be found, but there is no doubt that some patients should be treated primarily with radiation, others with surgery and still others with a combination of the two.

The selection of patients for radical surgery has already been mentioned. In general, only cases classified as Stage I or II are deemed operable. Stage III and Stage IV cases are not suitable since adequate dissection beyond the boundaries of tumor is not technically possible. The general status of the patient must be carefully evaluated, together with investigation of cardiac, pulmonary and renal systems. Obesity is a major factor in selection since it makes dissection in the deep recesses of the pelvis difficult and incomplete. Compensated heart disease, regulated diabetes, anemia and old age are not contraindications per se to radical surgery, but complete medical evaluation prior to surgery will prevent anesthetic, surgical and immediate postoperative accidents. The frequency with which cervical cancer affects the urinary tract makes complete evaluation of this system mandatory. This should include cystoscopy, excretory urography, determination of blood urea nitrogen, routine urinalysis and culture if indicated. The rectum and lower sigmoid should be carefully visualized by procto-sigmoidoscopy. A roentgenogram of the chest is routinely made and the cardiovascular potential determined. Electrocardiograms are performed on all patients over age 50 and a "metastatic series" of roentgenograms should be done to rule out involvement of skull, vertebrae and long bones by tumor. A hematologic profile including a determination of the blood volume should be done before surgery.

The operation embodies two separate aspects, the radical hysterectomy and the pelvic lymphadenectomy. The term *radical* implies the removal (in an en bloc dissection) of a wide parametrial, paracervical and paravaginal margin of tissue usually including both tubes and ovaries, the cervix and a wide cuff of vagina. (By contrast, a *simple total* hysterectomy includes only the uterine corpus and cervix.) The term *pelvic lymphadenectomy* implies the removal of all lymph nodes from the bifurcation of the aorta caudad and usually includes iliac, obturator, hypogastric and ureteral groups. The node dissection may be done separately or combined with the radical hysterectomy.

The operative mortality is less than 1 per cent in most series, but the morbidity rate averages 35–45 per cent. The most common complication is temporary paralysis of the urinary bladder and it has become evident that the more radical the surgery, the more serious will be the loss of bladder function. Although usually not permanent, the urinary stasis often results in chronic cystitis, ureteritis and pyelonephritis. Some patients have permanent bladder paralysis but learn to control micturition by developing a semi-automatic bladder which will empty itself with the aid of voluntary abdominal pressure. Another serious complication is the development of urinary fistulas, usually of the ureterovaginal type. These occurred in 7 per cent of the patients operated on by Meigs, in 19 per cent in Brunschwig's series and in 7.6 per cent of our own patients. The occurrence of urinary fistulas is believed not to be too high a price to pay if the patient can be cured of cancer, especially since most fistulas can be repaired later. Any surgeon contemplating this radical hysterectomy should be aware of the complications and competent to cope with them should they develop. Mitra has suggested treatment by a radical vaginal hysterectomy supplemented by extraperitoneal lymphadenectomy in a two-stage operation. He modified the original Schauta (radical vaginal) hysterectomy and has found involved nodes in over 25 per cent of patients. He states that this procedure is simpler, more radical and associated with less ureteral fistulas (one in 280 operations).

The most widely quoted five-year salvage figures following radical hysterectomy are those of Meigs and Brunschwig. Meigs operated on 66 patients with Stage I lesions and had an 81.8 per cent survival rate. Five of 12 patients with node involvement in this same stage survived five years (41.7 per cent). In Stage II the survival rate was 61.8 per cent in 34 patients but only one of 11 patients with involved nodes (9.1 per cent) survived five years. Brunschwig reported an 82 per cent five-year salvage in Stage I and 58 per cent in Stage II. Kistner and Duncan had a five-year survival rate of 84.7 per cent in 40 Stage I patients. Twombley and Taylor carried out a study of alternate Stage I and II cases in 1945 and 1946 in which one group of patients was treated with radiotherapy and another with radical surgery followed by external radiation. At the close of the study the results were: 70.4 per cent of those receiving radiotherapy survived five years; 79 per cent survived five years after surgery and irradiation. Some patients assigned to the surgical group were not operated on, however, because they were too fat, too old, too hypertensive or had rapid extension of disease while awaiting surgery. Thus, in order to secure a survival rate equal to that of the irradiated group, a process of extreme selection was utilized.

The results of radical surgery, even in centers where the operation is limited to carefully selected patients with Stage I and Stage II lesions and from a clinic in which an attempt is made to treat all patients surgically, are excellent. But the results have not yet demonstrated that highly competent and skilful surgeons can reduce the 20 per cent mortality in Stage I or the 35–40 per cent mortality in Stage II lesions. Thus the over-all survival rate in patients treated primarily by surgery has not as yet proved convincingly superior to a series of patients treated exclusively by radiation. The results of treatment of Stage I and Stage II carcinoma of the cervix by the various modalities of therapy are shown in Tables 4–6 and 4–7.

TABLE 4–6.—TREATMENT OF CARCINOMA OF THE CERVIX—STAGE I
14th ANNUAL REPORT—STOCKHOLM

METHOD	No. OF PATIENTS		5-YR. SURVIVAL–%
Radiation	7,133		72.0
Radiation & Surgery	4,621		78.2
Surgery Alone	391		71.8
Selected Surgery	2,052		74.0
Total	14,197	Average	74.0

TABLE 4-7.—TREATMENT OF CARCINOMA OF THE CERVIX—STAGE II
14th ANNUAL REPORT—STOCKHOLM

METHOD	No. OF PATIENTS	5-YR. SURVIVAL-%
Radiation	12,120	53.8
Radiation & Surgery	6,407	55.7
Surgery Alone	601	52.5
Selected Surgery	2,523	50.6
Total	21,651	Average 53.2

Since adequate methods of patient selection are not available, the student may be justly confused as to which course of therapy to select. Twombly has suggested a few commonsense rules and certain specific selective criteria. He advises: (1) to cure cancer surgically, go wide of the disease; (2) do not perform radical surgery for palliation; (3) fully irradiated cancer will not respond to further radiation. The patients he feels should be treated surgically are those with (1) carcinoma in situ, (2) cancer during pregnancy, (3) radioresistant cancer, (4) stage IV carcinoma involving rectum or bladder but without lateral spread, (5) radiation necrosis, (6) procidentia and cancer, and (7) fibroids and cancer. I would point out that an insufficient number of patients have been treated surgically during pregnancy to suggest that radical hysterectomy is superior to irradiation. We have reduced the procidentia and treated these patients radiologically without difficulty. Similarly, if fibroids are bothersome, myomectomies may be performed and radium and x-ray given shortly thereafter. Although the question of preoperative radiation is being debated, most series treated in this way do not show a significant difference. Therefore, beginning in 1969 patients treated at the Boston Hospital for Women were treated surgically without preoperative radium.

The surgical approach to the treatment of cancer has necessitated a revision of the staging. Patients should continue to be staged preoperatively according to generally accepted criteria. However, after the specimen is removed a more precise "pathologic classification" may be designated and prognosis more clearly envisioned. The classification suggested by Meigs and Brunschwig is given here.

Class 0 Carcinoma in situ, also known as preinvasive carcinoma, intraepithelial carcinoma or microcarcinoma.

Class A Carcinoma confined strictly to the cervix.

Class Ao No tumor in the cervix in the surgical specimen after a biopsy positive for infiltrating carcinoma.

Class B Carcinoma extending from the cervix to involve the vagina except for the lower third. The carcinoma extends into the corpus and may involve the upper vagina and corpus. Vaginal or uterine extension may be by direct spread or by metastasis.

Class C Carcinoma involving paracervical or paravaginal tissue by direct extension or by lymphatic vessels or in nodes within such tissue. Spread may be by vaginal metastasis or by direct extension into the lower third of the vagina.

Class D Lymph vessel and node involvement beyond paracervical and paravaginal regions, including all lymph vessels or nodes in the true pelvis, except as described in class C. Metastases occur to ovary or tube.

Class E Carcinoma that has penetrated to the serosa, musculature or mucosa of the bladder or to the colon or rectum.

Class F Carcinoma involving the pelvic wall or aortic nodes.

Although proper emphasis has been given to the generally poor prognosis associated with metastatic tumor in the excised pelvic lymph nodes, recent studies by Friedell and associates concerning blood vessel invasion may be of equal importance. These authors found blood vessel invasion by tumor in 39 of 58 patients in whom an exenteration had been performed and in 10 of 38 who had radical hysterectomy. Only four of nine patients treated by radical hysterectomy and having no node involvement but blood vessel invasion were alive after two years. In contrast, 21 of 24 patients without node involvement and without blood vessel invasion were alive and well two years after surgery.

In the exenteration group, three of 13 patients without node involvement survived two or more years after operation when blood vessel invasion was not present, whereas only two of 20 survived two or more years when blood vessel invasion was present. These figures suggest that blood vessel invasion has prognostic significance, particularly in patients without involvement of lymph nodes.

Cervical Cancer in Pregnancy

The problem of cancer of the cervix in pregnancy is not basically different from the problem of cervical cancer in general, the main facets being prevention, early diagnosis and optimum treatment during various stages of the disease. Pregnancy introduces another facet by posing two questions. Does pregnancy influence the behavior of the disease? What is the optimum method of treatment in each trimester?

In a review of 136 patients with cervical cancer in pregnancy (including the first four postpartum months), we noted that about 1 per cent of all cervical cancers occurred in pregnant women and that pregnancy is complicated by this disease once in every 2,000 cases. Average age is about 33 years and average parity about 5. Three-fourths of the patients in this series complained of persistent vaginal bleeding or staining, but 14 per cent had no symptoms whatever. Diagnosis is facilitated by speculum inspection, palpation, biopsy and cytology. Most of the cancers are squamous cell and moderately well differentiated. Carcinoma in situ may exist an an entity during pregnancy but definite treatment should await the outcome of studies done following delivery.

Treatment of invasive cancer is variable, depending on the particular trimester in which the diagnosis is made. During the first two trimesters radium and x-ray or radium followed by radical hysterectomy may be employed, depending on the clinical stage of the disease. If x-ray is given first during the first 12 weeks of gestation, spontaneous abortion will almost always occur and radium therapy can be started three weeks later. Preliminary curettage to produce abortion may theoretically increase the possibility of spreading cancer and is not recommended. In the second trimester treatment with intracervical and contracervical radium is initiated and abdominal hysterotomy is carried out one week later. After the uterine drainage is minimal, a second application of radium is given and followed in three weeks by external x-ray therapy. During the third trimester primary consideration must be given to the viable or near-viable fetus. I favor a classic cesarean section as soon as the fetus is believed to be viable followed by x-ray therapy and then two applications of radium at approximately three-week intervals. A low cervical cesarean section or a supracervical hysterectomy after cesarean section carries the possibility of cutting across and disseminating tumor. In selected cases a radical hysterectomy may be combined with a cesarean section, to be followed by x-ray therapy if the excised nodes show metastases.

The answer to the question regarding the effect of pregnancy on cervical cancer is given in the analyses of results. Five-year survival rates indicate that before the middle of the last trimester there is no appreciable difference in the pregnant compared to the nonpregnant state. The apparent cure rate when cervical cancer is discovered after the thirty-fourth week of pregnancy or in the first four months after delivery is poor. Hormonal alterations together with increased vascularity may be etiologic but, regardless of what the changes are, the crucial problem is earlier diagnosis and treatment.

It should be re-emphasized that there is no evidence that pelvic examination and speculum visualization of the cervix during early pregnancy, even in the presence of bleeding, can cause or precipitate abortion. Single or multiple cervical biopsies or even conization may be performed during pregnancy without affecting gestation.

Every pregnant woman should have a speculum and bimanual examination at the first or second visit. Schiller's test and biopsy of the cervix should be performed as indicated and cytology by aspiration of the cervix done routinely. If bleeding occurs, the examination and tests should be repeated. During the last trimester the cervix is again palpated and inspected. It is only by such complete prophylactic and diagnostic procedures that the tragedy of permitting cervical cancer to go untreated during pregnancy will be prevented.

CERVICAL CANCER COMPLICATING PROCIDENTIA

There is a somewhat diminished incidence of cervical cancer when uterine and cervical procidentia has occurred. No adequate reason is known for this diminution although excess keratinization, lessened vaginal secretions and inadequate blood and lymph supply have been suggested. The incidence of this combination was 0.1 per cent at the Boston Hospital for Women in 1929 but had risen to 1 per cent in 1954. The incidence of cervical cancer in women with nonprolapsed cervices is said to be about 2 per cent. The diagnosis is made by doing routine cytology and biopsies on all patients with procidentia. Direct smears may be made by cervical scrapings, but Schiller's test is frequently of no value because of the associated hyperkeratosis. Such studies will avoid the embarrassment of having the pathologist find invasive carcinoma in a vaginal hysterectomy specimen or, even worse, find cervical cancer after the performance of a LeFort or Manchester-Fothergill operation.

Treatment at the Boston Hospital for Women has been, with minor exceptions, with radium and x-ray. In most cases the procidentia may be reduced and boroglycerin tampons inserted to reduce edema. pHisoHex douches and sitz baths are used to clear up inflammation until radium may safely be administered. Usually sufficient fibrosis and fixation occurs from the irradiation so that further treatment for prolapse is unnecessary. Most patients having cervical cancer with procidentia are in the older age group and are not deemed good surgical risks because of associated medical diseases. In an occasional patient, particularly when obesity makes the administration of x-ray therapy inadequate, radical vaginal hysterectomy may be selected.

RECURRENT AND ADVANCED CERVICAL CARCINOMA

Cancer of the cervix usually recurs within two to three years of primary treatment although recurrence is frequently impossible to differentiate from persistence. Symptoms include vaginal bleeding, bloody discharge, hematuria, dysuria, constipation, melena, pelvic and leg pain and fistulas. If sacral backache or pain of sciatic distribution occurs, it is invariably due to invasion of the sacral plexus by tumor. Costovertebral angle and flank pain may herald the development of ureteral obstruction and pyelonephritis. There is usually associated lassitude, anorexia, weight loss and anemia. Diagnosis may be simplified by routine cytologic studies in follow-up examinations since tumor cells may be detected before symptoms develop. This, of course, is applicable to recurrence in the vagina and cervix only, since tumor in the pelvic nodes or broad ligament will not exfoliate tumor cells. In most cases the diagnosis depends on an evaluation of symptoms and a careful pelvic examination. Progressive firm nodularity in the paracervical and uterosacral areas, felt best on rectal examination, usually is pathognomonic of viable tumor. Abnormalities of the excretory urogram, such as the development of hydroureter and hydronephrosis, suggest periureteral compression by tumor although radiation fibrosis may produce the same condition. The differentiation between tumor and radiation fibrosis can only be made by laparotomy and biopsy of the periureteral tissue.

The treatment of advanced or recurrent cervical cancer depends on many factors and the most important aspect of the problem is that of individualization. A categorical statement that re-irradiation of treated patients is of no value has already been made. This presupposes, however, that complete x-ray and radium therapy has been administered. Review of the radiation equipment, dosage and amount of tumor roentgens delivered may reveal that inadequate therapy was given. Treatment in such a case is obvious.

Certain patients have areas of localized tumor recurrence in the endocervix, vaginal apex, or even lower down in the vagina as carcinoma in situ. We have treated such lesions by radical hysterectomy, pelvic lymphadenectomy and total vaginectomy. The usual type of recurrence, unfortunately, is more extensive and includes spread to vesicovaginal septum, bladder, rectum, pelvic lymph nodes, ureters and lateral pelvic wall. One or more fistulas may be present. This is the type of patient who should be considered for multivisceral pelvic resection, commonly known as an "exenteration."

The total pelvic exenteration, as suggested by Brunschwig, includes a radical hysterectomy and pelvic lymphadenectomy together with cystectomy, vaginectomy and removal of the rectosigmoid. A combined abdominoperineal or a single-stage abdominal approach is used.

Some selection must be exercised in the performance of this procedure. Distant metastases to bone or palpable liver metastases, involvement of the external iliac artery, iliopsoas muscle, lumbosacral plexus, para-aortic lymph nodes or serosal implants interdict surgery. The presence of indurated, painful and swollen legs usually indicates inoperability. It is equally important to consider the general medical condition of the patient, i.e., obesity, age, cardiovascular status and mental status. One cannot emphasize too strongly the importance of a complete understanding between the patient, the family and the surgeon concerning the magnitude of, and the anatomic deficit created by, such surgery. At the Boston Hospital for Women the surgeon prepares and evaluates the patient personally during the week or 10 days necessary for complete diagnostic work-up. She should be made aware that colonic and urinary diversion will be necessary and that collecting devices for these must be worn. Most patients will choose this ultraradical surgery, however, because of their debilitating symptoms, narcotic addiction and the fact that they feel a complete cure is still possible. That this is not false hope is borne out by the results of Brunschwig who originally performed exenterations for palliation only. He reported a 22 per cent two-year survival and a 15 per cent five-year survival in 111 patients. Brunschwig also had several 10-year survivals as of 1964.

The available figures from all sources suggest an operative mortality of 15–20 per cent. This varies with the type of patient, the preoperative preparation, the skill of the surgeon and anesthesiologist and postoperative care. The major causes of surgical mortality include hemorrhagic shock, peritonitis and sepsis, lower nephron nephrosis, intestinal fistulas and pulmonary embolism. At the Boston Hospital for Women a few patients have been selected for partial exenteration on the basis of localized bladder or rectal extension. There is no doubt that the best results will be obtained if there is only limited extension in the anteroposterior diameter without nodal involvement. Such patients are best treated by anterior or posterior exenterations. When there is disease in both rectum and bladder or when a good deal of lateral extension is present, a total procedure should be performed. We have recently attempted to stage these operations. The first stage is to divert the urinary stream into a segment of small bowel taken from continuity in the terminal ileum. This procedure is not shocking and allows a complete exploratory survey of the abdomen. The ileal conduits seem to have many advantages over ureteral anastomoses into intact bowel. Fecal reflux up the ureter is not possible and the incidence of pyelonephritis is therefore minimal if the anastomoses are technically and functionally good. Absorption of chlorides and nitrogen excretory products are minimal since the urine is not contained in the segment for any length of time. Hydroureter and hydronephrosis have actually been noted to disappear after the compressed ureter is dissected free and placed in the ileal segment.

The second stage of the exenteration is performed two to three weeks later after urinary function is well established. We have found it time-saving to have a "double team" set up, so that at the close of the abdominal procedure the entire specimen may be removed with ease through a perineal approach with excision of labia minora and anus.

ADENOCARCINOMA OF THE CERVIX

This malignant neoplasm arises from the columnar epithelium of the endocervix and constitutes 4–5 per cent of all cervical cancers. It usually arises in the endocervical canal and may be found localized to the isthmic region in an occasional hysterectomy specimen. Some adenocarcinomas may be seen to originate on the portio and probably do so in abnormal columnar epithelium of an eversion. Hellman and others have described various degrees of hyperplasia of the columnar epithelium during pregnancy, with adenomatous and anaplastic patterns. This same pattern may be reproduced to a lesser degree in normal postmenopausal women by the administration of estrogens in high dosage over three to four weeks. Rarely, a pattern of carcinoma in situ of the endocervical glands is noted adjacent to areas of obvious adenocarcinoma. The tumor usually assumes a papillary or ulcerative type of growth but on occasion the cancer invades the cervical stroma extensively without producing ulceration of the canal. The combination of rapid spread to lymphatics and minimal symptoms produces a rapidly lethal course. In some cases it is impossible to state whether the origin of the tumor was in the endocervix, isthmus or lower uterine segment because of the extent and undifferentiated pattern of the tumor.

The microscopic pattern is variable, resembling endocervical glandular, endometrial, tubal or bowel epithelium. Some present an extremely undifferentiated, anaplastic pattern and may be difficult to distinguish from metastatic carcinoma from the ovary or other structures.

Symptoms are similar to those of squamous cell cervical cancer but in some endophytic lesions the patient is asymptomatic and diagnosis is made by routine cytology or at the time of a diagnostic curettage. In the presence of suspicious or frankly positive vaginal smears and a normal-appearing portio epithelium, a "fractional" curettage is mandatory. In this procedure the entire endocervix is separately curetted with a small, sharp instrument before routine curettage of the corpus is performed.

The treatment of endocervical cancer does not differ from that of squamous cell carcinoma, with the possible exception that the lesion may have a higher incidence of radioresistance and thus indicate surgery as primary treatment more often. A survey at the Boston Hospital for Women revealed a five-year survival rate of only 18 per cent in this disease. This is due in large measure to the advanced stage of the disease when the patient is first seen rather than to difficulties of treatment. Haggard reported a five-year survival of 27.6 per cent in 137 patients, almost 50 per cent having stage III or IV lesions.

BIBLIOGRAPHY

Embryology and Anatomy

Curtis, A. H., and Huffman, J. W.: *A Textbook of Gynecology* (6th ed.; Philadelphia: W. B. Saunders Company, 1950), p. 32.

Fluhmann, C. F.: *The Cervix Uteri and Its Diseases* (Philadelphia, W. B. Saunders Company, 1961).

Hertig, A. T., and Mansell, H., in Anderson, W. A. D. (ed.): *Pathology* (3d ed.; St. Louis: C. V. Mosby Company, 1957), p. 1033.

Huffman, J. W.: Mesonephric remnants in the cervix, Am. J. Obst. & Gynec. 56:23, 1948.

Johnson, L. D., *et al.*: The histogenesis of carcinoma in situ of the uterine cervix. A preliminary report of the origin of carcinoma in situ in subcylindrical cell anaplasia, Cancer 17:213, 1964.

Meyer, R.: *Handbuch der Gynäkologie*, Stoeckel, W., (ed.) (München: J. F. Bergmann, 1926), Vol. 6, Part 1, p. 651.

Song, J.: *The Human Uterus. Morphogenesis and Embryological Basis for Cancer* (Springfield, Ill., Charles C Thomas, Publisher, 1964).

Wislocki, G. B.; Bunting, H., and Dempsey, E. W.: The Chemical Histology of the Human Uterine Cervix, with Supplementary Notes on the Endometrium, in Engle, E. T. (ed.): *Menstruation and Its Disorders* (Springfield, Ill.: Charles C Thomas, Publisher, 1950), p. 23.

Physiologic alterations

Coppleson, M., and Reid, B. L.: *Preclinical Carcinoma of the Cervix Uteri* (New York: Pergamon Press, 1967).
De Alvarez, R. R., *et al.*: Long range studies of the biologic behavior of the human cervix: III. Squamous metaplasia, Am. J. Obst. & Gynec. 75:945, 1958.
Glass, M., and Rosenthal, A. H.: Cervical changes in pregnancy, labor and the puerperium, Am. J. Obst. & Gynec. 60:353, 1950.
Hellman, L. M., *et al.*: Some factors influencing the proliferation of the reserve cells in the human cervix, Am. J. Obst. & Gynec. 67:899, 1954.
Nesbitt, R. E. L., and Hellman, L. M.: The histopathology and cytology of the cervix in pregnancy, Surg. Gynec. & Obst. 94:10, 1952.
Schneppenheim, P., *et al.*: Die Beziehungen des Schleimepithels zum Plattenepithel an der Cervix Uteri im Lebanslauf der Frau, Arch. Gynak. 190:303, 1958. Cited by Hamperl, H., and Kaufmann, C.: The cervix uteri at different ages, Obst. & Gynec. 14:621, 1959.
Zondek, B.: Cervical Mucus Arborization as an Aid in Diagnosis, in Meigs, J. V., and Sturgis, S. H.: *Progress in Gynecology* (New York: Grune & Stratton, Inc., 1957), vol. III.

Pathologic alterations

Coppleson, M., and Reid, B. L.: *Preclinical Carcinoma of the Cervix Uteri* (New York: Pergamon Press, 1967).
Howard, L. Jr., Erickson, C. C., and Stoddard, L. D.: A study of the incidence and histogenesis of endocervical metaplasia and intraepithelial carcinoma, Cancer 4:1210, 1951.
Roblee, M. A.: Cervicitis clinic: Twenty-five years in review, Am. J. Obst. & Gynec. 71:660, 1956.
Song, J.: *The Human Uterus. Morphogenesis and Embryological Basis for Cancer* (Springfield, Ill., Charles C Thomas, Publisher, 1964).

Benign neoplasms

Greene, R. R., and Peckham, B. M.: Squamous papillomas of the cervix, Am. J. Obst. & Gynec. 67:883, 1954.
Kistner, R. W., and Hertig, A. T.: Papillomas of the uterine cervix: Their malignant potentiality, Obst. & Gynec. 6:147, 1955.
Marsh, M. R.: Papilloma of the cervix, Am. J. Obst. & Gynec. 64:281, 1952.

Premalignant neoplasms

Christopherson, W. M.: Concepts of genesis and development in early cervical neoplasia, Obst. & Gynec. Surv. 24:842, 1969.
Conference on early cervical neoplasia, American Cancer Society, Obst. & Gynec. Surv., Special Issue, 24:677–1048, Part 2, 1969.
Epperson, J. W. W., *et al.*: The morphologic changes in the cervix during pregnancy, including intraepithelial carcinoma, Am. J. Obst. & Gynec. 61:50, 1951.
Griffiths, C. T., and Younge, P. A.: The clinical diagnosis of early cervical cancer, Obst. & Gynec. Surv. 24:967, 1969.
Johnson, L. D.: The histopathological approach to early cervical neoplasia, Obst. & Gynec. Surv. 24:735, 1969.
Kirkland, J. A.: The study of chromosomes in cervical neoplasia, Obst. & Gynec. Surv. 24:784, 1969.

Malignant neoplasms

Barber, H. R. K. and Brunschwig, A.: Results of the surgical treatment of recurrent cancer of the endometrium, in Lewis, Wentz, & Jaffe (Eds.): *New Concepts in Gynecological Oncology* (Philadelphia, F. A. Davis Company, 1966).
Broders, A. C.: Carcinoma grading and practical application, Arch. Path. 2:376, 1926.
Brunschwig, A. and Daniel, W.: Evaluation of pelvic exenteration for advanced cancer of the cervix, Surg. Gynec, & Obst. 103:337, 1956.
Cancer Facts & Figures, American Cancer Society, 1968.
Cherry, C. P., *et al.*: Observations on lymph node involvement in carcinoma of the cervix, J. Obst. & Gynaec. Brit. Emp. 60:368, 1953.
Christopherson, W. M. and Parker, J. E.: Relation of cervical cancer to early marriage and childbearing, New England J. Med. 273:235, 1965.
Coppleson, M., and Reid, B. L.: *Preclinical Carcinoma of the Cervix Uteri* (New York: Pergamon Press, 1967).
Fennell, A. H., Jr.: Carcinoma in situ of the cervix with early invasive changes, Cancer 8:302, 1955.
Fidler, H. K., Boyes, D. A. and Worth, A. J.: Cervical cancer detection in British Columbia: a progress report, J. Obst. Gynaec. Brit. Commonwealth 75:392, 1968.
Fletcher, G. H.: External Radiation Therapy in Cancer of the Uterine Cervix, in Lewis, Wentz, & Jaffe (Eds.): *New Concepts in Gynecological Oncology* (Philadelphia, F. A. Davis Company, 1966).
Friedell, G. H.: Terminology for epithelial abnormalities of the uterine cervix, Am. J. Clin. Path. 44:280, 1965.

Friedell, G. H., Hertig, A. T., and Younge, P. A.: *Carcinoma In Situ of the Uterine Cervix. A Study of 235 Cases from the Free Hospital for Women* (Springfield, Ill., Charles C Thomas, Publisher, 1960).

Friedell, G. H., Steiner, G. and Kistner, R. W.: Prognostic value of blood-vessel invasion in cervical cancer, Obst. & Gynec. 29:855, 1967.

Graham, J. B. and Graham, R. M.: The curability of regional lymph node metastases in cancer of the uterine cervix, Surg. Gynec. & Obst. 100:149, 1955.

Graham, J. B., Graham, R. M. and Schulz, M.: Cancer of the uterine cervix, Harvard study 1954 through 1956, Am. J. Obst. & Gynec. 89:421, 1964.

Gray, L. A. (ed.): *Dysplasia, Carcinoma In Situ and Micro-Invasive Carcinoma of the Cervix Uteri* (Springfield, Ill., Charles C Thomas, Publisher, 1964).

Greene, R. R., *et al.*: Preinvasive carcinoma of the cervix during pregnancy, Surg. Gynec. & Obst. 96:71, 1953.

Griffiths, C. T., Austin, J. H., and Younge, P. A.: Punch biopsy of the cervix, Am. J. Obst. & Gynec. 88:695, 1964.

Griffiths, C. T., Grogan, R. H., and Younge, P. A.: *Management of Normal and Abnormal Cytology as Practiced at the Parkway Division of the Boston Hospital for Women* (Boston, Nimrod Press, 1967).

Griffiths, C. T. and Younge, P. A.: The clinical diagnosis of early cervical cancer, Obst. & Gynec. Surv., 24:967, 1969

Gusberg, S. B., and McKay, D. G.: Lesions of the Cervix and Corpus Uteri, in Danforth, D.N. (ed.): *Textbook of Obstetrics and Gynecology* (New York and London: Hoeber Medical Division. Harper & Row, Publishers, 1966), p. 958.

Haggard, J. L. *et al.*: Primary adenocarcinoma of the cervix, Obst. & Gynec. 24:183, 1964.

Hamperl, H.: Definition and Classification of the So-called Carcinoma In Situ, in *Cancer of the Cervix: Diagnosis of Early Forms*. Ciba Foundation Study Group 3. (Boston: Little, Brown & Company, 1959).

Henrikson, E.: The lymphatic spread of carcinoma of the cervix and of the body of the uterus, Am. J. Obst. & Gynec. 58:924, 1949.

Hertig, A. T. and Younge, P. A.: A debate: What is cancer in situ of the cervix? Is it the preinvasive form of true carcinoma? Am. J. Obst. & Gynec. 64:807, 1952.

Heyman, J. Kottmeier, H. L., and Segerdahl, C. O.: An investigation of the reliability of stage-grouping in cancer of the uterine cervix, Acta obst. et gynec. scandinav. 32:65, 1953.

Horne, H. W.: Carcinoma of the cervix uteri, 1926–1948, Obst. & Gynec. 9:167, 1957.

Hurteau, G. D., Morris, J. M. and Chang, C. H.: Injuries related to radiation treatment of carcinoma of the cervix and complications of supplemental surgery, Am. J. Obst. & Gynec. 95:696, 1966.

Johnson, L. D., *et al.*: Epidemiologic evidence for the spectrum of change from dysplasia through carcinoma in situ to invasive cancer, Cancer 22:901, 1968.

Kistner, R. W.: Cervical carcinoma complicating procidentia, Obst. & Gynec. 10:482, 1957.

———, and Duncan, C. J.: An analysis of 105 radical hysterectomies at the Free Hospital for Women, Surg. Gynec. & Obst. 104:733, 1957.

———; Gorbach, A. C. and Smith, G. V.: Cervical cancer in pregnancy, Obst. & Gynec. 9:554, 1957.

———, and Hertig, A. T.: A correlation of histologic grade, clinical stage, and radiation response in carcinoma of the uterine cervix, Am. J. Obst. & Gynec. 61:1293, 1951.

Kottmeier, H. L.: Surgical & radiation treatment of invasive carcinoma of the uterine cervix, Acta obst. et gynec. scandinav. 43:1, (Supp.-2), 1964.

Masterson, J. G.: Analysis of Untreated Intraepithelial Carcinoma of the Cervix, in *Proceedings 3rd National Cancer Conference* (Philadelphia: J. B. Lippincott Company, 1957), p. 671.

McKay, D. G., *et al.*: The clinical and pathological significance of anaplasia (atypical hyperplasia) of the cervix uteri, Obst. & Gynec. 13:2, 1959.

Meigs, J. V.: Carcinoma of the cervix: The Wertheim operation, Surg. Gynec. & Obst. 78:1, 1944.

———: (ed.): *Surgical Treatment of Cancer of the Cervix* (New York, Grune & Stratton, Inc. 1954).

Mitra, S.: Radical vaginal hysterectomy and extraperitoneal pelvic lymphadenectomy for cancer of the cervix, J. Obst. & Gynaec. Brit. Emp. 62:872, 1955.

Naib, Z. M.: Exfoliative cytology of viral cervico-vaginitis, Acta cytol. 10:126, 1966.

Nolan, J. F.; Costolow, W. E., and DuSault, L.: Radium treatment of carcinoma of the cervix uteri, Radiology 54:821. 1950.

Okagaki, T., *et al.*: Diagnosis of anaplasia and carcinoma in situ by differential cell counts, Acta cytol. 6:343, 1962.

Peterson, O.: Spontaneous course of cervical precancerous conditions, Am. J. Obst. & Gynec. 72:1063, 1956.

Rawls, W. E., *et al.*: Herpesvirus type 2: Association with carcinoma of the cervix. Science 161: 1255, 1968.

Reagan, J. W. and Wentz, W. B.: Genesis of carcinoma of the uterine cervix, Clin. Obst. & Gynec. 10:883, 1967.

Richart, R. M. and Sciarra, J. J.: Treatment of cervical dysplasia by outpatient electocauterization, Am. J. Obst. & Gynec. 101:200, 1968.

Ruch, R. M. *et al.:* The changing incidence of cervical carcinoma, Am. J. Obst. & Gynec. 89:727, 1964.

Silbar, E. L., and Woodruff, J. D.: Evaluation of biopsy, cone, and hysterectomy sequence in intraepithelial carcinoma of the cervix, Obst. & Gynec. 27:89, 1966.

Song, J.: *The Human Uterus. Morphogenesis and Embryological Basis for Cancer.* (Springfield, Ill., Charles C Thomas, Publisher, 1964.)

Stern, E., and Neely, P. M.: Dysplasia of the uterine cervix: Incidence of regression, recurrence and cancer, Cancer 17:508, 1964.

Suit, H. D., Moore, E. B., Fletcher, G. H., and Worsnop, R.: Modification of Fletcher's ovoid system for afterloading using standard-size radium tubes, Radiology 81:126, 1963.

Walter, L., *et al.:* Assessment of response of cervical cancers to irradiation by routine histologic methods, Brit. M. J. 1:1673, 1964.

Wheeler, J. D., and Hertig, A. T.: The pathologic anatomy of carcinoma of the uterus: I. Squamous carcinoma of the cervix, Am. J. Clin. Path. 25:345, 1955.

Younge, P. A.: Cancer of the uterine cervix. A preventable disease, Obst. & Gynec. 10:469, 1957.

Younge. P. A.: Clinical Findings in Early Lesions of the Cervix, in Gray, L. A., (ed.) *Dysplasia, Carcinoma In Situ and Micro-Invasive Carcinoma of the Cervix Uteri* (Springfield, Ill., Charles C Thomas, Publisher, 1964).

Younge, P. A., Hertig, A. T., and Armstrong, D.: A study of 135 cases of carcinoma in situ of the cervix at the Free Hospital for Women, Am. J. Obst. & Gynec. 58:867, 1949.

CHAPTER 5

The Uterine Corpus

General Considerations

THE NOUN "uterus" is of Latin derivation and is synonymous with the lay term "womb." The Greek word *hystera*, however, has come to have wide acceptance, especially with regard to surgical terminology, and the word "hysterectomy" is well known to nonmedical as well as medical personnel. Hysteria was, at one time, believed to be of uterine origin since this organ was considered the anatomic site of the human mind. As far as is known at present, however, the uterus serves one function—childbearing. Menstruation occurs only when the process of ovulation is not followed by successful fertilization and should not be regarded as a primary function. Although suggestions have been made that the uterus secretes a hormone, there is no valid evidence to support this supposition.

The position and physiologic characteristics of the uterus lead to the development of numerous irregularities, mostly in the form of abnormal bleeding. Happily for the gynecologist, however, the uterine cavity is readily available for thorough investigation by dilatation and curettage, and this has become the most common of all gynecologic operations. Because of this facility for early and complete diagnosis, together with the intrinsic physical characteristics of the uterus, malignant disease of this organ is attended by a five-year survival rate of at least 60 per cent, a figure much superior to those for malignancy of the vulva, vagina, cervix, oviduct and ovary.

The field of endocrinology is intimately correlated with the normal and pathologic physiology of the uterus. The mucosal lining of the uterus, the endometrium, is a sensitive end organ which reflects both the effects of the ovarian hormones estrogen and progesterone and the stability of the hypothalamic-pituitary-thyroid-adrenal-ovarian axis. The secretions of these glands act in concert to produce a regulated, rhythmic pattern of endometrial change. Defects or deficiencies of any or all of these organs may result in abnormalities evidenced only as abnormal flowing, amenorrhea, or irregular ovulation. Diagnosis and treatment depend on a clear understanding of basic physiologic principles.

The uterus consists of two portions, the corpus and the cervix. Attention will be given in this chapter to diseases and physiologic aberrations of the corpus.

Anatomy

The uterus (Fig. 5–1) is a muscular, hollow organ which lies in the true pelvis between the bladder and rectum. Its measurements are usually stated to be: length 7–7.5 cm.; width 4.5–5 cm.; thickness 2.5–3 cm. The cephalic portion of the corpus is known as the *fundus* and is characterized by lateral flarings known as horns or *cornua*. The oviducts enter the fundus in the region of these cornua and demarcate the fundus from the main body of the uterus. As the corpus approaches the cervix it becomes narrowed, giving a somewhat triangular appearance when viewed from both the front and the side. This constricted area separates the corpus from the cervix and is known as the *isthmus*. The cavity of the corpus is continuous with that of the endocervix and vagina and has an average depth of about 6 cm. and a capacity of 3–8 cc. When the cavity is viewed in frontal section it appears triangular, with the base at the fundus and the two corners extending toward the orifices of the oviducts. In sagittal section the uterine cavity appears as a narrow cleft, whereas in transverse section it has the outline of a flattened ellipse.

The corpus possesses anterior and posterior surfaces, both of which are covered by visceral peritoneum. The anterior surface is slightly convex and, in the normally situated uterus, lies in contact with the most cephalad portion of the urinary bladder. As the uterine peritoneum approaches the region of the isthmus on the anterior uterine wall, it is reflected ventrally onto the bladder and thence continues as the parietal layer. The narrow space between these layers of reflected peritoneum is known as the anterior cul-de-sac. A sagittal section through the normal female pelvis (Fig. 5–2) will show that the anterior surface of the uterine isthmus is not covered by peritoneum. This anatomic fact is utilized in the performance of the

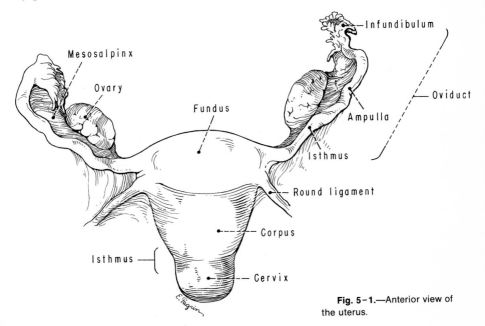

Fig. 5–1.—Anterior view of the uterus.

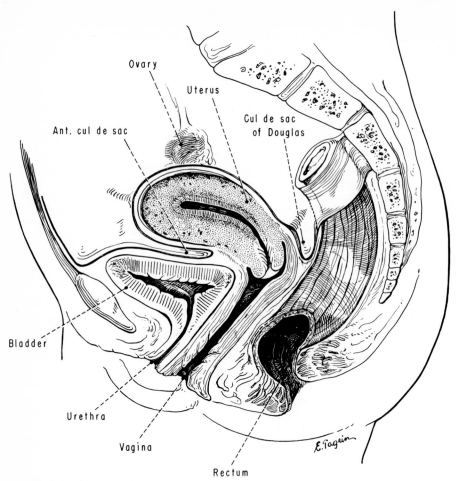

Fig. 5–2.—Sagittal section through normal female pelvis.

"extraperitoneal" cesarean section in grossly infected patients since an adequate approach may be made by reflecting the bladder inferiorly and the peritoneum superiorly. The posterior surface of the corpus is slightly convex and is completely invested with a peritoneal covering. Caudally this peritoneal envelope is continued over the uterosacral ligaments, cervix and upper portion of the posterior vaginal wall and is then reflected dorsally and cephalad over the rectum and lower sigmoid colon. The space between the reflected layers of peritoneum is known as the cul-de-sac of Douglas. It is of importance to the gynecologist for two reasons. (1) Blood or pus may be drained through the vagina by incising the posterior cul-de-sac, thus avoiding the major peritoneal cavity, and (2) various endoscopic instruments may be placed into this space through the vagina for a complete inspection of the oviducts, ovaries and posterior uterine surface (see culdoscopy).

The anterior and posterior peritoneal coverings of the corpus join at the lateral uterine margin and form the leaves of the *broad* ligament (Fig. 5–3).

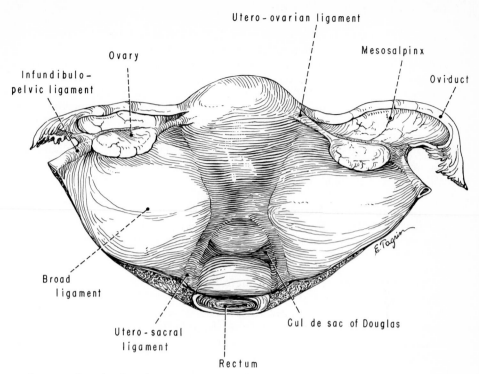

Utero-ovarian ligament

Ovary

Mesosalpinx

Infundibulo-
pelvic ligament

Oviduct

Broad
ligament

Utero-sacral
ligament

Cul de sac of Douglas

Rectum

Fig. 5-3.—Posterior view of uterus and adnexae showing the broad ligament.

The peritoneal surfaces are in close proximity except where they diverge slightly to invest the *round* and *infundibulopelvic* ligaments. The broad ligament is, therefore, a double layer of peritoneum which extends from the lateral surface of the uterus outward to the pelvic wall. Its upper border consists of the peritoneal fold over the oviduct and the lateral extension from the ovary encircling the infundibulopelvic vessels. The mid-portion encompasses the round ligament, and the most inferior portion is thickened and contains a condensation of connective tissue and muscle fibers called the *cardinal* ligament or ligamentum colli of Mackenrodt. The uterine vessels approach the lateral aspect of the cervix in the cardinal ligament, an anatomic point of importance in total hysterectomy.

The portion of the broad ligament between the ovary and the oviduct contains many small blood vessels and is termed the *mesosalpinx* or tubal mesentery. The vestigial remnants of the mesonephric tubules and duct are located within the leaves of the mesentery and are known as the epoophoron (lateral portion of the tubules) and the paraoophoron (medial portion of the tubules). All of these vestigial tubules are connected with the remnant of the mesonephric duct (Gartner's duct). The blind upper extremity of the duct is occasionally dilated into one or more cystic structures known as hydatids of Morgagni. Cysts may develop from the main duct or from one of the smaller tubules and may be confused with ovarian cysts at the time of pelvic examination. These will be discussed further in Chapter 6.

The round ligaments consist principally of bands of muscle tissue which extend laterally from the anterolateral aspect of the fundus. They leave the peritoneal cavity through the internal inguinal ring, traverse the inguinal canal to the labia majora and terminate by dissemination of fibers into the surrounding tissue. Although the round ligaments consist principally of muscle fibers prolonged from the uterus, there is also an admixture of fibrous and areolar tissue, blood vessels, lymphatics and nerves. The round ligaments are about 10–12 cm. long and 0.5 to 0.75 cm. thick and are covered by the anterior and posterior leaves of the broad ligament as far as the internal abdominal ring. In the fetus this duplicature of peritoneum is prolonged as a short tubular process into the inguinal canal (canal of Nuck). It is generally obliterated in the adult, but occasionally it may persist and be the source of benign cystic structures which are frequently mistaken for hernias. Rarely endometriosis occurs in this peritoneal projection.

The round ligaments were formerly believed to play a major part in uterine support, particularly the maintenance of the normal anterior position. Numerous operations have been devised which, in effect, shorten these ligaments with the hope that this will hold the fundus forward. The round ligaments may have some effect in returning the anterior uterus to its normal position after displacement by a full bladder or after pregnancy. They hypertrophy greatly during pregnancy and may be the source of localized lower-quadrant pain which may simulate that of acute appendicitis. The lymphatics that traverse the ligaments are occasionally the route of metastases to the groin from endometrial carcinoma.

The uterosacral ligaments arise from the posterior wall of the uterus at the level of the internal cervical os. They are made up of connective tissue and involuntary muscle and contain blood vessels, lymphatics and nerve filaments of the parasympathetic and sympathetic systems. Each ligament describes a posterior arc, passing dorsally around the rectosigmoid toward an insertion on the sacral wall at the level of the second and third sacral vertebrae. The peritoneum over the posterior uterine wall and cul-de-sac is reflected over the uterosacral ligaments throughout their course. The function of these ligaments is to exert tension on the cervix in a dorsal direction, in effect keeping the corpus anterior and the axis of the corpus and cervix at a right angle to the vagina. This prevents the uterus from assuming a position which would be in the axis of, and in direct line with, the vagina—a situation that is almost always associated with uterine prolapse.

The cardinal or transverse cervical ligaments (of Mackenrodt) have been mentioned as forming the inferior aspect or base of the broad ligament. They offer the chief support for the cervix and upper vagina and do so by integrating posteriorly with the uterosacral ligaments and anteriorly with the cervicovaginal portion of the endopelvic fascia. The cardinal ligaments are composed of muscle fibers and connective tissue which ensheath the uterine vessels, nerve fibers and lymphatics. As they fan out laterally, the tissues of the ligaments insert into the fascia overlying the obturator muscles and the muscles of the pelvic diaphragm and, as pointed out by Anson, follow the course of the major vessels as a supporting framework. Careful dissection has shown that the effective dorsal fixation of the ligaments is provided by the perivascular fibrous tissue of the hypogastric and iliac vessels.

The utero-ovarian ligament (suspensory ligament of the ovary) extends from the lateral aspect of the uterus (between the round ligament and the oviduct) to the inferior pole of the ovary. It consists of connective tissue and smooth muscle in a rounded cord and is ensheathed between layers of the broad ligament. It is not known whether or not this ligament is capable of altering tubo-ovarian position at the time of ovulation, but some observations would indicate that this occurs.

Uterine Structure.—The uterus is composed of three separate and distinct layers: (1) The perimetrium (serosa), an outer peritoneal covering; (2) the myometrium, an inner layer of smooth muscle, and (3) the endometrium, the mucous membrane lining the cavity (Fig. 5-4). The perimetrium is continued laterally as the leaves of the broad ligament and is continued anteriorly and posteriorly as bladder and rectal reflections. The myometrium is composed of three rather indistinct layers of smooth muscle fibers. In each layer there is an interlacing and intermixture of the nonstriated muscle cells which are held in juxtaposition by a connective tissue rich in elastic fibers. The outer muscular layer (stratum supravasculare) is chiefly longitudinal and is continuous with fibers entering the broad and round ligaments, whereas the middle layer is thicker and presents fibers in circular arrangement. The middle layer makes up the major portion of the myometrium and contains many blood vessels located between muscle bands (stratum vasculare). The inner layer represents an exaggerated muscularis mucosae and is composed of thin muscle strands arranged obliquely and longitudinally. The arrangement of the blood vessels between muscle bundles affords an ideal method for hemostasis following delivery. This is borne out clinically by patients whose uteri are atonic following parturition and in whom hemorrhage may at times prove fatal.

The endometrium is a soft inner layer of variable thickness made up of simple tubular glands, a stroma of resting cells in a fine connective tissue mesh and a sensitive vasculature. The histology and physiologic variations of this layer will be considered in the section on Menstruation.

Blood Supply.—The uterus possesses a dual blood supply, receiving branches from both the uterine and ovarian arteries. The uterine artery is

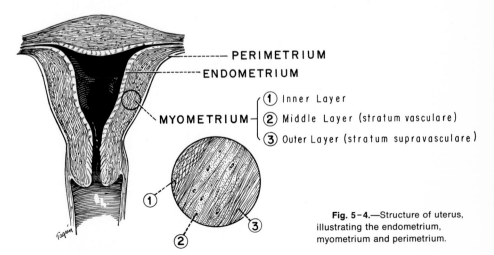

PERIMETRIUM
ENDOMETRIUM
MYOMETRIUM
1 Inner Layer
2 Middle Layer (stratum vasculare)
3 Outer Layer (stratum supravasculare)

Fig. 5-4.—Structure of uterus, illustrating the endometrium, myometrium and perimetrium.

derived from the hypogastric trunk (Fig. 5–5). It crosses over the ureter at the level of the internal os of the cervix and divides into ascending and descending limbs. The former runs tortuously upward between the leaves of the broad ligament, giving horizontal anterior and posterior branches to the cervix and corpus. As it reaches the cornu a branch is sent to the round ligament and then it is projected along the oviduct to anastomose with the ovarian vessels in the mesosalpinx. The descending branch of the uterine artery turns inferiorly and supplies the vagina from the lateral aspect. It anastomoses freely with the vaginal artery along its course.

The collecting veins from the corpus flow into two longitudinal trunks which are usually distinct. The anterior surface is drained by the anterior uterine vein situated anterior to the ureter and lateral to the uterine artery. This vein empties into the hypogastric vein. The posterior uterine surfaces, however, drain into a short and long trunk that pass posterior to the uterus and inferior to the uterine artery before joining either the hypogastric or obturator vein.

The processes of menstruation and pregnancy give singular importance to an understanding of the anatomic vascular pattern of the endometrium. As previously mentioned, a series of *radial* arteries are given off at right

Fig. 5–5.—Divisions of the hypogastric artery.

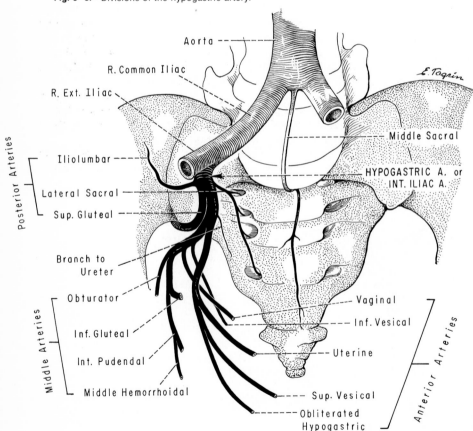

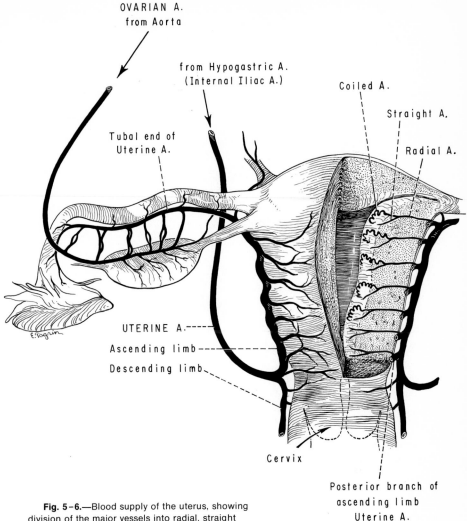

OVARIAN A.
from Aorta

from Hypogastric A.
(Internal Iliac A.)

Coiled A.

Straight A.

Radial A.

Tubal end of
Uterine A.

UTERINE A.

Ascending limb

Descending limb

Cervix

Posterior branch of
ascending limb
Uterine A.

Fig. 5-6.—Blood supply of the uterus, showing division of the major vessels into radial, straight and spiral (coiled) arteries and arterioles.

angles from the uterine artery as it courses along the corpus (Fig. 5-6). These radial arteries branch in the inner third of the myometrium into *straight* and *spiral* (coiled) vessels. The straight arteries pass only as far as the basal layer of the endometrium and terminate in capillaries in that region. The spiral arteries, however, follow a coiled course throughout the thickness of the endometrium, give off a few branches in the endometrium, then fork and give rise to superficial capillaries just below the surface epithelium. These capillaries form plexuses in the stroma and a meshwork around the glands. In the superficial layer of the endometrium the capillaries form sinus-like dilatations known as "lakes." The blood is returned via small veins which drain these vascular lakes and capillary plexuses. It should be remembered that the vascular pattern is a dynamic one with

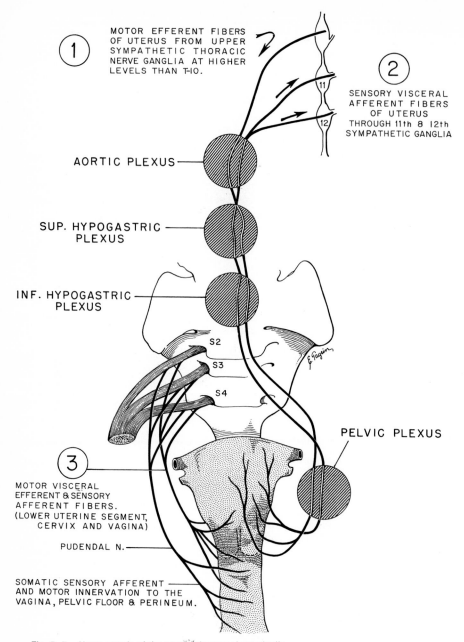

MOTOR EFFERENT FIBERS OF UTERUS FROM UPPER SYMPATHETIC THORACIC NERVE GANGLIA AT HIGHER LEVELS THAN T-10.

SENSORY VISCERAL AFFERENT FIBERS OF UTERUS THROUGH 11th & 12th SYMPATHETIC GANGLIA

AORTIC PLEXUS

SUP. HYPOGASTRIC PLEXUS

INF. HYPOGASTRIC PLEXUS

S2
S3
S4

PELVIC PLEXUS

MOTOR VISCERAL EFFERENT & SENSORY AFFERENT FIBERS. (LOWER UTERINE SEGMENT, CERVIX AND VAGINA)

PUDENDAL N.

SOMATIC SENSORY AFFERENT AND MOTOR INNERVATION TO THE VAGINA, PELVIC FLOOR & PERINEUM.

Fig. 5-7.—Nerve supply of the uterus shown schematically.

constant proliferation and regression. The specific morphologic details are considered under Menstruation.

Although the prime function of the straight arteries is to supply the basal endometrium, they may also function to support regeneration of the lower portion of the functional layer. The coiled arteries alone supply blood to the superficial third of the endometrium and most of the blood to the middle third. Markee has shown in intraocular endometrial transplants, however, that some straight arteries may be converted into coiled ones and then later to the straight type. Thus it is possible that the blood supply of the endometrium could regenerate and develop specificity of function even after complete curettage.

The importance of the coiled arteries is not completely known. However, it should be pointed out that they are absent or not fully developed in areas where extensive cyclic variations do not occur. Thus, in the lower uterine segment and lateral recesses of the endometrium the vascular supply is mostly through straight arteries.

Nerve Supply.—The uterine extrinsic nerve supply is derived from three sources (Fig. 5–7). (1) *Motor* fibers from the upper sympathetic thoracic ganglia course through the aortic plexus and the celiac ganglion to the *superior hypogastric plexus.* Fibers then diverge as they pass caudally to form the *inferior hypogastric plexus,* thence forward over the lateral surface of the rectal ampulla to join the *pelvic plexus* or *cervical ganglion of Frankenhäuser.* From this plexus, fibers pass along the uterosacral ligament to the smooth muscle of the uterus. Clinical evidence indicates that the motor fibers to the uterus leave the spinal cord at levels higher than the tenth thoracic nerve. (2) *Sensory* fibers are special visceral afferents that run through the hypogastric and aortic plexuses, through the *eleventh* and *twelfth* sympathetic ganglia without synapse, into the dorsal spinal root ganglia of these segments, thence up the dorsolateral fasciculus to the thalamus. The sensory supply to the cervix travels through the sacral parasympathetic chain communicating with the second, third and fourth sacral nerves. (3) *Sensory and motor* fibers to the lower uterine segment and cervix are found in the sympathetic and parasympathetic plexuses, communicating with the second, third and fourth sacral nerves. Visceral efferent fibers believed to be motor to the longitudinal muscle of the lower uterine segment and the circular fibers of the cervix and possibly inhibitory to the uterine fundus travel in the parasympathetic chain.

It should be remembered that although the sensory nerve fibers course through pelvic, hypogastric and aortic plexuses before reaching the eleventh and twelfth thoracic nerves, they are functionally independent of the autonomic system. The sensory supply to the cervix, although traversing the sacral parasympathetics, is also functionally independent of the autonomic system.

Lymphatic Supply.—The lymphatics of the uterine corpus proceed in four or five channels through the broad ligament just below the oviducts, thence upward along the ovarian vessels. In the course of their passage through the parametrium and ovarian ligament, they communicate with the ovarian lymphatics to terminate in the lumbar lymph nodes found in front of the aorta from its bifurcation to the diaphragm. The lymphatics from the lower uterine segment anastomose with adjacent lymph channels from the cervix and drain to the obturator, iliac, hypogastric and sacral nodes. A third route of lymphatic drainage, especially from the fundal area, is via the round ligament to the superficial nodes.

Embryology

The normal uterus develops from the conjunction of two müllerian ducts of equal size, shape and growth potential. The midline, unpaired structure is evolved as a result of three well-defined growth phases. These are: (1) contact of the ducts, (2) fusion of the duct walls and (3) involution of the created septum. If the ducts are not of equivalent size or have varying growth rates, a *uterus unicornis* may develop. If an abnormality of fusion occurs, a *uterus bicornis* or *didelphys* may develop. If the midline septum is not absorbed, the uterine cavity may be divided into two parts, forming a *uterus septus duplex*. The major developmental abnormalities are depicted in Figure 5–8.

The lining of the prospective uterine cavity is columnar epithelium derived from the epithelium of the müllerian ducts. By a local downgrowth this epithelium forms the endometrial glands and these, in turn, provoke the development of an unusual stroma of a type found nowhere else in the body. Since organs (such as the uterus) derived from the müllerian duct

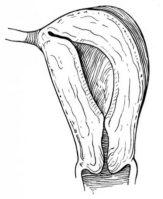

Uterus Unicornis

Fig. 5–8.—Major congenital anomalies of the uterus.

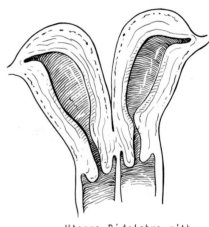

Uterus Didelphys with
Double Vagina

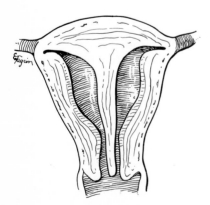

Uterus Septus Duplex

epithelium and duct wall originate from the same germinal layer, the stroma and epithelium are more closely related in the internal genitalia than in most other organs. This is evident in the disease known as adenomyosis, in which islands of benign endometrial tissue "invade" the myometrium and seem to function just as normally as if they were lining the uterine cavity.

Menstruation

Menstruation represents the effects of a fine interplay of gonadal and extragonadal hormones acting in concert on the endometrium in a sequential and cyclic fashion. It occurs usually about every 28 days, beginning at the menarche and continuing until menopause. It consists of the discharge from the uterus of fragments of endometrium, blood and mucus with an admixture of vaginal epithelial cells. In this chapter the term "menstruation" will be considered to be the result of sloughing of secretory endometrium, that is, an endometrium that has been acted on by progesterone subsequent to ovulation. Uterine bleeding from a nonsecretory endometrium is considered abnormal and will be discussed in the section on Dysfunctional Uterine Bleeding.

The age of onset of menstruation is variable, but in the temperate zone is usually between 10 and 16. A number of cases have been reported of so-called idiopathic precocious puberty, in which children begin to ovulate and menstruate between the ages of 2 and 8, and some of these have become pregnant. No apparent endocrinologic disorder has been found in these children, but in others pituitary, midbrain or ovarian tumors may bring about bleeding of an anovulatory nature. The onset of menstruation (*menarche*—month beginning) may be delayed in some individuals until age 19 or 20. In such patients it should be remembered that many factors such as climate, heredity, health and hygiene as well as social and economic background may delay the onset of the menses. It has been reported that warmer climates predispose to early menarche, whereas in extremely cold climates onset may be delayed. This, however, may merely be representative of variations in dietary and hereditary factors. Adolescents should not be subjected to vigorous hormonal treatment when the sole abnormality is the persistence of amenorrhea until age 18 or 19.

A plausible explanation of menstruation is now available from a study of current concepts of embryogenesis as well as a study of endometrial histology and biogenesis of steroids. The varying quality and quantity of the steroid hormones evoke growth and function of secretory tubules in endometrial tissue. These epithelial structures extend laterally, each joining its adjacent counterpart to form a complete lining of the uterine cavity. Under the influence of estrogen and progesterone an unbranched spiral artery of each endometrial segment expands into a terminal network of superficial capillaries. These arterioles, and associated venules, serve to make maternal blood accessible to the expectant trophoblast. The weak reticular matrix surrounding these vessels is converted into a buttressed tissue of contiguous stromal cells by their conversion into decidua, principally by the action of progesterone. Thus the endometrium is primed and prepared for the arrival of the trophoblast.

The physiologic and morphologic changes responsible for the process of menstruation are: (1) estrogen and progesterone withdrawal and slowed circulation, (2) vascular stasis and vasodilatation, (3) vasoconstriction and (4) menstruation. These processes are under precise hormonal control and specific conditions are essential for completion of endometrial sloughing. A reduction in the circulating levels of the endometrial-supporting steroids, estrogen and progesterone, precipitate the morphologic events culminating in menses. There are four important conditions that are essential for this terminal event: (1) the hormonal stimulus must have been sufficiently intense; (2) the stimulus must have been present for an adequate duration of time; (3) the stimulus must be withdrawn relatively suddenly; and (4) the decrease must be sufficiently great. These conditions operate in all normal menstrual cycles and are the basis of the commonly used substitutional therapeutic schedules.

In the absence of trophoblastic implantation, and as a result of diminishing levels of estrogen and progesterone, the prediciduum is deprived of nutriment. The decidual cells shrink, autolysis occurs and the tissue becomes thinner. The Smiths have suggested that a toxin derived from catabolism of stromal cells, causes or potentiates tissue autolysis and arteriolar contraction. Superficial capillaries become devoid of stromal support and undergo autolysis. The caliber of spiral arterioles is diminished due to hormonal withdrawal, and intermittent contractions of these vessels eventuate in recurrent foci of ischemia. This slowed circulation is followed by a decrease in the thickness of the endometrium, mainly as a result of a fluid shift wherein a loss of extravascular fluid occurs.

As stromal shrinkage continues, the coiled arteries show further buckling with increased stasis. In intraocular transplants, the erythrocytes may not move for 60 to 90 seconds and a distinct bluing of the transplants is observable with the naked eye. A similar bluing of the human endometrium has been observed during the premenstrual period. Vasodilatation is sometimes seen during the period of stasis. It has been suggested that arteriovenous anastomoses play a role in the production of the stasis that leads to necrosis and menstrual bleeding. This theory assumes that acetylcholine-type compounds act on nerve fibers to control the opening and closing of the anastomoses. The presence of arteriovenous shunts has been confirmed but that they play a physiologic role in the menstrual process is not certain.

Some hours before menstrual bleeding begins, there is constriction of the basal part of the spiral arteries. This constriction is limited to that part of the artery that is located in the deepest part of the basalis or in the adjacent myometrium. The vasoconstriction affects individual coiled arteries in a random fashion. When vasoconstriction occurs it results in blanching of that part of the endometrium supplied by the constricted vessel. The constriction of the coiled arteries persists throughout the period of menstrual bleeding, being interrupted in individual vessels for only short periods.

Menstrual bleeding occurs when a previously constricted artery relaxes and blood again surges through it and its branches. It may be assumed that some weakening of the vessel's walls may have accompanied vasoconstriction. Several types of bleeding have been observed: (1) arterial or capillary bleeding with the formation of a hematoma, (2) direct hemorrhage from arterioles through the surface epithelium, (3) diapedesis through capillary walls and (4) direct or retrograde blood flow from veins in the fields of previous hemorrhage and tissue destruction. Near the end of the first day of menstruation, fragments of endometrium slowly become detached and become part of the menstrual discharge.

The cessation of menstrual bleeding and endometrial desquamation usually occurs as the estrogen level begins to rise. Re-epithelization occurs relatively rapidly and the vascular bed is restored.

Recent evidence suggests that a hormonal substance, one of the prostaglandins known as $PGF_{2\alpha}$, is found in endometrial tissue in large amounts during the luteal phase of the cycle. This substance, one of 9 prostaglandins derived from a carbon 20 compound known as prostanoic acid, is similar to the 5 known prostaglandins derived from human seminal plasma. When $PGF_{2\alpha}$ is infused intravenously or directly into the uterine lumen of the rat a dramatic shift of the steroid pattern of ovaries occurs: progesterone levels are depressed whereas the 20-hydroxy-progesterone levels are elevated. It has been suggested that $PGF_{2\alpha}$, a potent venoconstrictor, results in venospasms all along the venous pathway until the venoconstrictor is diluted in an ineffective concentration by venocaval blood. But the proximity of the ovary permits direct action on the production of steroids of the corpus luteum, thus causing a luteolytic effect. Thus a feedback mechanism between ovary and endometrium is established: $PGF_{2\alpha}$ is produced in the endometrium as a result of the effects of estrogen and progesterone; when the levels of $PGF_{2\alpha}$ reach a critical level during luteal phase, production of estrogen and progesterone are diminished by the potent venoconstrictor substance; diminution of estrogen and progesterone permits endometrial sloughing, reduction of $PGF_{2\alpha}$, and release of the hypothalamic blockade. This most attractive theory would explain the limitation of life of the corpus luteum and support exists in cows, sheep, pigs, guinea pigs and rats, animals that have shared venous drainage between the ipsilateral ovaries and the uterine cornua. These animals exhibit a unilateral effect on the ovary when a unilateral hysterectomy is performed. Proof of this mechanism in the human female awaits confirmation.

The average menstrual cycle is from 27 to 30 days and about 95 per cent of ovulating women menstruate every 15 to 45 days. Therefore, if the cycle in a given individual is rhythmic (within a two- to three-day variation) and occurs within the interval mentioned, it should be considered normal. Bleeding at intervals of less than 18 or more than 42 days or with a total absence of rhythm should be considered abnormal and is frequently anovulatory. Menstrual flow usually lasts from three to six days although many women bleed for only a day and a half and then have a day or so of staining. Others flow heavily for seven days but have always done so. Such variations should not be considered abnormal. About 30–100 cc. of blood is lost during an average menstrual period, although many women may lose two to three times this amount and still have no physical or laboratory evidence of anemia.

Bleeding that is too profuse, too prolonged, or occurs at other than the usual regular intervals should be considered abnormal. Irregular or extremely long intervals are significant if they occur regularly. The degree of abnormality should be viewed in light of the patient's age. At the time of puberty or menopause the menstrual cycle is usually irregular—but only in respect to the length of intervals between periods. The duration and amount of bleeding should remain within the limits of 2 to 7 days and 4 to 5 pads a day. Prolonged or excessive bleeding is abnormal and should be investigated.

Menstrual discharge is characteristic in that it will not clot. This is probably due to a fibrinolysin and other factors prohibiting clotting rather than to the absence of some essential clotting factor, since if a small amount of menstrual discharge is added to fresh venous blood, clotting is speeded, then the clot dissolves. The average patient is aware of certain systemic changes for several days before the onset of flow. These include breast soreness or fullness, edema, backache and leg ache, or just a sense of depression or lethargy. This group of symptoms has been termed menstrual molimina (L., endeavor, effort).

HORMONAL ASPECTS OF MENSTRUATION

A major part of the known relationships between the pituitary gland and the ovaries has been derived from animal investigation and therefore much of what follows is merely an application of this knowledge to the human female. Quantification of serum levels of the various hormones would lead to a clearer understanding of the endocrinologic aspects of menstruation. Satisfactory methods for such analyses have recently become available.

The first day of the *menstrual period* is considered as day 1 of the *menstrual cycle*. As the process of endometrial sloughing continues, a gonadotropic substance known as the *follicle-stimulating* hormone (FSH) is elaborated by certain basophilic cells of the adenohypophysis in progressively increasing amounts. Studies of hormones isolated from sheep and swine pituitary glands have not succeeded in producing pure FSH since *luteinizing* hormone (LH) cannot be effectively separated. In general, however, FSH may be regarded as a glycoprotein with a molecular weight of about 67,000, containing 1.5 per cent hexosamine, 1.2 per cent hexose, 15.1 per cent nitrogen and 1.5 per cent sulfur. FSH brings about a proliferation of the granulosa cells and formation of an antrum in an undetermined number of ovarian graafian follicles. In the male FSH is a gametogenic agent, stimulating the seminiferous tubule system and spermatogenesis. The growth of the follicle prior to the antrum stage is controlled by extra-adenohypophyseal factors. The interstitial elements of the follicles are similarly stimulated to differentiate into the *theca interna* and the *theca externa*. Available evidence suggests that the theca cells, not the granulosa, secrete an *estrogenic* (causing estrus) substance, probably estradiol 17-β. FSH alone is unable to bring about this secretion of estradiol by the follicle but will do so in the presence of a small amount of luteinizing hormone, a substance secreted by another distinctive basophilic adenohypophyseal cell.

Luteinizing hormone (LH, ICSH) is responsible for luteinization of the theca interna and granulosa cells of the follicle. However, in recognition of this hormone's stimulating action on the interstitial cells of the testis, it is also appropriately called the interstitial cell stimulating hormone, ICSH.

In a number of important respects LH acts as a physiologic complement to FSH. LH, acting together with FSH, stimulates the follicle to full development and promotes the secretion of estrogen by the growing follicle. LH at optimal levels is essential for ovulation and, in a sense, could rightly be considered the ovulating hormone. Following ovulation, LH induces the qualitative transformation of the cells of the theca interna and granulosa layers of the follicle to lutein cells and promotes the formation of the corpus luteum. The maintenance and activity of the corpus luteum may be dependent upon a third gonadotropin, i.e., luteotropic hormone.

A pituitary luteotropic factor has never been chemically separated from lactogenic hormone preparations. Lactogenic hormone, one of the first anterior pituitary hormones to be isolated in pure form, is a protein or protein-like substance but unlike FSH and LH, does not contain a carbohydrate moiety. The molecular weight of lactogenic hormone preparations is about 26–35,000.

Lactogenic hormone stimulates the alveolar cells of the mammary gland resulting in the initiation and maintenance of milk secretion. Interestingly enough this hormone that plays such a vital role in the nuturing of all mammals has been extensively studied in such non-mammals as the pigeon. In fact, the most commonly used method for measuring potency of lactogenic hormone extracts is based on its ability to stimulate proliferation of the crop sac of squabs.

More recently lactogenic hormone has been shown to exert an effect on corpus luteum maintenance and secretion of progesterone. This corpus luteum stimulating effect resulted in the coining of the alternative name, luteotropic hormone (LTH).

The effects of estrogens are twofold. (1) The endometrium begins to show *proliferative* changes characterized by glandular growth, regeneration of surface epithelium and active mitoses in the stromal cells. These changes are considered in detail in the section on Dating the Endometrium. (2) A rise in the level of estrogen produces suppression of FSH, which is followed by a further rise in luteinizing hormone, perhaps stimulated by this particular level of estrogen. The normal range for estrogen production is usually between 60 and 200 μg. per day for the follicular phase of the cycle, between 150 and 300 μg. for the luteal phase of the cycle, and up to about 400 μg. during the ovulatory rise. In summary, relatively pure FSH brings about only follicular development, whereas FSH plus LH effectively result in the secretion of estrogen from the follicle.

The ovary can be divided into four anatomic and functional sub-units: the follicle, corpus luteum, stroma and hilus. Each is a sort of endocrine gland of its own within the ovary, producing its own spectrum of hormones and having its own characteristic response to gonadotropin stimulation.

The developing follicle produces a wide variety of steroid hormones on the basis of assays of the follicular fluid and the incubation of the follicular apparatus with steroid precursors in vitro. The steroids isolated from ovarian tissue and follicular fluid are listed in Table 5–1.

TABLE 5–1.—Steroids Isolated from the Human
Follicular Fluid, Ovarian Tissue and Corpora Lutea

Estrogens	Androgens	Progestins
Estradiol	Androstenedione	Progesterone
Estrone	Dehydroepiandrosterone*	20α-Hydroxypregn-4-en-3-one
Estriol*		17α-Hydroxyprogesterone

*Isolated predominantly from follicular tissue
(From Ryan, K. J. Biosynthesis and Metabolism of Ovarian Steroids, in Behrman, S. J., and Kistner, R. W. [ed.], *Progress in Infertility* [Boston, Little, Brown and Company, 1968], p. 277.)

These include estrogens, androgens and progestins, but the estrogens are quantitatively the most important constituents. Although not definitely established, it is assumed that well-developed and preovulatory follicles have the greatest steroid-producing potential. Isolation of these steroids from the ovary does not constitute proof of formation within the gland or follicle but is suggestive evidence due to the high concentration of hormones relative to other body fluids or tissues. It is evident that estrogens are the major hormones found, but progesterone, androstenedione, and even dehydroepiandrosterone are also formed.

Ryan has demonstrated that the granulosa cells can be separated from the theca cells of the follicle and has shown the capacity of each cell type in hormone synthesis. Both cell types have characteristic activity in steroid biosynthesis. The differences, thus far, seem more quantitative than qualitative but they may be of fundamental importance in the control of endocrine function. The granulosa has a clear superiority in progesterone accumulation. Ryan has also pointed out that in addition to their well-known histologic differences, the granulosa cell layer is an avascular tissue compared to the richly vascularized theca. Any hormone produced by the granulosa would no doubt have to traverse the theca before entering the blood stream. These observations are the bases for the so-called two-cell theory of hormone formation.

In summary, it has been demonstrated that the follicular fluid contains a wide variety of steroids, that the follicular wall can synthesize hormones in vitro, and that stimulation with gonadotropins results in increased follicular size and hormone production. The follicular phase of the cycle can be correlated with increased levels of estrogen in urine, and the absence of follicles in the menopause can be correlated with a marked decline in estrogens. Although the follicle normally produces progesterone, androgens and estrogens, its major secretory product appears to be estradiol.

Thus the stage is set for ovulation. An extremely delicate hormonal ovarian-pituitary relationship has brought a graafian follicle to the surface of the ovary where it appears as a blister-like elevation. Swelling of the entire structure occurs with expansion of the thinned granulosa and thecal elements. Simultaneously, the ovum is freed from its follicular attachment by the appearance of fluid in the cumulus cells. Within a short period thereafter the translucent edge of the follicle bulges from the ovarian surface as the *stigma* and, as a result of unknown factors, rupture occurs. This process is known as ovulation and usually occurs 14 plus or minus 2 days before the next expected menstrual period. The ovum is accompanied by the follicular liquor as it is released into the peritoneal cavity where it is enveloped by the fimbriated extensions of the oviduct.

The exact mechanism of ovulation is still unknown. Physical principles such as increasing intrafollicular tension, enzymatic destruction of the stigma and variations in the adjacent muscle and fibrous connective tissue have been considered as ancillary factors. The regulation of ovulation by hormonal changes must be considered in light of present evidence to follow the following pattern. (1) FSH and LH mature the graafian follicle by specific action (FSH on granulosa cells, LH on theca cells). (2) A fully developed theca interna secretes estrogen. (3) Low levels of estrogen stimulate FSH, thus increasing follicular growth. (4) Higher levels of estrogen and/or its oxidation products are intimately involved in both the stimula-

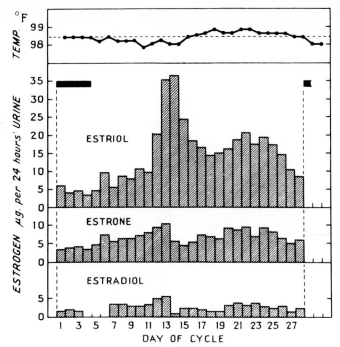

Fig. 5-9.—Daily urinary excretion of estriol, estrone and estradiol and basal temperature variation during a normal menstrual cycle. (From Brown, J. B.: Lancet 1:320, 1955.)

tion of the adenohypophysis and the release of LH (ICSH) from the pituitary gland. (5) Increased secretion of LH probably results in ovulation (definite lutein changes have been observed in the theca cells before ovulation, so the whole process is a gradual one). Since these preovulatory lutein changes may result in the secretion of small amounts of progesterone, the suggestion has been made that a proper balance of *estrogen* and *progesterone* effects adenohypophyseal secretion of LH through hypothalamic stimulation. This may be the final trigger mechanism necessary to rupture the stigma.

At the time of ovulation there is a slight decrease in circulating estrogen (Figs. 5-9 and 5-10). This drop coincides with the release of luteotropic hormone (LTH) from the pituitary. Under the combined stimulation of LH and LTH, the granulosa and theca cells undergo rapid luteinization.

Ovulation, in the human, usually occurs from only one ovary although more than one follicle may rupture at one time, resulting in dizygotic multiple pregnancy. There is no particular pattern of frequency as far as one ovary or the other is concerned, and studies in the monkey suggest a tendency for ovulation to occur in the proximity of the tubal end of the ovary and nearer the free edge than the hilum. Methods of detecting ovulation presently available are by direct observation at the time of laparotomy, by culdoscopy and by certain presumptive laboratory methods. Included in the laboratory procedures are endometrial biopsy, basal body temperature, exfoliative cytology, variations in hormone levels and changes in the cervical mucus. The effects of progesterone on the endometrium may be reliably assayed by biopsy and results of the assay afford a fairly accurate

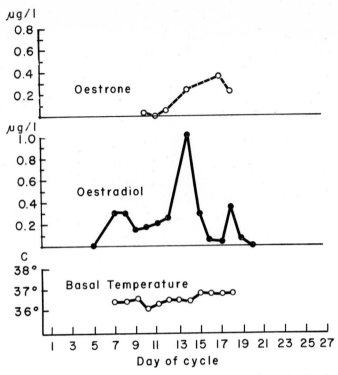

Fig. 5-10.—Plasma levels of estrone and estradiol during the normal menstrual cycle. (From Svendsen, R., and Sorensen, R.: Acta endocrinol. 47:245, 1964.)

estimate of the time of previous ovulation. Progesterone causes a rise in basal body temperature ranging between 0.4 and 1 degree F., which is usually maintained until menstruation. In general it is presumed that ovulation may be considered as occurring on or within two days before or after the day the temperature first rises. Exfoliative vaginal cytology is not as applicable to clinical gynecology for the determination of the time of ovulation as biopsy or temperature charts but it may serve as corroborative evidence. Progesterone produces a change in the cornification index of the squamous cells and, although the slides may be read rapidly, considerable training is necessary for correct evaluation. Hormone assays of estrogenic substances found in urine reveal two peaks, the first just before ovulation and the second four to six days after ovulation. Studies on plasma progesterone indicate that free progesterone appears 24–48 hours before, or coincidental with, a prominent rise in waking temperature. Progesterone is excreted in the urine, in part, as pregnanediol, and current evidence indicates that the pregnanediol level rises significantly approximately 24 hours after ovulation (Figs. 5–11 and 5–12).

The functional *corpus luteum* secretes both estrogens and *progesterone*. It usually lasts for about 14 days but begins to show degenerative changes from the ninth to twelfth days. If pregnancy supervenes, the corpus luteum is maintained in an active state by gonadotropins derived from the cyto-

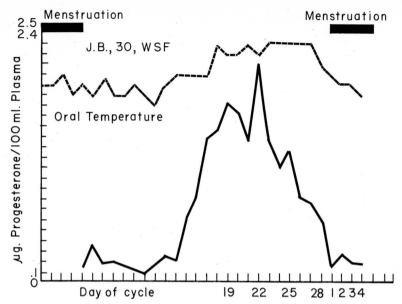

Fig. 5-11.—Plasma progesterone levels during the normal menstrual cycle in micrograms per 100 ml. (From Woolever, C. A.: Am. J. Obst. & Gynec. 85:981, 1963.)

trophoblastic cells of the chorion. In the human female this state of pre-servation approximates 70–90 days.

The released ovum and its attached cells are about 150μ in diameter, just visible to the unaided eye, and undergoes rapid degeneration in about 24 hours unless fertilized. The process of fertilization is said to occur in or near the fimbriated portion of the oviduct. Transfer of the fertilized human ovum along the oviduct usually takes about three days and implantation of the blastocyst occurs on the sixth or seventh day after fertilization.

The corpus luteum (yellow body) is formed from the remaining cells of the ovulated follicle. Following closure of the stigma, and as a result of increasing amounts of LH and LTH, the granulosa cells enlarge, assume a polygonal shape with vesicular nuclei and contain lipid vacuoles. They are now called "granulosa-lutein" cells. The theca interna cells assume an epithelial appearance and migrate along newly formed vascular channels into the granulosa-lutein layer. The theca-lutein cells also contain lipid vacuoles and droplets and are believed to be the source of both estrogen and progesterone. Only small amounts of steroidal substances have been demonstrated in the granulosa-lutein cells during the active stage of the corpus luteum. Certain specialized and darker-staining cells derived from the theca interna (K cells) have been demonstrated among the luteinized granulosa cells. They contain a high concentration of steroid substance and it has been suggested that they are a major source of progesterone.

Numerous investigators have reported the levels of progesterone in plasma to vary from 0.1 to 1.6 μg. per 100 ml. during the follicular phase of the cycle, and from 0.4 to 2.0 μg. per 100 ml. during the luteal phase. The secretion rate of progesterone has been calculated as varying between 2.3

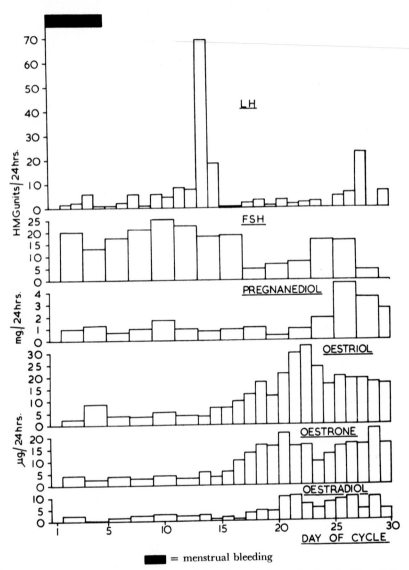

Fig. 5-12.—Hormone excretion pattern during the normal menstrual cycle. (From Bell, E. T., *et al.*: Acta endocrinol. 51:578, 1966.)

and 5.4 mg. per day during the follicular phase of the cycle and from 22 to 43 mg. per day during the luteal phase. A secretion rate of 1.3 mg. per day was calculated for ovariectomized females, the latter presumably of adrenal origin.

Direct assay of corpus luteum tissue has resulted in the identification of many of the same steroids isolated from follicular fluid. The main distinguishing feature is the predominance of progesterone in the corpus luteum. The presence of the corpus luteum has been correlated with elevated levels of pregnanediol in urine and progesterone in blood. Such studies provide confirmatory evidence for an endocrine function of the corpus luteum during the second phase of the cycle.

The corpus luteum can readily be separated from the remainder of the ovary, and many studies have been performed by incubation of this tissue with steroid precursors in vitro. The corpus luteum can synthesize progesterone, androgens and estrogens, but progesterone appears to be the major product. The estrogen produced during the luteal phase of the cycle is probably also produced by the corpus luteum but could in part be a product of developing follicles.

The ovarian stroma and hilus can be considered together since they are essentially a continuum of ovarian tissue devoid of follicles and corpora lutea. The hilus is distinguished by greater vascularity and the presence of a Leydig-cell type which sometimes forms the locus of an androgen-producing hilar cell tumor. The stroma and hilus can produce steroids in vitro with a spectrum of hormones qualitatively similar to those formed in the follicle and corpus luteum. In contrast to these other ovarian sub-units, the stroma produces largely androgens. In the postmenopausal period, and when follicles are atretic, the stroma may be the site of significant hormone production. There is no evidence to suggest that these tissues are important during the normal cycle when either the follicle or the corpus luteum is active, but their role in this circumstance remains to be defined.

The effects of increased estrogen and progesterone secretion on the endometrium are discussed in detail in the next section. In general, there is an increased volume of blood carried to the glandular capillaries with the development of glycogen formation in the gland cells. This is followed by release of glycogen into the gland lumen—the "secretory" phase of the cycle. Stromal edema occurs at the midportion of the secretory phase and is followed by the collection of predecidual cells around the spiral arterioles.

Increased secretion of progesterone by the corpus luteum is probably responsible for the disintegration of that structure beginning about day 22 or 23 of the cycle. Progesterone has the ability to augment the conversion of estradiol to estrone and estrone to estriol and thus inhibits the formation of oxidation products of estrogen. It has been postulated by the Smiths that these oxidative products of estrogen (and not unchanged estrogen) are responsible for the release of LH and LTH. It becomes evident, then, that as the oxidative products diminish, LH and LTH are reduced and the corpus luteum begins to disintegrate with a resultant reduction in estrogen and progesterone secretion. Thus the support of the endometrium is withdrawn and within a few days bleeding—menstruation—occurs from the secretory endometrium.

The changes which take place in the endometrium have been studied by Markee in his classic experiments on transplanting monkey endometrium to the anterior chamber of the eye and observing the physiologic process with a dissecting microscope. He found that, following estrogen-progesterone withdrawal, the spiral arterioles underwent a process of constriction followed by dilatation. In addition, the number of capillaries supplying blood to the stroma decreases and the flow rate through these capillaries diminishes sharply. This is followed by a decrease in the total mass of endometrium with resultant increased stromal density. Shrinkage of the stroma withdraws lateral support from the coiled arterioles, causing them to buckle, and stasis results. This stasis is apparently caused by the increased resistance to flow resulting from the increased coiling of the arterioles. Stasis leads to diminished oxygenation of tissue with secondary necrosis. Tissue necrosis results in the production of *necrosin* which brings about constriction of the undegenerated part of the coiled arterioles. Vasoconstriction begins slowly, then one coiled artery after another contracts during a one- to five-hour period, until all of those in a particular transplant show constriction. This period of vasoconstriction precedes every menstrual period and always starts four to 24 hours before the onset of bleeding. When the amount of necrosin is reduced through diffusion, the coiled arteriole relaxes and hemorrhage occurs. Bleeding follows and continues as long as circulation through these arteries persists. These minute hemorrhages coalesce and grow and gradually effect a sloughing of the functional layer. The resultant endometrial slough, mucous secretion and glands, together with the focal areas of hemorrhage, constitute the menstrual discharge.

Dating the Endometrium

Specific changes occurring in the stromal and glandular elements of the endometrium during the menstrual cycle have been of interest to both pathologist and clinician. By close scrutiny of these changes it has been possible to "date" the endometrium (within a range of about 48 hours), particularly in the postovulatory phase of the cycle. This correlation between the date of the cycle and the histologic appearance of the endometrium has particular importance in the study of the infertile patient. For purposes of simplicity a 28-day cycle, with ovulation occurring on the fourteenth day, will be described. The first day of the menstrual period will be considered the first day of the cycle, with the menstrual flow lasting four days. The *proliferative* phase of the cycle then begins at the termination of the *menstrual* phase. The postovulatory phase or *secretory* phase in this cycle extends from day 14 to day 28. Thus it is evident that the proliferative phase may persist for an indefinite period but the secretory phase is a constant 14 (±2) days. It should be remembered that the changes to be described occur only in the functional layers of the endometrium and not in the basal layer or in the lower uterine segment. Biopsies of the endometrium therefore have significance only if an adequate amount of functional endometrium is obtained. It is recognized that all parts of the endometrium do not undergo simultaneous change since the tissue responsiveness may vary, depending on blood supply, adjacent leiomyomas, etc. However, in the normal cycle an approximation of dating within 48 hours is frequently of considerable help.

Proliferative Phase.—Under the stimulation of estrogen, the endometrium gradually rebuilds its substance. The *early* proliferative phase extends from the fourth through the seventh days, the *middle* proliferative phase extends from day 8 through day 10 and the *late* proliferative phase lasts from day 11 until the time of ovulation on day 14 (Fig. 5–13). The characteristic histologic pattern of each phase is as follows (modified after Noyes, Hertig and Rock):

Early proliferative phase (Fig. 5–14).—Glands: short, narrow, with mitotic activity (some glands remaining from menstrual phase may show secretory exhaustion). Surface epithelium: regenerating between openings of glands. Stroma: compact, few mitoses, cells stellate or spindle-shaped with scanty cytoplasm; nucleus large.

MIDDLE PROLIFERATIVE PHASE (Fig. 5–15).—Glands: longer with slight curved effect; beginning pseudostratification of nuclei (nuclei appear superimposed in layers but actually all cells are attached at same level). Stroma: edema of variable degree; numerous mitotic figures; scanty cytoplasm and edema gives "naked nucleus" effect. Surface epithelium: covered with columnar epithelium.

LATE PROLIFERATIVE PHASE (Fig. 5–16).—Glands: tortuous as a result of active growth; numerous mitoses; pseudostratification of nuclei. Stroma: dense with active growth pattern and numerous mitoses.

Fig. 5–13.—Changes in various morphologic features utilized in dating the endometrium graphed according to their appearance and disappearance during the menstrual cycle. (From Noyes, R. W.; Hertig, A. T., and Rock, J.: Fertil. & Steril. 1:3, 1950.)

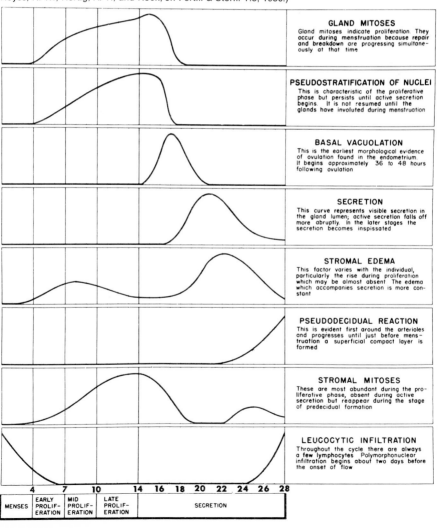

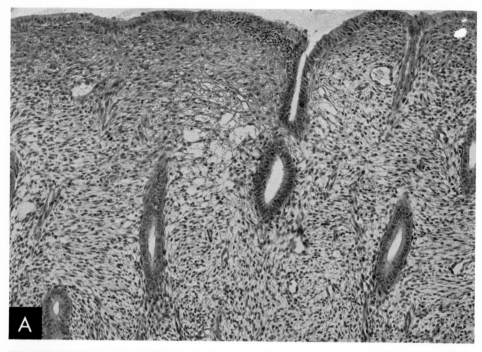

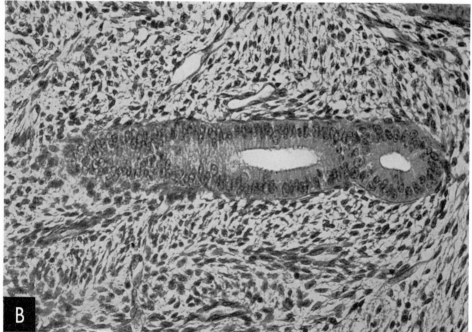

Fig. 5–14.—Early proliferative endometrium. **A,** surface epithelium thin; glands sparse, narrow and straight. **B,** few mitoses in glands and stroma; little pseudostratification of gland nuclei.

(Figures 5–14 to 5–24 from Noyes, R. W.; Hertig, A. T., and Rock, J.: Fertil. & Steril. 1:3, 1950. Low-power photomicrographs are all magnified ×150; high power, ×400.)

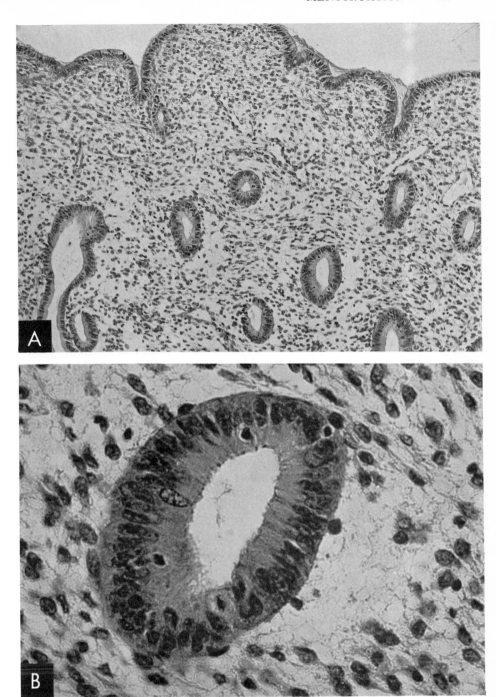

Fig. 5–15.—Endometrium showing intermediate degree of proliferation. **A,** glands slightly tortuous; tall columnar surface epithelium. Extracellular fluid is not always as marked as in this section. **B,** glands show numerous mitoses with pseudostratification becoming marked. Note the "naked nucleus" type of stromal cell with fine anastomosing processes.

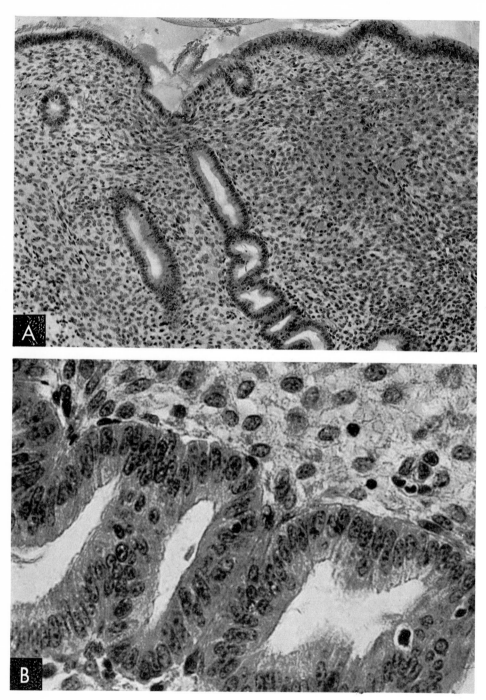

Fig. 5–16.—Late proliferative endometrium. **A,** glands tortuous; stroma usually quite dense. **B,** epithelial nuclei are pseudostratified and oval in shape.

Secretory Phase.—The changes after ovulation are due to the effects of estrogen and progesterone on an endometrium previously stimulated or "primed" with estrogen. As previously mentioned, this phase lasts about 14 days, the first seven of which are characterized by typical changes in the glandular epithelium. During the last seven days specific stromal changes occur which may be utilized for dating purposes.

15th day.—This is essentially a late proliferative pattern except for occasional vacuoles below the nuclei of the glands.

16th day (Fig. 5–17).—Basal vacuoles are seen in most glands; last day of pseudostratification; mitoses in glands and stroma.

17th day (Fig. 5–18).—Characteristic pattern of subnuclear glycogen vacuoles is evident, with homogeneous cytoplasm above nuclei of glands; position of nuclei rather regular; loss of pseudostratification of cells, with increase in diameter and tortuosity; mitotic figures in glands and stroma rare.

18th day (Fig. 5–19).—Subnuclear vacuoles appear smaller as nuclei move back toward base of cell; beginning secretion of glycogen into lumen of gland; no mitoses.

19th day—Few subnuclear vacuoles are seen; resembles day 16 pattern except for secretion in lumen of gland and absence of pseudostratification and mitoses.

20th day (Fig. 5–20).—Occasional subnuclear vacuoles; acidophilic secretion is prominent in gland lumen.

21st day.—Beginning stromal effects: cells of stroma have dark, dense nuclei with filamentous cytoplasm; beginning stromal edema.

22d day (Fig. 5–21).—Maximum point of stromal edema; thin-walled spiral arterioles may be seen. Secretion in gland lumen is active but subsiding and undergoing inspissation.

23d day (Fig. 5–22).—Edema of stroma persists but characteristic change is a condensation of the stroma around the spiral arterioles. This is due to an enlargement of stromal nuclei with an increase in cytoplasm and is called *predecidual* change.

24th day (Fig. 5–23).—Predecidual collections surrounding arterioles are marked; active stromal mitoses but lessening of stromal edema. The endometrium is now beginning to undergo involution unless maintained by pregnancy.

25th day (Fig. 5–24).—Predecidua is forming beneath the surface epithelium, and there is some edema around the arterioles; beginning lymphocytic infiltration of the stroma.

26th day.—Gradual increase in predecidua is seen throughout stroma, with infiltration of polymorphonuclear leukocytes.

27th day.—Predecidua is prominent around blood vessels and under surface epithelium; marked infiltration of polymorphonuclear leukocytes.

28th day.—There is beginning focal necrosis of the predecidua with small areas of stromal hemorrhage. Stromal cells are clumped together; extensive polymorphonuclear leukocytic infiltration. Tortuous glands appear to have undergone secretory "exhaustion."

Certain specific changes in glands and stroma may be considered to indicate physiologic changes occurring in the endometrium. Thus, *gland mitoses* indicate active proliferation and growth and may be found from day 3 or 4 of the cycle until day 16 or 17. *Pseudostratification* of gland

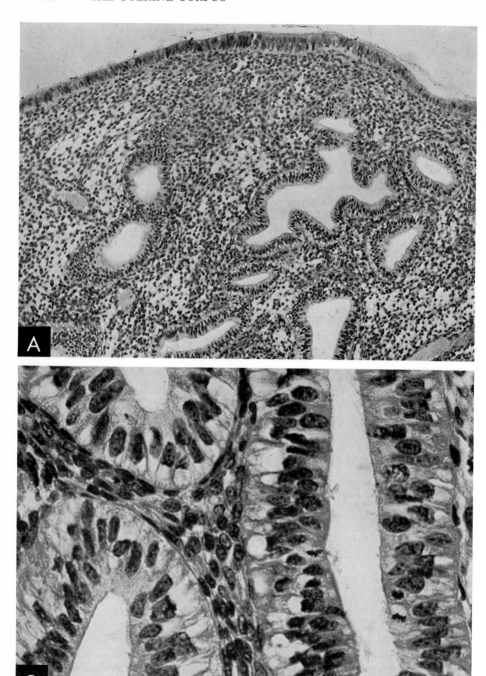

Fig. 5–17.—Second postovulatory day. **A,** glands tortuous; stroma dense; cells consisting of nearly naked nuclei. **B,** gland mitoses very numerous; pseudostratification of nuclei exaggerated by subnuclear vacuoles.

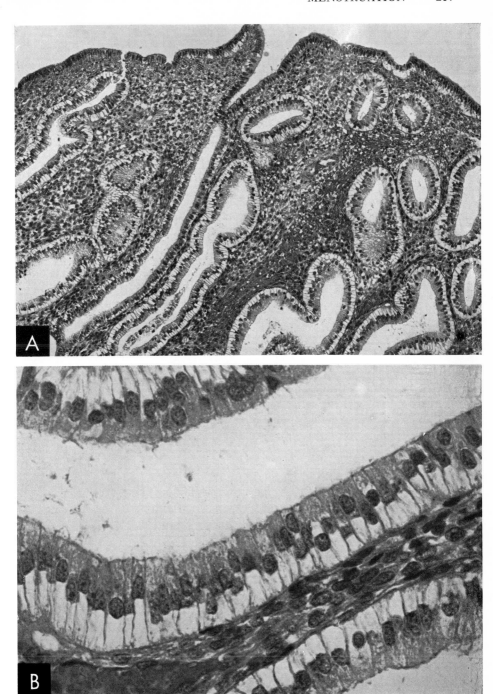

Fig. 5-18.—Third postovulatory day. **A,** gland nuclei are pushed to the center of the epithelial cells with cytoplasm above and vacuoles below them. **B,** gland mitoses rare; pseudostratification decreasing.

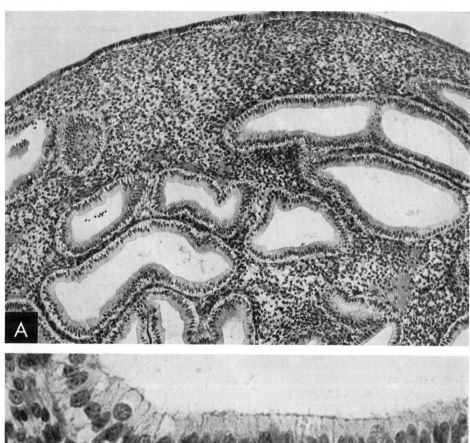

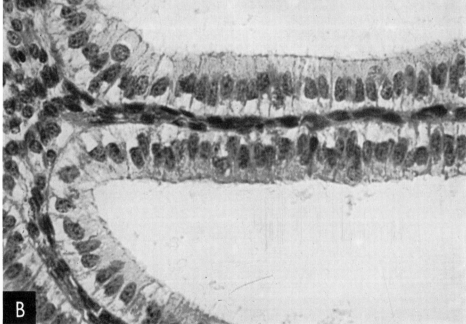

Fig. 5–19.—Fourth postovulatory day. **A,** gland nuclei are returning to base of cells. Wisps of secretory material are present in lumina. **B,** some vacuoles are pushed past the nucleus on their way to empty glycogen into the lumen. Mitoses and pseudostratification of nuclei absent. This is the stage of arrival of ovum in the uterus.

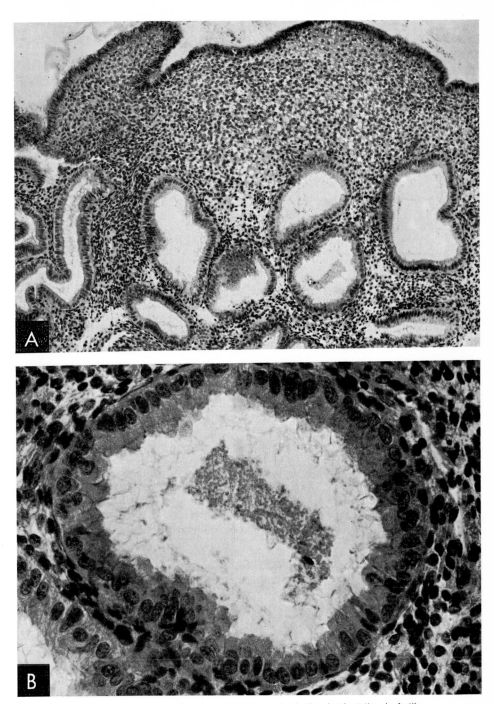

Fig. 5–20.—Sixth postovulatory day, corresponding to beginning implantation in fertile cycle. **A,** secretion in gland lumen at peak; beginning of accumulation of extravascular fluid in stroma. **B,** subnuclear vacuoles rare; nuclei round and basally located.

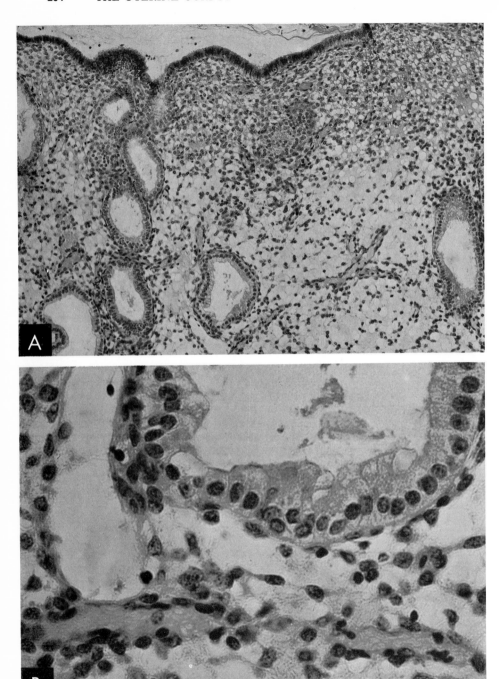

Fig. 5–21.—Eighth postovulatory day. **A,** extracellular fluid maximal. Walls of spiral arterioles are not prominent. **B,** stromal cells still appear as small dense "naked nuclei" widely separated by extracellular fluid. Glandular secretion still active but subsiding.

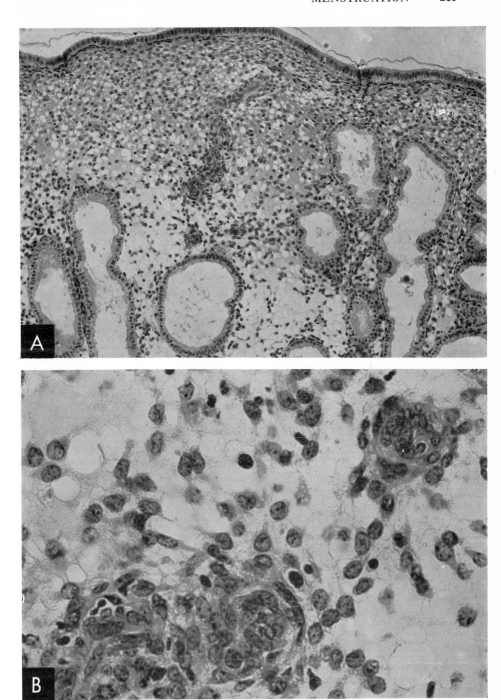

Fig. 5–22.—Ninth postovulatory day. **A,** spiral arterioles become prominent due to condensation of surrounding stroma. **B,** both nuclei and cytoplasm of periarteriolar stromal cells are enlarging. This is the earliest predecidual reaction.

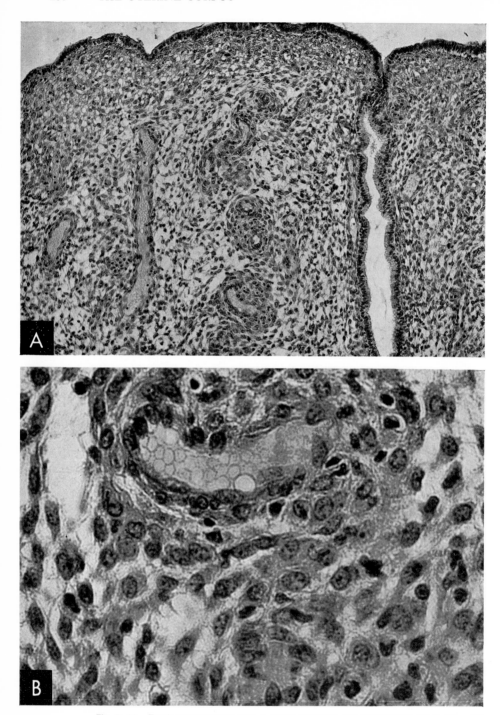

Fig. 5–23.—Tenth postovulatory day. **A,** spiral arterioles and surrounding predecidua still more prominent; extracellular fluid subsiding. **B,** thickening of periarteriolar predecidual cuff; stromal mitosis evident.

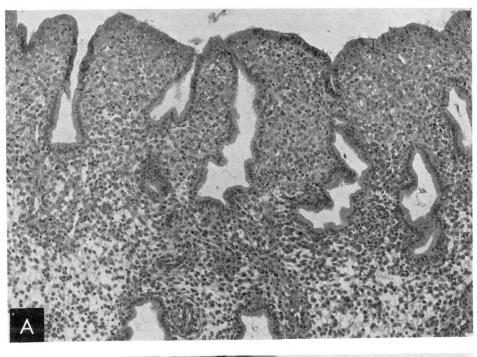

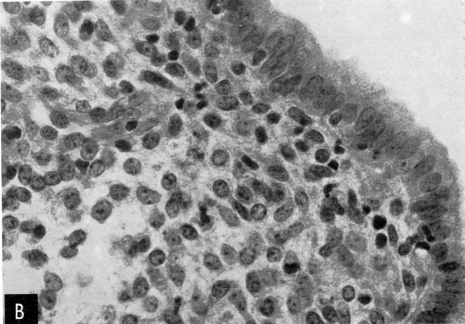

Fig. 5-24.—Eleventh postovulatory day. **A,** pseudodecidua begins to differentiate under surface epithelium. Stroma of the stratum spongiosum still contains extracellular fluid except in areas near a spiral arteriole. **B,** round cell infiltration accompanies predecidual differentiation. Stromal cells swell to become predecidual in type.

nuclei begins after the postmenstrual involution and usually disappears by day 17. It is an indication of proliferative glandular growth and its appearance is due to crowding of nuclei when the gland is sectioned transversely. *Basal vacuolation* is the earliest morphologic evidence of ovulation discernible in the endometrium. Although occasionally one may be seen in the absence of progesterone, basal vacuoles are usually identified between day 15 and day 19, the glycogen being pushed into the gland lumen about day 19 or 20. The characteristic lining up of the nuclei above the vacuoles is best seen on day 17 and is an excellent indication of recent ovulation.

The secretory function of the glands is evident from day 18 until day 22 by the appearance of loose, feathery material in the lumina. If the blastocyst implants itself on the surface of the endometrium about six days after ovulation it would appear that morphology and function were well correlated, since days 20 to 22 would be critical ones from the standpoint of nutrient materials. The *edema* of the stroma, most striking between days 22 and 23, may represent an effort of the endometrium to simplify the implantation process by lessening tissue resistance. Periarterial *predecidual reaction* is evident beginning about days 23 and 24 and may represent a protective mechanism against premature vascular disruption. The predecidua is looked on as providing a supporting framework for newly developed blood vessels to aid in their increased load should pregnancy supervene. These changes in morphologic features are graphically summarized in Figure 5–13.

SYSTEMIC CHANGES ASSOCIATED WITH THE MENSTRUAL CYCLE

Certain phases of water and electrolyte balance occurring during the menstrual cycle have been studied using I^{131} isotope-dilution technics which measure total exchangeable body sodium. No evidence of a cyclic change in sodium balance or sodium retention was found in these experiments. This is at variance with previously accepted ideas of premenstrual sodium and water retention which have been correlated with the syndrome of premenstrual tension. In other studies estrogenic substances have been shown to cause a *limited* storage of sodium and chloride together with an increase in the volume of extracellular fluid. A direct effect of estrogen on renal tubular reabsorption is believed to be the mechanism of this storage. Cyclic premenstrual edema in some individuals may represent a form of secondary aldosteronism. Antidiuretic hormone shows no variation during the menstrual cycle, and progesterone has been shown in castrate animals to increase urinary output.

The hematocrit declines and blood volume increases slightly at the end of menstruation. Plasma ester cholesterol diminishes at the time of ovulation and immediately before menstruation. The eosinophil count drops at the time of ovulation, with total counts being lower in the luteal than in the follicular phase.

Certain clinical correlations have been made by Rogers between diseases and menstruation. Thus, it has been noted that appendicitis rarely occurs during menses, whereas about three-fourths of women who contract poliomyelitis do so a few days postmenstrually. Porphyria may show an exacerbation at the time of menstrual flow and may be brought on by exogenous progesterone. Epistaxis, nasal hyperemia, sinusitis, rhinorrhea, asthmatic bronchitis and epilepsy have been noted as being brought on or worsened by menstruation. Several studies in penal institutions have shown that women in the childbearing age committed major crimes, including murder, most frequently during the premenstrual phase. Most females in this age group who attempt suicide do so during the postovulatory phase of the cycle.

The effects of impaired nutrition on the menstrual cycle, with the development of amenorrhea, have been observed and studied extensively. As a direct result of a diminished caloric intake, a lowering of FSH excretion is first observed, with subsequent hypothyroidism and hypoadrenocorticism. Although the release of gonadotropins into the circulation is restricted, the gonadotropic-hormone content of the adenohypophysis is normal or even increased. Obesity is similarly associated with abnormalities of menstruation, particularly amenorrhea, and weight reduction appears to effect resumption of normal menses in about half the patients. It has been suggested that both obesity and amenorrhea are symptoms of emotional disease that respond simultaneously to psychotherapy. It is also possible, however, that obesity is similar to inanition, both resulting in a diminished secretion of gonadotropin.

The Thyroid.—Disturbances of menstrual function may be associated with aberration of thyroid metabolism although the precise pathophysiologic mechanisms are unknown. Thyrotoxic females may have perfectly normal menstrual cycles but, if untreated, may progress to states of oligomenorrhea and amenorrhea. Observations in the rabbit have indicated that thyroid hormone decreases FSH content and increases LH content of the pituitary, a possible explanation for the amenorrhea. In states of severe hypothyroidism, such as myxedema, variations of dysfunctional uterine bleeding may occur, with the development of subsequent endometrial hyperplasia. The administration of thyroid hormone to such patients will usually result in normal ovulatory cycles. The anovulation of myxedema may result from persistent FSH stimulation without the interplay of LH since, in thyroidectomized animals, estrogen is not effective in suppressing pituitary activity. When, however, thyroid is administered, FSH is diminished and LH is increased.

This effect of hypothyroidism, i.e., anovulatory ovarian function, is of great clinical significance since a number of important gynecologic problems may be associated with it. Amenorrhea, oligomenorrhea and hyper- and polymenorrhea have all been associated with anovulatory ovarian activity. Obviously, ovulatory failure also leads to infertility.

The gynecologist's investigation of the cause of menstrual dysfunction should always include a thorough evaluation of thyroid function. In the true hypothyroid patient replacement therapy produces very dramatic results. However, such patients are rarely seen in gynecology. More often the gynecologist is confronted with a patient complaining of menstrual dysfunction with only minimal symptoms of thyroid deficiency and laboratory findings that are somewhat equivocal. In such instances a so-called trial course of thyroid medication is often used. If the patient's gynecologic problem does not improve, the conclusion should not be drawn that she did not require thyroid medication. If the anovulatory pattern has not reached an irreversible stage, restoration of normal menstrual cycles may follow treatment. This appears to occur more often in the younger patient or where the dysfunction has existed for a relatively short time. On the other hand, if anovulatory ovarian function has existed for months or years, an irreversible stage of polycystic ovarian disease may develop. In such cases thyroid medication may improve the general health of the patient but have little or no effect on the menstrual dysfunction.

Other experiments have suggested that thyroid may have a peripheral effect in decreasing the sensitivity of the ovary to the effects of adenohypophyseal hormones. The fine balance of such relationships has been reflected in the age-old custom of administering thyroid hormone to women who had noted irregularities of menstruation, infertility, or both. Recent controlled investigations in euthyroid subjects have proved the fallacy of this reasoning, so that at present there is no valid reason for giving thyroid preparations to such patients.

The Adrenal.—It has been known for some time that the adrenal gland played an integral part in the process of menstruation, and it was demonstrated recently in adrenalectomized rats that exogenously administered gonadotropins evoked no ovarian response. Gray and associates studied the aldosterone secretion rates, excretion of pregnanediol and urinary sodium/postassium ratio during the menstrual cycle of 13 normal women. They found the mean value of aldosterone secretion to be 140 μg. during the follicular phase and 233 μg. per day during the luteal phase. This increase in the aldosterone secretion rate during the luteal phase was observed in subjects taking a diet unrestricted in sodium, as well as in subjects with a controlled high sodium intake. When ovulation was suppressed with an estrogen-progestin combination, the rise in aldosterone secretion observed during the second half of the cycle was abolished.

Clinical evidence is seen in patients with Addison's disease who have persistent amenorrhea. Similarly, in the adrenogenital syndrome amenorrhea is a common symptom, and it has been postulated that the cause is an increased secretion of adrenal androgens and estrogens which suppress the formation and secretion of adenohypophyseal gonadotropins. In such patients the administration of cortisone (or cortisone-like preparations) depresses ACTH production and results in a diminution of secretion of adrenal androgens and estrogens with increased secretion of FSH and LH. Ovulation and menstruation subsequently occur. The basic defect in this situation is thought to be an enzyme insufficiency in the adrenal zona reticularis, whereby there is a failure of hydroxylation of the 11 and 21 positions of a C^{21} steroid. Thus, instead of formation of 17-hydroxycorticosterone there is produced an excess of 17-hyroxyprogesterone. Metabolites of 17-hydroxyprogesterone are not only androgenic (androsterone and etiocholanolone) but are unable to inhibit ACTH. There is thus set up a vicious circle, with further stimulation of the adrenal to produce more 17-hydroxyprogesterone. Cortisone inhibits the production of ACTH and removes the stimulus for the basic hyperplasia.

The Liver.—The liver is known to be an important site for the inactivation of estrogenic hormone. Thus, in animals estrus may be prevented by transplanting the ovaries into the mesentery or spleen. Estrogens are conjugated in the liver and apparently thereby inactivated. Progesterone is probably also similarly inactivated. Certain endocrine changes occurring in the premenopausal female with liver disease have therefore been attributed to delayed or incomplete estrogen deactivation. These are hypermenorrhea, polymenorrhea, endometrial hyperplasia, spider angiomas and palmar erythema. Whether these are brought about by a specific vitamin B deficiency of the liver or by the effects of concomitant inanition has not been determined. In any event, administration of riboflavin, thiamine, protein or a nutritious diet will frequently bring about clinical improvement in the symptoms of estrogen derangement.

Diabetes Mellitus.—Although diabetes mellitus in the adult female may cause oligomenorrhea, amenorrhea, diminished libido and infertility, the introduction and proper use of insulin has made these symptoms relatively uncommon. Menstruation has been noted to aggravate existing diabetes and several reports have pointed out the relation of the menstrual period to an increased incidence of acidosis. This may be due to lowered levels of estrogen. Diabetes occurring before and during the menopause has been shown to improve following the administration of estrogen. The author has noted this clinically in postmenopausal diabetic patients who were given large amounts of diethylstilbestrol because of disseminated mammary carcinoma. Animal experiments lend supporting evidence, in that diabetes induced in rats by subtotal pancreatectomy is made worse by oophorectomy. The mechanism by which estrogens improve diabetes is not known but two suggestions have been advanced. (1) Estrogen suppresses the growth hormone of the pituitary; (2) estrogen stimulates the islands of Langerhans to hypertrophy and hyperplasia. Progesterone or depo-medroxy-progesterone acetate, however, when administered to patients with disseminated endometrial carcinoma has been noted to increase the severity of diabetes and increase the need for insulin. Clomiphene citrate, however, when administered to similar patients has been noted to diminish the need for insulin.

Nervous System.—Epileptic seizures are more common at the time of the menses and serial electroencephalograms have demonstrated increased cortical instability at this time. Recent studies of body water and sodium have negated a long-held idea that this increased convulsive tendency was due to salt and water retention. Seizures are uncommon during the luteal phase and the increased incidence just before, during and after menstruation may be due to a lessened secretion of progesterone with its anticonvulsive effect. Migraine headaches may occur in association with the menses and are commonly relieved by periods of induced anovulation or by pregnancy. It has been suggested that the occurrence of migraine at the time of the menses is related to premenstrual retention of salt and water but recent studies indicate no correlation between fluid retention and headache. The suppression of ovulation by estrogen-progestin combinations in the oral contraceptives does not protect against migraine and some patients note aggravation of migraine subsequent to their use. The evidence suggests that the attack is related to *variations* in the levels of estrogen and progesterone rather than to excesses since the migraine headache seems to appear more frequently during the period when the oral contraceptive is *not* being taken. When these compounds are administered constantly, as in pseudopregnancy for endometriosis, migraine attacks are uncommon. Similarly, the use of a small amount of a synthetic progestin, administered constantly in a dose insufficient to suppress ovulation, is not attended by migraine attacks in women who experienced headache when the estrogen-progestin were used. This suggests an anti-estrogenic effect of the progestin on the cerebral vessels and there is evidence that a typical migraine attack may be initiated by the injection of estrogen in previously oophorectomized or postmenopausal females.

The Skin.—Acne vulgaris has been noted to become aggravated premenstrually, especially in adolescents. This is thought to be due to lowered estrogen and increased skin sebum. Improvement is frequently obtained by the administration of estrogenic substances. Chronic ulcerative vulvitis and stomatitis may relate to the menstrual cycle and mouth lesions such as Vincent's angina, aphthous stomatitis and pyorrhea alveolaris have been reported to be exaggerated premenstrually. Increased pigmentation of the skin around the eyes, nipples, and perioral area may be noted during the week prior to menstruation, an effect of variations in the release of melanocyte-stimulating hormone from the pituitary.

The Blood.—Thrombocytopenic purpura may be first evidenced by excessive uterine bleeding at the time of the menses. This is due to the rapid diminution in platelets and increased capillary fragility normally seen during the luteal phase of the cycle. Other blood dyscrasias which may result in hypermenorrhea are leukemia, erythrocytosis and pseudohemophilia. A simple screening method in the evaluation of patients with abnormal bleeding at the time of the menses is the performance of a blood smear, a platelet count and a determination of the bleeding time.

The Psyche.—Depression, irritability and occasionally aggression are commonly noted in the premenstrual phase of the cycle. Increased libidinous tendencies are frequently seen and crimes of violence committed by women are much commoner during this phase. These symptoms and the entity known as "premenstrual tension" have been attributed to progesterone deficiency, abnormal estrogen-progesterone relationship, abnormal sodium and water retention and abnormal psychodynamic processes. In the absence of a specific cause it is probably justified to consider these behavior patterns as abnormal manifestations of a normal physiologic process in susceptible or hyperreactive women.

Secondary amenorrhea is frequently psychogenic in origin and may be due to abnormalities of hypothalamic-adenohypophyseal function. Thus, LH may not be released or may not be sufficient to cause ovulation. Some patients with so-called hypothalamic amenorrhea may be resistant to exogenous estrogen and progesterone, suggesting a rapid neutralization or abnormal metabolism of these steroids. The gonadotropin excretion levels in psychotic patients have been found to be low, suggesting diminished pituitary function.

Hypermenorrhea may also occur in response to abnormal psychosomatic stimuli. Thus it may follow periods of depression, shock, anger, fright or similar stressful situations.

Uterine Retrodisplacement

The enthusiasm for surgical correction of uterine retrodisplacement so prevalent for many years has now abated. Gynecologists, especially those trained during the past decade, generally regard the operation as of no value. Many have completed recognized residencies without having performed a single suspension of the uterus. Similarly, the use of vaginal pessaries has received no more than token consideration.

We believe that there are certain patients with a particular symptom complex who may be helped by these simple gynecologic procedures. The selection of such a patient is difficult and necessitates taking a careful history and performing a meticulous examination, since studies in large gynecologic clinics have shown that approximately 20 per cent of women examined for gynecologic complaints have uterine retrodisplacement. In many, the malposition is asymptomatic and merely of statistical interest. In others, however, striking improvement may be brought about by an appreciation of a few principles of pelvic anatomy and physiology.

The intrinsic muscular tone of the uterus itself, together with its configuration and vascular status, may be causally related. The flabby, boggy uterus associated with the syndrome of pelvic congestion is frequently displaced posteriorly. The situation may be congenital—purely a physical derangement—incorporating a short anterior vaginal wall and an upward tilting of the cervix. The lateral cervical attachments (cardinal ligaments) are the main long axis support of the cervix and uterus. Weakening of these ligaments is probably the principal cause of prolapse, although the latter is almost always associated with some degree of retrodisplacement.

The round ligaments serve a definite function in retaining the normal anterior position of the uterus, although it is doubtful that they function alone. Even in severe retrodisplacement the round ligaments usually appear grossly normal. Given sufficient tension on the posterior aspect of the cervix by the uterorectosacral ligaments and normal intra-abdominal pressure on the posterior aspect of the fundus, the round ligaments aid in keeping the fundus anteflexed. Theoretically the round ligaments also function in the postpartum period of uterine involution to return the fundus to its anterior position. Similar function is presupposed after a full bladder has been emptied.

The uterorectosacral ligaments vary greatly in size, thickness and consistency, but serve a most important function in keeping the cervix directed posteriorly. When the combination of ligamentous support is deranged, either by physiologic changes such as pregnancy or by organic causes such as infection or endometriosis, retrodisplacement occurs.

Lastly, various tumors of the adnexa or bowel may displace the uterus from its normal position.

Uterine retrodisplacement may be considered under two general categories: (1) primary retrodisplacement which is associated with congenitally deficient supporting structures and/or a short anterior vaginal wall; (2) secondary retrodisplacement brought about by childbirth, pelvic infection, endometriosis or tumors.

Primary Retrodisplacement.—The uterus is always retrocessed and occasionally retroverted in infancy and childhood. At puberty it usually assumes an anteverted, anteflexed attitude, but when there are other stigmata of infantilism, such as a short anterior vaginal wall and short uterorectosacral ligaments, the uterus remains retroverted. Cases have been described of incomplete ovarian descent with shortening of the infundibulopelvic ligament and posterior pull on the uterus. Many nulliparous patients who undergo routine pelvic examinations have asymptomatic, retroverted uteri unassociated with pelvic pathology. In these women this may be a manifestation of a generalized diminution in intrinsic tissue tone as evidenced by renal and intestinal ptoses, leg and vulval varicosities, hemorrhoids, hernias and, occasionally, uterine prolapse.

Secondary Retrodisplacement (Ligamentous Relaxation).—As previously noted, secondary uterine retroversion is commonly associated with laxity of the pelvic supporting tissue, whether due to repeated childbirth or to vascular aberrations resulting in pelvic congestion. The rigors of pelvic delivery and the puerperium probably are the leading causes of secondary retroversion. Sustained hard physical work during the pregnancy and long hours without rest or support in the erect position early in the puerperium undoubtedly are contributing factors. Repeated pregnancies may cause a change in the normal musculature with an increasing amount of vasculature, subsequent congestion and, later, fibrosis. (Congenital factors must be considered as well, since many *grandes multiparas* have anteverted uteri.)

Postmenopausally this same uterine fibrosis occurs normally and results in atrophy and flaccidity. The uterus drops back and usually is found in the axis of the vagina—both anterior and posterior supports being, for the most part, inactive. The integrity of the cardinal ligaments and the pelvic diaphragm determines whether or not prolapse will occur at this stage.

Pathologic factors in retrodisplacement include endometriosis, pelvic infection and tumors. In endometriosis the uterus is not infrequently found in deep, fixed retroversion. This process, involving as it does the peritoneum of the cul-de-sac and uterosacral ligaments, frequently produces areas of scarring across the posterior aspect of the fundus. The rectal serosa occasionally is involved and the adnexa may be implicated, producing a fixed, tender pelvic mass. In a recent study of a large group of patients with pelvic endometriosis, uterine retrodisplacement was noted in 28 per cent.

The exudate of pelvic peritonitis may be etiologic in fixed retrodisplacement, since pelvic contour will cause such exudates to gravitate to the posterior cul-de-sac where organization and fibrosis occur. A large pyosalpinx is occasionally found anteriorly and adherent to the uterovesical space, with posterior displacement of the fundus. Postabortive, postpartum, tuberculous and gonorrheal infections are the major causes of such pelvic inflammation, although occasionally a ruptured appendix or diverticulum may produce the same situation.

Most adnexal tumors gravitate into the lateral pelvis or cul-de-sac and cause anterior rather than posterior displacement of the fundus. One exception to this is the dermoid cyst which frequently is found anterior to the broad ligament with the corpus posterior (Küstner's sign). Pedunculated uterine leiomyomas may reach sufficient size so that the fundus is displaced against the sacrum and may be independently palpated. Rarely, rectal carcinoma may force the cervix anteriorly with subsequent posterior displacement of the fundus.

The idea that retroversion of the uterus may be caused by falls, injuries or extensive athletic activity has generally been discarded by most gynecologists. Obviously, without a control examination before the accident or activity, conclusions would be hazardous.

Pathologic Physiology.—Following retrodisplacement of the uterine fundus, from whatever cause, vascular changes of great importance occur. The angles of entrance and exit of the uterine vessels are distorted, producing torsion and partial venous obstruction. The ovaries and tubes are drawn into a characteristic pelvic-wall prolapse attitude with increased pressure in the veins of the infundibulopelvic ligament. Laparotomy during the early puerperium strikingly reveals these changes, showing a large, congested, mottled, purple uterus, edematous tubes and varicosities of the veins of the broad ligament. Microscopically, the veins of the myometrium are dilated and congested.

The endometrium associated with symptomatic retroversion has not been studied extensively, but Derichsweiler noted edema and overfilling of the vessels of the mucosa. Taylor, in his study of pelvic vascular congestion and hyperemia, examined the endometrium in 17 cases. The findings were not unusual except for three cases of chronic endometritis. The ovaries are frequently involved, cystic degeneration being noted in more than physiologic degree. Cortical fibrosis has been described. Taylor noted ovarian edema and vascular engorgement with a tough, unyielding capsule. It has been suggested that long periods of congestion result in connective tissue hyperplasia of the ovarian cortex with subsequent interference with normal ovulation. In his study of 105 cases of chronic pelvic hyperemia and vascular congestion, Taylor noted retroversion of appreciable degree in one third of the cases. However, Cotte, by Lipiodol injection, demonstrated a reduction in uterine size following suspension of an enlarged, retroverted, congested uterus, so that there is adequate evidence for believing many of the changes are due to position alone.

Symptomatology.—Probably the most common symptom noted by patients with acquired retrodisplacement is sacral backache, although it should be noted at the outset that retroversion frequently causes no symptoms whatsoever. Why this should be so is not clear. Variations in pain threshold, mental tension and degrees of vascular abnormalities have been suggested as factors, but actually the physiopathology of this pain has not been adequately explained. In several series of cases of uterine retroversion the incidence of central, sacral backache has varied from 50 to 75 per cent. Backache usually is aggravated by long hours in the erect position and commonly is worse in the late afternoon and evening. A backache that is noted in the morning and that seems to lessen as the patient goes about her housework probably is not caused by uterine malposition.

Many women complain of pelvic pressure or a bearing-down feeling and are unable to delineate their discomfort further. Occasionally lower quadrant pain is noted or the patient describes a "soreness in the ovaries." About half the patients with symptomatic retrodisplacement describe definite aggravation of their difficulties just before or at the time of the menstrual period. The premenstrual tension syndrome is common. Irregularities of menstrual flow, increased flow at time of periods with passage of clots, constipation and leukorrhea may be associated with this syndrome. The leukorrhea is often due to an untreated cervical ectropion. Retroversion has been described as an etiologic factor in abortion, and King in an analysis of a large series of cases of spontaneous abortion found this statistically valid. Although retroversion is found in an appreciable number of cases of infertility, no conclusive evidence exists to support the idea that it is the position of the uterus which has prevented conception. The necessity for the cervix to "dip" into the seminal pool has received extensive consideration, but is apparently of minimum importance. Conception occurs whether the cervix is behind the symphysis, deep in the vault, or angulated forward or backward. As long as a film of seminal fluid with effective spermatozoa is placed across the os uteri, ascent into the uterine cavity will occur.

Treatment.—At the time of pelvic examination the ease with which the retroverted uterus may be replaced is usually determined. Frequently replacement may be accomplished by simple bimanual examination, exerting sufficient force against the cervix to lift the fundus with the abdominal hand. If replacement is not easy, strenuous efforts should not be exerted. The presence of pelvic infection, tumors or endometriosis, of course, contraindicates further palliative measures and necessitates surgical correction. Frequently the uterus is soft and boggy and the vagina tender. These patients are instructed in a course of pelvic depletion. This consists of daily, hot, 15-minute douches, sitz baths and knee-chest exercises for three or four weeks. At the end of this time replacement of the uterus usually is simplified, although occasionally it is necessary to use the tenaculum method of reposition. Should these methods prove unsuccessful,

Fig. 5–25.—Third-degree retroversion of the uterus replaced and held anteriorly by a Smith-Hodge pessary.

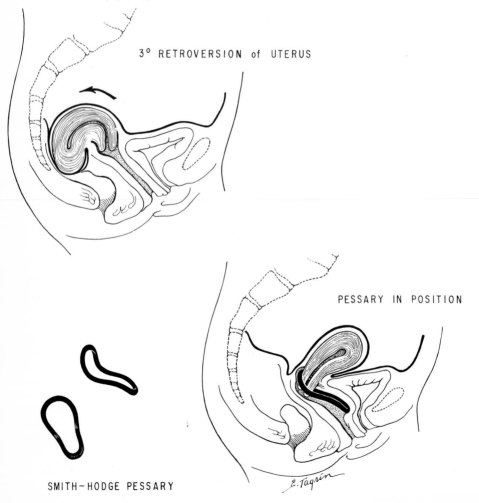

3° RETROVERSION of UTERUS

PESSARY IN POSITION

SMITH-HODGE PESSARY

E. Tagrin

correct positioning may be accomplished by inserting a pessary and then having the patient assume the knee-chest position. In this way air opens the vagina, and intravaginal manipulation can be used to replace the uterus and obtain a good application of the pessary. We have routinely used the Smith-Hodge or Hodge hard rubber pessary to correct retrodisplacement (Fig. 5–25.)

It is in the group of patients with "married woman's complaint" that marked symptomatic improvement may be expected. Such a patient is typically a hardworking housewife of moderate parity with one or more children under 4 years of age. Her complaints are those of backache, heaviness in the pelvis, aching thighs, vaginal discharge, chronic fatigue and dyspareunia. Cervical cauterization may be necessary in certain cases after adequate cytologic and biopsy studies. The pessary is kept in place for five to six months with monthly examination, removal and reinsertion. At the end of this time it may be removed and the patient observed for an additional two months. If symptoms recur and the fundus is again retroverted, re-treatment with a pessary may be tried. Uterine suspension occasionally may be considered, but is rarely indicated in this group of patients or as a primary surgical procedure. It is usually performed as part of a conservative laparotomy for infertility, endometriosis or the Stein-Leventhal syndrome. The use of estrogen-progestin combinations, particularly those containing a potent androgenic progestin with only 50 μg. of estrogen, has simplified the management of "married woman's complaint." After two or three cycles of therapy symptomatic improvement is usually noted. If the discomfort is exaggerated while taking these agents, adenomyosis or endometriosis should be suspected.

Infections

Infections of the uterine corpus are, for the most part, infections of the endometrium and are encompassed in the broad term *endometritis*. The most common etiologic factors are infected, usually criminal, abortions, parturition, gonorrhea and tuberculosis. Certain office gynecologic procedures may occasionally be followed by endometrial infection. These include biopsy and cauterization of the cervix, endometrial biopsy, hysterosalpingography and tubal insufflation. The use of a stem pessary for dysmenorrhea or insertion of gauze or radium into the uterine cavity may be followed by an acute or chronic endometrial inflammatory reaction. Cervical stenosis subsequent to conization, cauterization or irradiation may diminish or prohibit uterine drainage and be a predisposing factor in the etiology of pyometra.

Postabortal Infection

The most serious, and occasionally fatal, type of endometrial infection is that associated with a criminal abortion. The pathogenesis in this entity consists in the introduction of pathogenic bacteria into the uterine cavity by a catheter, bougie, sound, curet or pack. The conceptus and its coverings provide an ideal culture for growth of organisms, and the increased vascularity brought about by pregnancy permits rapid and widespread dissemination. The most common bacteria identified from cultures are the nonhemolytic, anaerobic streptococci, enterococci (Esch. coli, Pseudomonas aeruginosa, Aerobacter aerogenes) and Clostridium welchii. In the past few years, however, an increasing number of pathogenic staphylococci have been identified. These are presumably secondary invaders which follow preliminary control of the original organism by antibiotics. The pathologic process usually begins as a necrotizing endometritis and deciduitis at the placental site with spread along the decidua and into the myometrium. Microscopically there is an acute inflammatory exudate, the decidua contains leukocytes and plasma cells, and there are extensive necrosis and thrombosis of small vessels. The inflammatory process may extend into the myometrium, forming multiple small abscesses, and dissemination into small veins and lymphatics may be extensive. The myometrium appears pale and flabby and microscopically shows cytolysis and edema.

The symptoms of an infected abortion are severe, rather constant but occasionally crampy, pelvic pain, vaginal bleeding, chills and prostration. A history of one or more missed menses may be obtained, but rarely, if ever, is the historian rewarded by being informed that a criminal abortion has been performed. Examination reveals evidence of pelvic peritonitis with lower abdominal rigidity and rebound tenderness. The abdomen is usually distended due to ileus, and bowel sounds are hypoactive. Pelvic examination may disclose a foreign body (catheter or pack) in a cervical os which is soft and patulous. Occasionally necrotic decidua or membranes may be visualized coming through the cervix. The uterus is enlarged, soft and acutely tender and the broad ligaments feel thickened in the acute phase and ligneous in later phases of the process. The temperature is elevated, usually over 101 F., and there is tachycardia, leukocytosis and a moderate anemia.

In certain severe cases sudden hypotension occurs in the absence of blood loss and may rapidly result in death. The probable cause is the introduction of anaerobic, gram-negative organisms into the blood stream following a decidual and placental bacteremia. These bacteria are capable, under such circumstances, of liberating a potent endotoxin which possesses profound hemodynamic effects. The method of shock here has not been adequately explained but is probably correlated with a diminished peripheral resistance with visceral "pooling" and vascular sludging, together with a decreased cardiac output. Death may occur suddenly from shock or later from renal insufficiency.

Treatment.—Treatment of infected abortion cannot be didactically outlined—each case must be individually assayed. In general, however, the patient must be kept at complete bed rest and adequate hydration provided by intravenous fluids. Electrolyte balance should be maintained and anemia corrected by transfusions of whole blood. Culture specimens should be taken from the endocervix and from the blood and antibiotics administered in adequate dosage depending on sensitivity. Anaerobic cultures should be made to rule out Cl. welchii or anaerobic streptococci. It is our policy to give 2 Gm. of either tetracycline or chloramphenicol intravenously during the first 24 hours. This therapy is maintained until the drug can be taken orally but is changed if the sensitivities indicate that another antibiotic is preferable. The patient is kept in a mid- or high Fowler's position to promote the collection of pus in the posterior cul-de-sac. Repeated pelvic examinations are contraindicated; the patient's course may be followed by changes in temperature, pulse, sedimentation rate and white cell count. Adequate analgesia and sedation should be provided especially during the first 72 hours of illness. After five or six days, occasionally earlier, pelvic examination should be repeated in order to determine whether pus is localized in the posterior cul-de-sac. If so, it may be easily drained by posterior colpotomy. Postabortal infections usually spread laterally in the parametrial lymphatics, forming the typical "pelvic cellulitis," and in this way differ from gonorrheal infections. The latter frequently develop into tubo-ovarian abscesses which fill the cul-de-sac and make vaginal drainage quite easy and thus expedite convalescence. Postabortal phlegmons may occasionally form between the leaves of the broad ligament and then point above Poupart's ligament. These may be drained extraperitoneally, greatly aiding in resolution of the septic process. In long-standing cases of postabortal infection a thrombophlebitis of the pelvic veins may develop, with subsequent septic emboli. The diagnosis of this complication is difficult, but rapid and occasionally heroic treatment is necessary. Some authors suggest immediate ligation of the vena cava and infundibulopelvic veins and cite a low mortality rate and minimal morbidity with this procedure. In patients with seemingly irreversible shock, hysterectomy offers the only hope of salvage. Less radical treatment consists of complete and rapid anticoagulation and the use of antibiotics. Should embolization occur while the patient is on anticoagulant drugs, caval ligation remains as a life-saving procedure.

Anderson has noted a reduced mortality rate at the Los Angeles County General Hospital in patients with septic abortion since adoption of an aggressive therapeutic program. The regimen consists of massive doses of antibiotics, early curettage and administration of cortisone. Steroid therapy has replaced the use of vasopressors in patients exhibiting hypotension, since observations in animals showed that the highest mortality rate in endotoxemic shock occurred in animals treated with blood-pressure-raising agents.

The criteria for beginning antibiotic treatment are: (1) purulent material protruding through the cervix; (2) history of instrumentation; (3) signs of sepsis with no extrauterine source, and (4) shock out of proportion to blood loss. When the diagnosis is made, chloramphenicol, usually 500 mg., is given intravenously, followed by 1 Gm. in each liter of fluid given, so that 4 Gm. is given within a 24-hour period. Curettage is done immediately after the first injection. If shock is present or impending, 250 mg. of hydrocortisone is given. During the next 24 hours, 500 mg. of hydrocortisone is given in each liter of fluid, so that the patient receives a total of 1,750 mg. the first day. Antibiotics are specific in their activity and the use of a particular agent should be based on an explicit assumption, even though provisional, of the nature and etiology of the disease process. Intellectual discipline and medicolegal implications of criminal abortions suggest the wisdom of committing such an assumption to writing when initiating antibiotic treatment. A smear and gram stain of infected cervical or vaginal exudates often provide an immediate guide to specific therapy and may save days while waiting for cultures. Furthermore, these observations may indicate a predominant organism or may help to resolve a dilemma of antibiotic selection. In addition, a simple gram stain may suggest the need for special culture technics when fastidious organisms fail to grow or cultures have been improperly processed.

Bacteremia of unknown type, particularly if accompanied by "endo-toxin shock" is a specific indication for antibiotic combinations. The dosage schedules (assuming normal renal function) for adults are: (1) 8 to 12 Gm. cephalothin daily intravenously plus 5 mg. per kg. kanamycin every 8 hours intramuscularly; (2) cephalothin, kanamycin plus 0.8 to 1.0 mg. per kg. of polymyxin B every 8 hours intravenously; (3) cephalothin, plus polymyxin B or (4) 1 Gm. chloramphenicol every 8 hours intravenously plus 4 million units of penicillin G every 4 hours intravenously (or 1 to 2 Gm. ampicillin every 4 hours intravenously) plus polymyxin B. Clostridial infection is best treated with large doses of penicillin or tetracycline.

Vasopressors are used only if the blood pressure and urine output do not respond within six to eight hours. Antibiotics are continued until the patient has been afebrile for at least three days.

In severe cases or in patients not responding to these measures, hyster-ectomy is performed. Anderson has recommended that hysterectomy be performed under hypothermia (31° C.) on the grounds that it lessens the insult by reducing metabolism and interfering with bacterial metabolism.

TUBERCULOSIS

Tuberculosis of the female genital tract is not common in the United States and, when it does occur, is usually an incidental finding at laparot-omy for pelvic inflammatory disease or infertility. Its incidence, therefore, is somewhat higher in hospitals or clinics where these entities are fre-quently seen. The diagnosis may be made, also unexpectedly, by endo-metrial biopsy in the routine work-up of an infertility patient.

Genital tuberculosis is said to occur in from 3 to 8 per cent of patients with pulmonary tuberculosis and is usually found during the childbearing age, especially between 16 and 35. It is extremely rare in prepuberal and postmenopausal females. At the Boston Hospital for Women tuberculosis has been diagnosed in only 1.8 per cent of specimens removed surgically for salpingitis of various causes. This incidence is somewhat lower than the 5 per cent cited by Novak and is less than the 2–10 per cent cited in most pathologic reports. By comparison, in European countries tuberculosis may account for 20–50 per cent of all salpingectomies.

Tuberculosis usually involves the female genital tract secondarily, the most common primary sites being the lung and the gastrointestinal tract. Dissemination may occur from caseous lymph nodes via blood or lym-phatics or by contiguity from the peritoneal cavity. Primary tuberculosis of the vulva or cervix may be transmitted by coitus but this is extremely rare. The internal genitalia are then involved by direct ascending infection of the endometrium and oviduct. Proof of the primary site is lacking in well over one-half the patients with proved genital tuberculosis.

Pelvic tuberculosis is discussed at length in Chapter 6.

Benign Neoplasms

Benign neoplasms of the uterine corpus will be considered under two general headings: (1) those involving the myometrium and (2) those involving the endometrium. The disease entities most often involving the myometrium are adenomyosis and leiomyoma. Both are of major importance to the gynecologist because they are the major indications for hysterectomy during the premenopausal years.

ADENOMYOSIS

This is a serious, progressively disabling disorder of the premenopausal woman which has been described as "internal endometriosis" and is due to the presence of heterotopic endometrium in the myometrium. Such displaced endometrium must be at least two standard low-power fields beneath the endomyometrial junction and be associated with adjacent myometrial hyperplasia. It may occur focally or may be distributed throughout the uterus, producing generalized and symmetrical enlargement. Since the diagnosis is made almost exclusively by examination of excised uteri, the true incidence of the disease is unknown. Adenomyosis is found in 8–20 per cent of hysterectomy specimens in large gynecologic clinics, and its incidence at necropsy has been reported as high as 50 per cent.

Adenomyosis is a disease of the childbearing period, the incidence being greatest between ages 41 and 50. In most reported series about 80 per cent of the patients were multiparas and approximately 50 per cent had associated leiomyomas. Salpingitis isthmica nodosa is found in 20 per cent of these patients but simultaneously occurring endometriosis is uncommon. Benson, however, found endometriosis in 13 per cent of patients who had hysterectomy for adenomyosis. A recent study by Marcus lends support to the idea that adenomyosis is encountered more often in the uterus with carcinomatous endometrium than in one with benign endometrium. Similarly it was found that adenomyosis uteri and endometrial hyperplasia occurred or coexisted more frequently with endometrial carcinoma than with benign endometrium. These interrelations suggest that a common denominator, possibly hormonal, may exist in these three lesions.

The pathogenesis of this disease is unknown. Numerous theories have been suggested, the most acceptable being that of direct invasion or extension of basal endometrium into the myometrium. An opposite, and less tenable, explanation postulates invasion of the myometrium from the serosal surface by endometriosis. Dedifferentiation of myometrium, mesothelial metaplasia and misplaced müllerian or mesonephric duct tissue have also been suggested as possible etiologic factors. The stimulus for the benign invasion of glandular elements is unknown, although it has been suggested that this process is the result of an excess of normally present growth factor or an exaggerated response to this factor. Estrogen, being the essential hormone for endometrial and myometrial growth, has been implicated in pathogenesis. A certain modicum of support is lent to this idea by the cyclic response to estrogen which the adenomyotic glands demonstrate and by the symptomatic improvement which usually occurs with the menopause. Growth and migration of the glands may actually lag behind the spread of endometrial stroma into the myometrium, and there is some evidence that glandular "invasion" can occur only after the way has been "paved" by the fore-running stroma.

Diagnosis.—The clinical picture is difficult to evaluate, and correlation with the degree of adenomyosis is spurious because of associated leiomyo-

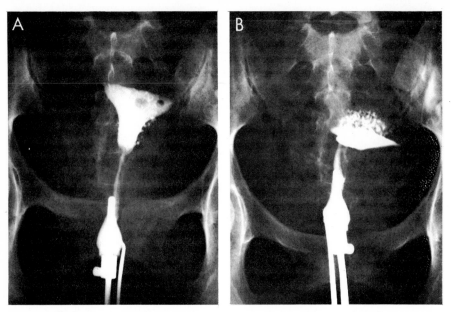

Fig. 5–26.—**A,** hysterogram showing adenomyosis in a 20-year-old infertile female. The diagnosis was later verified by biopsy at the time of hysterotomy. **B,** hysterogram of same patient with uterus anteverted showing extensive spread of radiopaque dye into areas of adenomyosis of the posterior uterine wall.

mas or tubal disease. However, in most patients without these disease processes, the most common symptoms are hypermenorrhea, acquired dysmenorrhea, polymenorrhea and premenstrual staining. Dyspareunia may be associated with a fixed third-degree uterine retroversion. The diagnosis should be suspected if one or more of these symptoms is described by a multiparous patient, aged 35–50, and pelvic examination discloses a moderately enlarged, globular, tender uterus which has a finely nodular surface. The tenderness seems to be increased if leiomyomas are present or if examination is done in the immediate premenstrual phase. In differential diagnosis, the entities to be considered are: (1) endometriosis, (2) multiple leiomyomas, (3) salpingitis isthmica nodosa with salpingitis, (4) idiopathic uterine hypertrophy of multiparity (fibrosis uteri) and (5) pelvic congestion syndrome. The diagnosis is not aided by uterine curettage but hysterography will occasionally show pathognomonic changes (Fig. 5–26). The symptoms of adenomyosis are exaggerated by estrogen-progestin combinations particularly if these are given constantly in the form of "pseudopregnancy.

Pathology.—The adenomyotic uterus is usually enlarged and heavier than usual, weighing about 125 Gm. (normal, 42 Gm.). Although symmetrical enlargement (Fig. 5–27) is the rule, focal adenomyomas may be found and these may occasionally protrude into the uterine cavity. When incised, the surface appears convex and bulging. The thickening of the uterine wall is seen to be made up of coarsely trabeculated areas, stippled or granular in appearance, with small yellow or darker cystic points which may contain serous fluid or old blood. Close inspection of the cut surface will frequently reveal an irregularity of the endomyometrial junction with foci of down-dipping basalis. While the pathologist usually has no difficulty in making a diagnosis of adenomyosis by gross examination of the cut specimen, the surgeon cannot approach this degree of accuracy with the uterus "in situ." He may, however, suspect the disease if a focal area of adenomyosis is mistaken for a leiomyoma and a myomectomy attempted. Areas of adenomyosis do not shell out or lend themselves to easy excision.

MICROSCOPIC APPEARANCE.—The pathognomonic feature of this disease is the occurrence of endometrial tissue, glands and stroma within the myometrium (Fig. 5–28), at least one low-power field (some authors demand two) from the endomyometrial junction. The misplaced endometrial tissue is similar to that of the basalis of the endometrial cavity and therefore does not always respond to hormonal stimulation. Occasionally, however, secretory change may be noted or there may be cystic or adenomatous hyperplasia. In several studies, a functional response in the aberrant endometrium was found in only about 50 per cent of the cases in which the normally located endometrium was functional. Decidual changes in the stroma of adenomyotic areas have been noted during pregnancy and spontaneous ruptures of these areas have been reported. Symptoms of dysmenorrhea or constant pelvic pain might be anticipated if areas of adenomyosis demonstrated functional capacity, with edema and bleeding. The cause of symptoms in patients whose uteri do not show functioning areas of adenomyosis is unknown.

Malignant neoplasia may rarely occur in either the glands or stroma or both, about 30 malignant adenomyomas having been reported. These may be in the form of adenocarcinoma, sarcoma or carcinosarcoma.

The myometrium is usually altered in uteri with extensive adenomyosis so that a surrounding zone of hypertrophy-hyperplasia is usually recogniz-

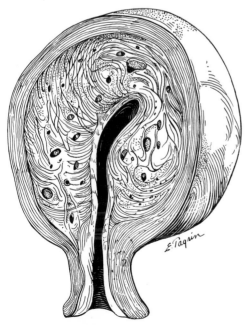

Fig. 5-27.—Adenomyosis.

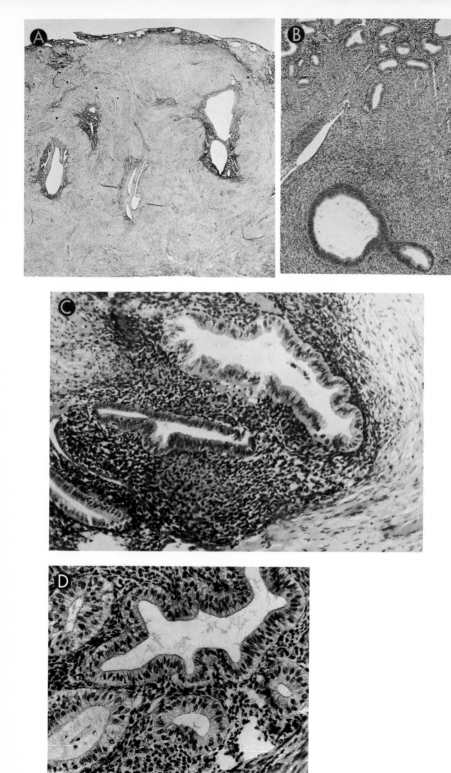

Fig. 5-28.—See legend on facing page.

able. Phagocytized hemosiderin may be seen deep in the myometrium, indicating previous extravasation of blood.

If the process of adenomyosis has extended into the cornua of the uterus and then laterally into the isthmic portion of the oviduct, a process may develop which is indistinguishable from salpingitis isthmica nodosa, except that inflammatory cells are usually present in the latter condition.

Correlation of Symptoms with Pathology.—It has been axiomatic to consider adenomyosis as the most probable diagnosis when dysfunctional uterine bleeding and increasingly severe dysmenorrhea accompany an enlarging, firm, tender uterus in a woman of moderate parity in the 40–50 age group. Yet this disease remains the most overdiagnosed when not present and the one most commonly missed when the process is moderately extensive. In the latter case the preoperative diagnosis is almost always "fibroids."

Ovarian dysfunction has been suggested as the major etiologic factor in the abnormal bleeding associated with adenomyosis. This has not been substantiated by pathologic studies, since there has been no evidence of ovarian failure, unusual cyst formation, stromal change or "overactivity." Secretory endometrium is found in most cases and attests to the ability of the ovaries to ovulate normally even though many of these patients are in the late forties or early fifties.

The vascular supply to the uterus has been shown to be appreciably increased in adenomyosis and enormously so when the disease is extensive. Interference with myometrial contractility and subsequent inadequate vascular control of myometrial and endometrial vasculature have been advanced as a possible cause of the abnormal bleeding associated with adenomyosis. Overdistention of the uterine wall by this increased vascularity during the menses would also explain the dysmenorrhea. Both of these explanations would be more acceptable if a closer correlation with symptoms could be elucidated. Unfortunately, many patients with extensive anatomic findings are symptom-free whereas others, with minimal or nonfunctional adenomyosis, are incapacitated by pain.

Treatment.—The definitive treatment for adenomyosis should be total hysterectomy, with or without ovarian conservation. Various hormonal regimens have been tried but have been uniformly unsuccessful. The use of various progestational agents as a "pseudopregnancy," has resulted in an actual increase in pelvic pain. This was due, in all probability, to marked edema and distortion of the areas of adenomyosis with subsequent increased uterine motility. Androgens have not proved advantageous in adenomyosis. Since most patients are in the late thirties or early forties and have completed their childbearing function, the loss of the uterus is not

Fig. 5–28.—**A,** typical adenomyosis in the wall of the uterus. Foci of basal type endometrium are located deep in the myometrium. The myometrium surrounding the areas of adenomyosis shows a whorled appearance similar to that seen in leiomyoma. (From Hertig, A. T., and Gore, H. M.: *Tumors of the Female Sex Organs: Part 2. Tumors of the Vulva, Vagina and Uterus,* sec. IX, fasc. 33 of *Atlas of Tumor Pathology* [Washington, D. C.: Armed Forces Institute of Pathology, 1960].) **B,** higher power of an area of adenomyosis showing cystic dilatation. The basal endometrium is at the top. **C,** adenomyosis in which the glandular element at the top right has undergone anaplasia. The glands are surrounded by typical endometrial stroma. **D,** adenomyosis showing secretory effect.

looked on with disfavor. If the patient has only minor complaints and a curettage has eliminated the possibility of endometrial abnormalities or a submucous leiomyoma, the use of analgesic agents together with explanation may be successful.

LEIOMYOMA

A leiomyoma is commonly but incorrectly termed a "fibroid." It is a well-circumscribed but nonencapsulated benign tumor composed mainly of muscle but with varying amounts of fibrous connective tissue. Synonymous descriptive terms are fibroma, fibromyoma and myoma. Although the absolute incidence of leiomyoma is difficult to determine, varying reports suggest that they occur in from 4 to 11 per cent of all women and comprise about 30 per cent of the specimens seen in large gynecologic pathology laboratories. This lesion is most frequently found during the fourth and fifth decades of life and it has been estimated that approximately 40 per cent of women age 50 or over harbor these tumors. They have not been reported before the menarche, and the incidence is three to nine times higher in the Negro race.

Numerous theories of histogenesis have been advanced but none has been adequately proved. It has been suggested that leiomyomas arise from totipotential primitive cells that normally give rise to muscle cells, connective tissue cells and blood vessels. Other studies have indicated that the tumor may arise from adult muscle cells or from stromal connective tissue cells. Still other investigators have suggested that leiomyomas arise from the adventitial cells of the blood vessels or from the muscle cells of the arterioles and larger veins. A definite correlation with the presence of estrogen has been noted, since these tumors seldom, if ever, occur before the menarche and tend to disappear after the menopause. Further, leiomyomas make their appearance during the years of maximum ovarian activity, enlarge during pregnancy, grow rapidly when exogenous estrogen is administered and are often found in association with hyperplasia of the endometrium and with granulosa-thecal cell tumors of the ovary. Miller has suggested that these tumors occur in susceptible women who have a high incidence of anovulatory cycles with prolonged estrogen stimulation. He believes they arise from small, immature muscle cell nests in the myometrium.

There are three major types of leiomyomas—submucous, subserous and intramural (Fig. 5–29). The subserous variety may be attached by a broad or narrow base and is commonly pedunculated. Occasionally an intramural leiomyoma may extend laterally into the leaves of the broad ligament, in which case it is known as an intraligamentary tumor. The cervix may be involved, although this occurs in less than 5 per cent of the total. A leiomyoma may become detached from its source and secure its blood supply from neighboring organs or omentum, in which case it is known as a "parasitic" myoma.

These tumors usually begin as minute seedings which may be seen scattered throughout the myometrium, each tumor measuring 3–4 mm. in greatest diameter. They may grow to rather large proportions and some may weigh as much as 10 or 15 lb. The largest on record at the Boston Hospital for Women weighed 30 pounds. The position of the leiomyoma is of

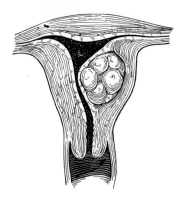

① SUBMUCOUS LEIOMYOMAS

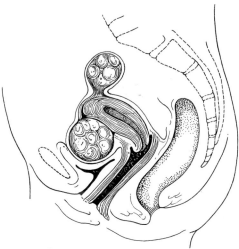

② SUBSEROUS LEIOMYOMAS

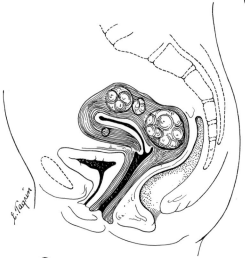

③ INTRAMURAL LEIOMYOMAS

Fig. 5–29.—Leiomyomas classified according to location.

clinical importance since a tumor that occludes the ostium of the oviduct may be an important factor in infertility, and one that projects into the endometrial cavity may be a predisposing factor in habitual abortion. Similarly, the submucous variety is associated with abnormal bleeding, usually hypermenorrhea. Pressure symptoms may result from growth anteriorly or posteriorly, affecting the bladder or rectum.

Pathology.—The gross appearance of a leiomyoma is somewhat variable, but in general the tumor is circumscribed and well demarcated from the surrounding muscle. A pseudocapsule is present which is merely flattened uterine muscle that has become compressed as the tumor increases in size. The consistency is usually firm or actually hard except in cases in which degeneration or hemorrhage has occurred. The color is light gray or pinkish white, depending on the degree of vascularity. When the leiomyoma is cut across, the tissue will usually project above the level of the surrounding myometrium. When viewed in the fresh state, the smooth muscle bundles can usually be identified in a pattern of intertwining or whorl-like arrangement.

The microscopic appearance of a leiomyoma is usually rather characteristic, in that the nonstriated muscle fibers are arranged in bundles of varying sizes running in multiple directions (Fig. 5–30), giving the pattern noted grossly. High-power examination reveals the spindle-shaped cells to have elongated nuclei which are, for the most part, of uniform size and staining quality. Connective tissue elements of varying amounts may be noted between the muscle cells. In certain tumors the amount of the connective tissue element may be excessive, in which case the term *fibromyoma* may be more descriptive.

Degenerative changes may occur, the most common being hyalinization and cyst formation. These changes are due to diminished vascularity of the connective tissue element, so that the detail of connective tissue fibers is lost. The hyalin material presents no cellular detail, stains deeply with eosin and may show remnants of muscle bundles interspersed between the homogeneous matrix. If the hyalinized connective tissue undergoes liquefaction necrosis, cystic degeneration then occurs. The cysts may then become filled with a gelatinous material which oozes forth when the tumor is cut across. This may be followed, especially in long-standing cases, by focal areas of calcification. In postmenopausal women these calcified leiomyomas may be evident on x-ray examination. Another type of degeneration is that known as acute red degeneration, occasionally seen as a complication of pregnancy. In this situation the cut surface simulates raw meat, this carneous change being due to hemorrhage into a partially hyalinized leiomyoma. This hemorrhagic complication is the result of accumulation of blood in the tumor because of venous obstruction and may occur during the rapid growth associated with pregnancy or immediately post partum when the venous drainage is occluded.

Sarcomatous change may occur in a leiomyoma (Fig. 5–31) but is extremely rare, the incidence being somewhere between 0.1 and 0.6 per cent. This malignant change should be suspected if a myoma undergoes rapid enlargement, especially after the menopause, or if postmenopausal bleeding occurs in the presence of known leiomyomas. During pregnancy a certain degree of pleomorphism which simulates the morphology of leiomyosarcoma is seen in 10–15 per cent of excised tumors. Although the

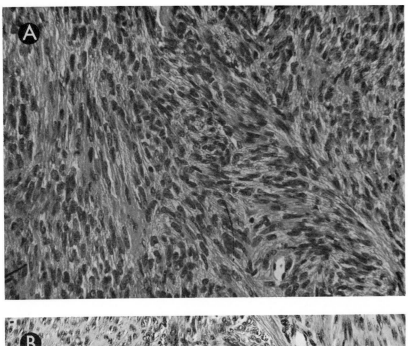

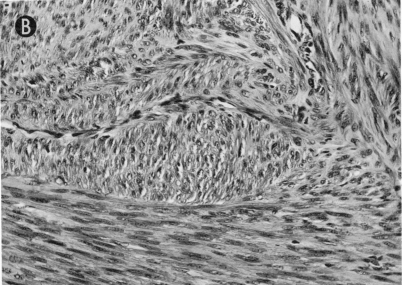

Fig. 5-30.—A, high-power view of leiomyoma, showing typical structure. The tumor is composed of groups and bundles of smooth muscle cells arranged in twists and whorls in an interlacing pattern. It is relatively avascular. **B,** higher power shows cellular detail. The smooth muscle fibers in the central portion have been cut across their long axis. Note uniform appearance and lack of mitoses.

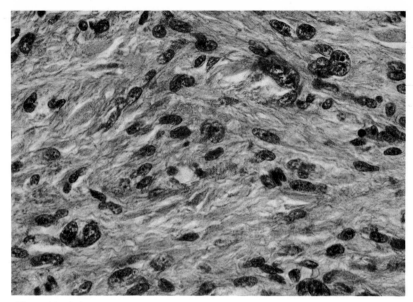

Fig. 5-31.—Leiomyosarcoma, showing resemblance to cells in Figure 5-30, *A* and *B*, but with pleomorphism and variation in size and staining density.

tumor may appear very fleshy and microscopically appears quite cellular, the cells are all of equal size, mitotic figures are absent and giant cells are not prominent.

Symptomatology.—The most important symptom associated with uterine leiomyomas is abnormal bleeding. This is usually in the form of hypermenorrhea and may be associated with the passage of large clots. Secondary anemia may therefore be present. The myoma per se does not cause bleeding. This is usually due to an abnormal endometrial pattern, frequently hyperplasia, overlying a submucous tumor. Bleeding may occur from the thinned endometrium overlying an intracavitary, pedunculated myoma. The presence of the tumor in the endomyometrium may so affect the normal hemostatic mechanism that extensive flow occurs. It is important to remember, however, that bleeding from other sources, such as carcinoma of the endometrium or cervix, may co-exist and definitive therapy should not be carried out until malignancy has been excluded. If the bleeding is intermenstrual or postcoital, carcinoma should be strongly suspected even though extensive myomas are present.

If a myoma reaches a size such that it practically fills the pelvic cavity, it may by encroachment on other organs cause certain pressure symptoms. Pressure on the bladder may be evidenced by suprapubic discomfort, frequency, urinary retention or overflow incontinence. If the rectosigmoid is encroached on by the growing tumor, constipation may result. A generalized feeling of discomfort, edema of the legs or increased varicosities may result from an enlarging tumor. In many patients no symptoms are noticed until the mass becomes sufficiently large to become an abdominal structure. The patient may then notice a firm, nodular mass or may simply complain of an increase in abdominal girth. Myomas usually do not produce pain unless they become twisted or undergo degeneration with subsequent hemorrhage and infection. When pain does occur in the presence of a myoma, it is likely to be caused by other pathology, e.g., tubal inflammation, endometriosis, diverticulitis or even ovarian cancer.

Diagnosis.—A presumptive diagnosis of a leiomyoma of the uterus may be made by abdominal palpation if the uterus is displaced out of the pelvis or if the tumors are large. They may be palpated as firm, irregular nodules or masses arising from the pelvis and extending into the lower abdomen. Usually these masses are movable without causing pain. Occasionally a firm, nodular mass may be felt almost to the level of the umbilicus without any symptoms having been noted by the patient. Bimanual pelvic examination is more helpful in making the diagnosis since the uterus can usually be outlined easily and the distortion of its normal contour is readily appreciated. The myomas may be small irregularities on the surface of the uterus, no larger than 1 cm., or they may incorporate and distort the fundus to such an extent that separation of tumor from uterus is impossible.

The differential diagnosis is not always easy. During the childbearing period an intrauterine gestation should always be suspected particularly if some degree of diminished flowing has occurred. A leiomyoma may occasionally be soft and the associated pelvic congestion may produce softening of the cervix. Conversely, an early intrauterine pregnancy may exist without softening of the cervix and when a leiomyoma occurs in a pregnant uterus it may undergo softening and enlargement. When in doubt a pregnancy test should always be obtained.

Another aspect of pregnancy may interfere with accurate diagnosis. During the early weeks of pregnancy the uterus may enlarge asymmetrically and if there is a tendency toward a bicornuate development, there will be a pronounced enlargement of one uterine horn. This may be mistaken for an ovarian mass or a myoma. Moderate degrees of this asymmetrical enlargement are normal in all pregnancies, presumably due to lateral placental implantation. Such a growth pattern is known as Piskacek's sign. Similarly, pregnancy occurring in the interstitial portion of the oviduct may give rise to an asymmetric enlargement of the uterus which may be confused with a myoma or ovarian lesion.

A subserous, pedunculated myoma is frequently mistaken for an ovarian tumor, either a fibroma or dermoid cyst, particularly if the pedicle has become elongated. Such leiomyomas are generally freely mobile, but careful examination will usually reveal an attachment to the uterus. In such patients it is important that the ovary be palpated and differentiated from the myoma since surgical exploration is indicated for an enlarged, solid ovarian mass whereas observation is suggested as optimum therapy if the mass is a simple, uncomplicated myoma. Frequently a parasitic or intraligamentous myoma cannot be delineated adequately since such lesions are usually fixed and may coalesce with the adnexal structures.

Other pelvic masses which may be mistaken for myomas are: (1) a redundant or distended cecum filled with feces, (2) a redundant sigmoid, (3) appendiceal abscess, (4) diverticulitis, (5) carcinoma of the sigmoid. Cleansing enemas and radiographic studies of the bowel will assist in diagnostic precision. Occasionally a pelvic kidney may rest close to the uterus but urography will detect this congenital abnormality. X-rays of the urinary tract are also indicated if a myoma is intraligamentous in order to ascertain ureteral deviation prior to surgery. A full bladder or urachal cyst may rarely be mistaken for a myoma but routine voiding prior to pelvic examination will eliminate this obvious error. Cystograms are indicated if bladder involvement is suspected. As a matter of fact, the radiologist is frequently suspicious of a myoma by the indentation it and the uterus make on the dome of the bladder as seen on the intravenous urogram. Calcification in a myoma may also be detected on the same films.

A pedunculated submucous myoma may be evident as a mass which protrudes through the cervix as a gray-pink smooth mass. The usual submucous myoma may be detected at the time of curettage or by hysterogram.

Treatment.—The treatment of uterine leiomyomas cannot be standardized. Each patient presents individual variations which must be assayed before suggesting extirpation. If the tumor is discovered at routine pelvic examination, is asymptomatic and not of excessive size, no specific treatment is indicated. This is especially true if the patient is premenopausal since the tumor will diminish in size after the menses cease. Close observation is suggested with pelvic examinations at about six-month intervals. Surgery is sometimes advisable on the basis of size alone, but exact measurements cannot be given. In general, if the leiomyoma fills the true pelvis, that is, it equals or exceeds the size of a 12-week gestation, surgery is usually indicated.

Conservative measures may also be followed if symptoms are minimal. Thus if the patient has noted only slight hypermenorrhea or pressure symptoms and is nearing the menopause, treatment may include oral or intramuscular administration of iron, vitamins and a high-protein diet. The use of androgenic substances has been suggested but should not exceed 300 mg. per month. If there is associated anovulatory bleeding with endometrial hyperplasia, treatment with an androgenic progestin (Norlutate, 10 mg. daily for 20 consecutive days) may reduce the amount of flowing and this may be continued indefinitely if successful. This has proved to be effective temporizing therapy in preparing patients for hysterectomy in whom blood loss has been excessive. Medroxyprogesterone acetate (Depo-Provera) has been used similarly in a dose of 100 mg. intramuscularly every 3 to 5 days while the patient is being prepared for surgery. In a few patients in whom hysterectomy was contraindicated because of serious medical disease, I have used Depo-Provera in a continuing dose of 200 mg. per month for as long as 3 years until the patient entered menopause and spontaneous regression of the myomas occurred. Oxytocic substances have little, if any, effect on the bleeding associated with leiomyomas.

Surgery is indicated in the following situations: (1) excessive size or excess rate of growth except during pregnancy; (2) submucous location if associated with hypermenorrhea; (3) if the tumor is pedunculated; (4) if the bladder or rectum is encroached on to a degree that produces pressure symptoms; (5) if the tumor is intraligamentous or if differentiation from an ovarian mass is not possible; (6) if there is associated pelvic pathology such as endometriosis or pelvic inflammatory disease; (7) if infertility or habitual abortion seems due to the anatomic location of the tumor.

Conservative surgery for leiomyomas may be performed in younger women if there is no other indication for removal of the uterus. However, the mere presence of a myoma that does not compromise tubal function or the integrity of the endometrial cavity should not be an indication for myomectomy. Uterotubograms may be utilized to demonstrate distortion of the endometrial cavity or obstruction of the intrauterine ostia of the oviducts. Preliminary curettage may reveal endometrial hyperplasia or polyps. Large cervical myomas may produce distortion and tortuosity of the cervical canal with obstruction to spermatozoa. In addition, before a planned laparotomy for a myomectomy, the cervix and endometrial cavity should be adequately studied by cytology and biopsy to rule out malignant or premalignant disease. If a myomectomy is planned because of infertility, the husband should have been studied thoroughly, the patency of the oviducts determined and the endometrium biopsied to make certain of ovulation and to exclude endometrial disease.

Myomectomy may be single or multiple. Pregnancies have followed the removal of large, solitary tumors that completely distorted the endometrial cavity as well as the removal of multiple small tumors. The incidence of pregnancy following myomectomy approximates 40 per cent. The patient should be informed, however, to attempt pregnancy soon after surgery, since the recurrence rate of leiomyoma is considerable, in some series being as high as 10 per cent.

The morbidity and mortality after myomectomy are minimal if the usual care is given to secure hemostasis and prevent infection. Delivery following myomectomy need not be by cesarean section unless the endometrial cavity was entered at the time of original surgery or the postoperative course was febrile and the myometrial scar possibly weakened.

Technique of Myomectomy.—The uterine fundus is grasped with double hooks or traction sutures and drawn toward the abdominal wound in such a position as to expose the myoma to be removed. An incision (Fig. 5–32, A) is made through the wall of the uterus parallel with the axis of the uterus over the most prominent part of the tumor. Hemostasis may be aided by placing a tourniquet such as a small Penrose drain around the uterus at the level of the uterine vessels. This can be done simply by merely piercing the broad ligament bilaterally and clamping the tourniquet posteriorly. The local injection of Pitocin or Neo-Synephrine has also been advocated for securing hemostasis. We have not utilized these methods if the myomas are small but have found them advantageous in the treatment of large and multiple leiomyomas. The incision is then carried down to the surface of the myoma (Fig. 5–32,B) which can be readily recognized by the difference in the direction of its fibers.

When the surface of the myoma is exposed the tumor is grasped either with a double hook or by a traction suture placed through its substance. With firm traction the tumor can be readily shelled out by means of blunt dissection, exposure being provided by placing Allis clamps on the lateral aspects of the myometrium (Fig. 5–32,C). The individual blood vessels are then clamped and ligated as necessary. The enucleation should be done carefully to prevent excessive laceration of the uterine wall and to avoid opening the uterine cavity if possible. If the tumor is an adenomyoma, it will not shell out with this facility and sharp dissection will be necessary.

Careful control of the bleeding is then important, and all bleeding points should be isolated and ligatured as completely as possible. The tourniquet may be released intermittently in order to identify such vessels. The dead space brought about by the removal of the tumor is obliterated by approximating the myometrium with interrupted (Fig. 5–32,D) or figure-of-eight sutures of chromic catgut. The peritoneum is then closed with sutures of fine catgut (Fig. 5–32,E) or by a subserosal continuous suture. When it is found necessary to remove a large number of myomas, it is important to make the incision in the uterine wall in such a way that multiple tumors may be removed through the same incision. Following the myomectomy, a suspension operation should always be performed to prevent the possibility of an adherent retroversion. If the myomectomy incision has involved the posterior wall of the uterus, adhesions to ileum or sigmoid colon are quite common. This complication may be

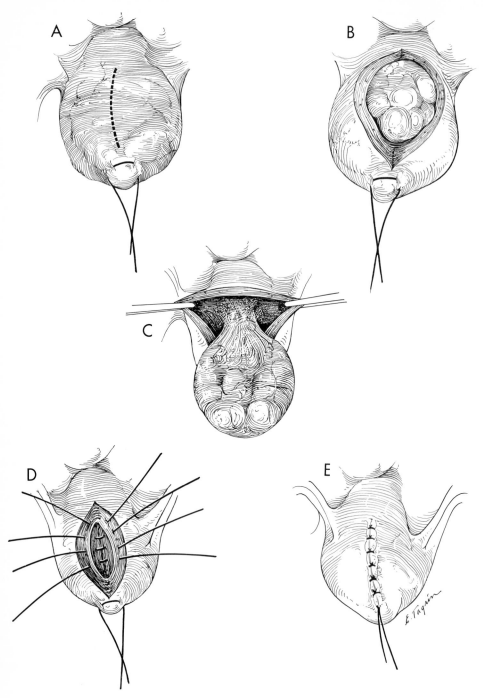

Fig. 5–32.—Technique of myomectomy.

prevented by meticulous closure of the uterine serosa or by attaching an omental graft to the uterine wall.

Hysterectomy.—Simple total hysterectomy is, in the hands of the well-trained specialist, a safe operation. Numerous reviews published during the past decade cite morbidity rates varying from 10 to 48 per cent. The extreme variation depends on whether or not the author has adhered to the strict interpretation of minor febrile reactions or has reported only what he considers to be morbid states. Mortality rates reported in these same reviews approximate 0.3 per cent with variation from 0.1 to 0.9 per cent. Most of the serious complications were caused by inadequate hemostasis, ureteral, bladder and rectal trauma and pulmonary disease. Methods of preventing the first two categories are outlined herein.

Two basic surgical principles are of major importance in the performance of the abdominal hysterectomy. They are good visualization and adequate hemostasis. The former is provided by a combination of proper positioning of the patient, well-chosen incisions and relaxing anesthesia. The latter is a result of careful dissection in proper cleavage planes, meticulous ligature of major vessels and elimination of needless steps. The actual procedure of removal of the uterus should never be started until the operative field has been freed of adhesions and the specimen mobilized.

Technique of Hysterectomy.—POSITION.—Most gynecologists prefer a modified Trendelenburg position of about 25 to 35 degrees for pelvic surgery. When spinal anesthesia is utilized lesser degrees are usually provided but because of excellent muscular and intestinal relaxation this seems adequate. Our own preference is for so-called "accentuated" Trendelenburg positioning of about 45 to 55 degrees with the table being broken at knee level. This has been used continuously for over 60 years at the Boston Hospital for Women, and recent surveys of morbidity have not indicated a greater incidence of pulmonary complications following its use. This position greatly facilitates visualization of the pelvic viscera.

INCISION.—Several large clinics have recently published data citing the advantages of the transverse incision over the midline or paramedian approach. Again it seems to be a matter of habit and training of the individual operator, and if he performs the transverse incision with ease and rapidity this is then superior for him. The amount of visualization and facile approach to the pelvic viscera with the transverse incision certainly equals and frequently exceeds that obtained with a vertical one especially if the recti muscles are divided. The cosmetic result is better, wound healing is improved, physiological stress patterns are diminished and postoperative hernias are extremely rare. The sole disadvantage seems to be that its opening and closure takes somewhat more time although this should not be a serious deterring factor. A retrocecal appendix may also be more difficult to mobilize but in most cases appendectomy is not hindered.

I have, in the past, utilized a left paramedian or midline incision for most hysterectomies but during the last several years have frequently employed the transverse approach with satisfaction.

HEMOSTASIS.—The principles of securing hemostasis have been previously noted but reiteration of one point is essential: the uterus and adnexa are completely mobilized before actual removal of the specimen is begun. Occasionally this entails more ingenuity and surgical skill than the hysterectomy itself but is rewarding by prevention of ureteral, bladder and rectal injury. In extensive pelvic inflammatory disease the adnexa must be dissected from their attachment to the posterior peritoneum and serosa of the rectosigmoid. Frequently this may be carried out by blunt finger dissection but if a good cleavage plane is not available sharp dissection with good visualization of the posterior pelvis is mandatory. This will prevent penetration of the rectosigmoid by the exploring finger. It has been found valuable to divide the uterosacral ligaments in such cases (after the rectum has been displaced) before actually starting the hysterectomy since the entire uterus then "rides up" into the superior strait of the pelvis and makes approach to the lateral ligaments easier.

In endometriosis of severe degree extensive uterine fixation frequently exists. Division of the posterior peritoneum and uterosacral ligaments will secure a line of cleavage inside the endopelvic fascia which will enable the operator to perform a total hysterectomy in almost every case.

THE LIGAMENTS.—The ligaments opposite the operator are usually ligated and divided first and these may be put on stretch by removing the retractor on the surgeon's side and exerting strong traction on the uterine fundus by means of a toothed hook. This may be done by the second assistant on the operator's side while the opposite retractor is held directly over the ligaments to be divided. Many authors have suggested starting the operation by clamping and dividing the round ligaments, then perforating the posterior leaf of the broad ligament with the finger and mobilizing the infundibulopelvic ligament in this fashion. They place two clamps across this ligament and replace each with a ligature of no. 0 or 00 chromic catgut. An alternative, and perhaps simpler method is to place a suture around the infundibulopelvic ligament first (if the ovaries are to be removed) without clamping and tie it. (A half-length Kelly clamp has previously been placed adjacent to the corpus and lateral to the ovary to prevent backflow. This clamp also includes the round ligament at its uterine margin.) Using the same suture the needle is placed directly through the round ligament and the suture tied in such a fashion as to include the infundibulopelvic ligament, thus securing it for the second time. The needle is then placed through the broad ligament about one-half centimeter below the round ligament. As the round ligament is divided the anterior peritoneum is easily picked up and a transverse incision carried halfway toward the midline (Fig. 5–33, A–C).

Following bilateral ligation of the round and infundibulopelvic ligaments, attention is usually turned to the uterine vessels and there is general agreement that they should be dissected cleanly of all adjacent areolar tissue and peritoneum. If this is carefully done the vessels may be secured by one or two ligatures without clamping. One important point that has not received adequate attention is the division of the posterior peritoneum and the uterosacral ligaments prior to uterine vessel ligation. This is usually carried out by cutting transversely with the scalpel beginning at the peritoneal edge developed by division of the round ligaments and exposure of the uterine vessels and continuing across the uterosacral ligaments superior to their insertion into the uterovaginal fascia. These ligaments usually do not need clamping and ligation. The posterior leaf of fascia, together with the uterosacral ligaments, is dissected or pushed off the posterior aspects of the cervix thus opening the posterior fascial envelope around the cervix. This also serves the important function of displacing the ureter posteriorly so that ligation of the uterine vessels is accomplished without danger (Fig. 5–33, D).

BLADDER PERITONEUM.—After the round ligaments have been divided bilaterally and the medial extension of the anterior peritoneum brought to the midline, the anterior peritoneal dissection is complete. Scissor dissection in the areolar tissue above the uterovaginal fascia serves to displace the bladder from the vagina for a distance of two to three centimeters. It is then technically easy with the thumb above the cervix and two fingers under it to displace the bladder digitally below the level of the cervicovaginal junction. If the bladder peritoneum is then sewed to the abdominal wall and retractors are placed *inside* the bladder peritoneum, ready access to the vessels and cervix is easily obtained. Whether the dissection of the anterior peritoneum is done before that of the posterior peritoneum or after is not important. The importance lies in preparing the uterine vessels for complete ligation (Fig. 5–33, E and F).

UTERINE VESSELS.—As previously noted, the uterine vessels may be either doubly

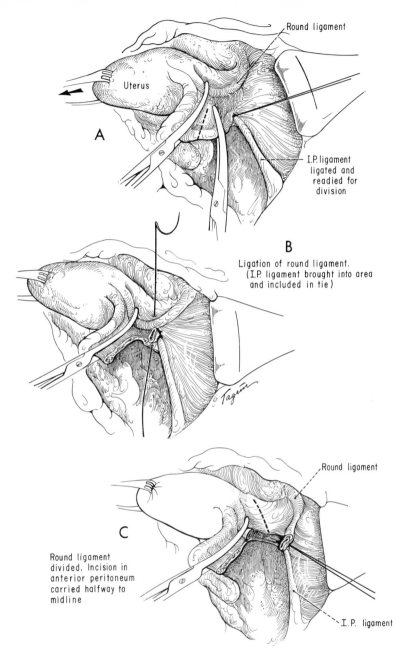

Round ligament

Uterus

A

I.P. ligament
ligated and
readied for
division

B

Ligation of round ligament.
(I.P. ligament brought into area
and included in tie)

Round ligament

C

Round ligament
divided. Incision in
anterior peritoneum
carried halfway to
midline

I.P. ligament

Fig. 5–33.—A, a Kelly clamp is placed over the round and infundibulopelvic ligaments to control backflow bleeding; a suture is placed around the infundibulopelvic ligament and a second Kelly clamp is applied medial to the suture; the infundibulopelvic ligament is then divided between the clamps. **B,** after division of the infundibulopelvic ligament, a suture is placed through the round ligament and tied so that the infundibulopelvic ligament is brought into proximity; the same suture is then placed through the broad ligament caudad to the round ligament as shown; when this suture is tied it encompasses the infundibulopelvic ligament thus doubly securing it. **C,** the round ligament is divided and the incision is continued through the anterior leaf of the broad ligament curving toward the midline. *(Continued.)*

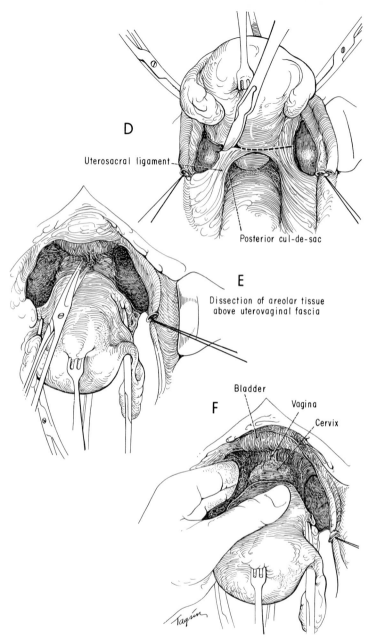

Fig. 5–33 *(cont.).*—**D,** after the posterior leaf of the broad ligament has been divided and the uterine vessels exposed and skeletonized, the posterior peritoneum and uterosacral ligaments are divided with a knife. **E,** the anterior peritoneum of the vesico-uterine fold has been completely divided and the vesico-cervical ligaments are divided; note that the scissors are turned away from the bladder; dissection should be in the plane of the areolar tissue between the fascial layers. **F,** traction cephalad is placed on the uterus and two fingers are placed below the cervix; a gentle rolling motion with the thumb displaces the bladder below the cervico-vaginal junction. *(Continued.)*

clamped, divided and ligated or simply ligated without preliminary clamping. Various technics of management of the anterior leaf of the uterovaginal fascia (pubovesicocervical fascia) have been published during the past decade. It has been suggested that this fascia be divided transversely, split through three-quarters of its circumference, or incised in the form of an inverted T. The advantages cited are: (1) by any of these technics the cardinal ligaments may be clamped and divided *inside* the endopelvic fascia, thus protecting the ureter, and (2) the resulting fascial envelopes may be utilized for vaginal closure and support. These fascial technics, while anatomically sound, have been found by others to be unnecessary and time-consuming.

A simplified method of management has been described which merely includes the endopelvic fascia (cardinal ligament) in the clamp on the uterine vessels. Thus if the ureter is well displaced by the development of the posterior peritoneum and subjacent fascia and the bladder is adequately advanced beyond the cervix, the first clamp on the uterine vessels can be placed much lower than usual. This clamp is placed at the level of the uterosacral attachment posteriorly, then swings anteriorly biting into and including a good portion of the anterior and lateral expanse of the fascia (Fig. 5–33,G). A second clamp is placed above the first and the usual backflow clamp is applied. The vessels and fascia are then divided and the suture ligatures placed so that the needle enters the medial portion of the fascia (Fig. 5–33,H). Double ligation is recommended.

This step secures the cardinal ligament in apposition to the vessels, eliminates the fascial incisions (which sometimes bleed), and makes separate bites of para-cervical tissue for the most part unnecessary. It seems to aid in hemostasis since the uterine vessels are anchored securely.

ENTERING THE VAGINA.—Anterior, lateral and posterior entrance have all been suggested and each author cites reasons why his particular method seems easier for him. For most gynecologists, however, it seems reasonably simple to identify the anterior longitudinal striations of the vagina, elevate them with a Kocher clamp in the midline and make a transverse thrust into the vaginal space with a knife just above the clamp. If another Kocher clamp is placed on the anterior lip of the cervix the incision may be everted so that by simply laying the curved scissors against the cervix it may be easily "circumcised." Kochers may be placed at each angle and in the midline posteriorly as the specimen is removed. Care should be taken to include the vaginal mucosa in the angle clamps since, if it pulls away, postoperative hemorrhage from the cuff may occur (Fig. 5–33, *H*–*K*).

TREATMENT OF THE VAGINA.—Review of recent literature on hysterectomy reveals that most authors favor closure of the vaginal cuff with catgut sutures with considerable importance being given to everting the vaginal mucosa into the vaginal space. The bothersome vascularity at the angle is usually managed by a figure-of-eight suture, which frequently serves the double purpose of securing the cardinal ligament to the vaginal cuff as a major means of support. If the fascial envelopes have been developed, they are frequently brought together over the closed cuff and closed with a running transverse suture. This, it is felt, adds further support to the vaginal apex.

Another group favors leaving the vagina open and simply running a hemostatic suture around the periphery of the cuff making certain to include a good bit of the mucosa with every bite (Fig. 5–33, L). Before placement of this stitch an important figure-of-eight suture is utilized to close the angle. This suture begins posteriorly, picking up the divided uterosacral ligament, goes obliquely through the posterior vaginal wall and also through the anterior vaginal wall (and its fascia) somewhat more medially. It is then looped around the angle clamp and is directed laterally through the posterior and anterior vaginal walls. As it is tied the loop incorporates the uterine vessels and the cardinal ligament. This places a third tie around these important vessels and secures the cardinal ligament to the vagina for support. The proponents of the open vagina feel that it results in a longer, more functional structure than if closed, that less granulation tissue develops and that early bleeding is

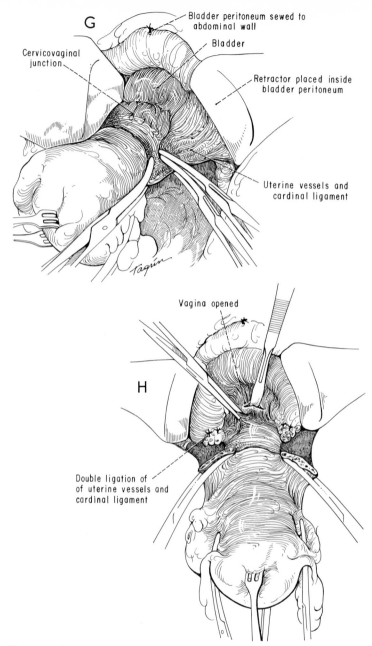

Fig. 5–33 *(cont.)*.—**G,** the bladder peritoneum is sutured to the abdominal wall and retractors are placed inside the reflected bladder; the lower clamp incorporates the lateral aspect of the endopelvic fascia as it is placed over the uterine vessels; a second clamp is placed over the vessels and they are divided with care to include some of the endopelvic fascia in the medial aspect; each clamp is replaced with a suture. **H,** unless the cervix is elongated a separate division and ligation of the cardinal ligament is not necessary; a Kocher clamp is placed across the vagina at the cervico-vaginal junction and the vagina is entered with a knife; a second clamp then picks up the lower vaginal edge. *(Continued.)*

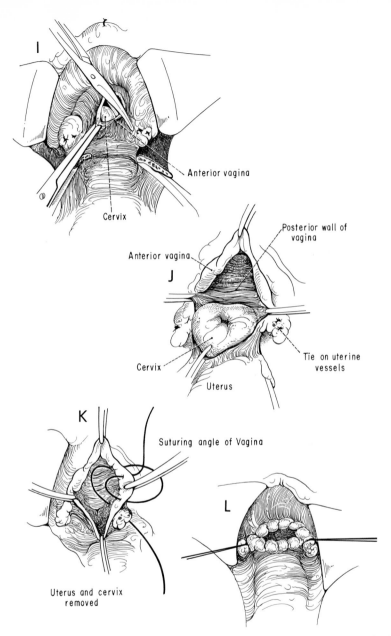

Fig. 5–33 *(cont.).*—**I,** with medial traction on the vaginal edges, the vagina is incised with a scissors directed toward the lateral angle. **J,** Kocher clamps are placed at each vaginal angle and the cervix is drawn cephalad; the posterior vaginal wall is divided under direct vision. **K,** the vaginal angle suture is placed through the uterosacral ligament, posterior vaginal wall, anterior vaginal wall and then is looped around the lateral clamp; the suture is then brought through the posterior and anterior vaginal walls lateral to the first loop; when the suture is tied the loop lateral to the vagina encircles the uterine vessels thus placing a third tie around them. **L,** the angle sutures are held with clamps and provide traction; a running, unlocked suture is begun in the midline of the posterior vaginal wall and is carried around the circumference of the vagina for hemostasis; the vagina is left open for drainage.

easily diagnosed and treated. Pelvic retroperitoneal hematomas are said to be less common. Advocates of the closed vagina state that by this method hemostasis is superior, support is better and, if care is taken with the mucosal edges, granulation tissue is minimal.

THE OVARIES.—The problem of ovarian salvage at the time of hysterectomy for benign conditions has not been satisfactorily solved. It is generally agreed that when extensive endometriosis or pelvic inflammatory disease exists and the uterus is removed the ovaries should be extirpated. If the patient is over the age of 45, many gynecologists prefer to remove what are apparently "normal" but nonfunctioning ovaries. It is now known that even after bilateral oophorectomy at this age measurable amounts of estrogenic substances continue to be excreted in the urine. This is presumably of adrenal origin since bilateral adrenalectomy will result in a marked diminution or total absence of such material as measured by present methods. Under the age of 45, or as long as the patient is having apparently normal ovulatory cycles, most authorities favor leaving one or both ovaries. However, a recent report from a large Boston clinic favors bilateral oophorectomy with every hysterectomy (regardless of age) with immediate postoperative replacement therapy. This management was based on a study in which 6 per cent of patients who had apparently "normal" ovaries left in at the time of hysterectomy had subsequent symptoms referable to the remaining ovary, and 3 per cent had later oophorectomy because of recurrent pain. An additional group had severe mastodynia with retained ovaries, and of major interest was the fact that the patients whose ovaries were left in had a greater incidence of vasomotor symptoms (flushes and sweats) than those who had bilateral oophorectomy and who received adequate replacement therapy.

If the ovaries are left in it seems wiser not to fix the round and utero-ovarian ligaments to the lateral aspect of the vaginal vault since this may drop the ovary into the posterior cul-de-sac and result in dyspareunia. It is also possible that by stretching the infundibulopelvic ligament the ovarian blood supply may be compromised. If the ovaries are removed and the untied infundibulopelvic and round ligaments are loose and long they may be tied into the vaginal angle suture. This simplifies peritonization but does not increase support of the vaginal vault to any degree. If the ligaments are short they are best left in position and peritonization begun by carefully picking up the lateral peritoneal edges with a running suture of no. 00 or 000 chromic catgut. Most of our ureteral injuries and angulations have occurred at this point and during this step the ureter should be visualized on the medial leaf of peritoneum with every bite.

ENDOLYMPHATIC STROMAL MYOSIS

This disease process should be differentiated from adenomyosis since there is evidence that it may have malignant potential. It has been called variously stromatous endometriosis, perithelioma, hemangiopericytoma, and stromatoid new growth of the uterine wall. It consists pathologically of strands and masses of noncollagenous connective tissue which is usually regarded as being of endometrial origin. The disease is found most often during the fourth and fifth decades of life and is associated with symptoms of menorrhagia, metrorrhagia or postmenopausal bleeding. Other symptoms include dysmenorrhea and weight loss. The one constant physical finding is a diffuse uterine enlargement.

The pathogenesis of endolymphatic stromal myosis is unknown but three theories of development have been advanced. The generally accepted concept suggests direct extension or invasion of stroma from the basal endometrium. Other theories indicate that the tissue develops from undifferentiated cells between myometrial fibers or from lymphatics and/or blood vessels of the endometrial stroma. Recent investigation lends strong support to the theory that the tumor arises from "vasoformative cells" such as pericytes, and therefore the term "hemangiopericytoma" has gained prominence in recent literature. The fact that late recurrence of endolymphatic stromal myosis has a pattern similar to the original tumor strongly supports this concept.

Gross examination of the uterus reveals diffuse enlargement, usually symmetrical, with white or yellow rubbery masses extending throughout the myometrium. Small yellow nodules may occasionally project above the cut surface or section of the freshly cut specimen. Occasionally the tumor masses may extend into the endometrial cavity as polypoid excrescences.

Microscopically, the tissue is made up of round or oval cells of uniform and moderate size (Fig. 5–34). The cells resemble endometrial stromal cells of the mid-to-late proliferative phase. The cytoplasm is scanty and irregular. Mitotic figures are rare and vascularity is variable. In some cases the tumor cells blend into the myometrium and its limits may be determined only by special stains.

Novak interpreted endolymphatic stromal myosis as a stage in the development of uterine malignancy. The simple infiltration of the myometrium by glands and stroma is represented by adenomyosis. A more advanced phase embraces endolymphatic and extravascular extension (endolymphatic stromal myosis), and a third group, more advanced, resembles endometrial stromal sarcoma.

The treatment of this unusual process usually consists of total hysterectomy and bilateral salpingo-oophorectomy. In most cases, this treatment has already been completed by the time diagnosis is made. There is no evidence at present that postoperative x-ray therapy increases the survival rate.

The prognosis is good if the above treatment is carried out and dissemination has not already occurred. The five-year survival rate in most series has approximated 85 per cent. Metastases have occurred to the lungs, peritoneum and ovary. Pleomorphism and mitotic activity indicate an increased liability to recurrence but an inactive histologic appearance is no guarantee against recurrence.

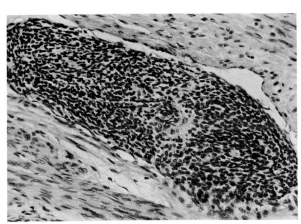

Fig. 5–34.—Endolymphatic stromal myosis, showing a lymphatic space in the uterine wall filled with benign endometrial stroma.

ENDOMETRIAL POLYPS

Endometrial polyps are hyperplastic overgrowths of the glands and stroma of rather localized extent that form a projection above the surface. Such polyps may be sessile or pedunculated and rarely show foci of neoplastic growth. These tumors are relatively common and usually occur between ages 29 and 59, with the greatest incidence after age 50. Symptoms are variable and, since polyps may exist with other abnormalities, are difficult to ascribe to the polyp per se. In general, the patient may note intermenstrual spotting or, more commonly, a postmenstrual staining of four to five days' duration. Usually this discharge is dark brown and somewhat mucoid. In postmenopausal patients irregular staining and bleeding may occur. Occasionally a history of oral ingestion of estrogenic substances for months or years may be elicited. It should be remembered that many unsuspected and asymptomatic polyps are discovered by the pathologist when hysterectomies are performed for other indications, such as leiomyomas or adenomyosis. This is particularly true in the postmenopausal patient who undergoes a vaginal hysterectomy for uterine prolapse. Similarly, approximately 10 per cent of uteri of postmenopausal women examined at autopsy harbor asymptomatic, benign polyps.

The diagnosis should be strongly suspected if a premenopausal patient notes recurrent postmenstrual staining without other symptoms of dysfunctional bleeding. Hysterograms will frequently demonstrate large polyps but smaller ones will not be visualized. Endometrial biopsy is inadequate for complete diagnosis since the polyp moves about so easily it may be brushed aside by the curet. A thorough uterine curettage is necessary for diagnosis and the operator should assiduously curet all portions of the endometrial cavity and then explore further with a polyp extractor, a modified placental forceps which grasps the polyp securely. Most gynecologists have had the experience of performing a "thorough" curettage prior to hysterectomy only to be surprised when the opened specimen is shown by the pathologist. Large, fleshy polyps are easily missed if not sought for repeatedly. If bleeding persists following a curettage for dysfunctional uterine bleeding, the physician should assume that a polyp remains in the endometrial cavity.

Gross examination of the excised polyp reveals a smooth, usually red or orange, velvety mass varying from 0.3 to 12 cm. in diameter, although most have a diameter of 2–4 cm. Although usually solitary, polyps may be multiple, especially if exogenous estrogen has been administered for long periods. Most polyps arise in the fundal region and extend downward (Fig. 5–35), occasionally prolapsing through the cervix. Since the base of the polyp is located high in the corpus and is broad and vascular, removal should not be attempted in the office or clinic. In this respect endometrial polyps differ from those arising in the endocervix.

Microscopically, most endometrial polyps show a histologic pattern of basal endometrium of an immature type usually not reactive to hormonal stimuli. The great majority are composed of cystically dilated glands lined by a single layer of flattened cells surrounded by relatively inactive stroma. The typical polyp found in the senescent uterus is of this type (Fig. 5–36). The thin-walled, cystically dilated glands may represent foci of previous hyperplasia, the "retrogressive hyperplasia" of Novak and Richardson. In

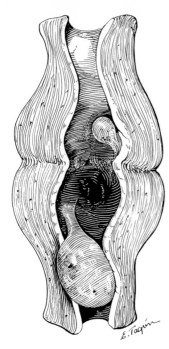

Fig. 5–35.—Endometrial polyps. The uterus has been bivalved to show interior of cavity.

Fig. 5–36.—Endometrial polyp in a postmenopausal uterus. The glands within the polyp show cystic dilatation, whereas the glands of the endometrium are senescent and inactive.

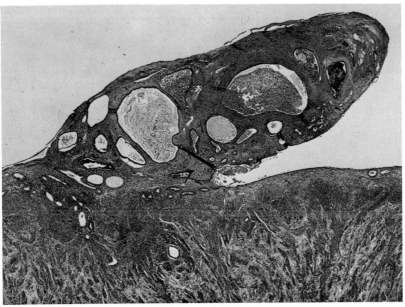

some polyps, the stroma shows extensive fibrosis and hyalinization, representing a diminution in vascular supply following the onset of the menopause. Other polyps demonstrate much more epithelial activity, with rather extensive cystic hyperplasia and foci of adenomatous hyperplasia as well. The stroma here is loose and edematous, and mitotic figures are common. These are frequently seen and associated with extensive cystic and adenomatous endometrial hyperplasia. A third type, which poses problems for both clinician and pathologist, demonstrates a mixture of hyperplasia, carcinoma in situ and questionable areas of invasive carcinoma. The accompanying endometrium may be perfectly normal so that, in most cases, cure is brought about by removal of the polyp alone. One should remember, however, that up to 15 per cent of women with endometrial cancer will also have polyps in the endometrial cavity at the time of hysterectomy. This finding makes thorough curettage mandatory in this particular age group.

Polyps are generally believed to develop as the result of prolonged anovulation together with persistent estrogen stimulation. Yet polyps are frequently found at autopsy in the uterine cavity of many women who have not taken estrogenic substances and whose ovaries are atrophic. The epithelium may, in patients who ovulate irregularly, exhibit secretory change on the surface. The finding of unequivocal invasive carcinoma in a polyp is extremely rare, especially when the remainder of the endometrial cavity is free from malignancy. Peterson and Novak found acceptable evidence of carcinoma in only 0.36 per cent. Hertig and Sommers noted that in 31 per cent of patients with invasive endometrial cancer, polyps had been discovered at prior curettage. This does not necessarily implicate polyps as being premalignant since these findings were based on a selective group of patients in a retrospective study. In general, polyps do not recur and most patients proceed through menopause without further difficulty. As previously noted, about 10 per cent of all uteri examined at autopsy show asymptomatic benign polyps.

Management.—The majority of patients with endometrial polyps are cured by thorough curettage. This is particularly true in the postmenopausal group. Therapy must be guided by the histologic pattern of the polyp itself as well as by that of the endometrium. If the polyp contains areas of anaplasia or carcinoma in situ and the endometrial curettings show a similar hyperplastic pattern, hysterectomy may be performed if the patient is beyond the childbearing age. An equally acceptable, although more conservative approach, would be to await another episode of abnormal uterine bleeding or to perform a second curettage within six months.

Since the changes in the polyp and the endometrium may represent only a temporary derangement of pituitary-ovarian function at menopause, with prolongation of estrogen stimulation and absence of progesterone differentiation, a single curettage may prove curative. Continued secretion of estrogenic substances by ovarian tumors of the granulosa-thecoma group would result in recurrence of the hyperplastic process and abnormal bleeding. In the postmenopausal patient, recurrence of uterine bleeding following removal of a benign polyp is an indication for hysterectomy. Uteri removed for this reason frequently show other polyps, missed at the first curettage, as well as foci of endometrial hyperplasia and rarely a minute area of carcinoma in a relatively inaccessible position. Such areas are in the fundus near the junction of the oviduct or behind a submucous leiomyoma. One should make certain, however, that the bleeding has its origin in the endometrial cavity and is not due to senescent or inflammatory vaginitis. Furthermore, it is imperative that the patient be questioned about the use of estrogenic substances in the form of tablets, injections, vaginal creams or suppositories and the use of the popular "hormonal" face creams.

Treatment in younger patients may be both expectant and hormonal. If the basic problem is one of anovulation or oligo-ovulation, adequate investigation of the causes of these problems should be performed. Therapy will depend on the specific endocrine derangement. (See chapter on Endocrine Disorders.) In certain patients, no cause for ovulatory failure can be found, but episodes of hypermenorrhea, irregular flowing and endometrial hyperplasia may be avoided by continued cyclic use of estrogen-progestin combinations. This therapeutic regimen, although administered solely for the relief of symptoms, is occasionally followed by a return to normal ovulatory cycles. Furthermore, it prevents the prolonged growth stimulation of the endometrium by estrogens, adds the differentiating effect of progesterone and allows for regular shedding of the glands and stroma.

Endometrial Hyperplasia

Endometrial hyperplasia includes a varied group of histologic patterns characterized by overgrowth of glandular and stromal elements together with increased vascularity and lymphocytic infiltration. The process may be generalized throughout the uterine cavity or localized to one or more areas. It may occur in any age group and is occasionally seen in teen-age patients who have persistent estrogen stimulation without intermittent progesterone. Similarly, it is commonly observed during the menopause when the process of ovulation is waning. It is obvious, then, that hyperplasia is seen frequently at the two extremes of the reproductive period and is associated with the clinical entity called dysfunctional uterine bleeding.

Endometrial hyperplasia may be produced in animals (monkey, hamster, rabbit) and in human subjects by the administration of estrogenic substances for prolonged periods. We produced varying degrees of hyperplasia (including anaplasia) in normally ovulating females by administering a synthetic estrogen for periods up to 90 days. This process was temporary, however, since the endometrium returned to normal as soon as the estrogen was discontinued and ovulation permitted to occur. Prophylactically, therefore, it is important to preserve the function of ovulation and the differentiating effect of progesterone.

Pathology.—Grossly, the appearance of the endometrial cavity containing hyperplastic tissue is quite variable. In some cases it is markedly thickened or polypoid (Fig. 5–37) and large quantities of tissue may be removed at the time of uterine curettage. This gross appearance is occasionally confused with that of the very thick and succulent endometrium removed on day 27 or 28 of a normal secretory cycle. In some patients, particularly menopausal ones, the curettings may be scanty and only a small focus will be found to contain areas of hyperplasia, and very often if a hysterectomy is performed within a few days or weeks after the curettage, the uterus will be found to harbor only atrophic endometrium. Thus, it is

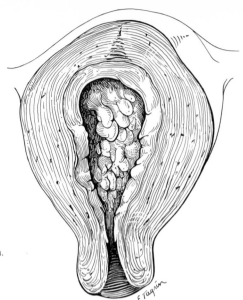

Fig. 5-37.—Endometrial hyperplasia.

possible, at least temporarily, to remove all hyperplastic endometrium by curettage. However, in this older age group one should strongly suspect that invasive carcinoma may be present in an area adjacent to the hyperplasia.

HISTOLOGIC PATTERNS.—Three major types of endometrial hyperplasia are recognized histologically. These are the cystic, the adenomatous and the anaplastic. Mixtures of all three frequently coexist in the same endometrial cavity and may coexist in the curettings. The typical hyperplastic pattern which follows estrogen therapy in the human female is of the cystic variety. This usually takes four to six weeks to develop and will do so only if moderately large doses of estrogens are administered. Cystic hyperplasia is characterized by a glandular pattern that resembles Swiss cheese, that is, irregular enlargement and dilatation of some glands and preservation of normal architecture in others (Fig. 5-38). The epithelium lining the dilated glands is usually cuboidal or cylindrical, with darkly stained nuclei and scant cytoplasm. The smaller glands are usually of proliferative type with numerous mitoses and pseudostratification of nuclei. The stroma is quite cellular and dense and the stromal cells show extensive mitotic activity. Aggregates of lymphocytes are frequently found in the stroma, together with dilated and engorged vascular spaces. It is not difficult in the usual case to distinguish cystic hyperplasia from a cystic gland that occasionally results from obstruction of the gland lumen or from one that is lined by atrophic flat cells found in the endometrium of the postmenopausal patient.

Adenomatous hyperplasia is characterized by an increased number of glands (Fig. 5-39), many of which have small outpouchings or budlike glandular projections into the stroma. A typical finger-in-glove appearance frequently results, and eventually these outpouchings become pinched off and lie in groups with a back-to-back pattern and very little or no inter-

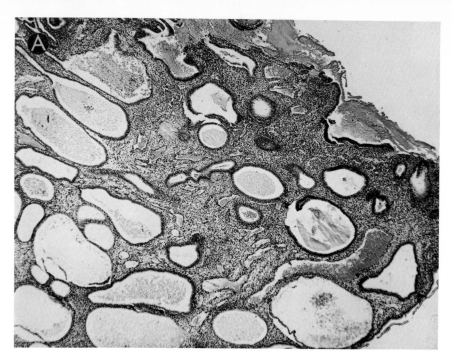

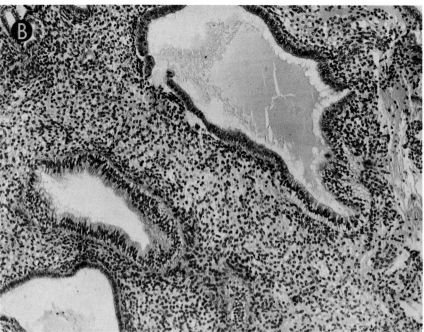

Fig. 5–38.—A, cystic hyperplasia of the endometrium, showing cystic dilatation of glands and an increase in the number and size of the blood vessels. (From Kistner, R. W., and Smith, O. W.: Fertil. & Steril. 12:121, 1961.) **B,** cystic endometrial hyperplasia showing secretory effect 10 days after administration of a single dose (100 mg.) of medroxyprogesterone acetate. The dilated gland at top right is lined by tall cells of high cuboidal and columnar type, but the lower-most fragment shows subnuclear vacuoles, the effect of the progestin. The gland at lower left shows pseudostratification with extensive subnuclear vacuoles. In this postmenopausal patient endometrial hyperplasia resulted from the administration of estrogens.

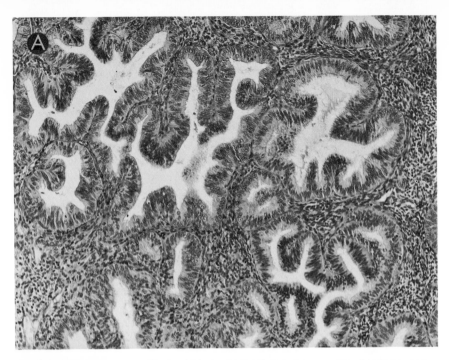

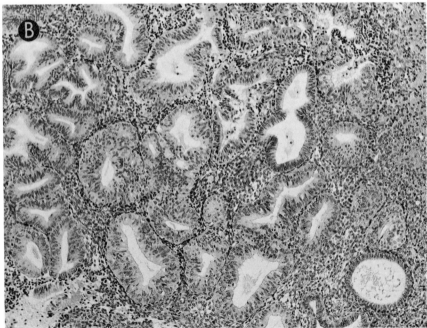

Fig. 5-39.—Adenomatous hyperplasia of the endometrium. In **A,** note outpouching of glands into a dense stroma. The epithelium lining the glands is of active proliferative type and tends to form budlike projections which may be pinched off to form small nests of closely packed glands. These do not vary in staining qualities from the surrounding proliferative endometrium. Specimen was obtained by curettage from a woman, 42, who had received exogenous estrogens for several years. (From Kistner, R. W., and Smith, O. W.: Fertil. & Steril. 12:121, 1961.) **B,** focal carcinoma in situ in central area of adenomatous hyperplasia. (From Kistner, R. W.: Cancer 12:1106, 1959.)

vening stroma. The nuclei are usually darkly stained and the cytoplasm is scant.

Anaplasia, or lessened differentiation, has a typical histologic appearance. The lining cells of the glands exhibit a pronounced variation in size, shape, cytoplasmic staining and polarity. Similarly, the nuclei are usually irregularly shaped and show marked variation in size and staining qualities. There is a generalized pallor of the cells but this may not be uniform.

Symptomatology.—The usual symptom associated with the process of endometrial hyperplasia is that of irregular, occasionally profuse, uterine bleeding. There may be lower abdominal, cramplike pain which is due to the accumulation of blood in the endometrial cavity. This pain is usually relieved by the expulsion of several large blood clots. Endometrial hyperplasia may exist in the teen-age patient due to constant estrogen stimulation. This process disappears as soon as cyclic ovulation and menstruation begin. In the middle-aged patient hyperplasia is associated with an interruption of ovulation either because of intrinsic disease (granulosa cell tumors, thecomas, Stein-Leventhal syndrome, adrenocortical hyperplasia) or because of constant administration of estrogenic substances. The history in these patients reveals an interruption in cyclic menses, usually with skips and delays of flow or with prolonged periods of amenorrhea. The usual premenstrual moliminal symptoms are absent. In postmenopausal patients endometrial hyperplasia is characterized by postmenopausal bleeding. If ingestion of exogenous estrogenic substances has been excluded, hyperplasia is due, in most patients, to ovarian lesions which are presumed to secrete steroidal substances of varying estrogenic potency. These lesions are cortical stromal hyperplasia, thecomatosis (thecosis), granulosa-theca tumors and gynandroblastoma.

Management.—The management of endometrial hyperplasia is similar to that outlined for endometrial polyps. Of prime importance are the age of the patient and the histologic pattern of the hyperplastic process. It is obvious that treatment of the teen-age girl with cystic hyperplasia will always be conservative, whereas, in the postmenopausal patient adenomatous or anaplastic hyperplasia is usually treated by hysterectomy and bilateral salpingo-oophorectomy. Between these two extremes there exist multiple variations of therapeutic regimens. They depend, in large measure, on the relationship of hyperplasia to carcinoma of the endometrium, unfortunately an unsettled and frequently disputed correlation.

It has been suggested that if ovulation could be brought about in certain patients who have a syndrome of obesity, hypertension, diabetes and endometrial abnormalities, the eventual development of carcinoma in such patients might be avoided. Hertig has stated that optimum treatment for these patients is ovulation, menstruation and pregnancy; most patients in this particular group never accomplish this goal.

The association of hyperplasia and carcinoma of the endometrium was first noted by Backer in 1904, but prior to the report of Taylor in 1932 the simultaneous occurrence of these two lesions was believed to be one of chance alone. The review by Taylor and that by Novak and Yui in 1936 suggested that a definite correlation between these entities did exist and, further, that estrogenic substances might, under favorable circumstances, be carcinogenic. Larson reviewed the literature on the relationship of estrogens in endometrial hyperplasia to carcinoma in 1954 and was able to formulate five distinctly different points of view held by various groups of investigators. Briefly, these are as follows.

1. Endometrial hyperplasia does *not* have any tendency toward malignant change in the *reproductive* years but when it occurs as a result of postmenopausal estrogenic stimulation of the endometrium, it *may* predispose toward malignant disease (Novak).

2. Endometrial hyperplasia (and hence excess estrogen) predisposes to carcinoma at any age (Dockerty *et al.*, Morrin and Max).

3. Endometrial hyperplasia and cancer are not associated but ". . . the unopposed action of estrin, with its resultant effect on the endometrium, is the basic principle at work in the development of malignancy of the endometrium of those individuals who possess the genetic factor necessary for the development of cancer" (Herrell).

4. Endometrial hyperplasia may be followed by anaplasia, carcinoma in situ and adenocarcinoma of the uterus, but "no convincing studies are available to show that estrogen stimulation alone will produce this picture, and many excellent estrogen studies failed to mention such histological changes" (Hertig and Sommers).

5. Neither hyperplasia nor prolonged estrogen stimulation is associated with corpus cancer other than on a chance basis (Fahlund and Broders; Jones and Brewer).

The available data from human material would suggest that: (1) there is little, if any, evidence that estrogenic substances are carcinogenic in the premenopausal woman; (2) only meager evidence is available to indicate that cystic (Swiss-cheese) hyperplasia is causally related to endometrial carcinoma; (3) in *predisposed* individuals, the unopposed action of estrogenic substances for considerable periods of time will result in endometrial adenomatous hyperplasia, anaplasia, carcinoma in situ and eventually carcinoma. We produced varying degrees of hyperplasia and anaplasia in young, normally menstruating women by the administration of an estrogen for 45–100 days. After the exogenous estrogen was stopped, all patients subsequently had normal menstrual periods and normal endometrium as determined by biopsy. Gusberg classified "atypical" hyperplasia as being histologically identical with adenomatous hyperplasia, carcinoma in situ and Stage 0 cancer. He followed 64 patients with this entity for five years and subsequently found invasive cancer in only three, or 4.6 per cent. In a later study Gusberg noted that carcinoma developed in 12 per cent of patients with atypical hyperplasia treated only by curettage and followed for at least five years. He concluded that adenomatous hyperplasia might be present in the same endometrium with adenocarcinoma or might be a precursor to cancer.

The specific morphologic changes preceding the development of carcinoma of the endometrium are not completely known. Some evidence has already been advanced by the work of Hertig and Sommers, based on retrospective study of prior curettings, that adenomatous (atypical) hyperplasia precedes carcinoma. However, there is also evidence to support the fact that adenomatous hyperplasia does not *always* proceed relentlessly toward unequivocal carcinoma, and the prediction of which hyperplasia will and which will not become malignant is presently impossible. It is probably true, however, that many of endometria in which there is carcinoma have passed through the various phases shown in Figure 5–40. On the other

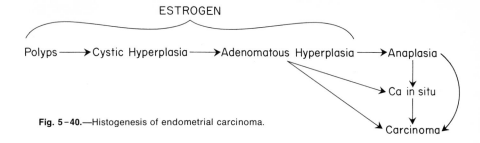

Fig. 5-40.—Histogenesis of endometrial carcinoma.

hand, carcinoma of the endometrium has been found in a few women who have had bilateral oophorectomy many years prior to diagnosis and in whom estrogenic substances had not been administered. In some instances endometrial carcinoma seems to arise in an atrophic endometrium, in a patient whose ovaries are also atrophic. Yet how can one be certain that the area of carcinoma was not an area of carcinoma in situ or atypical hyperplasia five years previously. Areas of carcinoma are occasionally found in basically secretory or proliferative endometrium, but I know of no endometrial carcinoma which co-existed with an intra-uterine pregnancy.

Our recent studies indicate that cystic and adenomatous hyperplastic glands may undergo regression and actively growing stroma may be converted to decidua by the action of synthetic progestational agents. These changes are noted even in the usually stable basal layer of the endometrium and are more pronounced after prolonged, constant therapy. In the younger patient optimum treatment would seem to be the cyclic administration of these newer progestins in the regimens outlined for dysfunctional uterine bleeding. Similarly, in older patients who are not good candidates for surgery, constant administration of large doses of either 17-alpha-hydroxyprogesterone caproate (Delalutin) or medroxyprogesterone (Depo-Provera) for periods of up to six months will bring about adequate hemostasis and endometrial atrophy. A succinct summary by Speert emphasizes the importance of an evaluation of prospective as well as retrospective studies: "Glandular hyperplasia of the endometrium was a common precursor of carcinoma, but carcinoma occurs in only a small proportion of women with endometrial hyperplasia." Therefore, because of the reversibility of glandular changes which heretofore were thought to be premalignant, the often quoted dictum of Halban, "Nicht Karzinom, aber besser heraus!" (not carcinoma, but better out!) is not wholly acceptable.

Premalignant Neoplasms

CARCINOMA IN SITU

The earliest stage of endometrial carcinoma, which is not invasive, has been termed "carcinoma in situ." Although this term is not acceptable in many clinics throughout the country, it has been so designated for a specific lesion, first described by Hertig, in the Pathology Laboratory at the Boston Hospital for Women since about 1940. The diagnosis is based on the presence of glands composed of large eosinophilic cells with abundant cytoplasm (Fig. 5–41). The nuclei tend to be pale with small chromatin

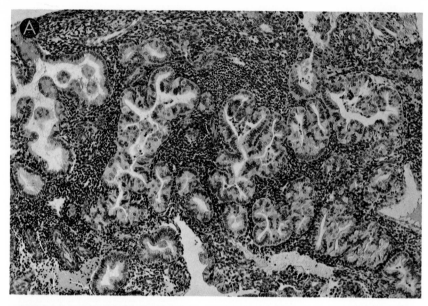

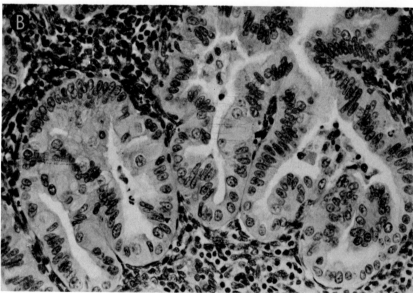

Fig. 5–41.—A, carcinoma in situ of the endometrium. The glands are composed of large cells with abundant, clear, eosinophilic cytoplasm. The nuclei are pale, with fine granular chromatin and slightly wrinkled or irregular nuclear membranes arranged in irregular palisades. **B,** higher power shows cellular disorientation and dyspolarity with intraluminal tufting. Carcinoma in situ is often sharply demarcated and easily distinguished from adjoining normal, senescent or hyperplastic glands. There is moderate crowding of affected glands but not necessarily a back-to-back pattern or invasion or displacement of the endometrial stroma. (From Kistner, R. W.: Cancer 12:1106, 1959.)

granules and slightly irregular, folded or scalloped nuclear membranes. Cytologic anaplasia is present, but there is no stromal invasion. The region of carcinoma in situ is usually focal, sharply in contrast in morphology and staining with neighborhood unaffected glands. In other clinics this same histologic picture has been designated as atypical hyperplasia or carcinoma Stage 0.

There is no characteristic symptom associated with carcinoma in situ of the endometrium other than that of irregular bleeding in the premenopausal woman or postmenstrual staining in the older patient. It is occasionally described as an incidental finding in endometrial hyperplasia or invasive carcinoma. Until 1960 it was believed that endometrium with this particular histologic picture did not revert to normal, hyperplastic or senescent endometrium and that, unless completely removed or destroyed, it would be followed in time by invasive endometrial carcinoma. The highest incidence of carcinoma in situ was noted in the three to five years before invasive cancer. The impact of the retrospective study of patients with invasive carcinoma has prevented adequate observation of the life history of this lesion in our clinic. Thus, Steiner and Craig have reviewed the material on 222 patients in whom a diagnosis of carcinoma in situ of the endometrium was made. Two hundred were treated by hysterectomy and only 15 were followed. Seven were lost to follow-up. Only two of the patients who were followed without further therapy developed invasive carcinoma and in one other patient the hysterectomy specimen showed a "questionable invasive" lesion. Invasive carcinoma was not found in any of the 200 hysterectomies done for carcinoma in situ of the endometrium.

Active therapeutic measures should be instituted without delay in the treatment of the adolescent female whose endometrium shows evidence of hyperplasia, anaplasia or carcinoma in situ (Fig. 5–42). An effort should be made to secure ovulation and cyclic secretory differentiation followed by shedding. It is important to ascertain the precise etiology of the anovulatory process by a complete diagnostic survey. Subsequent therapy with cortisone, progestins, clomiphene or wedge resection should be selected depending upon the diagnosis. Ovarian wedge resection should be the last, not the first, therapeutic measure employed in patients having Stein-Leventhal syndrome since the ovary in this disorder seems unusually responsive to clomiphene. If ovulation cannot be regularly established, substitutional therapy may be administered in the form of cyclic or constant progestins. The clinician should realize that the situation is not acute and that immediate hysterectomy is neither necessary nor indicated. This is of particular importance in the young, infertile female. It is imperative, however, that a thorough curettage be performed in all patients prior to therapy in order to exclude the presence of simultaneously occurring endometrial carcinoma. Although the progestins are capable of bringing about striking changes in the morphology of the endometrial glands, they should not be regarded as a panacea and should not be used as a substitute for usual and accepted diagnostic procedures and appropriate therapy.

Since it is impossible for the pathologist, at present, to predict the malignant potential of atypical endometrium, it is necessary that the clinician select the optimum method of therapy on the basis of other factors. The presence of other pathologic processes involving the internal genitalia or the inability to follow the patient adequately are valid reasons for hyster-

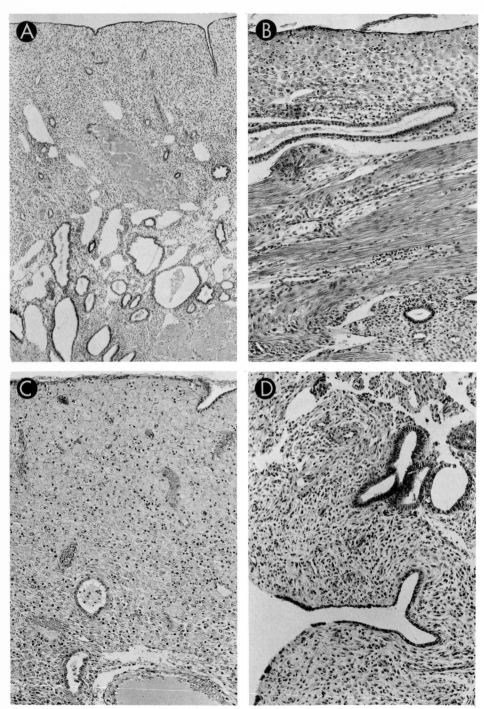

Fig. 5–42.—Effect of progestational agents on endometrial hyperplasia and carcinoma in situ. **A,** hysterectomy specimen from patient with carcinoma in situ after 44 days' therapy with

ectomy. In the young, the infertile, or the very old patient with serious medical disease, a more conservative approach is now possible. Although the patient most likely to benefit from a conservative regimen is the young female with irregular or absent ovulation, it should also be remembered that the endometrial hyperplastic process may occur in women approaching the menopause as a result of constant estrogen stimulation.

The following recommendations for therapy can be made. In the premenopausal or menopausal patient with adenomatous hyperplasia, in whom carcinoma has been excluded by uterine curettage, cyclic progestins may be given for 6 to 12 months. An androgenic-type progestin should be selected which will result in scanty flow and eventual endometrial atrophy. In patients having carcinoma in situ, constant intramuscular progestins may be given for 6 to 12 months. Hysterectomy may subsequently be performed depending upon the age of the patient, her medical status, and the response of the endometrium noted at the time of curettage. I have not seen persistence of the carcinoma in situ process when therapy has been given for at least 6 months. The medications used for constant therapy are as follows: depo-medroxyprogesterone acetate (100 mg. weekly for 4 weeks, followed by 400 mg. monthly for the next 5 months); 17-alpha-hydroxy-progesterone caproate (500 mg. daily for 2 weeks, followed by 2 Gm. weekly for 6 months).

Malignant Neoplasms

ADENOCARCINOMA

Adenocarcinoma of the body of the uterus is a common disease. In the past it was said to occur only about one-eighth to one-tenth as frequently as cervical carcinoma. In recent years, however, particularly at the Boston Hospital for Women, there has been a marked increase in the incidence of carcinoma of the corpus and a marked decrease in the incidence of cervical cancer. Adenocarcinoma is a malignant neoplasm arising from the epithelial elements of the endometrium. Although it is usually glandular, squamous metaplastic elements occasionally are noted and rarely the lesion may be of a pure squamous cell type. In an analysis of the incidence of various cancers in the female in the state of New York, Corscaden reported an incidence of 11.9 cases per 100,000 female population for corpus

---

Enovid. In the superficial endometrium the glands are small, circular and lined by a single layer of cuboidal epithelium. Glands are inactive in a layer of dense decidual stroma. Cystically dilated glands in an edematous stroma are seen in the basalis but even here the epithelium is inactive. A portion of the myometrium is seen at lower right. **B,** hysterectomy specimen obtained after 80 days of continuous therapy with Enovid in a patient with carcinoma in situ (seen in Fig. 5–41). There is an extremely thin layer of endometrium with decidual effect. A single, thinned-out basal gland is seen with intraluminal secretion. **C,** another section of endometrium from same specimen as B. The compact and superficial layers show well-preserved decidua. Two inactive glands of the basalis are seen below and to the left of a dilated blood vessel. (A–C from Kistner, R. W.: Cancer 12:1106, 1959.) **D,** curettage specimen from a patient with extensive carcinoma in situ of the endometrium obtained after 55 Gm. hydroxyprogesterone caproate was given over nine months. Only scanty curettings were obtained and the glands were inactive. Focal decidual reaction is seen in the stroma. (From Kistner, R. W.: Clin. Obst. & Gynec. 5:1178, 1962.)

cancer and a comparable figure of 34.3 for carcinoma of the cervix. During the interval 1957–1967 the number of patients admitted to the Boston Hospital for Women with endometrial cancer was 404 and the number with cancer of the cervix was 400, a 1:1 ratio. This is in marked contrast to the ratio of 6:1 noted in this hospital during the interval 1930–1940. The cause for the increasing incidence of endometrial carcinoma is unknown but may be due to improved diagnostic methods, more precise histologic criteria or simply an aging population. Increased use of estrogenic hormones during the last 20 years is not believed to be significant as far as an etiologic factor is concerned. Speert reviewed the nine major series of endometrial carcinoma reports in 1948 and noted that the mean age varied from 54 to 58.6 years, with an average of 55.5. At the Boston Hospital for Women, Hertig found the mean age to be 57.2 years in a study of 500 patients. The range was 25 to 88 years with a peak incidence of 40.6 per cent in the sixth decade.

Pathology.—Adenocarcinoma (Fig. 5–43) may arise from any part of the uterus and has been separated into two major anatomic types, the diffuse and the localized. In addition, invasive carcinoma has been described in the tip of an endometrial polyp.

The discrete or circumscribed variety of endometrial carcinoma may arise anywhere in the cavity but is generally believed to be found more commonly on the posterior wall. This form may merely represent an earlier variety of the disease than the extensive, diffuse form. The lesion may be papillary, polypoid or only slightly raised from the surrounding endometrium. Frequently it can be diagnosed only by microscopic examination and may then be called a "microcarcinoma." Although the discrete variety may be localized to the endometrium, more often it has invaded the myometrium to a rather considerable degree. Despite this fact, as pointed out by Javert, tumor tends to remain localized in the myometrium in slightly over one-half the cases, and this particular feature accounts in large measure for the relatively good prognosis. In many patients the disease process is so localized that it is entirely removed at the time of curettage, the subsequent hysterectomy specimen being completely devoid of tumor. Needless to say, the prognosis in such a patient is excellent. Minute focal carcinomas are occasionally found in the region of the cornua and these are notoriously difficult to diagnose by routine curettage. Approximately one-fifth arise in the isthmus or lower uterine segment and frequently spread to the endocervix. It is for this reason that a "fractional" curettage is done routinely at the Boston Hospital for Women in an effort to localize the tumor, since endocervical involvement makes it mandatory to treat the patient as if she had primary cervical cancer.

The diffuse form of endometrial carcinoma may be quite superficial and may be difficult to distinguish from polypoid hyperplasia. Grossly, however, the carcinoma is paler, firmer, more friable and less likely to have a glistening mucosal surface. Since this tumor is notoriously slow to invade the myometrium and since it invades the stroma before spread to the myometrium, prognosis is proportionately better than for other genital cancers. In patients with tumor localized to the endometrium, only 1 of 51 had metastases within a five-year follow-up. Javert reported that usually the tumor grows out into the uterine cavity as a cauliflowerlike mass faster than it invades the myometrium. In some cases ulceration may be extensive and it is then difficult to make a definite diagnosis from the curettage since only

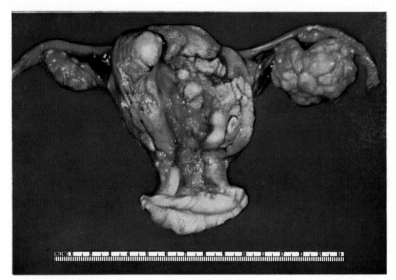

Fig. 5-43.—Endometrial carcinoma of the uterine fundus. (From Benson, R.: Carcinoma of the endometrium, Ca—A Cancer Journal for Clinicians, 18:11, 1968.)

necrotic tissue is recovered. In advanced cases the endometrium is markedly thickened with large exophytic masses protruding into the cavity of the uterus and invasion of the muscular wall and the serosa is frequently obvious. The cervical canal may be blocked by the extension of tumor, with resulting pyometra. Since many endometrial carcinomas produce excessive mucus it is not unusual to find a blood-stained mucoid vaginal discharge as a distinctive sign. The finding of pyometra with endometrial carcinoma alters the prognosis significantly, not only because of the intrinsic septic nature of the pyometra but also because of the more extensive lymphatic permeation of the cancer. In fact, pyometra as the primary cause of death was noted by Henriksen in 28.8 per cent of 208 patients with pyometra complicating uterine cancer.

The microscopic picture varies considerably according to the degree of malignancy and the gross extent of the tumor. All grades of undifferentiation are seen, from a simple increase in the number of glands to extensive arborization of solid tumor. Usually the diagnosis can be made on low-power examination simply by the obvious glandular pattern. Examination of the specific epithelial cells shows various changes, and in the low-grade type the cells grow regularly in a single layer, are larger and stain more deeply than normal cells and there is an increase in the number of mitotic figures. All degrees of undifferentiation beyond this simple picture are seen, with extensive piling up of cells in layers even filling the lumina of glands and invading the stroma. It should be remembered that although the disease fundamentally is an adenocarcinoma, in approximately 20 per cent of the cases there is an accompanying squamous element, such tumors being called *adenoacanthomas* (Fig. 5-44). In the latter the glandular carcinoma is usually fairly well differentiated but seems to be less malignant. The squamous element is usually well differentiated also and is not necessarily microscopically malignant. However, it is an integral part of the tumor, as

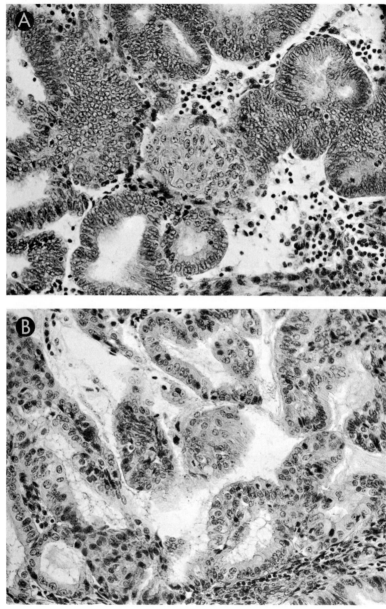

Fig. 5–44.—A, adenocarcinoma of the endometrium with squamous metaplasia, also called adenoacanthoma. **B,** adenocarcinoma showing a secretory pattern. Note the pale vacuolated cells and intraluminal secretion. Secretory adenocarcinomas are uncommon and frequently appear innocuous morphologically. However, they are capable of extension and metastasis. Occasionally a corpus luteum may be found in the ovary in such cases.

is indicated by the fact that metastases show both glandular and squamous elements.

Carcinoma of the endometrium does not lend itself well to strict microscopic grading because of the extreme variability of the tumor in different areas of the endometrial cavity. In general, however, it may be said that the prognosis is much better in well-differentiated tumors. Several series have indicated a survival rate of approximately 75 per cent in grade I tumors, with a gradual decline to approximately 25 per cent in grade IV tumors. The five-year survival is also correlated with the clinical staging of the disease, and it is obvious that undifferentiated tumors are found more commonly in patients with Stage III and Stage IV disease.

The following classification has been recommended by the International Federation of Obstetrics and Gynaecology.

CLINICAL STAGES OF CARCINOMA OF THE CORPUS

Stage I	The carcinoma is confined to the corpus.
Stage II	The carcinoma has involved the corpus and the cervix.
Stage III	The carcinoma has extended outside the uterus, but not outside the true pelvis.
Stage IV	The carcinoma has extended outside the true pelvis, or has obviously involved the mucosa of the bladder or rectum

NOTE: On occasions, it may be difficult to decide whether the cancer actually is of the endocervix or a carcinoma of the corpus and endocervix. If a clear differentiation is not possible from the findings at fractional curettage, then those which are adenocarcinoma should be classified as carcinoma of the corpus, and any epidermoid carcinoma as carcinoma of the cervix.

Three major lymphatic channels have been described by Henriksen as draining the corpus uteri. One of these effects drainage from the lower uterine segment and midportion of the corpus into the same lymphatic channels as those from the cervix; the second channel, mostly from the fundus of the uterus, drains through the broad ligament and the infundibulopelvic ligament to hypogastric, external iliac, common iliac and aortic nodes. The third channel drains along the course of the round ligament and into the superficial and deep inguinal nodes (Fig. 5–45). It is primarily because of this lymphatic drainage that surgical treatment of carcinoma of the endometrium by radical hysterectomy and lymph node dissection is not looked on with favor. Distant metastases occur in approximately 40 per cent of patients, and the organs most commonly involved are the lungs, liver, peritoneum, ovary, bowel, pleura, adrenal and bones. The peritoneal implantations are the result of direct extension of the tumor cells to the peritoneal cavity by way of the oviduct, whereas ovarian metastases, occurring in approximately 4 per cent of cases, are usually due to lymphatic spread.

Certain histochemical features have recently been described in carcinoma of the endometrium and may bear some relation to methods of treatment, particularly as regards progestational agents. Studies have been reported by Atkinson, Hall and McKay. Alkaline phosphatase reaches a peak in the cytoplasm during the proliferative phase of the cycle and has been described in endometrial hyperplasia and well-differentiated carcinoma. It seems to be correlated with growth patterns and differentiation. Glycogen is scanty during the proliferative phase but increases markedly in the progestational phase of a normal cycle. Glycogen has been found to be

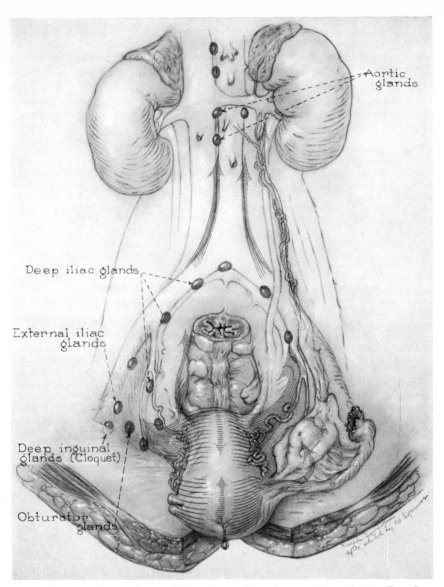

Fig. 5–45.—Lymphatic spread of carcinoma of the uterine cervix and fundus. (From Benson, R.: Carcinoma of the endometrium, Ca—A Cancer Journal for Clinicians, 18:10, 1968.)

scanty and variable in distribution in both hyperplasia and carcinoma in situ, whereas in actual adenocarcinoma all variations of glycogen content have been described. Ribonucleic acid has been found in large amounts in both hyperplasia and carcinoma. During the progestational phase of the normal cycle, ribonucleic acid progressively declines. Acid phosphatase is minimal in the proliferative phase of the normal cycle but increases during the progestational phase. It is present in rather marked degree in carcinoma in situ but its amount in invasive carcinoma is variable.

Recent studies have indicated a variation in content of deoxyribonucleic acid (DNA) in presumed precursors of endometrial carcinoma. Wagner and associates carried out microspectrophotometric measurements of Feulgen-stained gland-cell nuclei in 16 patients with presumed precursors (six cystic hyperplasia, 10 adenomatous hyperplasia) and six adenocarcinomas of the endometrium. In all patients with cystic hyperplasia a diploid to tetraploid DNA distribution was found which was indistinguishable from that of a normal proliferating endometrium. The same diploid to tetraploid DNA distribution was found in eight of the ten adenomatous hyperplasias. Only two cases of adenomatous hyperplasia had an aneuploid DNA distribution pattern and this was similar to that of invasive carcinoma. The six patients with adenocarcinoma had aneuploid DNA-distribution. Since every group of precursor lesions in other organs studied in a similar way have been reported to have aneuploid DNA-distribution patterns, the results of this study suggest that most of the lesions now diagnosed as precursors of endometrial carcinoma either deviate from the pattern of other epithelia or that the morphologic criteria which traditionally are used in the diagnosis of these lesions are insufficiently precise.

Vaginal metastases from adenocarcinoma of the endometrium have been described in from 10 to 15 per cent of patients. These metastatic areas are frequently found on the anterior vaginal wall, usually in the suburethral area. Although it has been felt that vaginal metastases were due to implantation of tumor cells at the time of surgery, in all probability they represent lymphatic permeation.

Pathogenesis.—Although the precise etiology of endometrial cancer is unknown, considerable evidence from clinical, endocrinologic and pathologic studies has accumulated which indicates that the lesion develops as a result of long-continued estrogen stimulation without the interposition of progesterone. This general concept is true in the young patient under age 35 with a history of dysfunctional bleeding, in the premenopausal patient with a similar history and even in the postmenopausal patient with a granulosa cell tumor of the ovary or thecomatosis.

Other stigmata of endocrine dysfunction in these patients are the increased incidence of obesity, diabetes, thyroid malfunction, breast cancer and infertility. As described in the section on Endometrial Hyperplasia, there may be a gradual progression through the various processes of cystic hyperplasia, adenomatous hyperplasia, anaplasia, carcinoma in situ and finally invasive carcinoma. Any one of these particular entities may regress at any time if the constant stimulation of estrogen is removed or if the differentiating effects of progesterone or pregnancy supervene. It is true that a carcinoma may arise in the endometrium in a young patient who is cyclically ovulating and who may have menstrual endometrium adjacent to the cancerous area. It is probable that such carcinomas originate in a focus of hyperplasia or a polyp which does not respond to the secretory stimulation of progesterone.

A gradual morphologic transition from benign hyperplasia to neoplasia has been observed in sequential biopsies and also in multiple curettings obtained at the same time from the same endometrium. As long ago as 1923, Meyer emphasized that the morphologic differences between hyperplasia and cancer were those of degree only and described the concomitant finding of hyperplasia and cancer in the same tissue sections.

The studies of Wagner and associates suggest, therefore, that the endometrial lesions conventionally regarded as being precursors to endometrial adenocarcinoma may be divided into two types—a unimorphous type and a polymorphous type. Unimorphous hyperplasia is seen commonly in patients to whom estrogenic drugs have been administered for relatively long periods and in anovulatory patients. The association between this type of alteration with estrogenic states and the epidemiologic studies suggesting the possible association of estrogenic hormones with endometrial carcinoma suggests a tentative hypothesis for the development of endometrial carcinoma in which estrogen may be regarded as an essential co-carcinogen which produces true hyperplasia which is diploid in character. This hyperplasia may progress to a true neoplasm by the continual action of another carcinogen or, in the absence of such additional stimuli, may remain unaltered. Our reports of the successful treatment of patients with adenomatous hyperplasia or carcinoma in situ by the administration of progestins suggests that some of these lesions may be reversible. It seems entirely possible that the reversible cases might fall into the unimorphous or diploid class.

Since an aneuploid DNA distribution, found in all other recognized groups of in situ neoplasms in other epithelia, was found in only two of ten patients reported by Wagner, one must conclude that adenomatous hyperplasia deviates from this general pattern or that the usual morphologic criteria for diagnosis are insufficiently precise. This failure of differentiation would place both benign abnormalities and pre-invasive neoplasms in the same diagnostic category. Such a mixture of hyperplastic and neoplastic lesions in the same diagnostic group might account for the relatively low incidence of invasive carcinoma eventually found in those patients followed without therapy. It remains to be determined, however, either by prospective or retrospective studies of patients with adenomatous hyperplasia whether the prognosis is truly different in the subdivisions of this group as defined by DNA content. Even if such a difference can be demonstrated, the clinical application may be difficult because of the coexistence of both types of adenomatous hyperplasia in the same patient and the notoriously inadequate sample of the endometrium obtained by biopsy or curettage.

We have been able to produce invasive carcinoma of the endometrium in the rabbit by the insertion of a cotton string impregnated with a known carcinogen, 3-methylcholanthrene. But it is necessary to leave the string in place for at least a year to produce cancer. A control of the experiment was made possible by the use of a string coated in bees-wax and placed in the opposite uterine horn. The tendency to carcinogenesis was absent in the control uterine horn. The necessity of estrogen in the experiment was emphasized by repeating the same plan in oophorectomized rabbits. No cancer developed in these animals. Based on the work of Wagner, it might be con-cluded that the addition of 3-methylcholanthrene to the estrogen-stimulated endometrium was sufficient to convert DNA distribution from a diploid or tetraploid pattern to the aneuploid pattern. Furthermore, when endogenous estrogen was removed by oophorectomy the DNA distribution of the atroph-ic endometrium was not affected by the carcinogen. Finally, the adminis-tration of synthetic progestins to rabbits with intact ovaries significantly inhibited the carcinogenesis in the methylcholanthrene uterus and caused regression of established carcinomas. We have theorized that the progestin, acting locally as an anti-estrogen and producing glandular atrophy, acts in the same fashion as oophorectomy.

Symptomatology and Diagnosis.—The commonest symptom is that of intermenstrual bleeding. Occasionally this may be profuse, although at the outset symptoms may be those of excessive flow at the time of the normally expected period and some bloody discharge, frequently mucoid, between the flows. After the menopause, irregular bleeding or just spotting may be the primary symptom; as the tumor becomes more extensive and necrotic, there is a constant bloody discharge.

Fractional uterine curettage and microscopic examination of the curet-tings is the only acceptable method of diagnostic survey in endometrial carcinoma. Although the disease may be suspected by positive results of cytology and even diagnosed by endometrial biopsy, a thorough curettage is mandatory for proper management. It has been customary at the Boston Hospital for Women to perform a so-called fractional curettage in these patients. The endocervix is first thoroughly curetted and this tissue placed in a separate fixative. The cervix is then carefully dilated and the uterine cavity is sounded to determine its extent and direction. Following this, the entire endometrial cavity is systematically and thoroughly investigated and special attention is paid to the uterine cornual areas since corpus carcinoma may be hidden in these areas. If pyometra is discovered at the time of cervical dilatation, drainage is instituted and the purulent material is cultured. Fractional curettage may be done later, following treatment with an appropriate antibiotic. Accidental perforation of the uterus in elderly women should lead to a suspicion of endometrial carcinoma. Occa-sionally leiomyomas are so situated that the curet cannot reach the malig-nant area, but fortunately such cases are rare. At the conclusion of the curettage polyp forceps should be used since the sharp curet may miss a polyp harboring carcinoma.

It should be emphasized that the size of the uterus is no absolute criterion for the presence or absence of carcinoma. In the average case the uterus is larger when tumor is present, but a well-developed cancer may be found in a small or even atrophic uterus. Tissue removed from the uterus may be screened through a gauze sponge which has been soaked in saline solution, since frequently the fragments of tumor are small and mixed with blood. With such a maneuver the tissue fragments will remain on the sponge and the liquid blood will drain through. If no readily discernible tissue is identi-fied, we routinely fix the entire sponge in Bouin's solution. The fixed tissue is then removed by the pathologist. Although we do not routinely perform frozen section for diagnosis at the time of curettage, this method will obviate a second anesthesia if intracavitary radium therapy is planned. In general, there is an error of about 5 per cent with frozen-section diagnosis, but this error may be reduced practically to zero by the use of rapid semi-permanent or permanent sections utilizing polychrome methylene blue stain. If this technique is perfected, diagnosis may be made at the time of the original curettage and immediate therapy carried out. As previously mentioned, the use of endometrial or suction biopsy is advantageous provided carcinoma is found, but it is of no value as negative evidence since a good-sized area of tumor may be missed. It has been my experience that when nothing but necrotic tissue is obtained, carcinoma of the endometrium is usually present and the patient should be treated accordingly. If hyperplastic endometrium is removed, the operator must decide whether hyperplasia is present alone or is accompanied by carcinoma or whether the hyperplasia is related, especially in the postmenopausal patient, to a tumor of the ovary. If endometrial tissue of any extent is removed in the postmenopausal patient, exclusive of a solitary polyp, the presence of a thecoma or granulosa-thecoma is strongly suspected and immediate hysterectomy may be carried out at this time. It seems unwise to advocate routine hysterectomy in all patients who have postmenopausal bleeding simply on the supposition that since cancer is frequently a cause it is better to operate rather than run the risk of causing metastases by doing a curettage.

The differential diagnosis includes dysfunctional (endocrine) uterine bleeding, submucous leiomyomas of the uterus, carcinoma of the cervix, polyps of the cervix and endometrium and ovarian tumors. Cancer of the endometrium is exceedingly rare before age 40, only 5 per cent of cases occurring prior to that age. Sixteen per cent of endometrial cancers occur before age 50. It is imperative, therefore, that curettage be done in all patients between age 35 and 50 who are suspected of having ovarian dysfunction as the cause of abnormal bleeding. Hormonal therapy administered prior to precise diagnosis may seriously delay early cancer detection.

When excess bleeding or bloody mucoid discharge occurs after the menopause, it indicates that cancer is present somewhere in the genital tract in about 50 per cent of cases.

The postmenopausal patient in whom careful examination and curettage fail to reveal a cause for the bleeding should be followed and, if bleeding recurs, should undergo hysterectomy. A neoplasm of the endometrium, oviduct or ovary may be present which cannot be demonstrated by other methods. One should never be satisfied, particularly in the postmenopausal patient, to assume that the bleeding is due to a senescent vaginitis or a cervical polyp even if these have been demonstrated. Many postmenopausal patients may have bleeding as a result of overenthusiastic use of various estrogenic preparations given for menopausal symptoms. Hysterectomy is not indicated in such patients, in the absence of carcinoma, since the iatrogenically induced hyperplasia will disappear after the exogenous use of estrogens is discontinued.

A thorough curettage should always precede a pelvic operation, whether it be performed via the vaginal or abdominal route, in order to exclude cancer of the endometrium before proceeding with the definitive procedure. However, if one swipe of the curet produces obvious endometrial carcinoma further curettage is not necessary and may disseminate tumor cells. Clusters of metastatic tumor cells are frequently seen on the ovarian surface when surgery is deferred for 3 weeks after curettage and radium treatment. If a diagnosis of carcinoma has been made by prior endometrial biopsy a subsequent curettage is unnecessary but the endocervix should be adequately sampled. Tissue which is suspicious should be given to the pathologist and an immediate frozen section performed. This is particularly true when vaginal plastic operations or combined procedures such as the Manchester-Fothergill operation are to be performed.

Vaginal cytology may prove to be a valuable aid in diagnosis of early carcinoma of the endometrium, but owing to the rather high incidence of false-negative results vaginal smears should never be relied on as final diagnostic tests. The diagnostic accuracy of cytologic examination may be greatly improved by the use of endometrial suction or endometrial lavage.

The commonest errors in diagnosis of endometrial carcinoma have been summarized as follows by Finn: (1) failure to investigate irregular bleeding in a woman who is still menstruating, (2) correction of only the obvious causes of postmenopausal bleeding, (3) failure to curet when a cervical stenosis is dilated and hematometra is drained, (4) disregard of the significance of perforation in an older woman, (5) reliance on cytologic smears alone to detect endometrial carcinoma, (6) complete reliance on endometrial biopsy to detect endometrial carcinoma, (7) inadequate curettage.

Treatment.—The basic and fundamental treatment of carcinoma of the endometrium is surgical, but various combinations of x-ray and radium have been used as adjunctive measures by most gynecologists throughout the country. Several clinics, however, have continued to utilize surgery alone, whenever this is possible, and report five-year cure rates from 47 to 66 per cent. It is obvious that the cure rate will depend on the clinical stage of the disease, and therefore if a particular clinic is fortunate enough to have most of their patients in Stage I or Stage II the cure rate by surgery alone should approach 60–70 per cent. With newer techniques of radium and x-ray administration followed by hysterectomy and bilateral salpingo-oophorectomy, five-year salvage rates from 75 to 94 per cent have been reported. In these later series an average of 84 per cent salvage was secured. It is important to realize that, because of the complicating factors of obesity, hypertension, diabetes and heart disease, death due to causes unrelated to the malignancy will occur in about 15–20 per cent of patients. During the years 1955 through 1960 at the Boston Hospital for Women nine different treatment methods were utilized in the management of patients with endometrial carcinoma. It is difficult to standardize treatment in a disease of this type, yet it is not adequate to state simply that treatment should be individualized in each patient.

If the diagnosis is made at the time of curettage, the generally accepted plan has been to insert intracavitary radium at this time and to do a total hysterectomy and bilateral salpingo-oophorectomy in approximately three weeks. Beginning in 1945 a so-called modified radical hysterectomy was introduced. This consists of removal of the external iliac, hypogastric, obturator and periureteral lymph nodes together with the adjacent areolar tissue. The ureters are not usually dissected although if the patient is in good general condition and is not too obese, the ureters may be displaced and a wide parametrial and cervical cuff removed, together with the upper third of the vagina. If the excised lymph nodes contain tumor or if there is extension of tumor to the oviduct, ovaries, outer portion of the myometrium or uterine serosa, postoperative x-ray therapy is administered.

It has been suggested that if the uterus is small and the contained tumor minute, intracavitary radium need not be administered. However, it is impossible to know how extensive the tumor is; also, if the uterine cavity is capacious, all parts of it may not receive the same intensity of radiation. This argument may be overcome, to a certain extent, by the use of multiple, small radium tubes together with adequate packing. The presence of submucous fibroids will distort the contour of the uterine cavity and will also prevent the full application of radium to the tumor area. Despite these difficulties it is believed that irradiation appreciably decreases the size of the tumor and the uterus, reduces congestion and probably devitalizes a certain number of cells so that there is less chance of spreading viable tumor cells during operation. Previous studies have indicated that residual carcinoma is found in approximately 50 per cent of uteri at hysterectomy after at least 3,600 mg./hr. of radium. With the use of Heyman capsules the incidence of tumor in removed uteri has been reduced to approximately 25 per cent.

A further reduction in the incidence of residual tumor may be obtained by the adjunctive use of progestational steroids with radium. For the last 10 years it has been my policy to give medroxyprogesterone acetate for 3 weeks prior to surgery beginning at the time radium is inserted. The following regimen is used: 400 mg. intramuscularly daily for 7 days (2800 mg); then 400 mg. 3 times weekly for two weeks (2400 mg.) If the excised specimen shows viable tumor beyond the inner third of the myometrium, medroxy-progesterone acetate is given along with Cobalt therapy in the following regimen: 400 mg. daily for 7 days; then 400 mg. 3 times weekly as long as x-ray therapy is given. Figure 5–46 illustrates the morphologic changes effected by the progestational agent.

Austin and MacMahon reviewed all cases of invasive carcinoma of the uterine corpus admitted to the Boston Hospital for Women between 1920 and 1959. Cases of in situ cancer were not included. During this interval 941 patients were classified as having invasive cancer but 180 were excluded because of prior treatment, lack of histological confirmation, mixed tumors and lack of follow-up. A total of 761 patients were then available for analysis. For the series as a whole, the crude five-year survival rate was 67.3 per cent, and the relative survival ratio was 76.5 per cent. Among patients in Stage I, the assignment of nuclear grade appeared to have considerable prognostic value since the survival was 93.3 per cent in well-differentiated nuclear grade I tumors but only 39.8 per cent in grade IV. This differential was maintained in patients not classified in Stage I. Clinical and postoperative staging were highly correlated with the probability of survival. Of the 761 patients clinically staged, 86 per cent were in Stage I, and 70 per cent remained in Stage I after examination of the excised uterus. The five-year survival in this group was 89.9 per cent. Austin and MacMahon noted no significant difference in survival based on uterine size if the enlargement was due to tumor. The five-year-survival rate was 94.1 per cent in patients without uterine enlargement due to tumor and 87.4 per cent in patients with enlarged uteri. Involvement of the myometrium was significant only if the tumor invaded deeply, since 91.2 per cent survived 5 years if only the endometrium was involved and 81.2 per cent survived if deep myometrial involvement was noted. Patients having an adenoacanthoma had slightly better survival rates than those with adenocarcinoma, 79.8 per cent of 191 patients with adenoacanthoma surviving

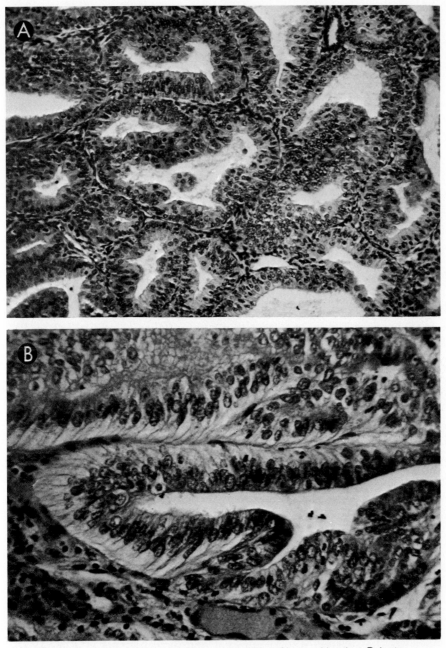

Fig. 5-46.—**A,** adenocarcinoma classified as grade III in a 61-year-old patient. **B,** hyster-ectomy specimen in patient noted in **A** after four days of intrauterine medroxyprogesterone acetate. The glycogen secretion in the glands of the basal endometrium simulates 17-day secretory pattern. (From Kistner, R. W., Griffiths, C. T., and Craig, J. M.: Use of progestational agents in the management of endometrial cancer, Cancer 18:1563, 1965.)

5 years as compared to 75.2 per cent of 570 patients with adenocarcinoma. The crude cumulative survival rate for the 761 patients diminished from 68.8 per cent at 5 years to 36.5 per cent at 20 years, but the *relative* cumulative survival rate dropped only from 76.5 per cent at 5 years to 70.8 per cent at 20 years.

It has been shown that patients who do not have residual carcinoma in the cavity of the uterus at the time of hysterectomy have a better prognosis. In certain clinics preoperative external irradiation has been utilized in all patients with operable endometrial carcinoma. This has been found to be a valuable adjunct to surgical treatment in these series, the reported five-year survival rate being 89.6 per cent. Surgery is usually performed approximately six weeks after the conclusion of external x-ray therapy and this combined method has not increased the incidence of postoperative fistulas. Not only has the over-all five-year survival rate been increased, but the incidence of recurrences seen in the vagina has been reduced from an average of 15 per cent to less than 1 per cent.

There has been some effort to treat endometrial carcinoma by a radical surgical approach in exactly the same manner in which cervical cancer is treated. The results, however, have not warranted a continuation of this program. Unfortunately this disease occurs in the later decades when obesity and cardiorenal disease are common. These factors and the number of inoperable cases reduce the total number which can be treated by surgery. Furthermore, several studies have indicated that the operative mortality rate and postoperative morbidity rate preclude the usual radical hysterectomy for this disease.

At the Boston Hospital for Women radical hysterectomy and pelvic lymphadencectomy is not utilized in the treatment of endometrial cancer unless the cervix is involved. In a series of 78 patients previously treated by this method between 1945 and 1959, 10 patients were found to have positive lymph nodes and only 2 of these survived 5 years. During the same period of time, however, two operative deaths occurred as a direct result of the radical procedure.

When surgery is strictly contraindicated, the patient is usually given two applications of intracavitary radium followed by full x-ray therapy, the external irradiation being administered to four pelvic ports, with the beams angled so that the body of the uterus is in the center of the cross-fire. If radium and x-ray are used without surgery it is essential to do.a thorough curettage about six months following first treatment to determine the presence of persistent disease. If disease is present, the patient may have become operable either by reduction in size of the pelvic organs or by an improvement of her general condition.

Kottmeier has recently reported on 1,123 patients treated by primary radiotherapy. The 5-year-cure rate in 864 patients in Stage I was 71 per cent; in 103 patients in Stage II it was 44 per cent; in 135 patients in Stage III the survival was 19 per cent and in 21 patients in Stage IV the 5-year salvage was also 19 per cent. The overall 5-year-cure rate was 61 per cent.

Since 1960 I have treated patients in the inoperable group by adding medroxyprogesterone acetate to the radiation plan. There is evidence, not as yet conclusive, that the progestin may increase the sensitivity of the tumor cell to radiation. The above progestin is given in the following regimen: 400 mg. intramuscularly daily for 7 days beginning at the time of the first radium insertion; then 400 mg. is given 3 times weekly during the next two weeks, giving a total "loading dose" of 5200 mg. during the first 3 weeks. During the period of x-ray therapy the same progestin is continued in a dose of 400 mg. weekly. If a repeat curettage fails to reveal viable tumor, progestin therapy is discontinued. However, if tumor remains or if there is evidence of distant metastases, the progestin is continued indefinitely in a dose of 400 mg. monthly.

Recurrent endometrial carcinoma is found in approximately 15 per cent of all patients treated, the rate of recurrence being directly proportional to the histologic grade of the carcinoma. In patients with undifferentiated cancers the recurrence rate is about five times as high as in those with well-differentiated cancers. The most common sites of recurrence are the remaining pelvic organs, the vagina, the bladder, the ureters, the pelvic lymph nodes and the pelvic peritoneum. The incidence of recurrence is high during the first three years following initial treatment, but thereafter approximates 1 per cent annually. The curative effect of x-ray or radium irradiation on recurrences has not been encouraging. In specific cases extensive pelvic surgery for solitary, localized recurrences has shown encouraging results, even though the number of patients treated has been small.

Approximately 25 per cent of all carcinomas of the endometrium in metastatic sites will respond to the use of 17-alpha-hydroxyprogesterone caproate (Delalutin) or medroxyprogesterone acetatè (Depo-Provera). Dramatic results have occurred in some patients, with complete disappearance of lesions in the vagina, mediastinum, pelvis and lung parenchyma (Fig. 5–47). Biopsy material, when available, has shown increased differentiation of tumor cells together with secretory activity as a result of the progestational agent in those patients with objective remissions. Sub-

Fig. 5–47.—**A,** roentgenogram of chest in an 82-year-old patient with metastatic foci of endometrial carcinoma in both lung fields. The larger lesions in the midthoracic area are noted by arrows. **B,** roentgenogram showing almost complete resolution of pulmonary metastases. The patient had received between 400 and 700 mg. of medroxyprogesterone acetate (Depo-Provera) weekly for three months and during this interval had marked subjective and objective improvement.

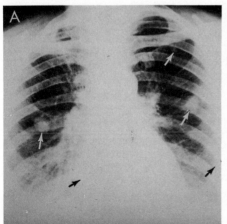
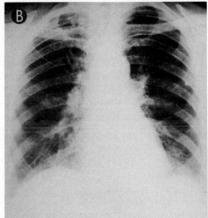

jective remissions have occurred in approximately 75 per cent of patients. The exact mode of action of progestational agents in endometrial carcinoma is not known but it is surmised that, because endometrium is a tissue normally under strong progestational control, endometrial carcinoma (and its metastases) may also have such sensitivity. It is important that such patients be treated with rather massive doses of 17-alpha-hydroxy-progesterone caproate, that is, from 3 to 7 Gm. weekly. The steroid substance is without toxic effects, and in some instances remissions have lasted for over 6 years. Well differentiated lesions in patients in whom there has been a long hiatus between original treatment and the discovery of the metastases will respond with lower doses, whereas maximum amounts should be given to other patients. The optimum dosage of medroxy-progesterone acetate for endometrial carcinoma seems to be in the range of 400–1,000 mg. monthly as a maintenance dose. Our results, however, indicate that an original loading dose of 3 to 5 Gm. given during the first 3 weeks of therapy is advisable. This may be accomplished by giving 400 mg. of depo-medroxyprogesterone acetate daily for 7 days, then 400 mg. three times weekly for the next 2 weeks. Therapy should be given for at least 6 weeks before a decision is reached regarding the presence of an objective response. If a remission is obtained it should be continued indefinitely and not diminished in amount. We have advised a maintenance dose of 400 mg. monthly although several authors have suggested doses in the range of 2 Gm. per month. In a few patients recurring carcinoma, while receiving progestins, has responded to the use of estrogen or an alkylating agent given along with the progestin.

The mechanism of action of progestational agents in effecting remissions has not been precisely defined. There is evidence to favor a local effect as a result of the marked changes brought about by the direct instillation of progestins into a vaginal metastasis or endometrial cavity. (see Fig. 5–46). It has been suggested that the progestins alter the receptor site in the endometrial cell for estrogen thus diminishing its potential for growth.

Sarcoma

Sarcoma may occur in the corpus of the uterus and may arise in the muscle tissue, in the connective tissue between the muscle or in the connective tissue of the endometrium. Further, it may originate per se in leiomyomas. Sarcoma occurs five times as often in the corpus as in the cervix. In general, it constitutes about 3 per cent of all malignant diseases of the uterus. The highest incidence is in the sixth decade and therefore it may be said to be a disease of the postmenopausal female.

There is always much speculation as to whether the sarcoma has actually arisen in a leiomyoma or in the normal tissues of the uterus, especially when the disease is extensive. Although different authors have a variance of opinion in regard to the percentage of leiomyomas that become sarcomatous, the average has been somewhere between 0.4 and 0.8 per cent. In a series of 5,000 leiomyomas at the Boston Hospital for Women the incidence of sarcomatous change was quoted as 0.81 per cent. The variation in incidence is due to a disagreement among pathologists as to the exact criteria for sarcoma. If a leiomyoma is rapidly growing and if the nuclei are rather closely packed together, a mistaken diagnosis of sarcoma may be

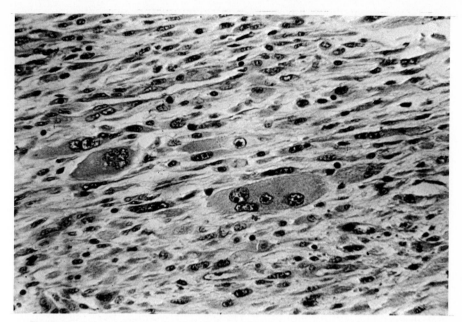

Fig. 5-48.—Leiomyosarcoma showing pleomorphism of muscle cells and multinucleated giant cells.

forthcoming. Various changes of a degenerative nature occur in leiomyomas, and sarcomatous change occurs most often at the center of the tumor. It has been described as having a raw-pork appearance in the early stages when the whorl-like arrangement of the fibers is lost. Eventually the tumor becomes necrotic and softened, with cavities formed by liquefaction of tissue.

A leiomyosarcoma may arise either in a pre-existing leiomyoma or in the uterine wall or from muscle or connective tissue in either site. It has recently been suggested that some tumors of this type may actually arise in the muscle and connective tissue of the uterine blood vessels. The gross appearance of a leiomyosarcoma is extremely variable and may be that of a simple, solitary nodule which cannot be distinguished from an ordinary leiomyoma. Occasionally the tumor may extend through the serosa and be adherent to the omentum and intestines. In other types, growth has occurred beneath the mucosa with actual projection into the endometrial cavity. Grossly the cut surface of the leiomyosarcoma may be difficult to distinguish from that of an ordinary leiomyoma. Usually, however, when the surface is cut the tumor area bulges above the surrounding tissue, loses its whorl pattern and appears homogeneous in color, with some mixture of pink and gray. Vascularity is prominent and there is no sharp line of demarcation between the tumor and the myometrium.

Microscopically a leiomyosarcoma presents the characteristic spindle, round or giant cell types (Fig. 5-48). In some areas the cells blend with mature muscle cells, and frequently more than one type of tumor cell is present. Prognosis depends on the "mitotic activity," and evidence has shown that when counts exceeded 2,000 mitoses/cu. mm. of tissue the patients died, whereas they survived when counts were less than 800/cu.

mm. Novak pointed out that when mitotic counts were over 30/high-power field the patient died and, in general, that low mitotic counts were usually found in sarcomas arising in a leiomyoma.

Endometrial Stromal Sarcoma.—This is a sarcoma which apparently arises from the stromal cell of the endometrium. Grossly these tumors are polypoid, fleshy masses which arise from the uterine fundus. Invasion of the myometrium often occurs despite the endometrial origin. Microscopically, endometrial stromal sarcomas are made up of spindle-shaped cells with varying amounts of cytoplasm, so that the cells frequently resemble the stromal cells of the proliferative phase of the menstrual cycle (Fig. 5-49). In other cases the cytoplasm is abundant and a resemblance to decidual cells is striking. Tumor giant cells are commonly seen since the tumor cells themselves exhibit marked pleomorphism. They may be confused with placental-site giant cells or even foreign-body giant cells. The degree of malignancy of the tumor depends on the number of mitoses identified.

There are no characteristic symptoms, most patients having episodes of irregular bleeding and abdominal or pelvic pain. A mass is frequently palpable and surgery carried out for this reason.

The only known treatment for endometrial stromal sarcomas is complete hysterectomy and bilateral salpingo-oophorectomy. X-ray therapy has not been of value except for palliation. The prognosis is poor, five-year survival rates being in the range of 14–16 per cent. By comparison, five-year survival rates for sarcomas arising in leiomyomas have ranged from 15 to 75 per cent.

Fig. 5-49.—Endometrial stromal sarcoma. This is a well-differentiated tumor showing neoplastic endometrial stroma with whorled pattern, pleomorphism and giant cells scattered about normal proliferative glands. (From Hertig, A. T., and Gore, H. M.: *Tumors of the Female Sex Organs: Part 2. Tumors of the Vulva, Vagina and Uterus,* sec. IX, fasc. 33 of *Atlas of Tumor Pathology* [Washington, D.C.: Armed Forces Institute of Pathology, 1960].)

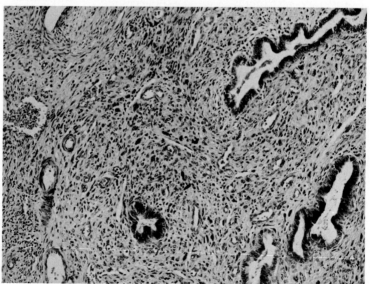

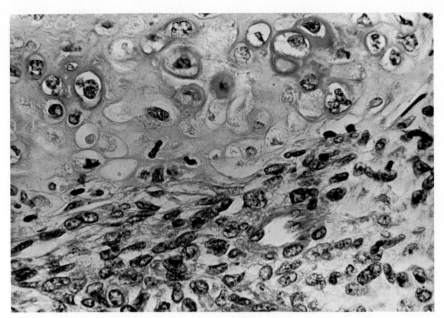

Fig. 5-50.—Mixed mesodermal tumor of the endometrium. This is predominantly a sarcoma of endometrial origin showing the tendency of the tumor to form cartilage in this area.

Mixed Mesodermal Tumor.—This is an uncommon tumor of endometrial stromal origin containing both sarcomatous elements of mesenchymal origin and carcinomatous elements of müllerian potential. Some doubt has been cast on the validity of these tumors as a biologic entity and they have been explained as originating: (1) as a "collision" tumor from two independent lesions invading one another; (2) as a "combination" tumor resulting from two blastomatous elements derived from one stem cell, or (3) as a "composition" tumor resulting from blastomatous conversion of stroma and parenchyma. Synonyms for this tumor are carcinosarcoma, combined mesenchymal sarcoma-carcinoma of the uterus, and the preferred description, *malignant mixed mesodermal tumor.*

Eleven patients with this lesion have been treated at the Boston Hospital for Women. All were postmenopausal and five gave a history of artificial induction of menopause by radiation. The uterus is usually enlarged and filled with multiple polypoid masses which are attached by broad masses to the endometrium. Such masses have been described as having a phallus-like appearance contained in the endometrial cavity. Microscopically, these polypoid masses are made up of intermingled carcinomatous and sarcomatous elements with varying degrees of differentiation. The carcinoma is usually an adenocarcinoma, but occasionally squamous elements may be found. There is frequently a tendency to form thin-walled blood vessels with associated areas of hemorrhage and necrosis. In some tumors striated muscle fibers, osteoid elements or cartilage may be identified (Fig. 5–50).

The treatment of this lesion is total hysterectomy and bilateral salpingo-oophorectomy followed by x-ray therapy. The value of adjunctive x-ray therapy is unknown, since most patients do not survive two years. Chemotherapeutic agents have not increased the length of survival of patients with this lesion.

BIBLIOGRAPHY

Anatomy and Physiology

Allan, F. D.: The Embryology of the Reproductive System, in Velardo, J. T.: *Endocrinology of Reproduction* (New York: Oxford University Press, 1958).

Anson, B. J., and Curtis, A. H.: Anatomy of the Female Pelvis and Perineum, in Curtis, A. H. (ed.): *Textbook of Gynecology* (Philadelphia: W. B. Saunders Company, 1946).

Gillman, J.: The Development of the Gonads in Man, with a Consideration of the Role of Fetal Endocrines and the Histogenesis of Ovarian Tumors, in *Contributions to Embryology* (Washington, D.C.: Carnegie Institute, 1948), vol. 32.

Gruenwald, P.: The relation of the growing müllerian to the wolffian duct and its importance for the genesis of malformations, Anat. Rec. 81:1, 1941.

————: The development of the sex cords in the gonads of man and mammals. Am. J. Anat. 70:359, 1942.

Koff, A. K.: Development of the Vagina in the Human Fetus, in *Contributions to Embryology* (Washington, D.C.: Carnegie Institute, 1933), vol. 24.

Velardo, J. T.: The Anatomy and Endocrine Physiology of the Female Reproductive System, in Velardo, J. T. (ed.): *Endocrinology of Reproduction* (New York: Oxford University Press, 1958).

Menstruation

Bartelmez, G. W.: Menstruation, Physiol. Rev. 17:28, 1937.

————: The phases of the menstrual cycle and their interpretation in terms of the pregnancy cycle, Am. J. Obst. & Gynec. 74:931, 1957.

————: Factors in the variability of the menstrual cycle, Anat. Rec. 115:101, 1953.

————: Premenstrual and menstrual ischemia and the myth of endometrial arteriovenous anastomosis, Am. J. Anat. 98:69, 1956.

Barlow, J. J.: Estrogens, in Behrman, S. J., and Kistner, R. W. (ed.): *Progress in Infertility* (Boston: Little, Brown and Company, 1968.)

————, and Logan, C. M.: Estrogen secretion, biosynthesis and metabolism: Their relationship to the menstrual cycle, Steroids 7:309, 1966.

Brown, J. B.: Urinary excretion of oestrogens during the menstrual cycle, Lancet 1:320, 1955.

Buxton, C. L., and Herrmann, W. L.: Effect of thyroid therapy on menstrual disorders and sterility, J.A.M.A. 155:1035, 1954.

Corner, G. W., and Allen, W. M.: Physiology of the corpus luteum: II. Production of special uterine reaction (progestational proliferation) by extracts of corpus luteum, Am. J. Physiol. 88:326, 1929.

Dignam, W. J.: Progestins, in Behrman, S. J., and Kistner, R. W. (ed.): *Progress in Infertility* (Boston: Little, Brown and Company, 1968.)

Goss, D. A.: Methods of gonadotropin assay, in Behrman, S. J., and Kistner, R. W. (ed.): *Progress in Infertility* (Boston: Little, Brown and Company, 1968.)

Granum, J. S. L., Venning, E. H., and Henry, J. S.: Corpus Luteum Hormone in Gynecology, in Meigs, J. V., and Sturgis S. H. (eds.): *Progress in Gynecology* (New York: Grune & Stratton, Inc., 1950), vol. 2.

Gray, M. J., Strausfield, K. S., Watanabe, M., Sims, E. A. H., and Solomon, S.: Aldosterone secretion rates in the normal menstrual cycle, J. Clin. Endocrinol. 28:1269, 1968.

Hagerman, D. D., and Villee, C. A.: Effects of the menstrual cycle on the metabolism of the human endometrium, Endocrinology 53:666, 1953.

Hartman, C. G.: Studies in the Reproduction of the Monkey Macacus Rhesus, with Special Reference to Menstruation and Pregnancy, in *Contributions to Embryology* (Washington, D.C.: Carnegie Institute, 1932), vol. 23, no. 134.

Holmstrom, E. G., and McLennan, C. E.: Menorrhagia associated with irregular shedding of the endometrium, Am. J. Obst. & Gynec. 53:727, 1947.

Kistner, R. W.: The use of progestational agents in obstetrics and gynecology, Clin. Obst. & Gynec. 3:1047, 1960.

Markee, J. E.: Menstruation in Intra-Ocular Endometrial Transplants in Rhesus Monkeys, in *Contributions to Embryology* (Washington, D.C.: Carnegie Institute, 1939), vol. 28.

Noyes, R. W., Hertig, A. T., and Rock, J.: Dating the endometrial biopsy, Fertil. & Steril. 1:3, 1950.

Phelps, D.: Physiology of Menstruation and Ovulation, in *A.M.A. Council on Pharmacy and Chemistry: Glandular Physiology and Therapy* (5th ed.; Philadelphia: J. B. Lippincott Company, 1954).

————: Menstruation, in Velardo, J. T. (ed.): *Essentials of Human Reproduction: Clinical Aspects, Normal and Abnormal* (New York: Oxford University Press, 1958).

Rock, J.: Menstruation, its disorders and their treatment, New England J. Med. 233:817, 1945.
———; Garcia, C., and Menkin, M. F.: A theory of menstruation, Ann. New York Acad. Sc. 75:831, 1959.
Rogers, J.: *Endocrine and Metabolic Aspects of Gynecology* (Philadelphia: W. B. Saunders Company, 1963).
Ryan, K. J.: Biosynthesis and metabolism of ovarian steroids, in Behrman, S. J., and Kistner, R. W. (ed.): *Progress in Infertility* (Boston: Little, Brown and Company, 1968.)
Smith, O. W.: Menstrual Toxin: Experimental Studies, in Engle, E. T. (ed.): *Menstruation and Its Disorders* (Springfield, Ill.: Charles C Thomas, Publisher, 1950).
Svendsen, R., and Sorenson, B.: The plasma concentration of unconjugated oestrone and 17 β-oestradiol in plasma, Acta endocrinol. (Kobenhavn) 35:161, 1960.
Taymor, M. L., *et al.*: Menorrhagia due to chronic iron deficiency, Obst. & Gynec. 16:571, 1960.
———:, and Sturgis, S. H.: Synthetic progestins in the management of anovulatory dysfunctional bleeding, Obst. & Gynec. 17:751, 1961.
White, R. F., *et al.*: Histological and Histochemical Observations on the Corpus Luteum of Human Pregnancy with Special Reference to Corpora Lutea Associated with Early Normal and Abnormal Ova, in *Contributions to Embryology* (Washington, D.C.: Carnegie Institute, 1951), vol. 34, no. 224.
Woolever, C. A.: Daily plasma progesterone levels during the menstrual cycle, Am. J. Obst. & Gynec. 85:981, 1963.

Ovulation

Gemzell, C. A.: The Induction of Ovulation in the Human by Human Pituitary Gonadotropin, in Villee, C. A. (ed.): *Control of Ovulation* (New York: Pergamon Press, 1961).
———; Diczfalusy, E., and Tillinger, K. G.: Clinical effect of human pituitary follicle-stimulating hormone, J. Clin. Endocrinol. 18:1333, 1958.
———; Roos, P. and Loeffler, F. E.: Follicle stimulating hormone extracted from human pituitary, in Behrman, S. J., and Kistner, R. W. (ed.): *Progress in Infertility* (Boston: Little, Brown and Co., 1968).
Greenblatt, R. B.: Experimental studies using clomiphene citrate, in Behrman, S. J., and Kistner, R. W. (ed.): *Progress in Infertility* (Boston: Little, Brown and Co., 1968).
———; *et al.*: Induction of ovulation with MRL-41, J.A.M.A. 178:101, 1961.
Kistner, R. W.: Further observations on the effects of clomiphene citrate (Clomid) in anovulatory females, Am. J. Obst. & Gynec. 92:380, 1965.
———,: Induction of ovulation with clomiphene citrate (Clomid), Obst. & Gynec. Survey 20:873, 1965.
———, Use of clomiphene citrate, human chorionic gonadotropin, and human menopausal gonadotropin for induction of ovulation in the human female, Fertil. & Steril. 17:569, 1966.
———,: Induction of Ovulation-Clinical Aspects, in Balin, H. and Glasser, S. (ed.) *Human Reproductive Biology* (Amsterdam, Acta Obst. & Gynec., 1971.)
———, and Smith, O. W.: Observations on the use of a non-steroidal estrogen antagonist: MER-25, Surg. Forum 10:725, 1959.
Rock, J., *et al.*: The use of estrogens and gestogens to induce human ovulation, Fertil & Steril. 11:303, 1960.
Rogers, J.: *Endocrine and Metabolic Aspects of Gynecology* (Philadelphia: W. B. Saunders Company, 1963).
———, and Mitchell, G. W., Jr.: The relation of obesity to menstrual disturbances, New England J. Med. 247:53, 1952.
Smith, O. W.: Chemical induction of ovulation: Letter to the Journal, J.A.M.A. 179:99, 1962.
———; Smith, G. V., and Kistner, R. W.: Action of MER-25 and of clomiphene on the human ovary, J.A.M.A. 184:878, 1963.
Taymor, M. L.: Human menopausal gonadotropin, in Behrman, S. J., and Kistner, R. W. (ed.): *Progress in Infertility* (Boston: Little, Brown and Co., 1968.)

Uterine Retrodisplacement

Cotte, G.: Section des ligaments utéro-sacrés et résection du nerf pre-sacré-dans le traitments des plexalgies hypogastrigar, Lyon méd. 144:549, 1929.
Derichsweiler, H.: Über das Ödem des Endometriums, Arch. Gynäk, 155:408, 1934.
Holmes, W. R.: Endometriosis, in Meigs, J. V., and Sturgis, S. H. (eds.): *Progress in Gynecology* (New York: Grune & Stratton, Inc., 1950), vol. 2.
King, A. G.: Threatened and repeated abortion, Obst. & Gynec. 1:104, 114, 1953.
Taylor, H. C., Jr.: Vascular congestion and hyperemia, Am. J. Obst. & Gynec. 57:211, 637, 654, 1949.

Infections

Douglas, R. G., and Birnbaum, S. J.: Intrapartum and puerperal infection, Clin. Obst. & Gynec. 2:693, 1959.
Goodno, J. A.; Cushner, I. M., and Molumphy, P. E.: Management of infected abortion, an analysis of 342 cases, Am. J. Obst. & Gynec. 85:16, 1963.

Mead, P. B. and Louria, D. B.: Antibiotics in pelvic infections, Clin. Obst. & Gynec. 12:219, 1969.
Mickal, A., and Sellman, A. H.: Management of tubo-ovarian abscess, Clin. Obst. & Gynec. 12:252, 1969.
Neuwirth, R. S., and Friedman, E. A.: Septic abortion: Changing concept of management, Am. J. Obst. & Gynec. 85:24, 1963.
Snaith, L.: Chronic pelvic inflammation and infertility, Clin. Obst. & Gynec. 2:862, 1959.
Studdiford, W. E., and Douglas, G. W.: Placental bacteremia: A significant finding in septic abortion accompanied by vascular collapse, Am. J. Obst. & Gynec. 71:842, 1956.

Benign Neoplasms

Benson, R. C., and Sneeden, V. D.: Adenomyosis: A re-appraisal of symptomatology, Am. J. Obst. & Gynec. 76:1044, 1958.
Brown, A. B.; Chamberlain, R., and Te Linde, R. W.: Myomectomy, Am. J. Obst. & Gynec. 71:759, 1956.
Colman, H. I., and Rosenthal, A. H.: Carcinoma developing in areas of adenomyosis, Obst. & Gynec. 14:342, 1959.
Cullen, T. S.: Adenomyoma of the Uterus (Philadelphia: W. B. Saunders Company, 1908).
Davids, A. M.: Management of fibromyomas in infertility and abortion, Clin. Obst. & Gynec. 2:837, 1959.
Emge, L. A.: Adenomyosis, Western J. Surg. 64:291, 1956.
Finn, W. F., and Muller, P. F.: Abdominal myomectomy: Special reference to subsequent pregnancy and to the re-appearance of fibromyomas of the uterus, Am. J. Obst. & Gynec. 60:109, 1950.
Hertig, A. T., and Gore, H.: Tumors of the Female Sex Organs: part 2. Tumors of the Vulva, Vagina and Uterus, sec. IX, fasc. 33 of Atlas of Tumor Pathology (Washington, D. C.: Armed Forces Institute of Pathology, 1960).
Israel, S. L., and Mutch, J. C.: Myomectomy, Clin. Obst. & Gynec. 1:455, 1958.
———, and Woutersz, T. D.: Adenomyosis: Neglected diagnosis, Obst. & Gynec. 14:168, 1959.
Marcus, C. C.: Relationship of adenomyosis uteri to endometrial hyperplasia and endometrial carcinoma, Am. J. Obst. & Gynec. 82:408, 1961.
Novak, E. R.: Benign and malignant changes in uterine myomas, Clin. Obst. & Gynec. 1:421, 1958.
Pedowitz, P.; Felmus, L. B., and Grayzel, D. G.: Hemangiopericytoma of the uterus, Am. J. Obst. & Gynec. 67:549, 1954.
Peterson, W. F., and Novak, E. R.: Endometrial polyps, Obst. & Gynec. 8:40, 1956.
Roddick, J. W., and Greene, R. R.: Endometrial changes and ovarian morphology, Am. J. Obst. & Gynec. 75:235, 1958.
Rubin, I. C.: Uterine fibromyomas and sterility, Clin. Obst. & Gynec. 1:501, 1958.
Sehgal, N., and Haskins, A. L.: The mechanism of uterine bleeding in the presence of fibromyomas, Am. Surgeon 26:21, 1960.

Hyperplasia and Carcinoma

Anderson, D. G.: Management of advanced endometrial adenocarcinoma with medroxyprogesterone acetate, Am. J. Obst. & Gynec. 92:87, 1965.
Andrews, W. C.: Estrogens in endometrial carcinoma, Obst. & Gynec. Surv. 16:747, 1961.
———, and Andrews, M. C.: Stein-Leventhal syndrome with associated adenocarcinoma of the endometrium: Report of a case in a 22-year-old woman. Am. J. Obst. & Gynec. 80:632, 1960.
Atkinson, W. B.; Gall, E. A., and Gusberg, S. B.: Histochemical studies on abnormal growth of human endometrium: III. Deposition of glycogen in hyperplasia and adenocarcinoma, Cancer 5:138. 1952.
Austin, J. H., and MacMahon, B.: Indicators of prognosis in carcinoma of the corpus uteri, Surg. Gynec. & Obst. 128:1247, 1969.
Barber, K. W., Jr.; Dockerty, M. B., and Pratt, J. H.: A clinicopathologic study of surgically treated carcinoma of the endometrium with nodal metastases, Surg., Gynec. & Obst. 115:568, 1962.
Bateman, J. C.; Carlton, H. N., and Thibeault, J. P.: Chemotherapy for carcinoma of the uterus, Obst. & Gynec. 15:35, 1960.
Blaikley, J. B., et al.: Classification and clinical study of carcinoma of the uterus, Am. J. Obst. & Gynec. 75:1286, 1958.
Corscaden, J. A.; Fertig, J. W., and Gusberg, S. D.: Carcinoma subsequent to the radiotherapeutic menopause, Am. J. Obst. & Gynec. 51:1, 1946.
Cox, L. W., and Kirkland, J. A.: Effect of ethynodiol diacetate on endometrial cancer: Symposium on recent advances in ovarian and synthetic steroids, Sydney, Australia, 1964.
Dockerty, M. B.; Lovelady, S. B., and Foust, G. T., Jr.: Carcinoma of corpus uteri in young women, Am. J. Obst. & Gynec. 61:966, 1951.
———, and Mussey, E.: Malignant lesions of the uterus associated with estrogen-producing ovarian tumors, Am. J. Obst. & Gynec. 61:147, 1951.
Ehrmann, R. L.; McKelvey, H. A., and Hertig, A. T.: Secretory behavior of endometrium in tissue culture, Obst. & Gynec. 17:416, 1961.
Finn, W. F.: A clinicopathological classification of endometrial carcinoma based upon physical findings, anatomical extent, and histological grade, Am. J. Obst. & Gynec. 62:1, 1951.

Griffiths, C. T., *et al.*: Effect of progestins, estrogens and castration on induced endometrial carcinoma in the rabbit, Surg. Forum 14:399, 1963.

Gusberg, S. B.: Developmental stages of uterine cancer and their diagnostic appraisal, Clin. Obst. & Gynec. 1:559, 1958.

————: Precursors of corpus carcinoma: Estrogens and adenomatous hyperplasia, Am. J. Obst. & Gynec. 54:905, 1947.

————; Moore, D. D., and Martin, F.: Precursors of corpus cancer: II. Clinical and pathological study of adenomatous hyperplasia, Am. J. Obst. & Gynec. 68:1472, 1954.

————, and Hall, R. E.: Precursors of corpus cancer: III. The appearance of cancer of the endometrium in estrogenically conditioned patients, Obst. & Gynec. 17:397, 1961.

————: Standard practices at Sloane Hospital. The management of carcinoma of the corpus, Bull. Sloane Hosp. for Women 5:53, 1959.

————; Jones, H. C., Jr.; and Tovell, H. M. M.: Selection of treatment for corpus cancer, Am. J. Obst. & Gynec. 80:374, 1960.

————, and Kaplan, A. L.: Precursors of corpus cancer: IV. Adenomatous hyperplasia as Stage 0 carcinoma of the endometrium, Am. J. Obst. & Gynec. 87:662, 1963.

Hall, J. E.: Alkaline phosphatase in human endometrium, Am. J. Obst. & Gynec. 60:212, 1950.

Hertig, A. T., and Sommers, S. C.: Genesis of endometrial carcinoma: I. Study of prior biopsies, Cancer 2:946, 1949.

————, ————, and Bengloff, H.: Genesis of endometrial carcinoma: III. Carcinoma in situ. Cancer 2:964, 1949.

Heyman, J.: Improvement of results in treatment, with special reference to radium therapy and applicators for its use, J.A.M.A. 135:412, 1947.

Javert, C. T.: Prognosis of endometrial cancer, Obst. & Gynec. 12:556, 1958.

————, and Hofammann, K.: Observations on surgical pathology, selective lymphadenectomy and classification of endometrial adenocarcinoma, Cancer 5:485, 1952.

Kaufman, R. H.: Abbott, W. P., and Wall, J. A. The endometrium before and after wedge resection of the ovaries in the Stein-Leventhal syndrome, Am. J. Obst. & Gynec. 77:1271, 1959.

Kelley, R. M., and Baker, W. H.: Effects of 17-alpha-Hydroxy Progesterone Caproate on Metastatic Endometrial Cancer, in *Conference on Experimental Clinical Cancer Chemotherapy,* monograph 9 (Bethesda, Md.: National Cancer Institute 1960).

Kennedy, B. J.: Progestogen for treatment of advanced endometrial cancer, J.A.M.A. 184:758, 1963.

Kistner, R. W.: Carcinoma of the endometrium—A preventable disease?, Am. J. Obst. & Gynec. 95:1011, 1966.

————: The Effects of clomiphene citrate on endometrial hyperplasia in the premenopausal female. Proc. 5th World Congress on Fertility and Sterility. Excerpta Medica Foundation, 81, Nov. 1967. Stockholm.

————: Further observations on the effects of progestational agents on hyperplasia and carcinoma in situ of the endometrium. Symposium on Oral Gestogens and Their Uses in General Medicine and Public Health, Clinical Trials Journal. 5:57. 1968.

————: Treatment of carcinoma in situ of the endometrium. Clin. Obst. & Gynec. 5:1166, 1962.

————: Histological effects of progestins on hyperplasia and carcinoma in situ of the endometrium, Cancer 12:1106, 1959.

————, and Griffiths, C. T.: Use of progestational agents in the management of metastatic carcinoma of the endometrium, Clin. Obst. & Gynec. 11:439, 1968.

————; ————, and Craig, J. M.: The use of progestational agents in the management of endometrial cancer, Cancer 19:1563, 1965.

Kottmeier, H. L.: Individualization of therapy in carcinoma of the corpus, in The University of Texas M. D. Anderson Hospital and Tumor Institute: *Cancer of the Uterus and Ovary* (Chicago: Year Book Medical Publishers, Inc., 1969).

————: Carcinoma of the corpus uteri: Diagnosis and therapy, Am. J. Obst. & Gynec. 78:1127, 1959.

Larson, J. A.: Estrogens and endometrial carcinoma, Obst. & Gynec. 3:551, 1954.

McKay, D. G.: Ovarian Cortical Stromal Hyperplasia, in Meigs, J. V. and Sturgis, S. H. (eds.): *Progress in Gynecology* (New York: Grune & Stratton, Inc., 1957), vol. 3.

McKelvey, J. L., and Prem, K. A.: Adenocarcinoma of the Endometrium; in Meigs, J. V., and Sturgis, S. H. (eds.): *Progress in Gynecology* (New York: Grune & Stratton, Inc., 1957), vol. 3.

MacMahon, B., and Austin, J. H.: Association of carcinomas of the breast and corpus uteri, Cancer 23:275, 1969.

Meissner, W. A.; Sommers, S. C., and Sherman, G.: Endometrial hyperplasia, endometrial carcinoma and endometriosis produced experimentally by estrogens, Cancer 10:500, 1957.

Miller, N. F.: Carcinoma of the endometrium: Some facts, figures and fancies, Obst. & Gynec. 15:579, 1960.

Nolan, J. F., and Harrison, L. A., Jr.: Carcinoma of the endometrium and an evaluation of preoperative radiation therapy, Obst. & Gynec. 17:601, 1961.

Nordqvist, R. S. B.: Hormone effects on carcinoma of the human uterine body studied in organ culture. A preliminary report, Acta obstet. gynec. scandinav. 43:296, 1964.

Novak, E. R.: Relationship of endometrial hyperplasia and adenocarcinoma of the uterine fundus, J.A.M.A. 154:217, 1954.

————: Cancer of uterus, J.A.M.A. 135:199, 1947.

————, and Yui, E.: Relation of endometrial hyperplasia to adenocarcinoma of uterus, Am. J. Obst. & Gynec. 32:674, 1936.

Sommers, S. C.; Hertig, A. T., and Bengloff, H.: Genesis of endometrial carcinoma: II. Cases 19–35 years old, Cancer 2:957, 1949.

Steiner, G. J.: Kistner, R. W., and Craig, J. M.: Histological effects of progestins on hyperplasia and carcinoma in situ of the endometrium—further observations. Metabolism 14:356, 1965.

Taylor, H. C., Jr.: Endometrial hyperplasia and carcinoma of body of uterus, Am. J. Obst. & Gynec. 23:309, 1932.

Taymor, M. L.; Yahia, C., and Buytendorp, A.: Day-to-day variation in luteinizing hormone excretion in carcinoma of the endometrium and normal menopause. Squibb Symposium on Delalutin in advanced endometrial cancer in women, October, 1962.

Te Linde, R. W.: Jones, H. W., Jr., and Galvin, G. A.: What are earliest endometrial changes to justify diagnosis of endometrial cancer? Am. J. Obst. & Gynec. 66:953, 1953.

Truscott, I. D.: Treatment of endometrial cancer by the instillation of a progestational agent. Presented at a Symposium on recent advances in ovarian and synthetic steroids. Sydney, Australia, October, 1964.

Varga, A., and Henriksen, E.: Urinary excretion assays of pituitary luteinizing hormone (LH) related to endometrial carcinoma, Obst. & Gynec. 22:120, 1963.

Wagner, D.; Richart, R. M., and Terner, J. Y.: Deoxyribonucleic acid content of presumed precursors of endometrial carcinoma, Cancer 20:2067, 1967.

Wentz, W. B.: Effect of a progestational agent on endometrial hyperplasia and endometrial cancer, Obst. & Gynec. 24:370, 1964.

Yahia, C.; Benirschke, K., and Sturgis, S. H.: Carcinoma of the Endometrium in Meigs, J. W., and Sturgis, S. H. (eds.): *Progress in Gynecology* (New York: Grune & Stratton, Inc., 1963), vol. 4.

Sarcoma

Aaro, L. A., and Dockerty, M. B.: Leiomyosarcoma of the uterus, Am. J. Obst. & Gynec. 77:1187, 1959.

Bell, H. G., and Edgehill, H.: Sarcomas developing in uterine fibroids: Review of literature and presentation of 3 cases, Am. J. Surg. 100:416, 1960.

Radman, H. M., and Korman W.: Sarcoma of uterus, Am. J. Obst. & Gynec. 78:604, 1959.

Schwartz, A. E., and Brunschwig, A.: Radical panhysterectomy and pelvic node excision for carcinoma of the corpus uteri, Surg., Gynec. & Obst. 105:675, 1957.

Sternberg, W. H.: Clark, W. H., and Smith, R. C.: Malignant mixed müllerian tumor (mixed mesodermal tumor of the uterus): A study of 21 cases, Cancer 7:704, 1954.

CHAPTER 6

The Oviduct

Anatomy and Histology

THE OVIDUCTS (fallopian tubes) are paired muscular canals which extend from the uterus to the ovaries, each measuring about 12 cm. Since these structures transport the ova into the uterine cavity they may be considered as ovarian excretory ducts, but, unlike other efferent ducts, the oviduct is not in continuity with the ovary—it is only in apposition with it. Both tubes are covered with peritoneum and lined with mucous membrane and, except for a short intrauterine portion, are enveloped in the free margin of the broad ligament known as the mesosalpinx.

The oviduct emerges from the uterine wall at the junction of the corpus and fundus. The proximal segment arches laterally and posteriorly, adjacent to the lower pole of the ovary, then assumes a tortuous course along the mesovarial border of the ovary to the fimbriated end. At this point the tube is in direct relation to the medial ovarian surface. Normal variations from this description are common, especially if there is a marked uterine retroversion. In disease states such as gonococcal salpingitis, both tubes may be displaced behind the uterus into the posterior cul-de-sac, whereas with adhesions due to a ruptured appendix the oviduct may be displaced laterally and fixed to the lateral pelvic wall or cecum. In endometriosis the fimbriae are usually patent but the rest of the oviduct may be densely adherent to the ovary or to the posterior peritoneum.

Four subdivisions of the oviduct are described (Fig. 6–1). (1) The *interstitial* portion is short and begins at the superior angle of the uterine cavity, communicating with the latter by a minute ostium. It extends through the thickness of the myometrium, angulating through the fundus to exit at the uterine cornu just superior to the attachments of the round and utero-ovarian ligaments. (2) The *isthmic* portion is a relatively straight, narrow but thick-walled segment. It gradually increases in luminal diameter and shows a diminution in thickness of the wall as it progresses laterally. (3) The *ampullar* portion is the longest segment of the oviduct. In its normal state it is slightly convoluted and has a relatively thin, dilatable muscular wall. (4) The *infundibular* portion is the terminal portion of the oviduct. It is somewhat trumpet shaped at its ovarian end and is divided into numerous delicate folds or fimbriae which give a fringed appearance. One of these folds is prolonged and is attached to the mesosalpinx. Frequently it lies in apposition to the tubal pole of the ovary.

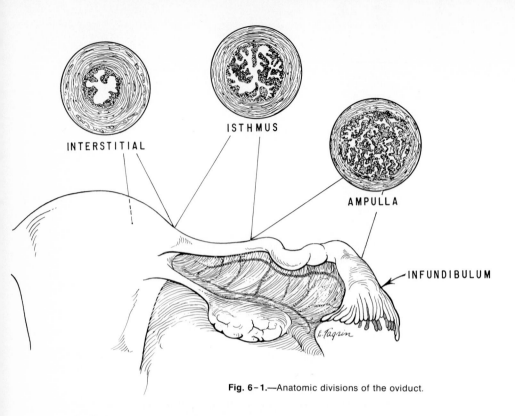

Fig. 6–1.—Anatomic divisions of the oviduct.

Fig. 6–2.—Normal oviduct. *(Continued.)*

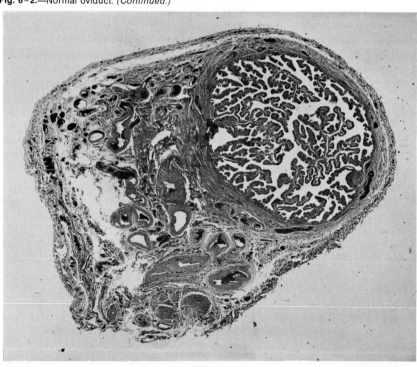

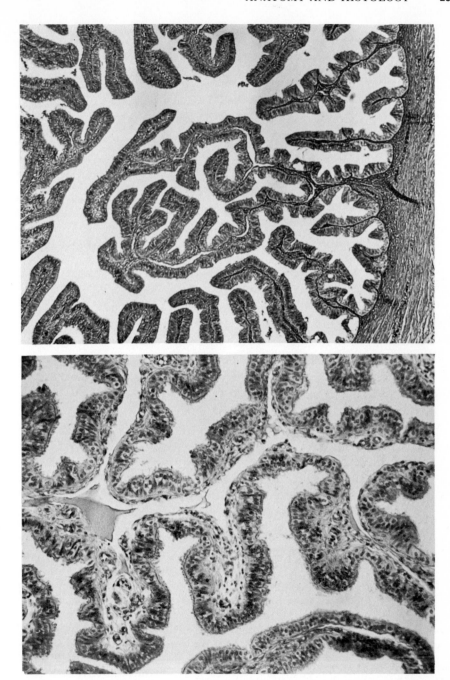

Fig. 6-2 *(cont.).*—**Above,** higher power to show epithelium in proliferative phase, **Below,** higher power to show epithelium in secretory phase. (From Hall, J. E.: *Applied Gynecologic Pathology* [New York: Appleton-Century-Crofts, Inc., 1963], p. 197.)

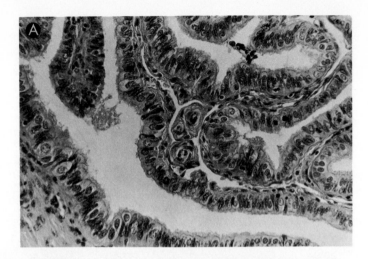

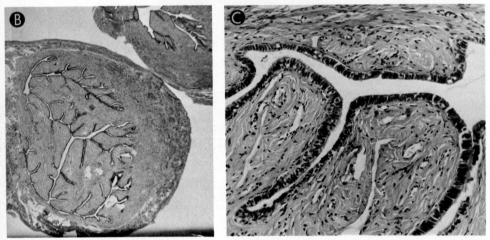

Fig. 6–3.—**A,** high-power magnification of epithelium covering the plicae of the oviduct. The darkly stained "peg" or intercalary cells are easily identified. **B,** cross-section through ampullar portion of a senescent oviduct. The epithelial element is sparse and there is extensive replacement by fibrous connective tissue. **C,** high power of senescent oviduct. The epithelium is flat and cuboidal, the tubal folds are rounded and ciliated cells are not present.

The wall of the oviduct consists of three layers, an external or serous, an intermediate muscular and an internal mucous layer. The serous covering is an extension of the broad ligament peritoneum and invests the tube completely except for the attachment of the mesosalpinx and the intrauterine portion. Beneath the mesothelial cells of the serosa is a connective tissue layer containing mostly blood vessels and nerves which intermingle with the subjacent muscular layer. The outer layer of the muscularis is arranged longitudinally whereas the inner layer is arranged circularly. The mucous membrane lining presents a characteristic folded, somewhat arborescent pattern which is most pronounced toward the fimbriated portion (plicae tubariae). These longitudinal folds begin as four duplications of the mucosa in the interstitial portion of the tube enclosing a small lumen. The lumen of the oviduct becomes larger as it approaches the fimbriated portion and thus affords added space for increased mucosal folding. As the ampullary portion of the tube is reached, the plicae are extremely complicated and present numerous reduplications and outpouchings (Fig. 6-2). The mucosa is lined with a columnar epithelium containing ciliated and nonciliated or "secretory" cells. Intercalary or "peg" cells are most easily identified in the premenstrual and menstrual period. The endosalpinx, like the endometrium, exhibits a cyclic morphologic variation depending on hormonal stimulation. During the proliferative phase of estrogen stimulation, the epithelium is uniformly tall with prominent ciliated cells and narrow nonciliated cells. During the late secretory phase the ciliated cells are much lower, and the secretory cells are quite prominent, giving a rather uneven surface to the mucosa. During the menstrual phase the epithelium is rather low, since the secretory cells have now been depleted of their cytoplasm. Intercalary cells (Fig. 6-3, A) are numerous during the menstrual phase and their appearance at this time suggests that they may merely be remnants of emptied secretory cells. The immediate postmenstrual phase presents a low epithelial surface in the oviduct, but regeneration is rapid during the proliferative phase.

During the postmenopausal period the epithelium is low and flat, the tubal folds become rounded and fibrous and their cilia disappear (Fig. 6-3, B and C). The tubal epithelium in patients with endometrial hyperplasia is usually high, with uniform, narrow cells, most of which are ciliated. This represents the effects of persistent estrogen stimulation without the normal cyclic intervention of progesterone. The hormonal effect is even more evident during pregnancy when a decidual reaction in the stromal cells may be extensive.

Embryology

The oviducts are formed by differentiation of the unfused paramesonephric ducts. (The fused portions form the uterus and a significant portion of the vagina.) The paramesonephric (müllerian) ducts arise early in the seventh week, lateral and parallel to the mesonephric duct, by a process of invagination of the celomic epithelium opposite the cranial end of the mesonephros. The solid portions of the ducts extend caudally through primitive mesenchyme and cross the mesonephric duct anteriorly at the level of the caudal end of the mesonephros.

The most common type of congenital anomaly of the oviduct is the absence of the ampullary portion (or a rudimentary one) which probably occurs because of torsion and subsequent ischemic atrophy. Supernumerary oviducts are rare, but duplication of the ampullary region and accessory tubal ostia are relatively common. Accessory tubes which arise along the course of the oviduct never communicate with the lumen but the accessory ostia located near the main ostium always do. Unilateral absence of the oviduct is uncommon but when it does occur it is associated with ureteral and renal abnormalities on the involved side. Bilateral tubal absence is rare and is usually associated with uterine and vaginal agenesis. In such cases, there may be normal ovaries which are attached laterally to the free edge of the empty broad ligament. Segmental atresia and persistence of the coiled fetal pattern are rare anomalies but may be seen occasionally when large numbers of laparotomies are done for so-called idio-pathic infertility.

Correlation of Structure and Function

Although it had generally been accepted that the human fallopian tube consisted of two layers of musculature between the serosa and the mucosa, work by Horstmann in 1952 revealed three distinct muscular layers. He described a subperitoneal layer running along the long axis of the tube, a middle or vasomotor layer with fibers paralleling the blood vessels which encircle the tube and an inner, spirally arranged layer which takes origin from multicentric areas in the tube. Stange recently described in detail the muscular arrangement of the fimbriated extremity. He noted that the sub-peritoneal fibers continue along to the fimbria and extend for greater lengths at the upper and lower tubal edge than on the sides. Thus a mech-anism for grasping is accomplished. These fibers are anchored to the sub-peritoneal blood vessels at the neck of the infundibulum, which in general is extremely well vascularized. The inner muscle layer also ends at the in-fundibulum with an intertwining of its fibers with the circular fibers of the vascular layer. In effect there is formed a functional sphincter at the fimbriated portion of the tube. Stange further suggested that the muscular component of the paraovarium actually lifts the ovary while the projected tubal frond (muscle attrahens tubae) brings the fimbriated end of the ovi-duct onto the ovary.

Westman has described the mechanism of ovum pickup in the rabbit and in the monkey. In these animals the fimbriated portion of the oviduct actually embraces the ovary. Decker observed this same phenomenon with the culdoscope and, in addition, described a shortening of the utero-ovarian ligament at this time. Doyle reported similar observations at culdotomy, noting a trumpet-shaped cone of contraction at the fimbriated opening. Both noted that the ovary and fimbriae were brought in close apposition to the uterus in a fossa on the posterior aspect of the broad ligament. Ovum pickup is probably assisted by tubal suction, since a current of fluid within the tube has been demonstrated by Von Ott, who recovered a dye from the cervix after placing it into the cul-de-sac, and by Decker, who made a similar observation using starch.

Ovum transport within the oviduct has been extensively studied in animals but only a few thorough investigations have been accomplished in women. It has been noted in animals that there is a rather striking in-crease in ciliary activity at the time of ovulation. Such action has also been described in the human oviduct, demonstrating that spermatozoa are dis-persed over the luminal surface by to-and-fro action of the cilia. Larger particles (such as the ovum) are permanently in contact with the mucosal cells, a steady movement toward the uterus being effected. An increase in muscular activity has been noted at the ovulatory phase of the menstrual cycle as well as slower, more uniform contractions during the premenstrual phase. These muscular contractions begin at the ampulla and proceed to the isthmus. Further, the frequency of the ampullary contractions is higher than those found in the isthmus. In all probability the action of the cilia provides the primary mechanism for ovum transport within the tube, aided and abetted by the muscular contractions.

It is known from studies of early implantation sites in the human subject that the fertilized ovum resides within the oviduct for approximately three days. The reason for this delay in transit is presently unknown. Although fertilized ova are retained in the ampullary portion of the tube in the rabbit, this is accomplished by a physiologic closure of the isthmus. There is no evidence of a similar mechanism in the human female. Furthermore, administration of estrogen to experimental animals will cause a diminution in the rate of descent of ova so that ovum retention may actually be produced in the absence of an anatomic occlusion of the isthmus. The delay in the oviduct is probably related to maturation of the ovum. Chang demonstrated a definite relation between the age of the ovum and the ability to implant. Thus, if rabbit ova were transferred from the oviduct to the uterus within 24 hours of fertilization, implantation did not occur. After 48 hours a small number of implantations occur, but the majority implanted when transfer was effected after three days.

After ovulation the ovum is surrounded by a mass of cells termed the *cumulus oophorus*. These cells may be made to disintegrate rapidly simply by exposing the freshly ovulated ova to spermatozoa in vitro. The *corona radiata,* however, is not removed by the exposure. There is evidence that complete dispersion of the corona radiata is brought about by some influence within the oviduct. Mansani and Mazzella found that either high hyaluronidase levels or semen merely loosened the cells of the cumulus oophorus, but that either of these combined with extracts of tubal mucosa caused complete denudation. This strongly suggests that a tubal enzyme is necessary for fertilization.

The morphologic variations that occur during the menstrual cycle have been described. Recent histochemical studies confirmed the earlier work and further demonstrated that PAS-reactive material (presumably glycogen) was present in the supranuclear and infranuclear areas of the ciliated cells. The supranuclear material disappears in the early luteal phase, coinciding with increased ciliary activity. Fredricsson has shown large amounts of PAS-reactive material in the tubal lumen in the mid-luteal phase. He postulated that this may provide the uterus with amylase to digest endometrial glycogen and nourish the newly implanted ovum.

There is evidence that early development of the ovum is greatly influenced by tubal environment. It has been known for years that in rabbits castrated shortly after ovulation the ova were fertilized but displayed degenerative changes after three days. Since the ova were lying free in the tubal lumen during this time, it was reasoned that the degeneration resulted from changed secretions of the tubal mucosa. Similar degeneration may be produced in rabbits by administering 5 μg. of estradiol daily, beginning an hour after mating. Such degeneration was coincident with a reduced deposition of mucin in the oviduct. Whereas progesterone increases the thickness of this mucin layer, the effect of estrogen is to reduce it. There is evidence also that the developing ovum is capable of incorporating specific substances elaborated by tubal mucosal cells. It has been demonstrated that a tubal fluid is secreted in the rabbit oviduct and that this fluid contains glucose, phospholipid and lactic acid. Castration reduces the rate of secretion but administration of estrogen causes a reversion to the precastration level. Progesterone brings about a diminished rate of secretion and during the first three days of pregnancy the secretion rate is diminished by one-half.

Present evidence strongly suggests that the oviduct functions in more than just a passive nature and serves as more than a simple conduit for ova and sperm. The changes in tubal morphology and fluid accumulation are obviously under hormonal regulation. The formation and elaboration of specific substances needed for growth and development of the ovum are similarly controlled by estrogen and progesterone.

Inflammation

SURFACE EXTENSION—GONORRHEA

Gonorrhea affects the oviducts as an infection ascending from the lower genital tract and is usually secondary to an acute infection of Bartholin's gland, the endocervix or the urethra. This organism has an affinity for glandular epithelium and therefore in its ascent through the female genital tract usually does not involve the squamous epithelium of the vagina or exocervix. Transient endometritis may occur but, because of the recurrent sloughing of the endometrium, the disease process usually extends into the oviduct where its most extensive manifestations occur. The physical force or trauma of intercourse may be sufficient to introduce the organism into the female genital tract and within a rather short period an acute inflammatory process may arise in the tubal epithelium. The initial infection may then extend to the ovary, resulting in an acute perioophoritis followed by a perisalpingitis.

In these earlier stages of the disease process the musculature of the oviduct is usually uninvolved. Grossly, the tube is slightly reddened or glistening with rather marked edema and fine, nonadherent adhesions of the tubal serosa to the ovary. The fimbriated portion of the oviduct may be similarly involved by edema and acute inflammation but the ostium is usually patent. With recurrent infection the tubal plicae adhere and form typical adenomatous spaces which may, on occasion, be confused with an early malignancy. The microscopic picture, however, is rather typical and has been termed follicular salpingitis. Eventually the entire tubal wall becomes involved, with subsequent occlusion of the fimbriated end as repeated exacerbations occur. Secondary bacterial invaders complicate the original gonococcal infection and lead to partial or complete sealing of the isthmus with subsequent retention of pus within the tubal lumen followed by varying degrees of distention.

At this stage the ovary is frequently involved in the total disease so that bilateral pyosalpinges very commonly embrace the ovary in a collective mass, the so-called tubo-ovarian abscess. It is probable that leakage of pus from the partially occluded ostium infects the contiguous ovary, the port of entry being provided by the periodic rupture of follicles. An enlarging ovarian abscess may eventually destroy all the normal ovarian parenchyma. Eventually, in the most advanced cases, the ovary is converted into a mass many times its original size. Further increase in the size of the abscess causes progressive thinning of the fibrous wall, which explains the ease with which these tubo-ovarian abscesses rupture. Similarly, the tube may become enormously distended, with extensive inflammatory involvement of the wall and subsequent ischemia (Fig. 6–4). This compromise of the vascular supply results in focal areas of necrosis and ultimate perforation. In long-standing infections the tubo-ovarian abscess may become

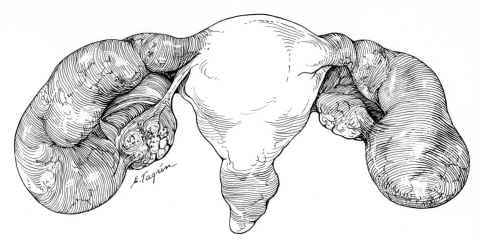

Fig. 6-4.—Gross appearance in acute pelvic inflammatory disease.

densely adherent to the bladder, rectosigmoid or vaginal vault, and perforation of the abscess with evacuation of the contents into these organs may occur. As might be expected, this frequently results in a dramatic relief of symptoms and eventual recovery.

These adnexal abscesses may rupture spontaneously or after trauma. In several cases rupture has been reported following the use of purgatives, too vigorous bimanual examination, coitus, uterine curettage and barium enemas. Although the etiologic agent in most cases of pelvic inflammatory diseases is believed to be the gonococcus, this organism is usually not found in cultures taken at the time of surgery for advanced inflammatory disease. As a matter of fact, positive culture results are found in less than 15 per cent of patients with ruptured tubo-ovarian abscesses and generalized peritonitis. While the positive organism of the primary infection is probably the gonococcus, in most cases secondary bacterial invaders are responsible for continued growth of the abscesses as well as the occasionally fatal peritonitis. Nonhemolytic streptococci and Esch. coli have been the organisms most often recovered from the peritoneal fluid and the abscess cavities.

A significant number of cases of acute pelvic inflammation have been noted following the insertion of an intrauterine device. Symptoms usually occur within one week of insertion and 10 deaths have been reported. After one month there is no conclusive evidence that the incidence or severity of inflammation is greater than in normal women. Fiumara believes that pelvic inflammation is aggravated in women using oral contraceptives because of increased vascularity.

Microscopically the acute phase of the salpingitis is characterized by edema of the plicae, the presence of polymorphonuclear leukocytes in the stroma of the plicae, leukostasis (stasis of leukocytes within the capillaries) and polymorphonuclear leukocytes in the tubal lumen (Fig. 6-5). When the inflammatory process is somewhat more intense there are leukocytic infiltration of the inner muscularis and necrosis of tubal epithelium. Depending on the length of time the tube has been involved in the inflammatory process, extension to the outer muscularis and serosa may be evident.

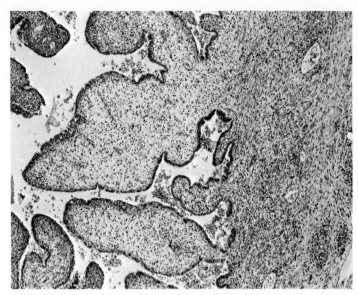

Fig. 6-5.—Acute salpingitis. Note edema of tubal plicae and inflammatory exudate. (Courtesy of Dr. J. D. Woodruff.)

During the acute phase, special stains will reveal bacteria in the tubal lumen, the plical connective tissue and muscularis.

Symptomatology.—The commonest symptom of acute salpingitis is that of pelvic pain. Although occasionally this is acute in onset and of a lancinating type, usually it is of a dull, aching variety more commonly described by the patient as discomfort. The pelvic pain may begin on one side with involvement of the opposite side within 24 or 48 hours. Frequently the onset is associated with a sensation of lassitude, occasionally with chills and low-grade fever. The pain frequently occurs in the immediate postmenstrual phase. It is usually exaggerated by intercourse and physical exertion.

Abnormal vaginal bleeding may occur in the form of intermittent staining of dark blood or spotting. Profuse vaginal bleeding is not common, although subsequent menstrual periods may be more profuse than normal if the disease process is protracted.

Involvement of the urethra and Bartholin's glands may result in urinary frequency and dysuria together with an increased vaginal discharge. The latter may also be associated with involvement of the endocervical glands by the offending organism.

The most constant clinical sign is abdominal and pelvic tenderness. Examination of the abdomen reveals tenderness in both lower quadrants on deep palpation. There is usually no rectus muscle rigidity or spasm even in the presence of a rather well-marked pelvic peritonitis. Although the disease process is usually bilateral, abdominal findings may be confined to the side more extensively involved. Pelvic examination may reveal a copious, yellow discharge, and pressure on the urethra will frequently bring forth purulent material from the urethral meatus and the periurethral glands. Speculum examination reveals an acutely inflamed cervix with a copious exudate from the glandular epithelium. Material should be obtained from the cervix and the periurethral glands and submitted for routine staining and culture in order to identify gram-negative intracellular diplococci. Occasionally there will be an acute bartholinitis and purulent material expressed from this gland should also be submitted for study.

The most common sign on pelvic examination is that of tenderness elicited on motion of the cervix. The uterus is usually of normal size and consistency but is also tender when manipulation is attempted. Adnexal tenderness is a characteristic finding but it varies in degree, depending on the duration and extent of the inflammatory process and on the pain threshold of the patient. In the early stages of the disease the tenderness may be elicited only on one side and the tube may be felt as a rubbery, cordlike structure with little, if any, fixation. As the disease process becomes more extensive and there is bilateral involvement with edema, the pelvic findings become more characteristic. At this stage, pelvic examination will reveal bilateral, tender, enlarged tubes which are found fixed in the posterior cul-de-sac.

During the acute phase of the disease and immediately following, there may be a slight elevation in temperature, usually not exceeding 101 F. There may be a moderate leukocytosis and a moderate increase in the erythrocyte sedimentation rate. It has been our custom to rely more on increases in the sedimentation rate since we have seen numerous patients with pelvic inflammatory disease, proved at surgery, who had normal white blood cell and differential counts. Similarly, after treatment has been initiated, the course of the disease may be followed by sequential sedimentation rates.

When the disease is more extensive, but still acute or subacute, the pelvic findings may be more characteristic. Thus, large tubo-ovarian masses may be palpated either posterior or anterior to the uterus. An intermittent fever of 101–102 F. may be present, together with rather marked leukocytosis and elevations of the sedimentation rate.

When an adnexal abscess leaks into the peritoneal cavity, a pelvic peritonitis or occasionally a generalized peritonitis results. If the perforation is small, adhesions may form around it and seal off the opening. This episode may be indistinguishable from an acute exacerbation of pelvic inflammatory disease. The patient usually has noted lower abdominal pain, weakness, rectal tenesmus and diarrhea. Examination reveals pelvic peritonitis with direct and rebound abdominal tenderness, and mild degrees of shock may even be present. On bimanual examination pus may be palpable in the posterior cul-de-sac or masses may be felt anterior or posterior to the uterus. Since these masses may be quite firm they are frequently mistaken for leiomyomas and the abdomen may be opened because of a mistaken diagnosis of "degenerating fibroids." Even in such cases the temperature may be normal but there is usually a moderate tachycardia. The examiner should reconsider carefully the diagnosis of uterine myomas if the history of intermittent pelvic pain and the palpation of tender masses are combined findings.

Massive perforation of an adnexal abscess gives a characteristic clinical picture. The onset is abrupt, with severe lower abdominal pain usually referred to the side of rupture. Within a short time the entire abdomen is involved because of the development of a generalized peritonitis and, especially if the amount of purulent material discharged is excessive, a rapid state of shock ensues. This may be initiated with symptoms of nausea and vomiting and the findings of extreme tachycardia, cold, clammy skin and hypotension. Abdominal distention secondary to paralytic ileus occurs rather rapidly and the patient appears severely ill or even moribund. Immediately following rupture of the mass the temperature may be normal or even subnormal. Within a matter of hours, however, it rises abruptly and may reach levels of 107–108 F. The resulting shock is due to a combination of peritoneal insult and endotoxemia. The hypotension therefore does not respond in full measure to the administration of blood or blood replacements or to corticosteroids. Pelvic examination may be important in that a previously described adnexal mass will no longer be palpable. As a matter of fact, such catastrophes may actually occur within two to three hours of repeated examination. Laboratory aids are of no help diagnostically since the white cell count may be markedly elevated to 30,000 or more or even depressed to 6,000 or less. At this stage of the disease the erythrocyte sedimentation rate is of no value in diagnosis.

Differential Diagnosis.—Pelvic inflammatory disease must be differentiated from ectopic pregnancy, septic abortion associated with an inflammatory process, torsion or rupture of an ovarian cyst, endometriosis, acute appendicitis and other acute inflammatory processes of the small and large intestine such as regional ileitis and diverticulitis.

Treatment.—Treatment of acute pelvic inflammatory disease is basically medical, with surgical procedures being reserved for the treatment of complications and sequelae. During the acute phase of the illness, especially if the gonococcus has been isolated, treatment should be supportive and should include bed rest, analgesics and antipyretics together with specific antibiotics such as penicillin or the tetracyclines. Penicillin is given in a dose of 2.4 to 4.8 million units intramuscularly and is repeated once. Benemid is effective in a dose of 0.5 Gm. for six doses. Coitus should be interdicted, and cultures should be repeated following completion of therapy.

When the disease process has become more extensive and may be termed subacute, the same treatment is indicated, but in addition the use of pelvic heat in the way of hot douches and hot sitz baths is advantageous. Since the gonococcus is usually not the offending organism at this time, the use of a broad-spectrum antibiotic such as chlortetracycline is usually more effective although in certain instances the specific gram-negative organism may be more susceptible to penicillin and streptomycin. It has been our routine to give 1,000,000 units of penicillin daily together with 0.5 Gm. streptomycin twice daily for five days. The streptomycin is then discontinued in order to reduce the risk of eighth nerve complications, but the penicillin is continued until the sedimentation rate becomes normal. The antibiotic of choice in Bacteroides infections is chloramphenicol, although erythromycin, tetracycline and lincomycin are also effective. For pseudomonas infections, colistin, polymyxin or gentamycin may be used. If renal disease complicates the pelvic infection, carbenicillin should be used for pseudomonas and proteus infections.

Large adnexal masses have been noted to decrease considerably during a therapeutic regimen of this type, although the functional integrity of the endosalpinx may never return to its normal state. During this so-called subacute phase of the disease the patient should be kept hospitalized and only minor activities permitted. Pelvic and rectovaginal examination should be done gently every three or four days to determine whether a cul-de-sac abscess has developed. Should one develop, drainage of the abscess by cul-de-sac incision will greatly expedite the recovery rate. When a posterior colpotomy is performed, a split Penrose drain should be placed in the posterior cul-de-sac to prevent premature closure of the incision.

Numerous strains of gonococci have become resistant to penicillin and therapy has assumed geographic limitations. For example, in California 60 per cent of gonococci are penicillin resistant whereas in Maine almost all stains are penicillin sensitive. Therefore, the tetracyclines are first choice in many areas of the United States and Asia. Vibramycin has been shown to be particularly effective in a regimen of 200 mg. to start followed by 100 mg. twice daily for five days. Acute gonococcal urethritis in males is usually cured by a single dose of 300 mg. of Vibramycin.

The treatment of ruptured adnexal abscesses is primarily surgical and the urgency and extent of the procedure will depend on the size of the perforation. Similarly, if a lack of response to conservative treatment is evidenced by persistent pelvic pain, fever, tachycardia, leukocytosis and particularly by elevation of the sedimentation rate, a small perforation with persistent leakage of an adnexal abscess should be suspected. Many of these patients may be managed by drainage of the abscess through a posterior colpotomy together with transfusions of whole blood, intestinal suction, supportive intravenous fluids and antibiotics. Following recovery from the acute phase, and with improvement of the patient's general condition, hysterectomy and bilateral salpingo-oophorectomy may be performed without unnecessary risk. Failure to operate at this time may be hazardous since subsequent rupture of the abscess will probably occur if the patient is exposed to repeated infections.

Treatment of large ruptures of adnexal abscesses demands immediate and major surgery. It has been shown that the interval between rupture of the abscess and operative treatment is an important factor in prognosis. The lowest mortality rate will obviously be associated when surgery is performed during the first six to 12 hours, and the sooner the better. If the offending organism is not known, penicillin, keflin and colymycin should be given; or keflin may be combined with gentamycin. If the organism is gram-negative, ampicillin plus kanamycin or gentamycin should be administered. Pedowitz and Felmus reported treatment of 19 patients without a single fatality and attribute their success to the combination of radical surgery, blood transfusions, excellent anesthesia and antibiotics. They pointed out that these patients do not respond to the usual remedial measures for shock, and recovery may be expected only when the source of contamination has been removed. They advise hysterectomy and bilateral salpingo-oophorectomy provided the technical difficulties are not too great. If it is necessary to do a supracervical hysterectomy, the cervix should be split or coned since drainage through the vagina will result in fewer postoperative complications. In some patients it may be technically easier to open the posterior vaginal wall behind the cervix and lead a rubber drain into the vagina. Surgical procedures for ruptured tubo-ovarian abscesses are difficult technically because of extreme edema, pus and distortion of structures. In order to prevent damage to the ureter, I usually open the retroperitoneal space bilaterally after dividing and ligating the infundibulo-pelvic ligaments. Both ureters are dissected free to the level of the uterine vessels. These vessels should be clamped, divided and ligated with the ureter in direct vision. In order to prevent postoperative hemorrhage due to tissue necrosis, I have taken advantage of the retroperitoneal approach to ligate both hypogastric arteries before beginning the hysterectomy. The mortality rate has been lower when both tubes and ovaries are removed than when residual infected material is allowed to remain. Oophorectomy also eliminates the need for subsequent surgery since, if recovery occurs, the ovary does not function normally and frequently becomes cystic.

The treatment of infertility caused by pelvic inflammation is discussed in Chapter 9.

Puerperal or Postabortal Salpingitis

The usual organisms causing this type of infection are the anaerobic streptococcus and the staphylococcus. Occasionally the offending organism may be Esch. coli, Cl. welchii, Proteus, Bacteroides or certain mycoses. These organisms are disseminated through lymphatics or thrombosed venous sinuses as well as by the interstitial tissues of the pelvic supporting structures. Occasionally beta-hemolytic streptococcal puerperal infection may spread via the mucosa of the tubes to the peritoneum. Before 1940 the commonest cause of this disease was an infection occurring during the early puerperium, and thus the term *childbed fever* was a common one. During the past two decades this type of salpingitis has occurred most frequently following septic, usually induced, abortion. In the fully developed state the gross appearance of the uterus and adnexal structures is characteristic. The uterus is softened and subinvoluted and may be focally necrotic and pultaceous. The tubal serosa is similarly involved because of the marked perisalpingitis, so that the peritoneal coverings of the uterus and tubes appear dull and are flecked with areas of thrombosis and subserosal abscesses. The cut surface of the uterus is boggy and gray, resembling certain sarcomas. There may also be multiple small abscess cavities. The vessels and lymphatics of the broad ligament are similarly involved. Microscopically the endometrium shows a mixture of an acute and chronic process with remnants of placental tissue and decidua. The superficial areas are completely necrotic and colonies of bacteria may be identified in the stroma and in perivascular spaces.

Symptomatology.—During the acute phase of postabortal salpingitis, symptoms of the acute process will be evident. The patient usually complains of constant or intermittent pelvic pain and irregular vaginal bleeding which may be dark brown and odorous. Backache, generalized lassitude and a chilly sensation or frank shaking chills frequently occur. There may be associated dysuria and a history of dyspareunia. The temperature is usually above 101 F. and may be as high as 106 or 107 F. If the offending organism is of the gram-negative variety, endotoxemic shock may occur. In this case the pulse will be rapid and thready, the blood pressure hypotensive and the urinary output minimal. If the abortion has been induced with a paste abortifacient, jaundice of severe degree may be noted. This results from the extravasation of certain soap contents into the generalized circulation with massive intravascular hemolysis. Clostridium welchii may occasionally be introduced into the uterine cavity during the performance of an illegal abortion. Owing to the biochemical characteristics of this organism, gas may form in and around the vagina and cervix, with large submucosal bullae resulting. Cases have actually been reported of massive collections of air and pus (pyophysometra), especially if drainage through the cervix is inadequate.

Pelvic examination reveals the cervix to be soft and frequently slightly patulous. Blood, seropurulent material or actual fragments of placental tissue or membranes may be seen protruding through the external cervical os. The uterus is usually subinvoluted and tender and both adnexal areas are acutely tender, with a doughy consistency. The characteristics of the pelvic examination will depend on the extent of the disease, the organism involved and the temporal relationship to the onset of infection and the type of treatment utilized. Thus, early in the disease process the tube feels edematous and is distinct from the ovary. After a week or 10 days, however, the entire lateral aspect of the broad ligament and paracervical areas takes on the characteristics of a soft tissue phlegmon. At this stage of the disease the tissues are firm and characteristically stony hard. It is difficult to distinguish the ovary from the tube.

The differential diagnosis is essentially the same as that noted under gonococcal salpingitis, but the precise diagnosis is usually simplified by the presence of placental tissue or membranes protruding through the cervix. Occasionally the patient will even volunteer the information that an abortion has been done or telltale marks of the tenacula may be seen on the anterior lip of the cervix.

Treatment.—Treatment consists in combating the infection with the appropriate antibiotic, supporting normal metabolic processes, correcting shock and evacuating the uterus at the opportune time. If the patient is not bleeding excessively and her general condition is good, initial therapy consists of either penicillin, streptomycin, chlortetracycline, cephalothin, kanamycin, polymyxin-B or combinations thereof, intravenous fluids and oxytocics. Anemia is corrected by transfusion and when the temperature has returned to normal and evidence of lateral infection has abated, a gentle uterine curettage is performed with extreme care taken not to perforate the wall of the subinvoluted uterus. Antibiotics should not be discontinued too quickly following curettage since residual infection frequently remains in the endometrium and in the perisalpingeal tissue.

Conservative management cannot be continued in the presence of hemorrhage, a lack of response to treatment or massive gram-negative endotoxemia. If bleeding is profuse and does not respond to oxytocic drugs, immediate curettage should be performed despite the presence of parametrial extension of the disease. This curettage must be gentle but thorough and uterine contractility may be improved by the use of a continuous intravenous drip of Pitocin or Methergine. At the same time ampicillin plus kanamycin or gentamycin is given. The latter is effective against all bacteria found in postabortal sepsis except group B streptococci. The uterine cavity should not be packed and rarely a hysterectomy may be necessary to control bleeding. Two other approaches have recently been suggested in an effort to save the uterus and to control uterine bleeding. These are (1) bilateral ligation of the uterine arteries by the vaginal approach and (2) bilateral ligation of the hypogastric arteries via an abdominal transperitoneal route or an extraperitoneal approach through an inguinal incision.

Hysterectomy may be the only procedure which will salvage a patient with overwhelming gram-negative endotoxemic shock from a persistent uterine focus. It has been suggested that, in such patients, the uterus is merely a "bag of pus" and the only certain method of cure is rapid hysterectomy. The patient must be supported before, during and after surgery with transfusions of whole blood since there is frequently intravascular hemolysis. Massive doses of antibiotics and potent vasopressor agents should be given to support the blood pressure and maintain cardiac output. In severely ill patients we have utilized combinations of antibiotics as follows: (assuming that renal function is normal) (1) 8 to 12 Gm. cephalothin daily intravenously plus 5 mg. per kg. kanamycin every 8 hours intramuscularly; (2) cephalothin plus kanamycin as in (1), plus polymyxin-B in a dose of 0.8 to 1.0 mg. per kg. every 8 hours intravenously; (3) penicillin G, 4 million units every 4 hours intravenously plus chloramphenicol, 1 Gm. every 8 hours intravenously plus polymyxin-B as above; (4) ampicillin, 1 to 2 Gm. every 4 hours intravenously.

TUBERCULOSIS

The incidence of pelvic tuberculosis varies considerably with the geographic location being studied and with the type of patient under consideration. Thus, in some areas of Scotland pelvic tuberculosis is discovered in 0.5-1 per cent of all female hospital admissions. When the incidence of pulmonary tuberculosis in a particular area is above normal, one may expect a high incidence of pelvic tuberculosis since it is found in approximately 10 per cent of patients with pulmonary disease. The incidence will also be higher in clinics where patients are studied extensively because of infertility. For this reason the Boston Hospital for Women, because of the association of the fertility and endocrine clinic, has a greater than normal incidence of pelvic tuberculosis. This increased incidence may be attributed in part to the large number of endometrial biopsies performed on infertile patients. Most patients with pelvic tuberculosis are in the childbearing age group, and the diagnosis in our clinic has often been made as a result of an unexpected finding in endometrium removed by biopsy or at the time of laparotomy for pelvic inflammatory disease.

The pathogenesis of the tuberculous process in the oviduct is usually believed to be via hematogenous spread, although occasional cases have been reported in which the infection is presumed to have been transmitted by the male. In the latter cases no extragenital site was discovered in the female and the male partner was known to have genital tuberculosis. It is believed that the oviduct is the primary site of genital tuberculosis and that subsequent spread is by direct continuity or via lymphatics. The endometrium is usually secondarily involved but is more resistant to extensive development of disease because of cyclic sloughing. The ovary is involved only when there is extensive salpingitis.

We have recently utilized progestational drugs to create a pseudopregnancy for two to three months in patients with suspected pelvic tuberculosis. This prevents the cyclic shedding of the superficial and intermediate layers of the endometrium, and subsequent endometrial biopsies have shown abundant tubercles when the previous material, obtained during the normal luteal or menstrual phase, gave negative findings. The resultant histologic picture is a most unusual one, since the progestational agent exerts its usual effect on the stroma and an extensive decidual reaction is formed. In addition, the glandular elements proceed through secretion and then begin to regress after approximately six to eight weeks of constant therapy. In some of the biopsies or curettages performed after such a pseudopregnancy abundant glandular atypia has been found. This is probably due to the inflammatory reaction set up by the tuberculous process. The routine use of such a procedure could conceivably increase the number of early diagnoses in infertile patients.

Pathology.—The gross findings are extremely variable, depending on the duration and extent of the disease. In early cases the oviducts may appear normal to gross inspection or only a few small, elevated tubercles may be identified on the serosal surface. When the disease is more advanced, the tube is markedly thickened and firm and there are numerous adhesions to adjacent bowel and ovary. At this stage a hysterectomy and bilateral salpingo-oophorectomy may be done under the mistaken diagnosis of postgonococcal inflammatory disease. In later stages the diagnosis is obvious, since the oviduct and ovary are usually involved in a conglomerate mass which is soft, pultaceous and tortuous with numerous gray nodulations on the surface (Fig. 6–6). The lumen of the tube contains caseous material and the peritoneum of the pelvis is usually involved with small white tubercles varying in size from 0.1 to 0.2 cm. The fimbriated portions of the oviduct are usually patent even in the extensive tuberculous process, but the peculiar eversion of the fimbria has an appearance that has been likened to a tobacco pouch.

Microscopically the tubal mucosa presents a rather typical follicular salpingitis in which the tubercles characteristic of tuberculosis are seen. In addition, when the disease is extensive, areas of caseous necrosis are common. The epithelium may on occasion exert an exuberant growth pattern, resembling the glandular arrangement seen in adenocarcinoma. However, the tubercles will usually distinguish the process as being nonmalignant.

Fig. 6–6.—Tuberculosis of oviduct. There is thickening of the serosa with tubercles scattered over the surface.

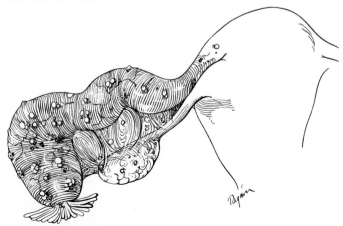

There are certain conditions which may mimic the microscopic picture seen in tuberculous salpingitis, and it is therefore mandatory that the organism be identified by specific staining technics and by culture. Culture may be done in tissue removed from the endometrium at the time of curettage, but the number of positive results will be greatly increased if the curettage is done just at or prior to the onset of the menstrual period. Although tuberculous peritonitis is a common complication of tuberculous salpingitis, rupture of the tube is uncommon. Tubal pregnancy in an oviduct showing tuberculous involvement is rare, fewer than 100 cases having been reported. Our study of 197 cases of tuberculous salpingitis at the Boston Hospital for Women during 54 years revealed ectopic pregnancy co-existing in only one patient. During this same period 313 patients were operated on for tubal pregnancy.

Diagnosis.—The pelvic examination in women having early tubal tuberculosis is usually completely normal. When the disease process has been present for some time, palpation of the abdomen may reveal a characteristic doughiness, a result of the matting together of the intestines and peritoneum from the tuberculous process. Ascites in young women is highly suggestive of tuberculous peritonitis. Bimanual examination may reveal the tube to be completely normal or slightly thickened. Occasionally large tubo-ovarian masses are present. If the introitus is virginal and bilateral tubo-ovarian masses are discovered, pelvic tuberculosis should be suspected.

To confirm the diagnosis of genital tuberculosis certain bacteriologic, roentgenographic and histologic examinations are necessary.

The tuberculin test should be performed routinely, except in the presence of fever, pregnancy, influenza or measles since these conditions produce a temporary false-negative reaction. A positive tuberculin reaction (an area of edema and redness measuring 5 mm. or more 48 hours after the injection) signifies only that the patient has been sensitized to the foreign protein of the tubercle bacillus. Therefore if the results are negative, except as noted above, one may be quite certain that the patient does not have pelvic tuberculosis.

An x-ray of the chest should be taken routinely although *active* pulmonary tuberculosis is not frequently associated with pelvic tuberculosis. Endometrial curettage is preferable to endometrial biopsy and should be performed in the immediate premenstrual phase of the cycle. Tissue obtained from the cornual regions is most likely to show tubercles. Endometrial biopsy may be performed, as noted previously, after creating a pseudopregnancy with progestational agents. Tissue removed at curettage should be inoculated into several culture mediums, into a guinea pig and the rest examined by a direct smear using the Ziehl-Neelsen method. Since it is necessary to wait six to eight weeks before a definite result is obtained from cultures and guinea-pig inoculation, it is important to prepare and examine numerous fragments of tissue by the Ziehl-Neelsen method.

Menstrual discharge has been collected in a plastic cup and submitted to routine culture. Halbrecht reported positive results in almost 90 per cent of patients when menstrual blood was cultured, compared with 63 per cent when an endometrial biopsy specimen was cultured.

Whenever the tubogram reveals evidence of blockage in the course of a sterility work-up, the physician should strongly suspect tuberculous sal-

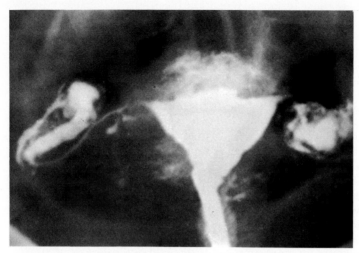

Fig. 6-7.—Tuberculosis of endometrium and tubes. Uterine shadow is surrounded by lymphatic extravasation of dye in a fine network. Both tubes have multiple sinus tracts, ragged contours, and terminal occlusion. (Courtesy of Dr. Alvin M. Siegler.)

pingitis. If the oviducts appear irregular or shaggy with multiple filling defects in the lumen, tuberculosis is suspect. In addition, especially in the disease process that has been present for some time, the oviducts are straight, rigid and have the appearance of a pipe stem. Calcified areas in the tubal lumen, pelvic lymph nodes, or in one or both ovaries, may also be visible and vascularization of the radiopaque material may occur in the uterine and ovarian vessels (Fig. 6-7). Culdoscopy is not particularly advantageous as a diagnostic adjuvant measure.

Treatment.—Schaefer has suggested the following summary of treatment. The optimum treatment for genital tuberculosis combines surgery with pre- and postoperative use of the antituberculosis drugs. When the patient is over age 40 complete removal of the uterus and adnexa serves the best interest of the patient. In selected cases in the younger woman, more conservative surgery may be indicated. Schaefer feels that once a tuberculous lesion has progressed to the stage of caseation, antibiotic therapy will not bring about a cure and such tissue should be completely removed. The radical extirpation of diseased tissue should be preceded by a course of streptomycin and para-aminosalicylic acid. The dose of streptomycin is 1 Gm. daily administered intramuscularly for two weeks and then 1 Gm. twice a week for six to eight weeks preoperatively. Para-aminosalicylic acid is given orally in doses of 12 Gm. daily in four divided doses. Postoperatively this medication is continued for three to four weeks or even longer, depending on the presence of active extrapelvic tuberculous lesions. Isonicotinic acid hydrazide in a dose of 100 mg. three times a day may be added to the streptomycin and para-aminosalicylic acid regimen.

The question of whether to do conservative or radical surgery is, to a certain degree, still unanswered. It has been shown that the effectiveness of streptomycin is in direct proportion to the blood supply of the lesion. Streptomycin produces temporarily excellent results in the earlier type of tuberculosis and in those lesions to which the blood supply is relatively good. Poor results have been obtained in the chronic fibrocaseous type of lesions, which are less vascular. Experiments with radioactive isoniazid, however, indicate that isoniazid and its metabolites diffuse into dense caseous lesions and are actually present there in high concentrations three to five hours after administration. It has also been noted that adnexal masses present before the start of chemotherapy may show no significant alteration at the termination of treatment. In certain cases, however, when unsuspected genital tuberculosis is found to be associated with infertility and no palpable adnexal lesions are present, chemotherapy should be instituted and the patient checked at intervals of three months for persistent activity of disease.

The indications for surgery are: (1) abdominal pain persisting during or recurring after treatment; (2) persistence or development of adnexal masses following treatment, and (3) recurrence of endometrial infection or excessive bleeding following treatment. Sutherland suggests admitting the patient to the hospital for one or two weeks prior to operation at which time a course of streptomycin, para-aminosalicylic acid and isoniazid is started. Surgery is timed for the middle of the ovarian cycle and a complete hysterectomy and bilateral salpingo-oophorectomy is performed whenever possible. Sutherland also suggests continuation of therapy for 6 months after surgery and for 1 year if the extirpated tissue shows active disease.

The chances of pregnancy and its normal progression to term are better in patients treated for tubal tuberculosis than in patients treated for endometrial tuberculosis. Prior to antibiotic therapy ectopic pregnancies were frequently reported (from areas where tuberculosis is common) in patients with active or even spontaneously healed tubal tuberculosis. Since the advent of antibiotics there has been an increase in both ectopic and intrauterine pregnancies, but the latter seldom reach term delivery. Before the use of antibiotics intrauterine pregnancies did not occur in patients with endometrial tuberculosis. Use of the newer drugs has brought about a small but appreciable increase in intrauterine pregnancies although early abortion is still common. Halbrecht and Blinick recently reported a full-term pregnancy after antibiotic treatment of proved endometrial tuberculosis and noted that four other instances had been reported in the literature up to 1960. In the series of 446 patients treated from 1950 through 1966 at the David Elder Infirmary in Glasgow, Scotland, Sutherland reported 34 pregnancies as having occurred in 23 patients. There were 15 ectopic pregnancies and nine abortions. Ten live babies were delivered including 2 to one patient. At the Boston Hospital for Women only 1 full term delivery has occurred subsequent to treatment but the incidence of tuberculosis of pelvic organs is only a fraction of that seen in Scotland.

Although there is still considerable disagreement as to whether all three drugs should be used simultaneously or whether a combination of any two is adequate, it is certain that short-term chemotherapy for pelvic tuberculosis is worthless. Schaefer showed evidence of tuberculosis in from 75 to 100 per cent of oviducts removed from patients who had received antimicrobial drugs for two to six months. Therefore, a period of therapy of at least one and probably two years is optimal. Schaefer suggests that all three drugs be used in treating advanced active disease and that the patient be examined every few weeks to note any change in the size of the ad-nexal masses. Some decrease in size will occur in six to eight weeks. Anti-microbial therapy should be continued for three to four months. Then, if further improvement has not occurred, surgery should be performed. If the patient is over age 40 a complete hysterectomy and bilateral salpingo-oophorectomy should be done. In younger women in whom it is desirable to retain childbearing function, or even menstrual function, the extent of the surgery must be governed by the extent of the pathologic findings.

In long-term treatment of minimal tuberculosis Schaefer has indicated a preference for isoniazid combined with streptomycin or PAS, or both. Since some patients will refuse to take streptomycin twice weekly for pro-longed periods, they may be continued on the other two preparations. Other patients cannot tolerate PAS and therefore may be carried on streptomycin and isoniazid. Although Halbrecht noted healing and cicatrization after antibiotic treatment in 80 per cent of the patients, the end results may show complete obliteration of the oviduct or other changes in the endosal-pinx that favor the development of a tubal pregnancy. Ryden has stated that tuberculous salpingitis produces lasting infertility in the vast majority of patients, particularly when the oviducts have been closed at the begin-ning of treatment. At the end of one year of therapy a repeat tubogram may be obtained to study the effect of the conservative program. Sutherland has recently reported the results of 80 patients utilizing the following triple therapy regimen: streptomycin, 1 Gm., PAS, 15 Gm., and isoniazid, 300 mg. daily for 120 days. PAS, 12 Gm., and isoniazid, 300 mg. daily are then con-tinued for 18 months. Of 69 patients having endometrial infection prior to treatment, 34 (49 per cent) had a persistently negative endometrium fol-lowing therapy—with an average duration of follow-up of 11 months.

If the diagnosis of genital tuberculosis is made at the time of surgery, and the disease is extensive, a bilateral salpingo-oophorectomy and hyster-ectomy should be performed and postoperative chemotherapy administered for 12 months or longer. If the uterus and adnexa cannot be removed because of technical difficulties, the abdomen should be closed and a course of chemotherapy be given for three to four months. The disease process may then abate so that complete surgery may be performed at a later date. Postoperative chemotherapy should also be given for 12 months as before.

Physiologic Salpingitis

In the course of routine examination of fallopian tubes removed at the time of hysterectomy at the Boston Hospital for Women, numerous cases of salpingitis associated with menstrual endometrium have been en-countered. While the inflammatory reaction was of the acute variety and was associated with an infiltration of polymorphonuclear leukocytes, it did not have the precise pathologic appearance of acute salpingitis due to bacterial infection. Nassberg *et al.* described this inflammatory process in 43 of 69 patients who had hysterectomy and salpingectomy at the time of menstruation. The inflammatory reaction was characterized by polymor-phonuclear leukocytes *within* the lumen of the tube (Fig. 6–8), in the stroma of the tubal plicae, but only rarely in the muscularis. The plicae

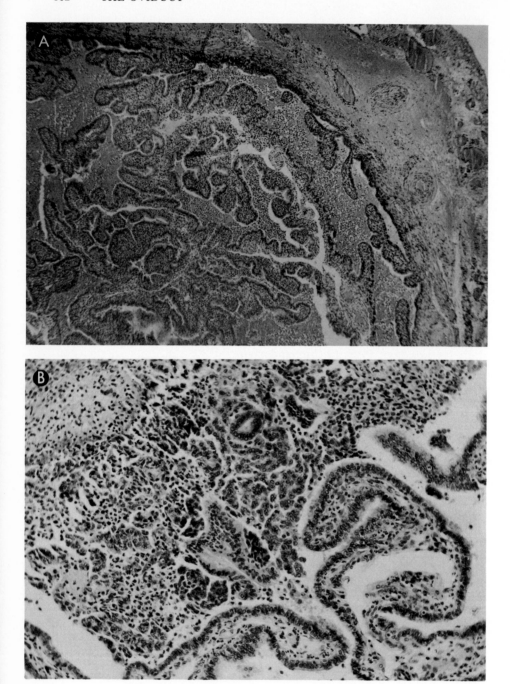

Fig. 6-8.—Physiologic salpingitis. **A,** low-power view. **B,** high power to show leukocytes and cellular debris in tubal lumen.

showed edema, stasis of leukocytes within their capillaries and dilatation of the lymphatics. The inflammatory process was confined to the mucosal part of the oviduct and the muscle walls were seldom involved. There was no associated evidence of healed follicular salpingitis as characterized by infiltration of lymphocytes, plasma cells or fusion of the tips of the plicae. No bacteria were demonstrated and the patients showed no evidence of infection clinically. Since the inflammation was superficial and submucosal and since endometrial debris as well as leukocytes and red cell debris were found in the lumina it was suggested that the cause of this reaction was related to the regurgitation of menstrual blood into the oviducts during the menstrual period. Although this inflammatory reaction appears to be quite severe, there is no evidence that residual damage to the tube occurs. Even during the acute phase neither necrosis nor destruction of any portion of the tubal structure is noted.

This same process had been produced by G. V. Smith by the injection of human menstrual discharge into one horn of a rabbit uterus. The histologic picture in this experiment and that seen in the human oviducts at the time of menstruation are practically identical.

Hellman described an acute salpingitis which appeared to be histologically identical with the morphology described by Nassberg. However, the oviducts studied by Hellman were obtained at the time of sterilization on various days of the puerperium. He found a nonbacterial, inflammatory reaction in approximately 30 per cent of the oviducts removed on the sixth to eighth puerperal day. It was rarely discovered during the first four days postpartum.

Since it has been previously demonstrated that the oviducts are the most sensitive of all the pelvic organs to pain stimuli, it is interesting to note that in Nassberg's series about 25 per cent of the patients complained of dysmenorrhea at the time of operation and several of these had had dysmenorrhea during previous menses. These observations suggest the possibility that the pain in certain cases of dysmenorrhea may be initiated by a transient acute physiologic salpingitis.

Nontuberculous Granulomatous Salpingitis

This is a rather common type of salpingitis which seems to be increasing in incidence because of the large number of salpingograms performed with iodine-oil preparations. The granulomatous lesion produced by the deposition of this oil in the tubal mucosa may simulate tuberculosis. However, the tubercle is atypical, organisms are not identified by proper staining and cultures are negative. Further, caseation necrosis is not seen.

Deposition of talc granules into the peritoneal cavity at the time of surgery may lead to a similar granulomatous salpingitis (Fig. 6–9). Apparently the talc granules are ingested by the fimbriated portion of the oviduct and become embedded in the endosalpinx. These are most commonly seen in the fimbriated and ampullary portion of the tube. Certain generalized diseases such as sarcoid or fungal infections such as actinomycosis may occasionally give rise to a granulomatous salpingitis which may be confused with that of tuberculosis.

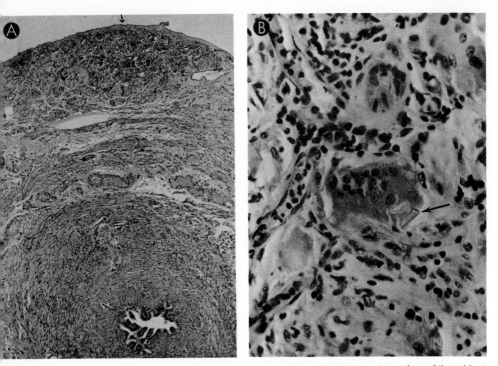

Fig. 6-9.—A, foreign-body granulomatous reaction from talc on the surface of the oviduct. **B,** higher power showing a crystal (talc) adjacent to the foreign-body giant cell.

Tubal Ectopic Pregnancy

Ectopic pregnancy continues to be a major diagnostic problem and is responsible for approximately 2-3 per cent of all obstetrically caused maternal deaths in the United States each year. The incidence of ectopic pregnancy is variable, depending on the type of hospital reporting the data. Thus, the incidence has been noted to be 0.6 per cent of all pregnancies at the Charity Hospital of New Orleans whereas at the Mayo Clinic it is 2.5 per cent. The use of antibiotics and conservative treatment of pelvic inflammation has undoubtedly increased the incidence of tubal gestation. The ages of patients with tubal ectopic pregnancy vary from 15 to 45, but in most reported series the average age is 30.

DIAGNOSIS

Presenting Signs and Symptoms. PAIN.—Pain is the most common and consistent symptom associated with ectopic pregnancy, but the type is variable depending upon the duration of the gestation and the extent of hemorrhage. Most of the patients with ectopic pregnancy complain of cramp-like pelvic or lower abdominal pain on the affected side early in the gestation. This pain may be due to uterine contractions and distention of the tubal serosa.

Lancinating pelvic pain associated with fainting is frequently seen in patients with acute rupture of an ectopic pregnancy whereas dull, aching pain occurs in those having an organized hematoma around an unruptured ectopic pregnancy. About 10 per cent of the patients have shoulder pain in addition to pelvic pain, an almost certain indication of intraperitoneal spill of blood and diaphragmatic irritation.

ABNORMAL VAGINAL BLEEDING.—A careful, accurate history of the recent menstrual periods is of extreme importance in diagnosis. The exact dates of the previous three bleeding episodes together with the character and duration of flow should be ascertained. Frequently, it will be discovered that the most recent bleeding did not occur at the expected time in the cycle and that it was slightly diminished in amount. In approximately 50 per cent of patients the menstrual history will be normal. However, most of these will have noted spotting or intermittent slight vaginal bleeding since the last normal menstrual period, and in about 10 per cent of patients the bleeding begins simultaneously with the onset of pain. Profuse bleeding with passage of large clots is not a common symptom unless the patient has associated leiomyomata. Continued diminished bleeding and the absence of large clots is helpful in distinguishing ectopic pregnancy from threatened or incomplete abortion.

Amenorrhea of two or three months' duration may be associated with an ectopic pregnancy occurring in the interstitial portion of the oviduct or in a rudimentary uterine horn since rupture in these areas is delayed.

PREGNANCY SIGNS AND SYMPTOMS.—Nausea, vomiting and breast engorgement are not usually seen because of the early termination of the gestation. They may be present in pregnancies occurring in the uterine cornua or interstitial portion of the oviduct.

Physical Examination. GENERAL.—The condition of the patient may vary from normal to one of extreme shock with pallor, clammy skin, sweating, tachycardia and hypotension. The majority of patients, however, do not present this typical "textbook" picture, which is associated with acute loss of blood into the peritoneal cavity. An exception to this is seen in rupture of a rudimentary horn or interstitial pregnancy. The intraperitoneal hemorrhage in these patients is massive because of the vascularity of the area and its double blood supply.

TEMPERATURE.—A ruptured ectopic pregnancy, even with a large pelvic hematoma, will cause only a slight elevation in temperature. In patients having acute rupture the temperature is frequently found to be subnormal and it is uncommon to find it exceeding 101 F. (38.3 C.). This characteristic of the temperature to remain subnormal or only slightly elevated is a valuable sign in differentiating pelvic inflammatory disease and septic abortion.

PULSE RATE.—The pulse rate is characteristically rapid when the ectopic pregnancy has ruptured but otherwise is normal.

BLOOD PRESSURE.—The blood pressure reflects both the acuteness of the process and the degree of blood loss. In patients with unruptured ectopic pregnancies as well as those with slowly leaking ruptures with hematoma formation, the blood pressure is normal. Systolic pressures below 80 mm. of Hg are seen in only about 10 per cent of patients.

ABDOMEN.—Examination of the abdomen is usually negative in patients with an unruptured or locally confined process. There may be lower quadrant tenderness if a large peritubal hematoma has formed. In the presence of massive intraperitoneal bleeding the abdomen is diffusely tender and presents typical muscular rigidity. If the intraperitoneal bleeding is of several days' duration, abdominal distention due to small bowel ileus may be noted. Occasionally a periumbilical blue discoloration is noted in patients with massive intraperitoneal bleeding (Cullen's sign).

PELVIC EXAMINATION.—Findings are extremely variable, depending upon the duration of pregnancy and the amount of intraperitoneal bleeding. The cervix and uterus are usually of normal size and consistency, but manipulation of the cervix causes pelvic pain in most patients if there is leakage of blood or rupture of the tube. In early unruptured tubal pregnancy, the tubal enlargement may be too slight to be detected by bimanual examination and is frequently missed. If the adnexa on the opposite side are normal to palpation, the chances of tubal pregnancy are greater. However, since chronic salpingitis is a predisposing factor to the development of ectopic pregnancy, the finding of contralateral disease does not eliminate the possibility.

After tubal abortion or rupture the adnexal area is exquisitely tender. If the tube has ruptured, it is apt to be less markedly enlarged than when tubal abortion has taken place. Liquid blood in the cul-de-sac produces a doughy or "full" feeling although frequently both adnexal areas will be thought to be normal even when bathed in liquid blood. After the blood has clotted it is easily felt as a soft, somewhat indefinite, tender mass in the cul-de-sac or adnexal region.

The importance of limiting bimanual examinations and observing extreme gentleness in doing this procedure must be emphasized. Examination under anesthesia is frequently desirable since the pain associated with manipulation of the internal genitalia limits the examiner considerably. Shock following a pelvic examination under anesthesia is suggestive of a ruptured ectopic pregnancy but may also occur subsequent to rupture of a tubo-ovarian abscess.

Diagnostic Procedures. LABORATORY. BLOOD EXAMINATION.—Determination of the leukocyte count is not of particular assistance. Approximately half of the patients with ectopic pregnancy have a white cell count below 10,000 and in three-quarters it is below 15,000. A leukocytosis exceeding 20,000 has been noted in only about 10 per cent of patients, and a persistent leukocytosis of this degree favors a diagnosis of pelvic inflammatory disease. There is an initial leukocytosis immediately following tubal rupture but this usually returns to normal within 24 hours unless there is recurrent bleeding.

The erythrocyte count and hematocrit reflect the extent of bleeding, but the initial determination is modified by pre-existing anemia and the state of hydration. In hospitals having a large indigent population, about 50 per cent of the patients have an erythrocyte count below three million prior to bleeding from ruptured ectopic pregnancy. Of more importance than the initial count are *sequential* determinations of the hematocrit and erythrocytes. A gradual decrease is frequently associated with persistent leakage of blood into a peritubal hematoma.

In patients with a chronically leaking ectopic pregnancy and gradual absorption of blood, the serum bilirubin and icteric index may be elevated.

BIOLOGIC TESTS FOR PREGNANCY.—These tests are negative in approximately half of the patients with ectopic pregnancy. When they are positive (as in tubal rupture or combined intra- and extrauterine gestation) they are indicative only of living trophoblastic tissue. The test is of no value in differentiating an intrauterine from an extrauterine pregnancy. These determinations are likely to be negative in patients with tubal abortion, particularly when the symptoms suggest recurring tubal bleeding with hemorrhagic disruption of the villi.

SURGICAL. EXAMINATION UNDER ANESTHESIA.—When this is performed the operating room should be ready for immediate laparotomy. Under anesthesia it is frequently possible to differentiate an early intrauterine pregnancy from an ectopic one by more detailed examination of the cervix, uterus and adnexa. The well-circumscribed outlines of the corpus luteum or follicular cyst are usually readily distinguished from the indefinite mass formed by the distended tube and adjacent hematoma. In many patients the localized enlargement of the oviduct may be delineated from the ovary even before rupture. However, in early tubal pregnancy more precise diagnostic methods such as culdocentesis, posterior colpotomy, culdoscopy or laparoscopy are necessary.

CULDOCENTESIS.—This procedure is of particular value if the cul-de-sac is bulging. It may be done without general anesthesia, using a long 15 to 18 gauge needle on a 10 or 20 cc. syringe. A dry tap is unusual and should warrant another attempt. The fluid obtained may suggest: (a) if clear, serous and straw-colored—a normal, negative pelvis; (b) if turbid but serous—pelvic inflammatory disease; (c) if blood-tinged and serous—ruptured ovarian cysts, ovulation bleeding or occasionally, pelvic inflammatory disease; (d) if bright red and grossly bloody—recently bleeding corpus luteum, recently ruptured ectopic pregnancy with fresh bleeding or a traumatic cul-de-sac aspiration; (e) if *old blood, brownish-colored*—ectopic pregnancy with intraperitoneal bleeding over a few days or weeks. *Blood does not clot*, or at times tiny clots may be aspirated.

POSTERIOR COLPOTOMY.—Colpotomy is safer than culdocentesis in patients without definite bulging of the cul-de-sac. If tubal abortion or rupture with intraperitoneal bleeding has occurred, usually sufficient blood is in the cul-de-sac to make it apparent as soon as the peritoneum is opened. When the vagina is roomy and the uterus is retroverted, visualization of the adnexa is easily accomplished. In other patients, with chronic salpingitis or previous pelvic surgery, adequate visualization is difficult or impossible. Culdoscopy is preferable in such cases.

CULDOSCOPY.—This procedure requires considerable experience and technical skill on the part of the operator but it is of extreme value in differentiating a corpus luteum or follicular cyst from an unruptured tubal pregnancy. If an organized blood clot is present in the cul-de-sac, culdocentesis may be negative, whereas the culdoscope will usually traverse the clot and the diagnosis can be made. If visualization by culdoscopy is not adequate, the incision may be extended and posterior colpotomy performed. If there is a large pelvic mass or obliteration of the cul-de-sac from endometriosis or inflammatory disease, culdoscopy is neither indicated nor advantageous. Moreover, injudicious attempts to introduce the trocar in such patients may result in damage to the rectosigmoid or small bowel. Laparoscopy is the optimum diagnostic procedure in such patients.

UTERINE CURETTAGE.—If chorionic tissue is found either grossly or microscopically, the presence of an intrauterine pregnancy is obvious. However, the rare combination of intra- and extrauterine pregnancy is still a possibility. If the curettings show only decidua, a diagnosis of ectopic pregnancy must be considered. However, it is possible to curette a pregnant uterus and miss the ovum so that only decidual tissue is obtained. Similarly, a decidual reaction in the endometrial stroma may be brought about by a corpus luteum cyst, a luteinized follicular cyst or granulosa cell tumor, or by the administration of potent synthetic progestational agents.

In general, it may be concluded that when decidua without chorionic tissue is found by curettage, there is a good possibility of an ectopic pregnancy, but the absence of decidua does not exclude tubal pregnancy, especially if the bleeding is of several weeks' duration. The endometrium in such patients may be secretory, proliferative or menstrual.

Specific morphologic changes in the epithelium of the endometrium have been described in association with either intra- or extrauterine pregnancy. This "Arias-Stella" reaction has been called an anaplasia of pregnancy and, if found, should alert the clinician to the possibility of an ectopic pregnancy. This morphologic pattern has not been described in the endometrium of patients receiving synthetic progestational agents for "pseudopregnancy."

Since the findings from curettage are equivocal in so many patients and since a normal intrauterine pregnancy may be interrupted, this procedure is not advised as a routine diagnostic procedure.

Treatment.—The optimum treatment for ectopic pregnancy is surgical removal. This should be performed as rapidly as possible after diagnosis has been made and supportive therapy, if necessary, should be administered in the operating room. Expectant treatment of ectopic pregnancy is extremely hazardous since the gestational sac and adjacent oviduct may rupture without warning and the patient die from massive hemorrhage. Despite inconvenience, it has been suggested that "the sun never set on a possible ectopic pregnancy." Transfusions of whole blood should be given to patients who are in shock, the patient transferred to the operating room as soon as possible and transfusion continued throughout the procedure.

The management of ectopic pregnancy demands that hemorrhage be

Fig. 6–10.—Anatomic sites of tubal ectopic pregnancies.

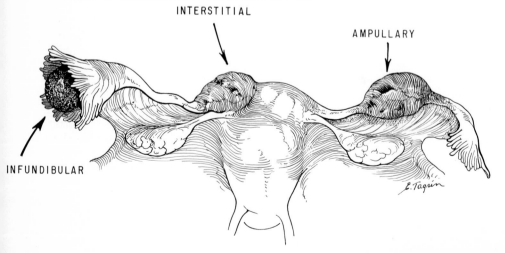

INTERSTITIAL

AMPULLARY

INFUNDIBULAR

E. Taquin

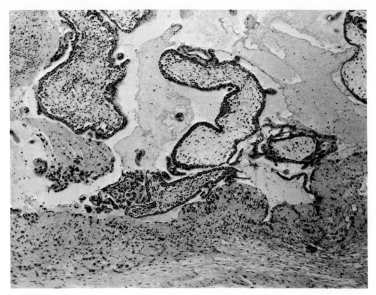

Fig. 6-11.—High power view showing chorionic villi and cytotrophoblastic cells in contact with tubal wall.

prevented or arrested. Therefore, treatment usually consists of excision of the involved tube. If the patient has been in shock or if there is massive intraperitoneal hemorrhage, operation should be limited to removal of the ectopic pregnancy and control of hemorrhage. In many patients who are operated on for ectopic pregnancy and whose condition is good, a hysterectomy may be indicated. This is true if one oviduct has been previously removed and the present ectopic pregnancy is in a part of the tube which cannot be salvaged. An ovarian neoplasm or an extensive inflammatory process involving the opposite tube is an adequate indication for hysterectomy at the time of surgery.

When the ectopic gestation involves the fimbriated portion of the tube or even the ampulla (Fig. 6-10), and particularly if a patient has been infertile, conservative procedures may help preserve the childbearing potential. Both lateral incisions of the tubes and salpingostomy have been suggested as methods of tubal preservation. With these operations a Silastic (silicone-dacron) tubule may be inserted into the repaired oviduct to maintain patency. The tubule is brought out through the ostium of the oviduct and is sutured to the anterior rectus sheath. It is left in place for 6 months, then removed through a small skin incision. After such a procedure the patient must be observed closely since the risk of repeat ectopic pregnancy is increased, both in the repaired and in the opposite tube, especially if follicular salpingitis is present.

Other ancillary surgical procedures may be performed without increasing morbidity if the patient's general condition is good and if massive intraperitoneal hemorrhage has not occurred. Appendectomy has been performed in many patients in this group and abdominal myomectomy has been carried out in a few nulliparous patients desirous of having children. Several studies have indicated that a patient who has an ectopic pregnancy has an increased potential for a second ectopic pregnancy, the incidence ranging from 5 to 11 per cent. It is important in performing a salpingectomy that the interstitial portion of the tube is removed to prevent implantation of a subsequent gestation in this particular area.

FERTILITY AFTER ECTOPIC PREGNANCY

There is no doubt that the occurrence of an ectopic pregnancy is a major accident for a patient who wishes subsequently to become pregnant. It has been estimated that only about one-third of such patients will ever succeed in delivering a living child. More than one-third will become pregnant but many will lose the gestation either by miscarriage or by recurrent ectopic pregnancy. It has been estimated that such patients are seven to eight times more likely to have a subsequent misplaced pregnancy than are women who have not had ectopic gestations. It is imperative therefore that every patient who undergoes surgery for an ectopic gestation be left with a normally patent residual tube. When infertility follows an operation for ectopic pregnancy, the possibility arises that the infertility is due to damage of the residual tube as a result of the surgical procedure itself. Grant suggests that the remaining tube is iatrogenically damaged by residual blood or subsequent infection in the peritoneal cavity in almost 50 per cent of cases.

In order to avoid this difficulty, Grant suggested the following principles: (1) early operation, (2) removal of the blood clot and the free blood from the peritoneal cavity, (3) conservation of the residual tube and (4) a patency test of the residual tube within a few weeks of operation. Grant emphasized the importance of removing the numerous blood clots and free blood from the peritoneal cavity since he feels that this may reduce the incidence of later adhesions. Further, it is suggested that a broad-spectrum antibiotic be administered routinely after surgery for a ruptured ectopic pregnancy. Grant also emphasized the importance of testing the residual tube for patency within one month of the operation. If it is found to be blocked, some nonsurgical therapy for tubal blockade may be instituted. Thus, repeated insufflations with carbon dioxide even at pressures exceeding 200 mm. Hg may be desirable. Recently hydrotubation with a solution of cortisone and antibiotics has been utilized successfully in a large number of patients.

Tubal plastic surgery for a tubal pregnancy is justified only when the opposite tube is absent or blocked. With our presently available techniques it is probable that tubal plastic surgery at the time of an ectopic pregnancy in a single residual tube is of greater psychologic than reproductive benefit to the patient. The pregnancy salvage is approximately 25 per cent, with a high recurrence rate of ectopic pregnancy. If the pregnancy is in the proximal half of the oviduct it seems advisable to excise the affected area and to reimplant the normal portion of the tube at a later date. Immediate tubal implantation into the uterus at the time of operation for ectopic pregnancy is time consuming and not advised.

It has been suggested that removal of the ovary on the side of the ruptured ectopic pregnancy at the time of salpingectomy results in a 12 per cent increase in the subsequent pregnancy rate. Although the placement of the remaining patent tube immediately adjacent to the only source of ova seems logical, it may occasionally result in a protest from the patient. It has not been our routine to remove the ovary on the side of the ectopic pregnancy unless that ovary is abnormal. In certain patients it may be a desirable procedure.

Combined Intra- and Extrauterine Pregnancies

The diagnosis of combined pregnancy should be considered if the patient gives a history of ectopic pregnancy or has unilateral lower abdominal tenderness with concomitant evidence of an intrauterine pregnancy. If the uterus is enlarged, the cervix closed and there is minimal vaginal bleeding the physician should always be suspicious of this combination. The persistence of lower abdominal pain following spontaneous abortion of an early uterine pregnancy should suggest that an ectopic pregnancy may coexist. The treatment for combined pregnancy should be a laparotomy with removal of the extrauterine pregnancy. Postoperative attention should be directed toward the preservation of the intrauterine gestation. Routine curettage in extrauterine pregnancy is not advised because of the possibility of interruption of an intrauterine pregnancy.

Salpingitis Isthmica Nodosa

Salpingitis isthmica nodosa is a disease process of unknown etiology, characterized by nodular thickenings in the intramural and isthmic portions of the oviduct. Microscopically the nodules are noted to be in the muscular wall of the tube and to contain nests of glandlike tissue. Frequently the lumina of these glands are connected to the central tubal lumen. This disease process is also known variously as diverticulosis adenomyosis of the tube, adenosalpingitis and endosalpingiosis. The incidence is variable and depends on the detailed examination of the pathologist and on the number of microscopic sections taken through this portion of the oviduct. The disease occurs most commonly between the ages of 25 and 50 with an average age of 35. It is more common among Negroes than among the white population.

The pathogenesis of this disease is controversial but several theories have been advanced as to its origin. The most commonly accepted suggests that this disease is the sequel of inflammation either of gonorrheal or of tuberculous type. The support for the inflammatory origin is provided chiefly by the fact that associated inflammation is found in 75–80 per cent of cases. Bilateral lesions are also quite common. Finally, certain patients who had grossly normal oviducts at the time of laparotomy later were found, following an attack of gonorrhea, to have typical salpingitis isthmica nodosa. It has been suggested that the islands of glandular tissue are formed as a result of an extension of the mucosa during the acute inflammatory process. Thus, minute intraluminal abscesses may rupture or dissect into the softened muscularis. This process is abetted by the absence of a typical muscularis mucosa in the oviduct. Some time later these fragments of displaced epithelium form glandlike spaces which subsequently undergo proliferation and set up an irritative process. Hypertrophy and hyperplasia of the muscle fibers result.

In several reports of patients with salpingitis isthmica nodosa, less than

50 per cent had an associated inflammatory process. In such patients the lesion was thought to be of noninflammatory origin, and it was suggested that the process arose from a proliferation or hyperplasia of the epithelial lining cells of the isthmus or possibly by a contiguous spread of uterine adenomyosis.

The congenital origin of salpingitis isthmica nodosa was championed by numerous authors at the turn of the century but recent studies have indicated many discrepancies in this theory of histogenesis. In the first place, the condition has been found only in the adult female and not in the fetus. Secondly, the connections between the glandlike spaces and the tubal lumen have definitely been demonstrated, proving that they are diverticula. Thirdly, the condition has been shown to be present only where there is evidence of a chronic inflammatory process. The German pathologist Robert Meyer also denied the congenital origin of this disease after he had examined 100 uteri from all ages of fetal development. He found adenomatous structures of this variety to be rare in the fetus, whereas in adults glandular proliferation in the oviducts occurred rather frequently.

The gross appearance of salpingitis isthmica nodosa (Fig. 6–12) is usually characteristic. The lesions are bilateral in about 35 per cent of patients. Usually the nodules are multiple and irregularly distributed, presenting a somewhat beaded appearance. The nodules vary in size from a few millimeters to 2.5 cm. in diameter and frequently are sharply circumscribed, firm, irregular but with a smooth surface. The mucosa and the serosa are generally smooth and essentially normal. On cut surface the nodules are seen to be white or brownish yellow, generally solid but occasionally with a central lumen.

The microscopic appearance of salpingitis isthmica nodosa (Fig. 6–13) is variable, depending on the duration of the lesion. In its earliest form there is a simple outpocketing of the tubal mucosa into the musculature. In its fully developed state glandlike spaces are scattered throughout the myosalpinx and are associated with hyperplasia and hypertrophy of the muscle fibers. The spaces are extremely variable in size and shape and some appear cystically dilated. The epithelial connection with the tubal lumen may or may not be apparent. The epithelium is usually cuboidal or columnar, of one-cell layer thickness, with cells typical of those ordinarily

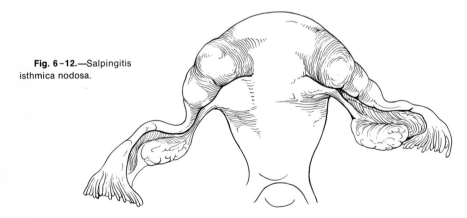

Fig. 6–12.—Salpingitis isthmica nodosa.

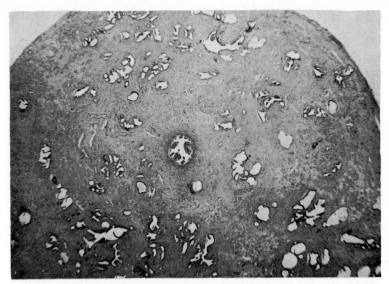

Fig. 6-13.—Salpingitis isthmica nodosa. Photomicrograph shows multiple islands of epithelium in tubal isthmus. The tubal lumen is evident in the center of the section.

seen in the normal oviduct. In cystically dilated glands there is flattening of the epithelium, whereas in the smaller glandular spaces the epithelium is a mixture of that seen in the tube and endometrium. The epithelium usually does not show the cyclic changes seen in the endometrium, but on occasion certain glands may simulate the secretory phase of the endometrial epithelium. There is a surrounding stroma of collagenous fibrous connective tissue which is usually infiltrated with plasma cells, leukocytes or eosinophils. In certain cases the stroma may closely resemble the stroma of the endometrium. In adjacent areas there may be evidence of a chronic salpingitis.

Diagnosis.—The diagnosis of salpingitis isthmica nodosa is usually made at the time of laparotomy for infertility or pelvic inflammatory disease. However, with the use of the culdoscope this diagnosis has been made in a large number of patients in our clinic prior to definitive surgery. In 1951 Bunster demonstrated that this lesion, which he called tubal diverticulosis, could be diagnosed by means of salpingography and he published hysterosalpingograms revealing such diverticula. Siegler, in 1955, was able to diagnose tubal diverticulosis in 1.6 per cent of 1,160 hysterosalpingograms performed on patients whose primary complaint was infertility. He suggested that the diagnosis should be suspected in a woman in the fourth decade of life who has had a history of unexplained involuntary sterility for five years or more and in whom no previous pelvic inflammatory disease had occurred. The temperature, leukocyte count and sedimentation rate are usually normal, and on pelvic examination adnexal masses are usually not palpable. Siegler further cautioned that the x-ray picture of tubal diverticulosis must be differentiated from that of tubal tuberculosis. In the latter condition, the oviducts are usually rigid, devoid of peristalsis and are often occluded at the proximal end of the ampulla.

However, fistulous tracts seen in tuberculosis may be confused with diverticulosis. Calcification of pelvic lymph nodes or calcified areas in the tubal lumen or in one or both ovaries are diagnostic of genital tuberculosis. The endometrial biopsy may reveal typical tuberculous endometritis.

Treatment.—The lesions per se are innocuous and require no specific treatment. The prognosis is good and might be compared to the prognosis in a nonspecific salpingitis. The lesion is not considered to be premalignant. If tubal diverticulosis is discovered as an incidental finding at laparotomy and the tubes are grossly normal, nothing need be done. However, a patient with a long-standing history of infertility who has bilateral isthmic occlusion due to diverticulosis could be considered a candidate for reconstructive surgery. In this case bilateral reimplantation of the oviducts would be the procedure of choice.

Benign Neoplasms

Benign tumors of the oviduct are rare entities, yet a large variety of neoplasms have been reported as having originated in the fallopian tube. Tumors may be located in the wall or within the lumen or occasionally may be pedunculated and project from the fimbriated portion of the tube. In a consideration of benign tumors of the oviduct, lesions such as salpingitis isthmica nodosa, endometriosis and adenomyosis should be excluded. Similarly, the hydatids of Morgagni are so commonplace that they should not be considered as a tumor mass. The following benign tumors have been reported in the literature: cystic and solid teratomas, papilloma, fibroadenoma, fibroma, leiomyoma, lipoma, hemangioma, lymphangioma, mesothelioma and mesonephroma.

Somewhat more common is the adenomatoid tumor (Fig. 6–14), sometimes called an angiomyoma or a reticuloendothelioma. This is a small circumscribed tumor of the tube usually confined to the muscle wall and found incidentally at the time of laparotomy. It has a characteristic microscopic appearance, being composed of small glandlike spaces lined by cells of mesothelial, endothelial or even epithelial appearance. Grossly the tumors appear as gray, gray-white or yellow, discrete nodules occupying the muscularis and rarely exceeding 3 cm. in diameter. Because of the glandular arrangement of the cells, the microscopic picture has occasionally been confused with a low-grade adenocarcinoma. The histogenesis of these tumors is not clearly defined. Hertig and Gore consider this tumor to be of peritoneal origin and therefore support its origin from mesothelial cells. It is not believed that these adenomatoid tumors possess malignant potential.

Leiomyomas of the tube are usually asymptomatic lesions which are discovered at laparotomy performed for another indication. Approximately 50 cases have been reported in the literature, but since these tumors are usually solitary and small it is entirely probable that many have been unreported. Occasionally they have enlarged and produced acute torsion of the oviduct, and degenerative changes similar to those occurring in uterine leiomyomas have been reported.

Approximately 35 cystic teratomas of the oviduct have been reported, most having been discovered accidentally. These cystic teratomas may

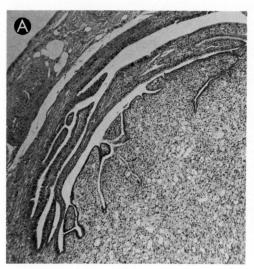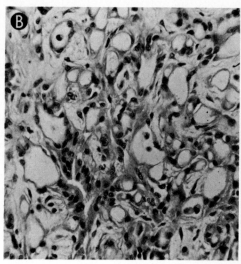

Fig. 6-14.—Adenomatoid tumor. **A,** low power. **B,** higher power.

become infected and give rise to a clinical situation simulating pelvic inflammatory disease. Intraperitoneal rupture may occur, producing the same clinical and pathologic picture as a ruptured dermoid cyst of the ovary. A few solid teratomas of the oviduct have been reported. In one, reported by Henriksen, the entire tumor consisted of adult thyroid tissue, a so-called struma salpingii. Hertig and Gore have suggested that these dermoid tumors of the oviduct arise from primordial germ cells that have been arrested in their migration from the mesentery of the gut to the ovary.

Malignant Neoplasms

PRIMARY CARCINOMA

The rarest carcinoma of the female genital tract is primary carcinoma of the oviduct. Since the report of the first patient in 1888, approximately 500 cases of this entity have been documented. In relation to the over-all incidence of genital cancer, the incidence of tubal carcinoma varies from 0.1 to 0.5 per cent. This is in marked contrast to carcinoma of the cervix which accounts for approximately 45 per cent and carcinoma of the corpus which accounts for approximately 30 per cent of the total. At the Boston Hospital for Women, Hu *et al.* found that tubal carcinoma constituted 0.31 per cent of all genital cancers. This was based on a report of 12 patients operated on between 1909 and 1948. An additional 26 patients with primary tubal carcinoma have been seen since 1948, a total of 38 cases in 52 years. At the state cancer hospital in Pondville, Mass., 18 cases have been seen (0.1 per cent incidence) and at the Massachusetts General Hospital 16 tubal carcinomas have been treated (incidence 0.4 per cent).

The age incidence has varied from 18 to 80 years, but most patients have been between 40 and 65, with an average of approximately 52 years. Infertility has been a common finding in patients with tubal carcinoma and, in a review by Wechsler, 32 per cent of the patients had never given birth to a full-term child. At the Boston Hospital for Women the incidence of sterility was 44 per cent.

Two factors have been suggested in the histogenesis of this tumor. Chronic salpingitis has long been held as a predisposing cause and tuberculosis has also been suggested as being a possible forerunner of the disease. At the Boston Hospital for Women during the past five years, three patients were found to have, as incidental findings, carcinoma in situ in the tubal mucosa. Neither tuberculosis nor chronic salpingitis was found in these patients. Crosson states that the "preceding chronic tubal infection is the most important single etiologic factor" in the development of this disease, whereas Ayre doubts the validity of this statement since salpingitis is so common and malignancy so rare. Hu *et al.* found that salpingitis was present in all but three of their 12 cases. Finn and Javert reported six cases and stated that the opposite tube was free from salpingitis in all five instances, one patient having bilateral carcinoma. In all probability the tumor itself produces a chronic inflammatory reaction which eventually seals off the fimbriated portion of the tube and actually may simulate a hydrosalpinx.

Diagnosis.—While there are no distinctive symptoms which might be called pathognomonic, the most consistent sign is a watery and frequently blood-tinged vaginal discharge. Intermittent or colicky, low abdominal pain associated with abnormal bleeding may also be present. The latter may be manifested as irregular bleeding or spotting during the postmenopausal era and as menstrual irregularities during the childbearing period. Occasionally the discharge may be profuse although the occurrence of *hydrops tubae profluens* as a characteristic symptom is quite rare. The latter may occur, with the release of a watery or blood-tinged fluid from a hydrosalpinx through the uterus and vagina, regardless of whether or not tubal carcinoma is associated.

The physical findings include abdominal enlargement, if ascites is present, and a palpable abdominal mass or more commonly a palpable, firm mass found during pelvic examination. The finding of a tubal carcinoma is so rare that it is only occasionally listed as the primary preoperative diagnosis. According to Martzloff, in only 6 per cent of the cases reported in the literature had the correct diagnosis been made preoperatively, and in the series at the Boston Hospital for Women only one patient had a preoperative diagnosis of tubal carcinoma. In postmenopausal patients the usual diagnosis is ovarian tumor, and in premenopausal patients the most common diagnoses are leiomyomas and pelvic inflammatory disease. However, if there is recurrent bleeding—or particularly a bloody, watery discharge—in a postmenopausal patient in whom biopsies of the cervix and endometrial curettage have given negative findings, the suspicion of tubal cancer should be strongly entertained. Vaginal smears may disclose neoplastic cells characteristic of tubal cancer, particularly when there is a loss of fluid from the uterus. Culdocentesis may also reveal suspicious or definite malignant elements. Occasionally hysterosalpingography has suggested a cancer of the tube and culdoscopy or culdotomy may verify the diagnosis. A dilatation and curettage may reveal tubal cancer metastatic to the endometrial cavity. In one of our patients the presenting complaint was that of an inguinal mass which on biopsy revealed an undifferentiated adenocarcinoma. Laparotomy subsequently revealed the primary carcinoma to be in the fallopian tube and the endometrial cavity was not involved.

Pathology.—The lesion is usually unilateral, only about 30 per cent of the patients having had bilateral tumors. If the fimbriated portion of the tube is closed, the gross appearance (Fig. 6–15) of the mass may simulate that of a hydro- or pyosalpinx. The serosal surface is frequently roughened and adherent to the large and small intestines. Lesions have been described as large as 17 cm. in diameter although the association of a pyo- or hydrosalpinx may make the gross appearance much larger. Cross-section of the tumor reveals granular tissue that is gray or yellow-tan in color, with a marked tendency to friability. The lesion is usually situated in the distal third of the tube, from where it may extend through the fimbriated portion. The tubal lumen is usually distended with fluid, and a papillary mass of friable or hemorrhagic tumor lines the mucosal surface.

The pathologic diagnosis of primary carcinoma of the oviduct is based on proof that the tumor arises from the endosalpinx. The criteria suggested by Hu for differentiating between primary and metastatic tumors are as follows: (1) Grossly, the main tumor is in the tube. (2) Microscopically the mucosa should be chiefly involved and should show a papillary pattern. (3) If the tubal wall is involved to a great extent, the transition between benign and malignant tubal epithelium should be demonstrated. The following microscopic classification of tubal carcinomas is used at the Boston Hospital for Women.

PAPILLARY (grade I): The pure papillary growth is confined to the tubal lumen and transition between normal and malignant epithelium is clearly seen. The cells are fairly well differentiated and columnar in shape, and there are scanty mitotic figures (Fig. 6–16, *A*).

PAPILLARY-ALVEOLAR (grade II): This group shows beginning glandular formation and invasion of the tubal muscularis. The cells are undifferentiated, with a moderate number of mitoses (Fig. 6–16, *B*).

ALVEOLAR MEDULLARY (grade III): The growth pattern is more solid, in contrast to the papillary type. The cells are arranged in medullary or glandular pattern and there is definite invasion of the tubal lymphatics. The cells are poorly differentiated, with vacuolation and abundant and atypical mitoses.

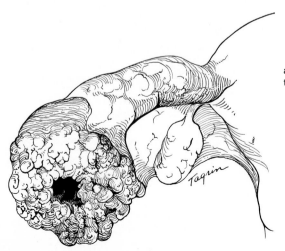

Fig. 6–15.—Typical gross appearance of carcinoma of the oviduct.

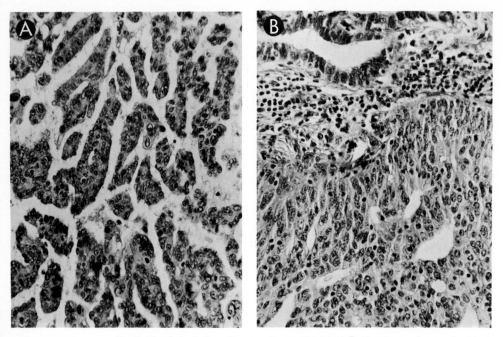

Fig. 6-16.—A, typical papillary carcinoma of oviduct. **B,** alveolar carcinoma of oviduct.

Fig. 6-17.—Carcinoma of the oviduct involving tubal mucosa.

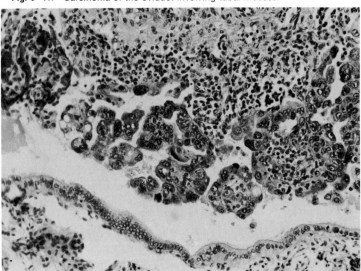

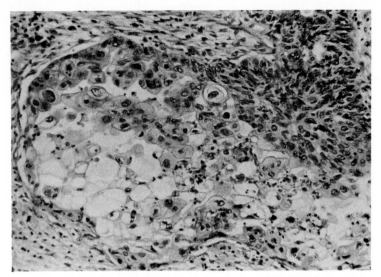

Fig. 6-18.—Carcinoma of the oviduct metastatic to peritubal lymphatic.

The usual method of spread of tubal carcinoma is via the lymphatics, but tumor growth may occur via the tubal lumen along the mucosal surface (Fig. 6-17). Generalized peritoneal implants are uncommon, due in all probability to closure of the fimbriated portion of the tube. The iliac, lumbar and preaortic nodes may be involved by lymphatic permeation (Fig. 6-18), and occasionally dissemination via the round ligament to the inguinal nodes may occur. Hematogenous spread accounts for metastases to the liver, lungs, stomach and supraclavicular lymph nodes. The ovary, uterine corpus and vagina may be involved by direct extension.

Treatment.—The optimum method of treatment is total hysterectomy with bilateral salpingo-oophorectomy followed by x-ray therapy. If there is extension to the endocervix or upper vagina a radical hysterectomy and pelvic lymphadenectomy is advisable. If a primary cancer of the tube is discovered early and removed promptly, the prognosis is good. Otherwise the prognosis is considered to be poor. The prognosis in general is considered to be poor although the five-year survival rate is directly related to the extent of disease. The prognosis is also worse in poorly differentiated lesions but it is in this particular group that metastases are found at the time of surgery. Prior to 1926 only three five-year survivals were reported in the first 200 cases in the literature. The five-year salvage rate has varied from 5 to 48 per cent, the latter figure being noted in the 38 cases from the Boston Hospital for Women in which a five-year follow-up was possible. The average five-year survival rate for primary fallopian tube cancer the world over is between 10 and 15 per cent. Alertness to the possibility of tubal cancer, prompt intervention and adequate treatment will improve this discouragingly low "cure rate." The precise value of postoperative x-ray therapy is difficult to determine since the number of cases in each series is too small and, in addition, x-ray has not been given to all patients who had a very localized lesion. In many instances x-ray therapy for palliation may be all that can be done for the patient with advanced disease.

Sarcoma

These tumors are extremely rare, less than 30 cases having been reported in the literature. The ratio of sarcoma to carcinoma of the oviduct is of the order of 1 to 25. The age incidence and clinical picture are similar to those in carcinoma of the tube. If the disease is extensive, the most common symptoms are pelvic pain, abdominal enlargement and malaise. Physical examination may reveal abdominal distention, a pelvic mass and emaciation. The tubal tumor varies in size from 2 to 20 cm. and the cross-section reveals a soft, papillary or pultaceous intraluminal mass. Microscopically the sarcoma is most commonly of the spindle-cell type but other variations such as round cell, myosarcoma, myxosarcoma, perithelioma and endothelioma have been described.

This most malignant tumor may spread via the blood stream, lymphatics or by direct extension to adjacent pelvic organs. The optimum method of treatment is total hysterectomy with bilateral salpingo-oophorectomy followed by x-ray therapy. The prognosis is poor and it is doubtful whether therapy of any type retards the eventual outcome in advanced cases.

Carcinoma Metastatic to the Oviduct

As might be expected, the two organs responsible for most metastatic lesions in the oviduct are the ovary and the endometrium. The method of spread may be either by direct extension or via the lymphatics. Carcinoma of the stomach and pancreas may also metastasize to the tube. The lesions may be unilateral or bilateral, and there is no characteristic gross appear-

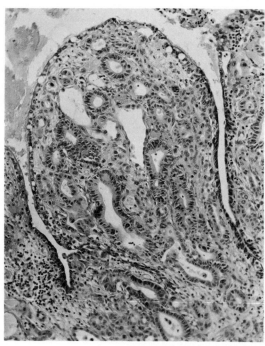

Fig. 6–19.—Carcinoma of the pancreas metastatic to the oviduct.

ance. Histologically the tumors are identical with the primary tumor (Fig. 6–19) and, in contrast to primary carcinoma of the tube, the serosa of the oviducts as well as the lymphatics of the muscularis and of the mesosalpinx are usually involved. The treatment is that of the primary disease, usually complete hysterectomy and bilateral salpingo-oophorectomy. Postoperative x-ray therapy is advisable but the prognosis for five-year survival is poor.

BIBLIOGRAPHY

Structure and Function

Borell, U.; Nilsson, O., and Westman, A.: Ciliary activity in the rabbit fallopian tube during estrus and after copulation, Acta obst. et gynec. scandinav. 36:22, 1957.
Chang, M. C.: Development and fate of transferred rabbit ova or blastocysts in relation to the ovulation time of recipients, J. Exper. Zool. 114:197, 1950.
Clewe, T. H., and Mastroianni, L.: Mechanisms of ovum pickup: I. Functional capacity of rabbit oviducts ligated near the fimbria, Fertil. & Steril. 9:13, 1958.
Decker, A.: Culdoscopic observations on the tubo-ovarian mechanism of ovum reception, Fertil. & Steril. 2:253, 1951.
Doyle, J. B.: Tubo-ovarian mechanism: Observation at laparotomy, Obst. & Gynec. 8:686, 1956.
Horstmann, E.: Uber die Bedeutung der Epoophoromuskulatur, Arch. Gynäk. 182:314, 1952.
Huffman, J. W.: in Curtis, A. H., and Huffman, J. W.: *Textbook of Gynecology* (Philadelphia: W. B. Saunders Company, 1950).
Kneer, M., and Cless, H.: Flimmerung und Stromung im menschlichen Eileiter, Geburtsh. u. Frauenh. 11:233, 1951.
von Ott, D.: Eine neue Methode zur Prüfung der Tubendurchgangigkeit, Zentralbl. Gynäk. 49: 546, 1925.
Seckinger, D. L., and Snyder, F. F.: Cyclic changes in the spontaneous contractions of the human fallopian tube, Bull. Johns Hopkins Hosp. 39:371, 1926.
Stange, H. H.: Zur funktionellen Morphologie des fimbrienendes der menschlichen Tube und des Epoophoron, Arch. Gynäk. 182:77, 1952.
Westman, A. A.: A contribution to the question of the transit of the ovum from ovary to uterus in rabbits, Acta obst. et gynec. scandinav. 5:7, 1926.

Inflammation

Hellman, L. M.: The morphology of the human fallopian tube in the early puerperium, Am. J. Obst. & Gynec. 57:154, 1949.
McGruder, C. J.: Surgical management of chronic pelvic inflammatory disease. Obst. & Gynec. 13:591, 1959.
Mead, P. B., and Louria, D. B.: Antibiotics in pelvic infections, Clin. Obst. & Gynec. 12:219, 1969.
Mickal, A., and Sellman, A. H.: Management of tubo-ovarian abscess, Clin. Obst. & Gynec. 12: 252, 1969.
Mishell, D. R., and Moyer, D. L.: Association of pelvic inflammatory disease with the intrauterine device, Clin. Obst. & Gynec. 12:179, 1969.
Mohler, R. W.: A study and classification of pelvic inflammatory disease, Am. J. Obst. & Gynec. 57:1077, 1949.
Nassberg, S.; McKay, D. G., and Hertig, A. T.: Physiological salpingitis, Am. J. Obst. & Gynec. 67:130, 1954.
Pedowitz, P., and Felmus, L.: Rupture of tubo-ovarian abscesses, Am. J. Surg. 83:507, 1952.
Schaefer, G.: Female genital tuberculosis: A review of the literature, Obst. & Gynec. Surv. 8:461, 1953.
Smith, G. V.: in Engle, E. T. (ed.): *Menstruation and Its Disorders* (Springfield, Ill.: Charles C Thomas, Publisher, 1950), p. 187.
Studdiford, W. E., and Douglas, G. W.: Placental bacteremia: Significant findings in septic abortion, accompanied by vascular collapse, Am. J. Obst. & Gynec. 71:842, 1956.
Sutherland, A. M.: The treatment of genital tuberculosis in women, Geneesk. gids 45:(20) 362; (21) 386, 1967.

Tubal Ectopic Pregnancy

Beacham, W. D.; Webster, H. D., and Beacham, D. W.: Ectopic pregnancy at New Orleans Charity Hospital, Am. J. Obst. & Gynec. 72:830, 1956.
Bender, S.: Fertility after tubal pregnancy, J. Obst. & Gynaec. Brit. Emp. 63:400, 1956.
Grant, A.: The effect of ectopic pregnancy on fertility, Clin. Obst. & Gynec. 5:861, 1962.
Halbrecht, I., and Blinick, G.: Full term pregnancy after antibiotic treatment of proved endometrial tuberculosis, Fertil. & Steril. 11:480, 1960.

Kistner, R. W.: Ectopic Pregnancy in Conn, H. F. (ed.): *Current Diagnosis* (Philadelphia, W. B. Saunders Co., 1966.) p. 668.
———; Hertig, A. T., and Rock, J.: Tubal pregnancy complicating tuberculous salpingitis, Am. J. Obst. & Gynec. 62:1157, 1951.
Malkasian, G. D.; Hunter, J. S., and ReMine, W. H.: Ectopic pregnancy: Analysis of 322 consecutive cases, J.A.M.A. 166:985, 1958.
Romney, S. L.; Hertig, A. T., and Reid, D. E.: The endometria associated with ectopic pregnancy, Surg., Gynec. & Obst. 91:605, 1950.
Vasica, A. I., and Grable, E. E.: Simultaneous extrauterine and intrauterine pregnancies progressing to viability, Obst. & Gynec. Surv. 11:603, 1956.
Word, B.: The diagnosis and treatment of ectopic pregnancy, Surg., Gynec. & Obst. 92:333, 1951.

Salpingitis Isthmica Nodosa

Bunster, E.: Trompa de falopio y estrilidad de causa tubaria (Buenos Aires: Kraft, 1951).
Schenken, J. R. and Burns, E. L.: Diverticula of tubes: Study and classification of nodular lesions; salpingitis isthmica nodosa, Am. J. Obst. & Gynec. 45:624, 1943.
Siegler, A. M.: Diverticulosis of the fallopian tubes, Fertil. & Steril. 6:432, 1958.

Neoplasms

Golden, A., and Ash, J. E.: Adenomatoid tumors of the genital tract, Am. J. Path. 21:63, 1945.
Green, T. H., and Scully, R. E.: Tumors of the fallopian tube, Clin. Obst. & Gynec. 5:886, 1962.
Grimes, H. G., and Kornmesser, J. G.: Benign cystic teratoma of the oviduct, Obst. & Gynec. 16:85, 1960.
Herbut, P.: *Gynecological and Obstetrical Pathology* (Philadelphia: Lea & Febiger, 1953).
Hertig, A. T., and Gore, H.: Tumors of the Female Sex Organs: Part 3. Tumors of the Ovary and Fallopian Tube, sec. IX, fasc. 33 of *Atlas of Tumor Pathology* (Washington, D. C.: Armed Forces Institute of Pathology, 1961).
Hu, C. Y.; Taymor, M. L., and Hertig, A. T.: Primary carcinoma of the fallopian tube, Am. J. Obst. & Gynec. 59:58, 1950.

CHAPTER 7

The Ovary

Revised by C. Thomas Griffiths, M.D.

Embryology

Both the male and female gonads arise from an undifferentiated structure and are morphologically identical up to a certain stage of development. Between the 5.3 and the 7 mm. embryonic stages, the surface layer of the gonadal anlage increases rapidly by mitoses and the cells invade the subjacent mesenchyme, forming solid masses of cordlike strands. The area of differentiation occurs on the mesial aspect of the urogenital ridge, anterior to the mesonephros, along the entire length of the ridge. At this stage of development, the "genital area" extends from the sixth thoracic to the second sacral segment. Later, however, the cranial portions degenerate, leaving the caudal three or four segments. Variations in growth processes or regressive changes may lead to abnormalities in size, shape and position of the gonads as well as to developmental abnormalities.

In the 11 mm. embryo the urogenital ridge develops a median and a lateral cleft which deepen and divide the ridge into a genital and a mesonephric portion. As these clefts deepen, the segments become further separated until they maintain contact along the lateral border only, the site of the future *mesovarium.*

In the 9 mm. embryo, radial strands or medullary cords can be distinguished extending from the surface into the mesenchymal tissue. These cords are composed of epithelial-like cells and their presence demarcates sharply the genital area from that of the mesonephros. At this stage the indifferent genital gland consists of a layer of superficial epithelial cells, the medullary cords and supporting mesenchyme. It was originally thought that all the cords extending toward the hilus were the result of active proliferation of the surface epithelium. These so-called Waldeyer or Pflueger cords actually consist of primordial egg cells and smaller, round, cellular masses, the prospective granulosa cells. The latter cells have been shown to originate in situ from the local mesenchymal tissue with the egg cells functioning as "organizers."

The primitive egg cells, originally thought to be derived from the surface or "germinal" epithelium of the gonad, originate in the dorsal part of the epithelial lining of the hindgut. These specialized cells are easily identified in the hindgut by their larger size and paler staining cytoplasm. They possess the propensity for ameboid motility and subsequently migrate to the posterior portion of the gonad (the prospective hilus) and invade the mesenchymal portion. The egg cells differ from somatic cells in size, shape, cytoplasmic structure and nuclear arrangement. They have almost 30 times as much cell body as nucleus; the nucleus is vesicular and has a distinctive chromatin arrangement with several nucleoli. The granular, pale-staining cytoplasm contains both yolk granules and mitochondria.

The first stage in ovariogenesis is thus represented by the formation of primary cell cords from the local mesenchyme following migration of the egg cells. Some time later additional aggregates of cells form from the surface epithelium which fuse with the locally produced primary sex cords. Gruenwald has called these "secondary sex cords." It is possible that the latter cells retain totipotential reactivity to estrogen and progesterone in the adult ovary, accounting for the coelomic metaplasia theory of the origin of endometriosis.

The next differentiating step in ovariogenesis is the partitioning of the germinal cords into islands, each containing two or more germinal cells. This segmentation is brought about by proliferation of nonspecific mesenchymal stroma and is completed when each oocyte is a potentially functional unit surrounded by a single cell layer of prospective granulosa cells. As the granulosa cells proliferate, the egg cell is displaced eccentrically. Cellular proliferation is followed by liquefaction, with formation of a cavity —truly now a follicular structure—eponymically called a graafian follicle.

Approximately 12–15 such follicles may be found in the fetal ovary during the thirty-sixth week of gestation. The mature follicle has a diameter of 8–9 mm., whereas larger follicles usually are degenerative, containing no oocyte.

Although the extragonadal origin of germ cells is now proved and accepted, it was not until 1931 that Dantschakoff demonstrated this fact unequivocally. She destroyed the region of the embryonal shield (containing the primitive germ cells) in the chick and found (1) that germ cells were not found subsequently in the gonad and (2) that the gonad did not develop normally. In addition, she found that if the gonadal anlage was transplanted before the arrival of germ cells, it failed to develop. However, if the gonadal anlage was transplanted *after* the appearance of primitive germ cells, a typical gonad developed in the new location. Dantschakoff thus proved beyond doubt that the gonad was definitely dependent on the primitive extraregional germ cells for its development. She called the germ cells "entodermal wandering cells."

The *hilus*, from which the connective tissue and vascular channels radiate, represents that portion of the gonadal anlage that is not separated by the development of the lateral clefts and is therefore in direct continuity with the mesonephric ridge. From this area a network of connective tissue arises which penetrates the gonad and is completely developed in the 180 mm. fetus. These fibers form a coarse mesh in the medullary region but are much finer in the cortex. Under the surface epithelium another layer of coarse connective tissue develops and extends parallel to the ovarian surface. Eventually this becomes the *tunica albuginea.*

During the third fetal month an epithelial protuberance develops and projects into the region of the mesovarium. This is known as the *rete ovarii.*

Eventually, connective tissue strands develop and radiate into the ovarian hilus. Such *rete cords* usually degenerate but occasionally are seen in the ovary of the newborn. In the 15 mm. embryo these rete cords extend into the stroma of the mesonephros and are in apposition with the glomeruli. Occasionally lumina develop in the rete cords. These have their blind end toward the ovary and their patent end toward the cranial glomeruli of the mesonephros. Rete tubules, composed of a single layer of cells, may persist in the newborn and give rise to hilus cysts, hilus cell tumors or other related neoplasms.

The ovary of the newborn, full-term infant shows evidence of continual development and degeneration of follicles. Thus all stages of maturation have been described, from primordial to ripe graafian follicles. Large follicular cysts have been reported as well as atretic follicles and corpora lutea.

Anatomy

The human ovary undergoes decided changes in size, shape and position during its lifetime in addition to the extensive histologic changes brought about by various endocrine stimuli. It is important to realize these extremes of normalcy in order to prevent undue trauma or extirpation performed for mistaken neoplasia. Ovarian asymmetry is common, the right ovary usually being larger than the left. Independent fragments of ovary may exist as a result of complete segmentation during embryonal development. Occasionally an isolated segment may be discovered retroperitoneally—a possible source of estrogen and progesterone after bilateral oophorectomy. Similarly, a portion of the left ovary buried deep in the mesentery of the sigmoid colon may be allowed to remain in situ at the time of extirpative surgery.

The ovary of the newborn is a delicate, elongated structure approximately 1.5 cm. long and 0.5 cm. wide and varies from 1.5 to 3.5 mm. in thickness. It weighs about 0.3–0.4 Gm. and is shaped like a three-sided prism with rounded edges. The ovarian surface is pinkish white, smooth and glistening. Occasionally, small cystic structures may be seen through the surface epithelium. The surface incisures vary greatly in number and depth and radiate toward the hilus. The ovaries in the fetus at term lie in the posterior segment of the false pelvis, directly adjacent to the posterior surface of the uterus.

The ovary gradually enlarges in size and changes shape and position between birth and pubescence. The ovary becomes almond shaped and enlarges to an average size of 3 × 1.8 cm. with a thickness of about 1.2 cm. It gradually moves into the true pelvis. The weight of both ovaries at puberty is between 4 and 7 Gm. The number of cystic structures seen on the surface also increases and the cut surface shows cysts from 2 to 3 mm. in diameter. Its color becomes more gray near puberty. In general, the gross description of the pubescent ovary is much like that of the Stein-Leventhal ovary of later life.

The onset of puberty brings about many changes in the histologic anatomy of the ovary which in turn alter the gross anatomic appearance. The organ now measures 2.5–5 cm. in length, 1.5–3.0 cm. in width and 0.6–1.5 cm. in thickness. It lies close to the lateral pelvic wall and is invested by peritoneum to the line of *Farre-Waldeyer*. This juncture, a linear zone near the hilus, encircles the ovary and represents the juncture of coelomic peritoneum and ovarian surface epithelium. The anterior margin of the ovary is thin, straight and attached to the posterior surface of the broad ligament by a fold of tissue, the *mesovarium*. The posterior, or free margin, is rounded, thick, convex and unattached.

The upper rounded pole of the ovary (tubal pole) is embraced by the fimbria of the oviduct and is attached to the suspensory ligament. The lower, more pointed pole is attached to the uterus by a fibromuscular cord, the utero-ovarian ligament. Blood vessels and nerves enter and leave the ovary by way of the hilus through the mesovarium. As the ovary is normally situated, it lies in a triangular fossa formed by the diverging folds of peritoneum covering the iliac vessels. It is bounded laterally by the iliac veins and ureter and anteriorly by the round ligament. The vertical position of the ovary is maintained by the infundibulopelvic ligament aided by the mesovarium and the utero-ovarian ligament.

Various functional activities impart to the ovarian surface an uneven, occasionally nodular surface. The persistence of fetal markings, scars of previous ovulation and atretic follicles produce anatomic variations. An ovary which has not been scarred by ovulation usually presents a smooth and glistening surface. Single or multiple reddish elevations represent recently ruptured follicles or very recent corpora lutea, whereas older corpora lutea are yellow. Normal corpora lutea are a few millimeters to several centimeters in diameter but occasionally a large, yellow corpus luteum occupies one-third of the ovarian structure. If the lutein structure exceeds 2.5 cm. it is termed a *corpus luteum cyst* since, in essence, all corpora lutea are cystic. A hemorrhagic corpus luteum is not always identified easily because the wall is thin and may have lost its yellow color.

The normal ovarian cortex is usually tense and elastic. When cut, fluid escapes from cystic follicles, exposing a pink, moist surface. Follicular cysts present smooth, thin-walled cavities and vary in size from 3 to 5 cm. Theca-lutein cysts present a crenated border with a yellow wall. Corpora albicantia are identified as white or slightly yellow, crenated, scarred structures which may be scattered throughout the stroma. They represent the final result of involution of corpora lutea and atretic follicles.

The arterial supply of the ovary is derived from an anastomosis of the ovarian and uterine vessels. The ovarian artery arises from the aorta and is enmeshed with its venous counterpart in the infundibulopelvic ligament. As it reaches the broad ligament it divides, giving off a branch to the oviduct. The main ovarian trunk runs in the folds of the broad ligament and mesovarium, then divides again to give off multiple branches that enter the hilus. At this point each artery is subdivided into two medullary branches which traverse the entire ovary. Each medullary artery runs in a straight-line fashion to the opposite pole of the ovary, giving off *cortical* branches during its course. The cortical vessels divide into arterioles, each of which supplies a group of follicles. A free anastomosis between cortical arterioles is present, and at the cortical margin the arterioles anastomose with the venules.

The venous drainage is similar to the arterial arrangement, the veins emerging at the hilus as two major vessels. These represent both the uterine and ovarian venous systems and in pregnancy or extreme venous congestion a pampiniform plexus is evident. At the time of cesarean section these venous channels are enormously distended and tear quite easily. Spontaneous rupture has been reported, and the author has seen enormous distention of these veins, each 2 cm. or more in diameter, in a patient whose right oviduct had been artificially implanted in the uterine cornu. In this procedure a portion of the mesovarium had been sutured into the implantation site, producing acute angulation and the varices described. Spontaneous rupture of such a venous plexus might easily result in massive hemorrhage and death.

The nerve supply arises from a sympathetic plexus intimately enmeshed with the ovarian vessels in the infundibulopelvic ligament. Its fibers are derived from branches of the renal and aortic plexuses as well as from the celiac and mesenteric ganglia. Nonmedullated nerve trunks accompany the arterial trunks. They then divide into terminal plexuses which surround the arterioles and extend to the follicles.

To secure a complete pelvic "denervation" for the relief of pain, the nerve supply to the ovary should be interrupted in addition to performing a presacral neurectomy. However, most gynecologists have not found this necessary for the relief of primary dysmenorrhea. In the conservative management of endometriosis its use has been suggested but an insufficient number of cases has been studied to permit adequate evaluation.

During pregnancy the ovaries are lifted out of the true pelvis by the enlarging uterus and during the early weeks of gestation the corpus luteum of pregnancy is large and protrudes above the ovarian surface. Many such ovaries have been removed by surgeons because of unilateral pelvic pain in early pregnancy, the extirpation being performed for a "cystic" ovary. Unfortunately, the many anatomic variations of the ovary representing physiologic processes have not received adequate study by most surgeons. At the time of cesarean section the ovaries are usually of normal size but covered with a pink, irregular frosting which is attached to, or is actually a part of, the surface epithelium. This tissue represents a pseudodecidual reaction in totipotential mesenchyme due to the prolonged and continuous stimulation of chorionic estrogen and progesterone. As previously mentioned, this mesenchyme may have been pulled into the ovary at the time the secondary cords developed.

During the puerperium the ovary diminishes in size and the pseudodecidual reaction disappears. The cystic follicles undergo atresia, and some time may elapse before gonadotropic function brings about follicular maturation and ovulation. During this stage the ovary seems to be in a resting state.

Postmenopausally the ovary undergoes rapid regressive changes. It becomes smaller and the surface becomes wrinkled, frequently resembling the gyri and sulci of the cerebrum. The color fades from gray to almost white. Perhaps the most striking change is in the size of the organ, since it may be only 2 × 1.5 cm. or less. In most postmenopausal patients the ovary is so small it cannot be palpated on pelvic examination. A disproportion in the amount of ovarian cortex to medulla is seen in a specific condition known as cortical stromal hyperplasia. This may be due to pituitary stimulation of the senescent ovary which has lost its potential to respond by ovulation. Grossly the ovary may be of normal size for the particular age of the patient, but on cross-section the cortex is greatly thickened and arranged in a whorl-like pattern. This process may often be diagnosed by viewing the hematoxylin-eosin stained slide grossly; the cortical hyperplasia is evident as dark-stained, curled masses, whereas the medulla is relatively sparse and pale staining.

Histology

A brief summation of the microscopic anatomy is outlined here, but specific details are described in the articles listed in the Bibliography.

In the newborn, *the surface epithelium* of the ovary is made up of a single layer of low cuboidal or cylindrical cells, each having a large nucleus. It is continuous over the entire surface but is demarcated from the peritoneal attachment at the Farre-Waldeyer line. Below the surface epithelium is a network of *transverse fibers*, arranged in fibrillar pattern, which later becomes part of the tunica albuginea. The *parenchymatous zone* is immediately subjacent to the fibrillar layer and its peripheral portion is composed almost entirely of primordial follicles. In the fetus at term a few "egg balls" and "egg cords" may still be present in the peripheral portion of the parenchymatous zone. The primordial follicle measures about 50–60 μ in diameter and is composed of an ovum surrounded by a single layer of follicular cells. A portion of the parenchyma around the follicle is differentiated into spindle-shaped cells and fibrils. The ovum measures about 18–24μ in diameter with a well-defined nucleus of 12μ. The chromatin network of the ovum is well defined, as is the nucleolus. Both are easily identified in a finely granular cytoplasm.

In proximity to the medulla is a zone of growing follicles and in the newborn and infant well-developed graafian and atretic follicles are seen. During infancy, growth of follicles and stroma is rapid; this rate of differentiation then tapers off until the time of pubescence when rapid development again occurs. The number of primordial follicles diminishes from birth and there is no evidence that formation of new follicles subsequently occurs. The number of ova in the newborn ovary has been estimated at 50,000 to 400,000. In the average female not more than 300–400 will proceed through ovulation and be released, with the potential of fertilization.

During pubescence the follicles of the hilus develop first. Initially there is an increase in size of the follicular cells as they become cuboidal with an increase in cytoplasm. There is also an actual increase in number of cells, so that three or four layers surround the ovum. Eventually the follicular cells become multilayered and a fluid—the *liquor folliculi*—accumulates eccentrically. The precise origin of this fluid is unknown in the human subject, but it is presumed to be a combination of cell secretion, cell degeneration and vascular transudate.

In follicles under 0.3 mm. the ovum is centrally placed, but in follicles 0.4 mm. or larger a vesicular form appears and the ovum is placed eccentrically. The follicle cells, now known as granulosa cells, are arranged about the ovum in a covering 8 to 12 rows in thickness. The mound of granulosa cells containing the ovum which projects into the cavity of the follicle is known as the *cumulus oophorus* or *discus proligerus*. As the growth of granulosa cells continues, the cumulus moves to a more peripheral position and the cells around the ovum increase in number. The layer of granulosa cells immediately adjacent to the ovum is known as the *corona radiata*.

These cells characteristically have dark-staining nuclei and granular cytoplasm. There is a gradual increase in cytoplasm of the ovum, so that a 2 mm. follicle will contain an ovum of 90–100μ. During this stage of development the *zona pellucida,* a hyaline band around the ovum, begins to appear.

Whereas the early primordial follicle is devoid of a connective tissue covering, the fully developed follicle has two. The inner layer, the *theca interna,* is made up of fine, fibrillar, connective tissue cells with abundant blood vessels (see Fig. 7–4). Between its fibrils, fat-laden or spiral cells appear. There is evidence that these cells contain steroid substances which probably are precursors in the production of estrogen and progesterone. The origin of the theca interna cells is still unsolved. Although they possess many of the characteristics of epithelial cells, most anatomists maintain that they are converted mesenchymal cells. The *theca externa* contains many coarse fibers which intertwine around the follicle and form a thick capsule. In its interstices are many lymphatics and blood vessels.

The medulla of the ovary contains numerous blood vessels with cellular tissue containing elastic fibers as a supporting structure. Follicles are usually absent. The remnant of the *rete ovarii* is found in the medulla and is identified as a group of irregular tubules lined with cuboidal, cylindrical or ciliated epithelium. A complex group of muscle fibers surrounds the vessels and extends for a distance into the mesovarium. Other fetal remnants have been described in the medulla and may be the source of specific ovarian tumors. They are: epoophoron canals, mesonephric rests, müllerian duct remnants, paraganglionic cells and adrenal rests.

The mature ovary does not differ appreciably from the description of the ovary at pubescence except for the changes associated with ovulation. The surface epithelium retains only a single layer of cuboidal cells but there are furrows and folds due to cicatrization in areas of previous ovulation. Occasionally the surface epithelium dips into the cortical area and may become pinched off, providing an etiologic mechanism for cyst formation. The tunica albuginea lies subjacent to the surface epithelium and is composed of interlacing, coarse fibers with minimum cellularity. Scattered throughout the parenchymatous zone are maturing follicles of all ages, together with atretic follicles and recent and old corpora lutea. Several ripe follicles may be seen at the surface just prior to rupture. They actually protrude a bit beyond the surface and may measure up to 20 mm. in diameter.

Ovulation and Corpus Luteum Formation

The precise physical and chemical factors initiating ovulation in the human are unknown, but recent investigation in the rat indicates that ovulation is not due to, or associated with, increased intrafollicular pressure. Similarly, the theory that ovulation is prevented by a thickened tunica albuginea (as found in the Stein-Leventhal syndrome) has been questioned by Greenblatt, who performed a unilateral oophorectomy in such a patient and noted subsequent ovulation from the remaining ovary.

Follicular rupture is associated with an escape of the liquor and a collapse of the walls with extrusion of the ovum and discus proligerus into the fimbria of the oviduct or into the peritoneal cavity. Following rupture, there is hemorrhage into the theca interna and the stigma is sealed by a blood clot from the thecal vessels as well as by a central coagulum in the cavity. Examination at this stage reveals active mitoses in both the granulosa and theca cell layers, and the structure is rapidly converted into the *corpus luteum.* It is possible, however, for ovulation to occur without release of the ovum. Ovarian pregnancies and certain cases of idiopathic infertility may be explained on this basis.

Four stages in the life cycle of the corpus luteum are recognized: proliferation, vascularization, complete development and regression. During the *proliferative* stage, both granulosa cells and theca cells show active mitotic activity, and growth is rapid. The theca cells enlarge even more than the granulosa cells and deposits of lipid are seen in the cytoplasm. Fibrils of theca interna cells then penetrate the granulosa layer and a capillary endothelium accompanies these cells. This stage lasts about four days and results in the formation of an epithelial gland with secretory activity.

The stage of *vascularization* is characterized grossly by the appearance of a raspberry-like protuberance on the ovarian surface. The dark red peripheral area surrounds a jelly-like core which is gray or pink, and the entire structure is friable and vascular. The endothelial capillaries now extend through the entire granulosa layer to the central coagulum. Eventually fibrin is deposited in the core and connective tissue cells begin to invade the coagulum. The stigma is healed by a similar process.

The stage of *full development* is evidenced by a moderate increase in size of the total structure, firmness of the central core and a scalloped border which assumes a brown or yellow color. Liquefaction of the central coagulum may give rise to cyst formation. At this stage the granulosa cells have a characteristic pale, clear cytoplasm and the theca cells are diminished in number and are arranged in groups between the granulosa cell columns and around the periphery of the granulosa layer (see Fig. 7-7).

The stage of *regression,* beginning about day 26 of a normal cycle, proceeds rapidly. The core becomes fibrotic, the granulosa layer diminishes in size and the cells become granular and vacuolated and lose their columnar arrangement. The theca cells are loosely arranged in groups, with dark nuclei and pale cytoplasm. There are progressive fibrosis and hyalinization of the core, atrophy of the lutein layers and crenation of the hyalinized connective tissue. The resultant scar, known as a corpus albicans, requires about 70 days to develop.

FOLLICULAR ATRESIA

Since all primordial follicles do not reach maturity, it is evident that the vast majority undergo a degenerative process known as atresia. This process has been noted in the ovaries of newborn infants and young children. The zona pellucida first becomes hyalinized and crenated; the germinal vesicle then demonstrates lysis of its chromatin and the ovum is invaded by round cells. After degeneration of the ovum the follicular epithelium begins to show specific necrobiotic changes. In a well-developed follicle there are resorption of the liquor folliculi and folding of the peripheral layers. Both the granulosa and the theca layers are replaced by fibrous connective tissue which is later hyalinized. The scar may persist for long periods and is known as a corpus fibrosum or corpus atreticum. Large follicles may not undergo complete regression and, if the liquor is not completely absorbed, a cystic process may develop. This is well demonstrated in the sclerocystic ovary syndrome in which cyclic ovulation does not occur.

THE POSTMENOPAUSAL OVARY

After cessation of menstrual cycles the ovary becomes quiescent and shrinks greatly in size. The remaining follicles undergo atresia, and it is unusual to find residual follicles after four or five years of menstrual inactivity in this age group. Occasionally, however, an episode of bleeding may occur in a postmenopausal patient and, if hysterectomy with bilateral salpingo-oophorectomy is performed for this reason alone, the operator may be surprised to find a recent corpus luteum in the ovary and secretory endometrium in the uterus.

The surface epithelium persists in the senile ovary as a single layer of flattened cells, and the tunica albuginea is composed of dense connective tissue cells and a few inactive spindle cells. Below the tunica are numerous corpora fibrosa and corpora albicantia, together with areas of hyalinization and calcium. The stromal cells are relatively inactive although groups of theca cells may persist near the hilus. The blood vessels show degenerative processes of the intima and media with focal calcareous deposition. Finally the ovary shrinks and becomes a firm structure less than one-third the size of the mature organ.

VESTIGIAL REMNANTS

The tubular system of the primitive mesonephros persists in the adult ovary as a series of convoluted tubules (Kobelt) which run radially from the hilus to the mesovarium. This structure is known as the *epoophoron* and may occasionally give rise to cystic or papillary growths known as Kobelt cysts. The caudal glomeruli of the mesonephros may persist as tubules between branches of the ovarian artery in the broad ligament. This is known as the *paraoophoron*, and the tubules may have a direct connection with the rete ovarii. The mesonephric excretory canal is represented by Gartner's duct which extends from the caudal pole of the ovary to the lateral vaginal wall. Cystic dilatation of this duct may occur, the structure presenting as an intravaginal cyst usually in the upper third of the vagina (see Fig. 3–10).

Ovarian Neoplasms

The ovary of the human female is an organ of extreme interest to the surgeon and gynecologist as well as to the pathologist, endocrinologist and general practitioner. It has been the subject of much speculation and the object of extensive biochemical investigation. As the target organ for pituitary hormones it may present marked variations in appearance that closely simulate malignant processes. It is imperative that the student and surgeon recognize the normal variations of growth of this organ, since therapy in many instances is expectant and overenthusiastic surgery may result in sterility or pelvic disability. Although precise criteria for the diagnosis of specific lesions cannot be outlined, an attempt will be made to provide means for adequate differential diagnosis of the common physiologic, benign neoplastic and malignant lesions.

Classification.—Numerous classifications of ovarian tumors have been advocated, each having certain advantages and disadvantages. An ideal classification would be one which related to the biologic behavior of the tumor as well as to its histologic appearance. Certainly those based on physical characteristics such as solid or cystic, or on gross appearance such as papillary or non-papillary, serve little practical purpose. Although falling short of ideal, classifications based on presumed histologic origin allow broad grouping into similar clinical and histologic types from which more specific subgroups may be derived. A histogenetic classification proposed by Hertig and Gore has been in use at the Boston Hospital for Women since 1945 and has been adopted by many other institutions.

CLASSIFICATION OF OVARIAN TUMORS

1. Gonadal stromal tumors
    a) Granulosa-theca cell tumor
    b) Arrhenoblastoma
    c) Gynandroblastoma
2. Germ cell tumors
    a) Dysgerminoma
    b) Choriocarcinoma
    c) Benign cystic teratoma
    d) Malignant teratoma
    e) Teratocarcinoma
3. Cystomas (germinal epithelial origin)
    a) Serous cystadenoma and cystadenocarcinoma
    b) Mucinous cystadenoma and cystadenocarcinoma
    c) Endometrial cystoma, benign and malignant
    d) Cystadenofibroma, benign and malignant
4. Congenital rest tumors
    a) Adrenal rest tumor
    b) Mesometanephric rest tumor
    c) Brenner tumor
    d) Hilus cell tumor
5. Nonintrinsic connective tissue tumors
6. Metastatic tumors

The prognostic usefulness of this type of classification is limited because of considerable variation in malignant behavior within many cell types. In addition, undifferentiated ovarian carcinomas which defy classification are common. Since these drawbacks apply primarily to germinal epithelial derivatives, a more precise classification of Hertig and Gore's cystoma group has been adopted by both the International Federation of Gynaecology and Obstetrics and the American College of Obstetricians and Gynecologists. This histologic classification allows for undifferentiated adenocarcinomas as well as for those tumors of indeterminate or borderline malignant potential.

Patients with borderline tumors have consistently demonstrated 5- and 10-year survival rates well in excess of patients with definite histologic malignancies, irrespective of the stage of disease or treatment employed. Histologically, a possibly malignant tumor is characterized by a proliferation and piling up of the epithelium lining the glandular and cystic spaces. Although varying degrees of nuclear pleomorphism and mitotic activity are present, the cells retain the morphology of differentiated columnar cells. Most important, there is no demonstrable evidence of infiltrative, destructive growth into the stroma of the tumor. Even with apparent malignant behavior, such as implantation on serosal surfaces, tumors in the intermediate group must be designated only as proliferative cystadenomas without stromal invasion (possibly malignant).

In defining the cell types listed in their proposed classification, the Cancer Committee of the International Federation used as type specimens tumors illustrated in Hertig and Gore's *Tumors of the Female Sex Organs: Part 3. Tumors of the Ovary and Fallopian Tube.* A mixture of different cell types may occur in the same tumor, but usually only one type predominates and this should determine the diagnosis. The histologic classification of the International Federation is as follows:

1. Serous cystomas
   a) Serous cystadenoma, benign
   b) Proliferating serous cystadenoma without stromal invasion (possibly malignant)
   c) Serous cystadenocarcinoma, all grades
2. Mucinous cystomas
   a) Mucinous cystadenoma, benign
   b) Proliferating mucinous cystadenoma without stromal invasion (possibly malignant)
   c) Mucinous cystadenocarcinoma, all grades
3. Endometrioid tumors
   a) Endometriosis
   b) Proliferating endometrioid adenoma and cystadenoma without stromal invasion (possibly malignant)
   c) Endometrioid adenocarcinoma, all grades
4. Undifferentiated carcinoma (cell type unknown)

Incidence.—The exact incidence of ovarian tumors is impossible to determine since it is obvious that all patients with these disorders do not undergo diagnostic or therapeutic surgery. Allan and Hertig reviewed the tumors of the ovary at the Boston Hospital for Women in 1949 and reported that 85 per cent of all ovarian enlargements over 5 cm. in diameter were benign. Enlargements of the ovary occurring in teen-aged girls or patients in their early twenties may in general be expected to be benign lesions and frequently are physiologic cysts of the follicle or corpus luteum. Stanley Way has reported that 90 per cent of ovarian tumors discovered in women between 20 and 30 are benign. However, between ages 50 and 70 the distribution of malignant and benign ovarian tumors is approximately equal. After age 70, benign ovarian tumors again become more common and comprise about 66 per cent of the total.

Dockerty has stated that 15 per cent of all ovarian neoplasms at the Mayo Clinic are of the benign serous type, and benign mucinous types comprise 20 per cent. At the Boston Hospital for Women, Allan and Hertig in studying 1,740 proliferative ovarian tumors, reported that the benign serous variety made up 20 per cent of the total and the ratio of serous to mucinous was approximately 1:1. Table 7–1 shows that the large majority of benign tumors are either (1) a cystadenoma of serous or mucinous variety, (2) a dermoid cyst (cystic teratoma) or (3) a fibroma. This is further

TABLE 7-1.—INCIDENCE OF OVARIAN TUMORS AT THE
BOSTON HOSPITAL FOR WOMEN, 1904-1952

	BENIGN		MALIGNANT		BENIGN AND MALIGNANT	
	No.	% OF TYPE	No.	% OF TYPE	No.	% OF ALL CASES
Serous	406	65.5	214	34.5	620	24.5
Pseudomucinous	420	88.0	57	12.0	478	18.9
Unclassified cystadenoma	42	–	–	–	42	1.7
Dermoid cyst	438	98.8	5	1.2	443	17.5
Granulosa cell	29	66.0	15	34.0	44	1.7
Fibroma	739	99.9	1	0.1	740	29.2
Brenner tumor	31	100	–	–	31	1.2
Thecoma	56	100	–	–	56	2.2
Arrhenoblastoma	1	–	1	–	2	0.1
Miscellaneous* benign	19	100	–	–	19	0.8
Undifferentiated carcinoma	–	–	30	–	30	1.5
Mesometanephroma	–	–	9	–	9	0.4
Endometrio- carcinoma	–	–	13	–	13	0.5
Dysgerminoma	–	–	2	–	2	0.1
Carcinosarcoma	–	–	2	–	2	0.1
Total	2181		349	(13.8)	2531	100

*Includes leiomyoma, adenoma, adenomatoid tumor, adenomyoma
and paraganglioma.

simplified by the fact that the vast majority of fibromas were accidental laboratory findings of small subclinical tumors of microscopic size.

The usual incidence of malignancy in ovarian tumors is approximately 15 per cent. At the Boston Hospital for Women 13.8 per cent were malignant, which compares favorably with the 14.9 per cent reported by Robert Meyer in 1930. Malignant serous tumors are more common than malignant mucinous types. Table 7-1 indicates a 3:1 ratio for serous to mucinous types, which compares with the ratio of 2½:1 reported by Barzilai. Furthermore, a serous ovarian tumor is more likely to be malignant than a mucinous one. Of our serous tumors, one-third were found to be malignant whereas only one of eight mucinous tumors was so classified. This latter ratio, however, is much greater than the 1 in 20 figure reported by Novak.

The incidence of granulosa cell tumors was found to be about 2 per cent, and approximately 30 per cent of these were malignant. Dockerty noted that the diagnosis of malignancy in granulosa cell tumors varied in different reports from 4.5 to 33 per cent. Although only a small number of cases show frankly malignant histology, microscopically benign appearing tumors often prove to be malignant subsequently. Only 5 of 443 dermoid cysts (Table 7-1) proved to be malignant, an incidence of 1.2 per cent. This closely approximates the 1.7 per cent reported by Robert Meyer in a study of 1,268 dermoid cysts.

The report by Allan and Hertig summarized the pathology of the ovarian material at the Boston Hospital for Women from 1904 through 1943. Kent and McKay reviewed the material from 1943 through 1952, adding 790 cases for a total of 2,531 (Table 7-1). One hundred and eleven of these additional patients had primary ovarian cancer. Grouping the two series together, Kent and McKay found that the largest percentage of all tumors (29.2 per cent) consisted of the fibroma, only 1 of 740 such tumors being malignant. Serous tumors comprised 24.5 per cent of the total with 34.5 per cent of these being malignant. Nineteen per cent of the entire series were of mucinous type, but only 12 per cent of these were malignant. The other major grouping was that of dermoid cysts which comprised 17.5 per cent of the total. Five of these were malignant, an incidence of 1.2 per cent.

About 4 per cent of ovarian neoplasms are discovered in children under 10, and approximately 50 per cent of these are malignant. These are usually solid teratomas or carcinomas but occasionally a dysgerminoma or granulosa cell carcinoma may be found. The benign varieties are usually dermoid or epithelial cysts.

SYMPTOMATOLOGY AND DIAGNOSIS

Symptoms.—Unfortunately, ovarian neoplasms are frequently asymptomatic, subjective complaints occurring only after complications arise or, in the case of carcinoma, after dissemination is widespread. Specific symptoms will depend on the size, location and type of the tumor as well as on the presence of complicating factors such as torsion, hemorrhage, infection or rupture.

The most common subjective symptoms are low abdominal pain or discomfort together with distention or the presence of an abdominal mass (Table 7–2). The pain is usually not of severe intensity and is frequently described as a mild discomfort localized in the hypogastrium or lower quadrants of the abdomen. Patients with extensive carcinoma of the ovary frequently visit the clinic or their physician only because of a gradually enlarging abdomen and perhaps slight indigestion. This combination of moderate anorexia or indigestion and abdominal enlargement should make the physician suspicious of ovarian cancer even if ascites or an ovarian mass are not readily discovered. Severe pain may occur but is usually secondary to acute accidents, such as rupture of an endometrioma or corpus luteum cyst, or to torsion of an ovarian tumor on an elongated pedicle.

The menstrual periods were abnormal in 34 per cent of the patients in the Boston Hospital for Women series who had operations for ovarian lesions. However, in many of these patients other lesions such as endometrial hyperplasia, polyps or leiomyomas were responsible for the abnormal bleeding. In other patients, no adequate reason could be given for the abnormal bleeding, although the possibility of increased estrogen production by the abnormal ovary has been suggested by Smith and Hughesdon. Dysmenorrhea may be a common complaint if the ovarian tumor is endometriotic in origin. Abnormal bleeding or secondary amenorrhea may occur in association with biologically active ovarian tumors of the granulosa-theca cell variety or with an arrhenoblastoma.

TABLE 7–2.—SYMPTOMS IN OVARIAN NEOPLASMS

SYMPTOM	NO. OF CASES	% OF CASES
Pain or discomfort	198	56.7
Distention or mass	177	50.7
Abnormal uterine bleeding	120	34.4
Urinary	59	16.9
Gastrointestinal	57	16.3

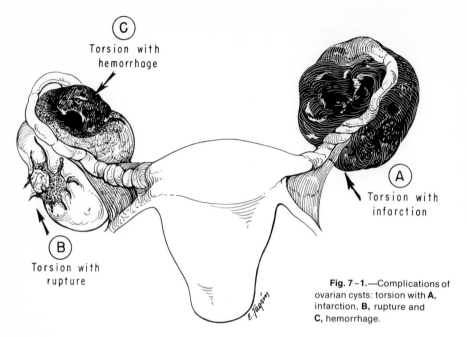

Fig. 7-1.—Complications of ovarian cysts: torsion with **A,** infarction, **B,** rupture and **C,** hemorrhage.

If the ovarian neoplasm has extended to adjacent structures, specific symptoms of pressure or pain may be related to involvement of the bladder, rectosigmoid or ureter. Rapidly growing ovarian tumors seem to produce symptoms earlier than those having a more leisurely growth pattern. In the series of patients reported by Kent and McKay the five-year survival rate was 42 per cent in patients who had symptoms for more than six months, whereas it was only 34 per cent in patients who had symptoms less than three months.

Specific complications of ovarian neoplasms have already been mentioned and, of these, a twisted ovarian pedicle is the most common. Dermoid cysts are particularly likely to undergo twisting because they reach a moderate size and are freely mobile and quite heavy. In addition, the pedicle is frequently long and slender and dermoids notoriously lie anterior to the broad ligament (Küstner's sign) where more mobility is afforded. A twisted ovarian cyst usually causes severe, localized pain, and the patient may note anorexia, nausea and vomiting. Physical examination reveals abdominal rigidity with rebound tenderness and pelvic examination may or may not reveal a cystic mass, depending on its size. Leukocytosis of moderate degree is usually present and the patient may be febrile although chills do not usually occur. If the torsion is incomplete, there is a partial occlusion of the blood supply with resultant venous stasis. Serum and blood eventually extravasate into the cyst cavity and the tumor becomes enlarged, edematous and cyanotic. If torsion is sufficient to produce obstruction of the arterial blood supply, gangrene of the tumor occurs. If infarction and necrosis are then extensive (Fig. 7-1), the entire mass may be ruptured during pelvic examination or at the time of laparotomy. It has been suggested that ovarian cysts with a twisted pedicle should not be unwound prior to removal because of the possibility of embolization.

Hemorrhage into an ovarian cyst is a rather common complication and it may occur spontaneously or as the result of torsion of the pedicle or physical trauma. The bleeding may be profuse, filling and enlarging a cystic cavity, as occurs with a hemorrhagic corpus luteum. Intermittent hemorrhage with slow growth and thickening of the capsule is common in endometriomas. Extensive hemorrhage may also be noted in soft, pultaceous tumors such as granulosa cell carcinoma. Thin-walled cysts of the corpus luteum or follicular variety may rupture into the peritoneal cavity, causing profound symptoms and shock. Ovarian cysts with thicker walls do not usually rupture, but occasionally rupture is seen in a large endometrioma following a fall or other trauma. Dermoid cysts may rupture into the peritoneal cavity, particularly after torsion with subsequent necrosis of the wall. A severe chemical peritonitis results due to the release of various lipids and hair into the peritoneal cavity.

Physical Signs.—The diagnosis of an ovarian neoplasm is usually made by bimanual pelvic examination. In order to outline these masses it is necessary that the bladder and lower bowel be empty and that good abdominal relaxation be obtained. Rectovaginal examination will add important information, especially if the mass is in the posterior cul-de-sac or happens to be adherent to the rectosigmoid.

Thin-walled physiologic cysts of the corpus luteum or follicular variety may be difficult to palpate especially if the patient is obese or if complete relaxation is not obtained. Such cysts may range in size from 3 to 6 cm. in greatest diameter and, because of their mobility, adequate delineation is not always possible. In our patients with ovarian carcinoma a pelvic mass was noted in 86 per cent and an abdominal mass in 76 per cent. Ascites was discovered in 30 per cent of patients with cancer, and 28 per cent of these had had excessive weight loss.

Diagnosis.—The precise preoperative diagnosis of ovarian neoplasm is not simple. Huge cysts that fill the abdomen are quite obvious and usually are mucinous or serous cystadenomas. However, even these have been confused with mesenteric cysts or cysts of the kidney or retroperitoneal space. Neoplastic ovarian tumors are usually more than 6 cm. in greatest diameter, although carcinoma of the ovary or even a granulosa cell carcinoma may be found in an ovary of normal size. Corpus luteum cysts or follicular cysts rarely exceed 6 cm. in greatest diameter but this is not an infallible rule. Simple cystomas and many mucinous cystadenomas have a perfectly smooth surface by both abdominal and pelvic examination. If irregular nodularities are felt on the surface a cystadenoma or carcinoma is suggested. Although most tumors are generally ovoid or spherical, extension or infiltration into adjacent structures may greatly modify the physical findings. Adhesions of the omentum or matted loops of small bowel will frequently mask the exact size and consistency of the ovarian mass. Although most physiologic or benign ovarian neoplasms are rather soft and flaccid they may on occasion become tensely fluctuant. Malignant tumors are more likely to have a solid or nubbly consistency, and firm nodularity in the posterior cul-de-sac in association with an ovarian mass strongly suggests endometriosis or metastatic carcinoma.

Except for dermoid cysts, most ovarian neoplasms are positioned lateral or posterior to the uterus, one notable exception is the dermoid cyst. A tumor which is situated in the posterior pelvis may displace the entire uterine corpus and cervix so that the cervical os may actually lie behind the symphysis pubis.

Unless they reach gigantic proportions, most ovarian tumors are quite mobile. If there is fixation the examiner should suspect malignancy, endometriosis, intraligamentary growth, simultaneous inflammatory processes or degeneration and adhesions.

Bilateral involvement suggests malignancy, cystadenomas or dermoid cysts. Thirty-two per cent of the ovarian carcinomas in the Boston Hospital for Women series were bilateral, a figure considerably lower than the 70 per cent reported by Montgomery. Mucinous carcinomas are least likely to be bilateral (only 15 per cent in our series), whereas the undifferentiated type of carcinoma is most likely to be bilateral (50 per cent in the series). Serous cystadenocarcinomas occupied an intermediate place (37 per cent).

Ascites may be of diagnostic importance when found preoperatively or at operation. In the Boston Hospital series it was found in 30 per cent of all patients and in 36 per cent of patients having a solid tumor. Ascites is found, however, in association with benign ovarian lesions, particularly papillary cystadenoma and fibroma. A pleural effusion suggests Meigs' syndrome, that is, a benign ovarian tumor with ascites and hydrothorax. A pleural effusion may similarly occur with metastatic ovarian carcinoma and therefore all pleural fluid should be submitted to cytologic examination and a cell block prepared for pathologic review. In addition, the fluid should be examined for tubercle bacilli by stain, culture and guinea-pig inoculation. Aspiration of fluid from the cul-de-sac by culdocentesis may be of value in the early diagnosis of ovarian carcinoma if experienced cytologists are available.

Additional procedures that may aid in the diagnosis of ovarian neoplasms are roentgenography, pneumoroentgenography and culdoscopy or posterior colpotomy. A flat plate of the abdomen should always be obtained before surgery since it may reveal foci of calcification or teeth, which are often seen in dermoid cysts. Also, the outline of the tumor may be determined and ascites or distended loops of intestine identified. A barium enema should be performed, especially if the patient has had intestinal complaints. This will frequently show evidence of extrinsic pressure on the colon or small intestine without constriction or deformity of the mucosa. If there is extensive involvement of the colon by ovarian cancer, definite filling defects with scalloped edges and mucous membrane destruction may be identified. It is important to know whether the carcinoma is primary in the sigmoid colon or in the ovary since subsequent treatment or chemotherapy will depend on the primary site.

Pneumoroentgenography may occasionally be of assistance in outlining the ovaries and determining symmetrical and unilateral enlargement. Irving Stein first suggested and popularized this method in 1931. Although his observations were made mostly in the diagnosis of the Stein-Leventhal syndrome, other ovarian lesions may be similarly demonstrated. Complete gynecography, as described by Stein, includes a pneumoperitoneum, using carbon dioxide injected intraperitoneally under manometric pressure, and hysterosalpingography with an opaque medium.

Culdoscopy is an important diagnostic procedure in the differential diagnosis of ovarian and tubal lesions. At the Boston Hospital for Women this procedure is performed in the operating room using hypobaric spinal anesthesia. Entrance through the posterior cul-de-sac is accomplished without difficulty unless cul-de-sac endometriosis or extensive pelvic inflammatory disease is present. This method affords an ideal means of differentiating between such lesions as an unruptured tubal ectopic pregnancy and a corpus luteum hematoma. However, we have also been able to diagnose endometriomas, fibromas, follicle cysts and ovaries of the Stein-Leventhal or agenesis type.

Posterior colpotomy is a valuable adjunctive measure in the diagnosis of ovarian lesions and has the added advantage of permitting therapeutic procedures to be performed as well. In many benign tumors and physiologic cysts, diagnosis may be made and immediate extirpation accomplished through a vaginal incision. If the gynecologist is accomplished in this particular phase of surgery, posterior colpotomy offers many definite advantages over laparotomy. Peritoneoscopy has recently been utilized in the diagnosis of "idiopathic" infertility problems and may be useful in the patient with a questionable ovarian lesion.

DIFFERENTIAL DIAGNOSIS

Before we proceed to the various lesions which may be confused with ovarian neoplasms, it should be emphasized that the most common midline "tumors" which on occasion may simulate an ovarian cyst are a distended urinary bladder and an enlargement of the uterus due to an intrauterine pregnancy or hydramnios. The urinary bladder that is tensely distended simulates a large cyst since it displaces the uterus backward, giving the impression of a mass anterior to the broad ligament. It is imperative, therefore, that all patients void or be catheterized before pelvic examination.

During the first 8 to 12 weeks of pregnancy the uterine corpus is smooth, soft, cystic and freely mobile. Since the lower uterine segment is particularly soft, the corpus may be palpated as a separate mass unless particular care is taken during examination. Similarly, if the pregnant uterus is in marked retroversion it may be mistaken for a posterior cul-de-sac cyst. Careful attention to the history, noting the presence of amenorrhea or shortened menstrual periods, together with nausea, lassitude, weight gain and breast soreness will aid in the proper diagnosis. The pelvic examination will often reveal the cervix to be soft and congested.

A sudden accumulation of amniotic fluid during the midtrimester of an unsuspected pregnancy has occasionally been misdiagnosed as an ovarian cyst. The aforementioned signs and symptoms of pregnancy or the demonstration of a fetal skeleton by x-ray will aid in the proper diagnosis.

During the early weeks of pregnancy the uterus may enlarge asymmetrically or, if there is a tendency toward a bicornuate uterus, there will be a pronounced unilateral enlargement. This may be mistaken for a cystic mass contiguous to a slightly enlarged uterus. Moderate degrees of this asymmetry are normal in all pregnancies and such a growth pattern is known as Piskacek's sign of early pregnancy.

Pregnancy occurring in the interstitial portion of the oviduct may give rise to an asymmetric enlargement of the uterus. This may be confused with an adjacent ovarian cyst but more commonly is confused with a leiomyoma of the uterus thought to occur with an incomplete abortion. Rupture of an interstitial pregnancy is usually delayed beyond that in ordinary

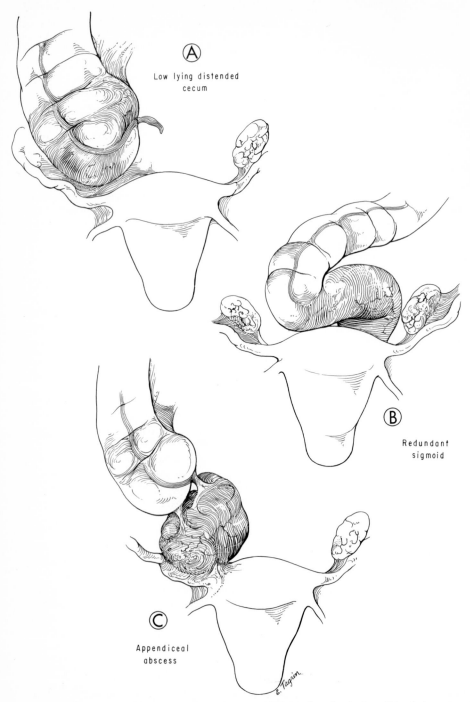

Fig. 7-2.—Differential diagnosis of ovarian lesions. **A,** redundant or distended cecum; **B,** redundant sigmoid colon; **C,** appendiceal abscess. (Continued.)

ectopic tubal pregnancy and may not occur until the third or fourth month of gestation.

Several conditions involving the pelvic colon are frequently confused with ovarian neoplasms. These include a low-lying or distended cecum, a redundant sigmoid colon, an appendiceal abscess, impacted feces in the rectosigmoid, carcinoma of the sigmoid and diverticulitis. Although the cecum usually occupies a position in the right iliac fossa, with its lowest point at the level of the midportion of the inguinal ligament, it occasionally hangs over the pelvic brim (Fig. 7-2, A) or rarely may be found within the pelvic cavity. A cecum that is distended with gas, particularly if there is associated pain, may be confused with a right ovarian cyst. Careful examination, however, will usually reveal the presence of fluid and gas on palpation, marked flaccidity and mobility and, of course, disappearance after catharsis or enemas. The sigmoid colon may present a similar situation. If this segment of the colon is redundant (Fig. 7-2, B) it may be filled with fecal material or gas and, because of its proximity to the uterine corpus, diagnosis may be that of a firm ovarian neoplasm. A thorough enema will clarify the diagnostic problem.

A localized abscess subsequent to rupture of the appendix (Fig. 7-2, C) may be confused with an ovarian neoplasm and may particularly suggest the possibility of hemorrhage, rupture or torsion. A previous history of upper abdominal or periumbilical pain associated with nausea, vomiting and subsequent localization of the pain in the right lower quadrant together with evidence of local peritoneal irritation will aid in diagnosis of a disease process in the appendix rather than in the ovary. Occasionally, however, the initial symptoms of acute appendicitis are minimal and the abscess develops gradually with the formation of a thick, adherent capsule. In such a case a correct preoperative diagnosis is almost impossible.

A firm, fixed mass in the left pelvis occurring in women over age 50 strongly suggests carcinoma of the ovary or sigmoid (Fig. 7-2, D). A history of altered bowel habits, constipation or diarrhea, pain of a colicky type, diminution in the caliber of the stool and melena suggests sigmoid cancer, and diagnosis is aided by rectal examination, sigmoidoscopy, barium enema and biopsy of the tumor mass. In some cases, however, the sigmoid colon and left ovary are so intimately adherent in a carcinomatous process that the pathologist finds it impossible to distinguish the primary site. X-rays also are occasionally misleading, since we have had several cases in which the radiologist interpreted the findings as indicating an extrinsic lesion of the bowel primary in the ovary, whereas in actuality the pathologist was able to determine just the reverse.

Diverticulitis of the sigmoid colon (Fig. 7-2, E) is a frequent cause for mistaken gynecologic diagnoses. Although many women over age 40 have uncomplicated diverticulosis which is usually asymptomatic, a mass in the left pelvis following rupture of a diverticulum may be difficult to distinguish from ovarian cancer. A typical attack of diverticulitis is manifested by intermittent cramplike abdominal pain, usually in the left lower quadrant, associated with diarrhea with mucus and small amounts of blood in the stool. There is associated evidence of peritoneal irritation together with leukocytosis and fever. Pelvic examination is not of great value in differentiation since a firm, localized mass may result from perforation and lodge

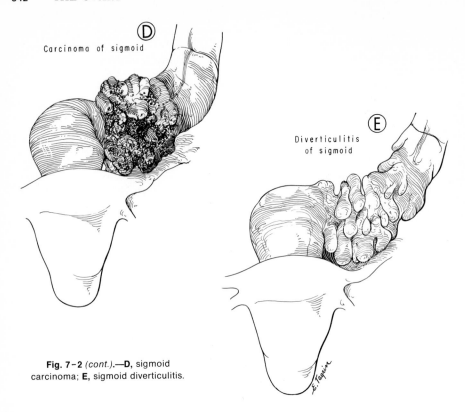

Carcinoma of sigmoid

Diverticulitis
of sigmoid

Fig. 7–2 *(cont.).*—**D,** sigmoid
carcinoma; **E,** sigmoid diverticulitis.

in the left pelvis. Exact diagnosis will depend on a barium enema which
should be done during a quiescent period of the disease. This will reveal
diverticula, an irritable colon and areas of stenosis.

Lesions of the oviduct or mesosalpinx may also give rise to cystic structures which must be differentiated from those arising in the ovary. A
paraovarian cyst may develop from the rudimentary structures in the mesosalpinx, the mass actually developing between the leaves of the broad
ligament. These cysts are usually unilateral, somewhat fixed, ovoid and
thin walled. Usually, however, the ovary may be felt separately from the
mass as a more solid structure. It is frequently difficult to differentiate a
paraovarian cyst from a cyst of follicular origin by pelvic examination
alone. An adenomatoid tumor of the oviduct is even more confusing, since
the tumor is quite solid and may reach a diameter of 6–8 cm. A tubal
ectopic pregnancy may closely simulate an acute accident arising in an
ovarian tumor, such as torsion. Symptoms suggesting pregnancy—a missed
period followed by irregular uterine bleeding, nausea, breast soreness—or a
history of a previous ectopic pregnancy will aid in the correct diagnosis.
The signs associated with a ruptured ectopic pregnancy may be exactly the
same as those associated with a ruptured ovarian cyst; in this case the
diagnosis can be made only by operative means.

One of the commonest lesions which may be mistaken for an ovarian
tumor is a pedunculated uterine leiomyoma. This is particularly true if the
fibroid is solitary and somewhat soft. Such fibroids are usually freely mobile,

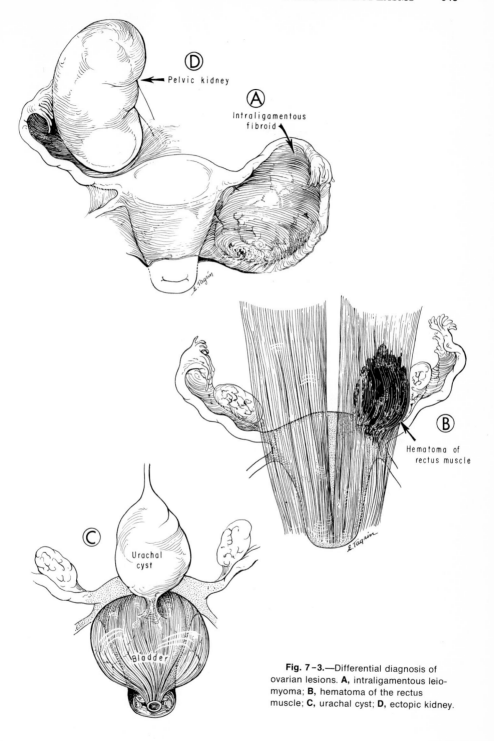

Fig. 7–3.—Differential diagnosis of ovarian lesions. **A,** intraligamentous leiomyoma; **B,** hematoma of the rectus muscle; **C,** urachal cyst; **D,** ectopic kidney.

but careful examination will reveal an area of attachment to the uterus. If the fibroid can be moved from the lateral position, the ovary can then be felt separately. It is impossible to delineate adequately a parasitic or intra-ligamentous fibroid (Fig. 7–3, *A*), since such lesions are relatively fixed and may be situated in areas directly adjacent to the ovary. If the pedicle of a pedunculated fibroid undergoes torsion, infarction may result, and the presenting signs and symptoms will be indistinguishable from those of a twisted ovarian cyst.

Other lesions which, although rare, may simulate ovarian tumors are a hematoma of the rectus muscle, a desmoid or urachal cyst, a pelvic kidney, a mesenteric cyst or polycystic kidney and a retroperitoneal neoplasm or abscess. A hematoma of the rectus muscle (Fig. 7–3, *B*) usually results from trauma or unusual strain on the rectus muscles, and if it happens to be localized in the lower abdomen a definite mass will be palpable. There may be an associated area of ecchymosis, but usually the thickness of the abdominal wall in such patients prevents this development. The super-ficial location may be demonstrated by tensing the abdominal muscles; however, in the postmenopausal patient the ovary cannot be felt distinctly by pelvic examination so that exact differentiation is not possible. A des-moid tumor may arise in the suprapubic portion of the anterior abdominal wall and in this location may closely simulate a fixed, firm ovarian mass lying anterior to the broad ligament. A urachal cyst (Fig. 7–3, *C*) may enlarge in the same area and show a similar clinical picture. An ectopic kidney (Fig. 7–3, *D*) which is situated in the true pelvis may be asympto-matic or may give rise to nonspecific symptoms attributable to an ovarian cyst. Pelvic examination reveals the lower end of the mass to be smooth, fixed, ovoid and of a rather rubbery consistency. The use of intravenous urograms before laparotomy for a suspected ovarian cyst is therefore of great importance in delineating the position of the kidneys and ureters. Retroperitoneal pelvic tumors such as fibromas, sarcomas, dermoids, malignant teratomas, metastatic carcinoma, osteochondromas and gangli-oneuromas may extend into the lower pelvis. Their presence may be sus-pected by intravenous urography but exact diagnosis can only be made after surgical exploration. Similarly, certain abscesses originating in the spine or perivesical areas may be confused with firm ovarian masses.

The accumulation of ascitic fluid within the peritoneal cavity may give the impression of a large, thin-walled ovarian cyst. In the presence of ascites, however, the small intestine is usually found to be located centrally, the tympanitic note of percussion therefore being located centrally, with shifting dullness observed in the flanks. In addition, a definite fluid wave should be present. By comparison, a large ovarian cyst will displace the small intestine laterally so that percussion reveals tympany laterally.

Non-neoplastic Cysts of Graafian Follicle Origin

In a consideration of ovarian neoplasms the student and clinician must be familiar with the physiologic variations of a normal ovulatory cycle which occasionally may result in a non-neoplastic ovarian cyst. By defini-tion these cysts are not capable of autonomous growth, but their clinical recognition as distinct from true ovarian neoplasms is frequently difficult on the basis of clinical signs and symptoms. The surgeon, however, should have had an adequate background in the pathologic differentiation of such cysts so that undue and irreparable harm will not result from his interference. It is true that cysts of graafian follicle origin may mimic true cystomas both grossly and microscopically. They may occur at any age before the menopause and, because of their hormonal activity, may disrupt or alter normal, physiologic menstrual function. Occasionally they arise as a result of persistent stimulation by chorionic gonadotropin from a normal or abnormal pregnancy. In these cases they may enlarge markedly, may become gangrenous and on occasion may even rupture.

A follicle cyst may arise during the evolution or during the involution of the graafian follicle. Its wall, therefore, may be composed either of granulosa or theca interna cells with or without luteinization, or of theca externa cells with or without hyalinization. Since the follicle undergoes cystic change as it develops normally, our pathology department has arbitrarily used a dimension of 2.5 cm. as the dividing line between a "cystic follicle" and a "follicular cyst." Usually an ovary which is enlarged by a single, large follicle cyst is asymptomatic or may give rise only to a sense of pelvic discomfort or heaviness in the involved side. The patient may also have noted some irregularity of the menstrual cycle, such as a delayed flow followed by irregular and intermittent staining. In the patient classified as an oligo-ovulator the ovary may show multiple cystic follicles each about 1–2 cm. in diameter which are thin walled, translucent and filled with watery fluid. These cysts may project just above the ovarian surface and, if opened, follicular fluid may spread out under pressure. This is not the typical ovary of the Stein-Leventhal syndrome which will be described later. These cysts have sometimes been called multiple follicle "retention" ovarian cysts (ovarian cystosis).

The normal ovary from a normally fertile patient may show eight to 10 follicles on midsagittal section, each varying in size from 3 to 5 mm. (Fig. 7–4). In the normal state these show varying degrees of congestion, hem-

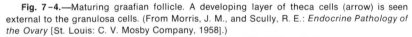

Fig. 7–4.—Maturing graafian follicle. A developing layer of theca cells (arrow) is seen external to the granulosa cells. (From Morris, J. M., and Scully, R. E.: *Endocrine Pathology of the Ovary* [St. Louis: C. V. Mosby Company, 1958].)

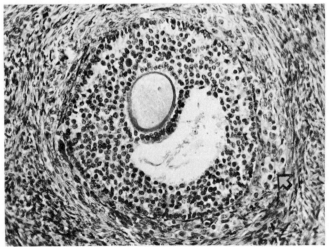

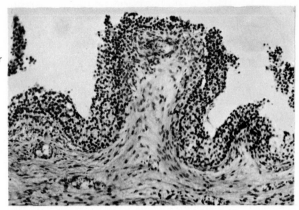

Fig. 7-5.—Wall of follicle cyst, showing pleomorphism of the inner granulosa cells and a moderately well-preserved theca layer. (From Hertig, A. T., and Gore, H.: *Tumors of the Female Sex Organs: Part 3. Tumors of the Ovary and Fallopian Tube*, sec. IX, fasc. 33 of *Atlas of Tumor Pathology* [Washington, D.C.: Armed Forces Institute of Pathology, 1961].)

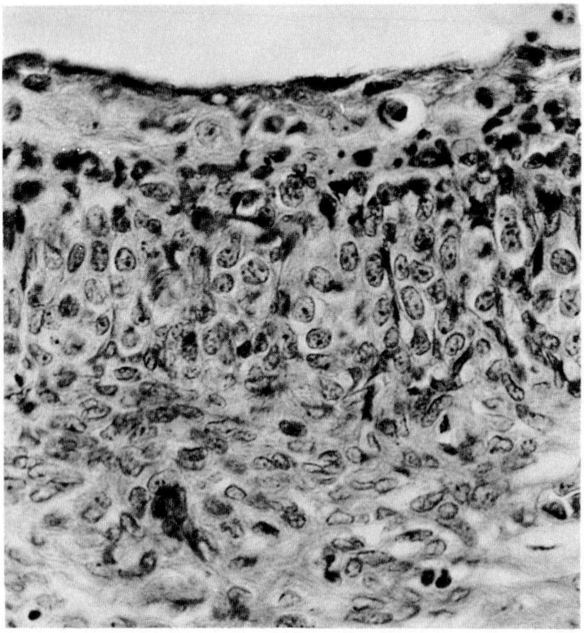

Fig. 7-6.—Luteinized follicle cyst. Note that most of the granulosa cells have disappeared but that the cells of the theca interna are prominent and luteinized.

orrhage and luteinization. The abnormal cystic follicles are similar to these in appearance but are closely crowded beneath the tunica albuginea, without adequate intervening stroma.

Microscopically the granulosa cells may show a good deal of pleomorphism with relatively large nuclei and moderate intercellular edema of the inner layer (Fig. 7-5). In cysts of the larger variety only a few granulosa cells may be identified, whereas cells of the theca externa are usually seen. These may show focal areas of luteinization or hyalinization depending on the age of the cyst (Fig. 7-6). *Hydrops folliculi* is a term used to describe unusual enlargement of a follicle cyst which occasionally may reach a diameter of 7-8 cm. At the time of surgery it may be difficult to distinguish such a cyst from a neoplastic serous cystoma. Occasionally blood from the vascularized theca cells may diffuse into the cavity of the follicle cyst. This will impart a bluish tinge to the contents. However, with more extensive bleeding a follicle cyst hematoma may occur. If this is not removed, the blood may become thick and brown, closely resembling the "chocolate cyst" of endometriosis.

Treatment of a follicle cyst should be conservative unless a specific complication warrants surgical intervention. If the cyst is 5 cm. or less in diameter the patient should have a pelvic examination every three or four weeks. If examination is performed after the next menstrual period, the previously palpable mass will often have disappeared. Should the cystic ovary persist through two or more menstrual cycles culdoscopy or laparoscopy is indicated. Since these cysts are dependent on pituitary gonadotropic stimulation, we have recently used progestational agents to hasten their disappearance. Administration of these suppressants of gonadotropic activity for 20 days will usually result in involution of the cystic mass.

CYSTIC STRUCTURES DERIVED FROM THE
NORMALLY RUPTURED FOLLICLE

It will be remembered from the discussion of the formation of a normal corpus luteum that the mature structure has a central core which is filled with blood. After resorption, the cavity may be distended with hemorrhagic or clear fluid. Thus, the corpus luteum itself is a cystic structure and a corpus luteum cyst therefore refers to an abnormal persistence or enlargement of this physiologic process. If the normal organization of the coagulum by fibroblasts is prevented or if there is extensive bleeding into the cavity, an abnormally functioning cyst will result. Such a *corpus luteum hematoma* may cause local pain, amenorrhea and signs closely resembling a tubal ectopic pregnancy. Although most hematomas of the corpus luteum do not exceed 7 or 8 cm., several as large as 11 cm. in diameter have been described. Following the resorption of the blood in such a hematoma a typical corpus luteum cyst may evolve.

The diagnosis cannot be made with exact precision but should be suspected in a patient who has noted delayed menses followed by irregular staining and a rather constant discomfort or sense of heaviness in one side of the pelvis. Endometrial biopsy may reveal atypical secretory endometrium showing the effects of progesterone as well as the effects of estrogen from a newly formed and growing follicle. This has been described ambiguously as irregular shedding of the endometrium. A positive diagnosis of a corpus luteum cyst or hematoma may usually be made by culdoscopy or posterior colpotomy.

A ruptured hemorrhagic corpus luteum will show all the signs and symptoms of massive intraperitoneal bleeding. Rupture may occur following pelvic examination, strenuous exercise or even coitus. The clinical picture includes lower abdominal pain, nausea and vomiting, rectus muscle spasm and rebound tenderness. Pelvic examination will reveal an enlarged, tender ovary or, if bleeding has been extensive, a doughy or fluctuant cul-de-sac. The temperature may be elevated to 100.4 F. and moderate leukocytosis is usually present. The blood loss occasionally is severe, exceeding 1,000 cc., and at the time of laparotomy there may be active bleeding at the site of rupture.

Gross examination of a corpus luteum cyst or hematoma usually reveals the yellowish color in the wall of the cyst. The wall is usually quite thin and the exact diagnosis is not possible until microscopic sections have been completed. Microscopically the typical cyst will show all of the elements of the normal corpus luteum (Fig. 7–7). Both granulosa- and theca-lutein cells will be found in the wall, together with organizing fibrous connective tissue and erythrocytes. If the corpus luteum hematoma has been small, spontaneous regression will occur, giving rise to a *corpus albicans cyst*. This characteristically presents a convoluted wall of the previously cystic structure composed of dense bands of fibrous connective tissue with hyalinized collagen.

The corpus luteum of early pregnancy is a cystic structure that occasionally gives rise to unilateral pain and is sometimes confused with an unruptured ectopic pregnancy. During pregnancy the corpus luteum functions for a variable time, usually six to nine weeks, occasionally somewhat longer. As the corpus luteum regresses, the cystic portion compresses and flattens the surrounding cellular elements. Following an early spontaneous abortion the corpus luteum of pregnancy may persist for varying periods, giving rise to dysfunctional uterine bleeding. Curettage does not reveal the retention of trophoblastic elements but only an atypical, somewhat hyperplastic, secretory endometrium.

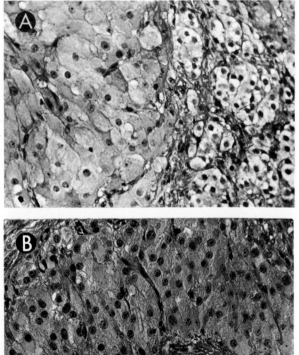

Fig. 7–7.—A, high power of mature corpus luteum. The larger, rounded cells at left are granulosa-lutein cells; the smaller, clearer cells are theca-lutein cells. (From Morris, J. M., and Scully, R. E.: *Endocrine Pathology of the Ovary* [St. Louis: C. V. Mosby Company, 1958].) **B,** wall of corpus luteum cyst, showing luteinized granulosa cells.

Physiologic ovarian cysts of rather large size may be associated with hydatidiform mole, chorioadenoma destruens or choriocarcinoma. They are due to the secretion of excess amounts of chorionic gonadotropic hormone by these tumors of the trophoblast. Bilateral lutein cysts occur in about one-third of these patients. Surgical extirpation of the ovaries is not necessary, however, since these lutein cysts gradually regress and the ovaries return to normal size and function after removal of the trophoblastic tissue. These cysts may reach rather large proportions, filling the pelvic cavity on both sides. Each large cyst is made up of multiple locules varying from 1 to 2 mm. in diameter. Each locule contains a clear yellow fluid and each cystic cavity is lined by luteinized theca interna cells which resemble the lutein cells of the corpus luteum. In certain instances luteinization of the granulosa cells as well as the cells of the theca interna have been reported.

Cystomas (of Germinal Epithelial Origin)

Most ovarian neoplasms may be classified under the major heading of cystomas of "germinal" epithelial origin. These include the serous cystad-

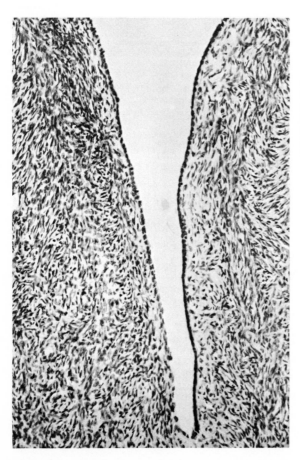

Fig. 7–8.—Histogenesis of ovarian tumors. Surface of ovary showing a groove lined by coelomic epithelium which has the potential to develop into serous, mucinous or endometrial epithelium. (From McKay, D. G.: Clin. Obst. & Gynec. 5:1188, 1962.)

enomas and cystadenocarcinomas, mucinous cystadenomas and cystadenocarcinomas, endometrial cystomas both benign and malignant, and
cystadenofibromas, benign and malignant. The surface epithelium of the
ovary is embryologically related to the embryonic pelvic peritoneum and
retains its potential for infolding and differentiation into varieties of specialized epithelium (Fig. 7–8). This accounts for the variety of benign and
malignant cystomas which arise from the surface covering of the ovary
(Fig. 7–9). Although this layer has been described as "germinal" epithelium, it is now evident that the primordial germ cells do not arise within it
and that the term is a misnomer. Thus, all stages in the histogenesis of
müllerian-type cystomas may be identified. A simple infolding of the surface epithelium may form a "germinal" inclusion cyst (Fig. 7–10). Separation of the epithelial element from this surface, together with formation of
a secretion in the lumen, gives rise to a simple serous cystoma. Occasionally all three cell types may be identified in one cyst, some areas showing
serous epithelium similar to that of the oviduct whereas in others the epithelium may be mucinous as in the endocervix or may even be endometrial,
with both glands and stroma. Thus it is the multipotentiality of the surface
epithelium that accounts for the mixed forms of cystomas and their malignant counterparts.

Fig. 7–9.—Schematic diagram of origin of ovarian cystomas from surface or "germinal"
epithelium. On the surface are a papillary outgrowth of germinal epithelium, an early infolding,
a later stage of infolding and a small focus of endometrial-type stroma lying beneath the germinal epithelium. A germinal inclusion cyst is lying within the cortex and is surrounded mainly by
ovarian cortical stroma and partly by endometrial stroma. The three main derivatives are
shown. (From Hertig, A. T., and Gore, H.: Rocky Mountain M. J. 55:47–50, 1958.)

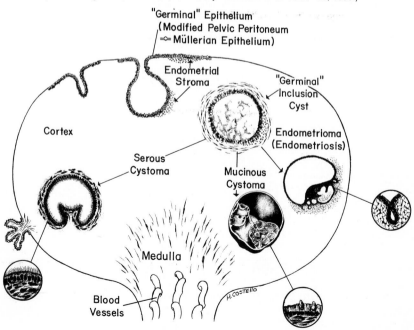

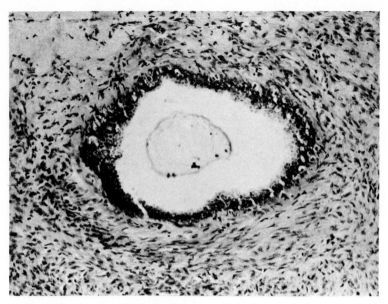

Fig. 7–10.—Histogenesis of ovarian tumors. Coelomic epithelial inclusion cyst formed by "pinching off" of epithelium noted in Figure 7–8. (From McKay, D. G.: Clin. Obst. & Gynec. 5:1118, 1962.)

SIMPLE SEROUS CYSTOMA

The simple serous cyst (serous cystoma) is a unilocular cyst lined by serous epithelium. It is thin walled and smooth surfaced with a gray-white or translucent appearance. Its size rarely exceeds 8–10 cm. and it is usually unilateral. It is filled with a clear, serous, watery or straw-colored fluid which is rich in serum proteins but lacks the viscid characteristic of mucinous fluid. The inner lining is smooth and glistening and does not show papillary infoldings.

Microscopically the lining of the cyst consists of characteristic serous epithelium, usually a single layer of cuboidal or low cylindrical cells with central dark-staining nuclei (Figs. 7–11 and 7–12). Cilia may be seen focally originating from these cells. The supporting tissue is fibrous and does not contain glandular structures. Although papillary projections are uncommon, occasionally a broad, solitary papilla may be seen, covered by a single layer of cuboidal epithelium similar to that which lines the cyst proper.

This neoplastic tumor is quite common, Randall having found that approximately 25 per cent of benign ovarian cysts and tumors, exclusive of follicle and corpus luteum cysts, could be grouped under this classification. Serous cystomas are most common between the ages of 20 and 50 years and reach their peak incidence in the third and fourth decades. Partial ovarian resection or oophorectomy is adequate therapy for neoplasms of this type. Over age 40, hysterectomy is recommended.

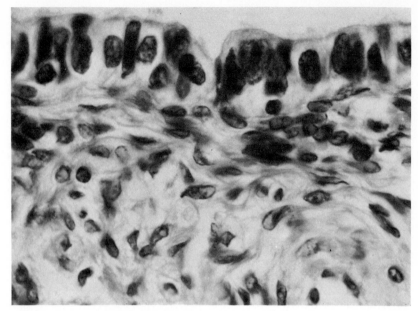

Fig. 7-11.—Tubal epithelium. Note ciliated cells, secretory cells and peg cells. The epithelium of serous cysts simulates this most closely.

Fig. 7-12.—Epithelium lining a serous cyst. Compare with Fig. 7-11. (From McKay, D. G.: Clin. Obst. & Gynec. 5:1189, 1962.)

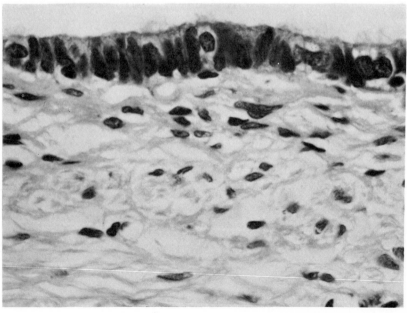

SEROUS CYSTADENOMA

These are unilocular or multilocular cystic neoplasms whose epithelium resembles the mucosa of the oviduct. They tend to be bilateral, often form papillary projections and may be clinically or histologically malignant.

In a series of 2,530 ovarian neoplasms of all types and degrees of malignancy examined from 1904 through 1952 at the Boston Hospital for Women, 24.5 per cent were benign and malignant *serous* tumors while 18.9 per cent were benign and malignant *mucinous* types. The incidence of serous and mucinous types in the benign group was approximately equal —about 24 per cent. Of the malignant tumors, however, the serous comprised 60 per cent, compared to 16 per cent for mucinous cystadenocarcinomas. Hence, the serous variety is more than three times as likely to be malignant as is the mucinous variety.

Serous cystadenomas, when multilocular, are quite irregular in shape but have a smooth surface that is frequently covered with fine blood vessels. The color may vary in individual locules, but in general the thickened fibrous wall appears grayish white. Hemorrhage of varying degrees into the individual locules may cause the cysts to appear brown, red or blue. Cross-section of the multilocular serous cystadenoma reveals numerous separate locules of different sizes. The grapelike cystadenoma is a variation of this classification and is characterized by multiple pedunculated cysts which project from the surface of the ovary and resemble a cluster of grapes. The fluid content of the various locules of the multilocular cystomas may vary from the typical thin, clear, serous type to a turbid, sticky variety with varying amounts of blood. Occasionally the fluid is slightly mucinous since not all of the epithelium is purely serous in type. Microscopically the acini and walls of the various individual cysts are lined by a typical single layer of cuboidal or low columnar ciliated epithelium. The stroma may vary from an edematous to a densely fibrous type.

Serous cystadenomas are benign neoplasms and therefore the usual treatment is unilateral oophorectomy. However, because of the propensity for bilateral involvement the opposite ovary should always be carefully inspected and even bisected to discover an unsuspected tumor. When this type of ovarian neoplasm is found as a unilateral tumor in a postmenopausal patient a complete hysterectomy and bilateral salpingo-oophorectomy is performed. Although a serous cystadenoma does not often become as large as the mucinous type, one occasionally may become enormous, filling the entire abdomen. Care should be exercised in removing the cyst to avoid spilling the contents.

Papillary serous cystadenomas are serous cysts which manifest intra- or extracystic papillary growths in addition to adenomatous proliferation of the epithelium. Grossly they resemble the serous cystadenomas and are commonly multilocular, spherical and lobulated. When the papillary projections are confined to the inner wall, the cyst is apt to be unilateral and to attain a large size. When external as well as internal projections are present, the ovarian masses tend to be smaller and are more frequently bilateral. The papillary projections may be striking and involve isolated segments of locules or the entire inner surface. A fine, granular surface may be due to papillae which have penetrated through the wall from the cyst lining. Pedunculated, branching papillae may coalesce and form large cauliflower masses of varying colors. Other discolorations of the papillary masses may be due to hemorrhage, edema or necrosis. Occasionally calcium deposits are found in the wall of the cyst, giving a sandy sensation when palpated.

Microscopic examination may be quite variable. The cyst wall itself is composed of fibrous connective tissue with the usual inner lining of serous epithelium. Most of the cells are low columnar or cuboidal, occasionally ciliated, with central vesicular nuclei. The presence of "peg" cells suggests a similarity to epithelium of the oviduct. Because of these cells the term "endosalpingioma" has been applied to serous epithelial ovarian cysts.

The papillae present a wide spectrum of architecture, including simple as well as arborescent patterns. The papillary projections may be covered with tall columnar ciliated epithelium or cuboidal non-ciliated cells resembling those of the cyst wall. The stroma may be dense, fibrous tissue similar to that in the tunica albuginea.

Symptoms associated with papillary serous cystadenomas are dependent on the size of the masses or on the presence of certain complications such as a torsion of the pedicle with infarction. Although the cyst may be asymptomatic, there is usually some local discomfort with pressure symptoms involving the urinary or intestinal tract. Ascites may occur, with subsequent abdominal enlargement. A pleural effusion is occasionally associated with a papillary cystadenoma as well as with the usual fibroma of Meigs's syndrome.

Although papillary tumors may be considered benign, most borderline serous carcinomas fall into this category. Therefore, multiple sections of representative areas of tumor should be examined to determine its relative benignancy or malignancy. Although external papillations or implants on peritoneal surfaces are considered evidence of malignancy, such implants associated with or due to papillary cystadenomas may be harmless mesotheliomata or benign endosalpingiosis. On the other hand, such implants may be metastases and after lying dormant for years sudden growth can be rapidly fatal. In certain instances the original histology of the tumor was apparently benign although spread to the surface of the ovary and metastasis to the omentum had already occurred.

At the time of operation, benignity is suggested if the cyst wall is thin and the papillary excrescences are small and discrete. If, however, bloody ascitic fluid is found together with peritoneal implants and there are solid areas of infiltration in the cyst wall or fixation of the neoplasm to neighboring structures, microscopic sections will undoubtedly prove malignant. It is important to remember, therefore, that even though the histology of the papillary serous tumor is benign a subsequent benign clinical course is not guaranteed.

The treatment will depend on many factors, the chief one being the age of the patient. In patients over 40 years of age a complete hysterectomy and bilateral salpingo-oophorectomy should be performed. Even in younger women the presence of bilateral involvement, peritoneal implants, ascites or external excrescences demands radical therapy. A conservative attitude may be adopted in the young patient, particularly a nullipara, in whom the ovarian mass is unilateral and has an intact capsule and sparse papillae. Rapid histologic sections are often unreliable and it is best not to make a decision on this basis. In some cases findings on the permanent sections will convince the surgeon to reoperate within a short period to remove the opposite ovary as well as the uterus. In certain cases where borderline tumors are accompanied by peritoneal implants, x-ray therapy is indicated postoperatively even though a frank diagnosis of invasive carcinoma has not been made.

PAPILLARY SEROUS CYSTADENOCARCINOMA

Papillary serous cystadenocarcinomas comprise about 60 per cent of the ovarian cancers reported in most series. The symptoms associated with papillary serous cystadenocarcinomas are, in general, the same as those listed for any other ovarian tumors. Unfortunately, signs and symptoms are completely absent in about 25 per cent of cases. The clinical picture can be said to be highly nonspecific and variable, involving such complaints as abdominal enlargement, abnormal uterine bleeding, nonspecific pain and constipation. It is important, therefore, that patients have periodic, routine pelvic examinations to determine the presence of ovarian enlargement or abnormal fixation. This is particularly necessary in women over 40 because of the high incidence of carcinoma in this group. In women under age 40 the incidence of malignancy in ovarian tumors is approximately 6 per cent; in the 40–50 age group it is 25 per cent, and in women over age 50, it is 40 per cent.

Pathologically the papillary serous cystadenocarcinomas are a heterogeneous group. About one-fourth are primarily cystic, two-thirds are semisolid and one-twelfth are entirely solid. The contour may vary from coarse lobulation to fine nodularity, depending on the number and size of the cavities. The external surface may be smooth or granular, the latter type being due to papillae arising in a firm or calcified base. Microscopically the epithelium of papillary serous cystadenocarcinomas shows varying degrees of differentiation (Fig. 7–13). In some instances the architecture may resemble the mucosa of the oviduct, being well differentiated and ciliated. Other areas in the same tumor may show nonciliated, pleomorphic and even very undifferentiated cellular patterns. Of particular importance is the presence of papillary processes of the epithelium in which stroma is scant or absent. In other tumors the epithelium is nonciliated but pseudostratified, resembling that seen in the endometrium. In the highly anaplastic serous cystadenocarcinomas (Fig. 7–13, D) the epithelial overgrowth may be so pronounced that the papillae are partially obliterated. In such cases the tumor may merely be called an adenocarcinoma of the ovary, but multiple sections will usually reveal the proper identity.

MUCINOUS CYSTADENOMA AND CYSTADENOCARCINOMA

The benign and malignant variants of this ovarian tumor will be discussed together, since there are gradual transitions between the obviously benign and obviously malignant forms. These unilocular or multilocular cystic ovarian neoplasms are of varied and sometimes uncertain origin but usually arise from the surface epithelium. In contrast to serous epithelial tumors, they are less likely to be bilateral (10 per cent) or papillary (10 per cent) and are rarely malignant (5–15 per cent). The term "pseudomuci-

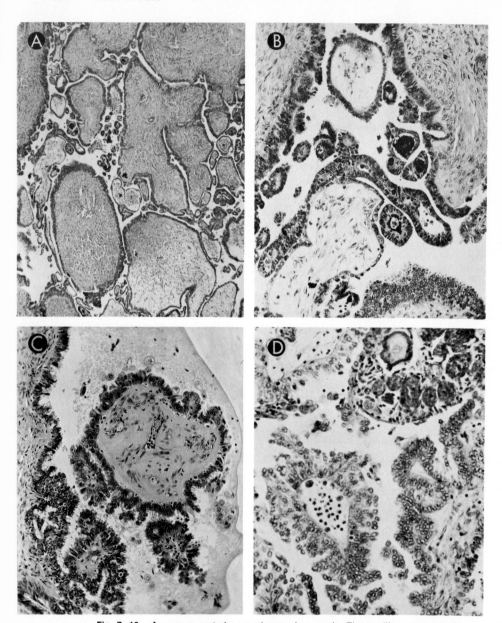

Fig. 7-13.—A, serous cystadenocarcinoma, low grade. The papillary processes have a fibrous stroma covered by well-differentiated but pleomorphic epithelium. Areas of calcification are seen in the central papillae. **B,** higher power of A to show pseudostratification of epithelium. **C,** papillary serous cystadenocarcinoma, showing marked epithelial overgrowth. The epithelium lining the cyst wall at left is well differentiated and ciliated, resembling that of the oviduct. **D,** papillary serous cystadenocarcinoma, anaplastic type. The epithelium covering the papillae is nonciliated, pleomorphic and appears malignant. (From Hertig, A. T., and Gore, H.: *Tumors of the Female Sex Organs: Part 3. Tumors of the Ovary and Fallopian Tube,* sec. IX, fasc. 33 of *Atlas of Tumor Pathology* [Washington, D.C.: Armed Forces Institute of Pathology, 1961].)

nous" has been applied to the stringy, viscid fluid found in the cystic spaces of these tumors. Although it differs from true mucin in that it is soluble in water and dilute acids, it is similar to mucin in that it is precipitated by alcohol. There is now general agreement that the prefix "pseudo" be dropped in favor of mucinous. These tumors represent a common type of ovarian cyst, occurring with slightly less frequency than serous cystadenomas. They are usually encountered during the reproductive years, being rare before puberty or after the menopause. In the report from the Boston Hospital for Women by Kent and McKay, mucinous tumors, both benign and malignant, accounted for 18.9 per cent of the total (478 of 2,530). In this same series serous cystadenomas and cystadenocarcinomas accounted for 24.5 per cent of the total. However, only 12 per cent of the mucinous tumors were malignant.

Although mucinous cystadenomas occur most often during the third to fifth decades, rare instances have been reported in infants and children. About 10 per cent are found in patients who are postmenopausal. The malignant variety is most common during the fourth to sixth decades and therefore either the benign or malignant form may be discovered during pregnancy.

A review of the histogenesis of this tumor has been presented by Dockerty and Reagan. Reagan favors the concept that this tumor originates from involuting microcystic graafian follicles. Dockerty has suggested that the tumors may arise from tubules in the epoophoron and rete ovarii since approximately one-third of Brenner tumors have associated mucinous cystomas. Reagan noted that the epithelium of this tumor is similar to other mucus-secreting epithelium and most closely resembles that of the intestine. Hertig has suggested that the tumor is derived chiefly from the surface or germinal epithelium (Fig. 7–14). He noted that cysts of surface epithelial origin may demonstrate all the müllerian elements in one cyst or in multiple cysts within the same ovary. In certain reports of mucinous tumors, up to 11 per cent showed a mixture of serous and mucinous elements. Hertig also accepts the theory that a few mucinous cystadenomas may be derived

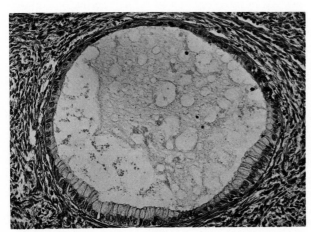

Fig. 7–14.—Early mucinous cystoma arising in a germinal inclusion cyst. Note tall columnar epithelium gradually merging into the indifferent cuboidal germinal epithelium of the cyst. (From Hertig, A. T., and Mansell, H.: in Anderson, W. A. D. [ed.]: *Pathology* [3d ed.; St. Louis: C. V. Mosby Company, 1957].)

from a monophyletic teratoma. This theory is based on the fact that mucinous cysts occur frequently in the walls of ovarian dermoids and intestinal enzymes have been demonstrated in these tumors. Hertig and Gore described one case in which a dermoid cyst was present in one ovary and an intestinal-type mucinous cystoma in the opposite ovary.

Grossly the outer surface of a mucinous cyst is generally smooth, lobulated, glistening and gray-white in color. These tumors, both benign and malignant, may be very large. Although some of the cysts are of microscopic size, the range has been given as 1–50 cm. in diameter, with most being between 15 and 30 cm. and weighing between 2,000 and 4,000 Gm. The largest tumor on record is said to have weighed 328 lb.

The malignant form of mucinous cystoma tends to be bilateral more often (15–23 per cent) than the benign variants (2–5 per cent). The serosal surface of the benign form is smooth, pink to gray, and does not possess extracystic growths. The serosal surface of the malignant form, however, may show extracystic growths which become densely adherent to adjacent structures, particularly the bowel and bladder. When invasion of the capsule is extensive, there may be rupture of the tumor. Benign tumors are not fixed to adjacent structures and therefore twisting of the pedicle with subsequent infarction is more likely to occur.

The consistency of these tumors is variable and depends on the number and size of cysts in relation to the amount of solid tissue. Occasionally there is hemorrhage into the cavity and the cut surface may then be dark red, brown or even black. If necrosis occurs, the color may be yellow or gray. The individual locules vary in size and contain a sticky, viscid, mucinous material. Almost 25 per cent of benign and a greater proportion of malignant tumors will present intracystic papillary projections. If section of an apparently benign tumor shows one or more papillary processes, the surgeon should regard this lesion with suspicion. Occasionally the tumor is quite bulky and solid, being composed of numerous minute compartments with a spongelike appearance. If there is cholesterol deposition into the wall, a greenish discoloration is evident.

Microscopically the connective tissue capsule is composed of an outer layer of dense fibrous tissue and an inner layer which is loose and quite cellular. Areas of degeneration may be noted with scattered foci of inflammation, necrosis and calcification. The inner zone of connective tissue is projected into the tumor, forming the dividing septa. The characteristic cell of the mucinous cystoma is a tall, columnar, picket cell which resembles closely the secretory cells of the endocervix (Figs. 7–15 and 7–16). These columnar cells have characteristic deep-staining basal nuclei and finely granular, acidophilic cytoplasm. Between the columnar cells actively secreting goblet cells may be identified. The secretory activity of the goblet cell is mainly of the merocrine type but occasionally it is holocrine, with destruction of the cell occurring on secretion.

In certain areas of a mucinous cystadenoma, intestinal-type epithelium such as Paneth cells may be identified. This histologic feature has led certain authors to suggest that this tumor is composed of one element derived from a teratoma, the other elements having been suppressed.

The symptoms associated with a mucinous cystadenoma are those generally seen with benign ovarian neoplasms, except that torsion of the pedicle is rather common, occurring in about 20 per cent of cases. Ascites is

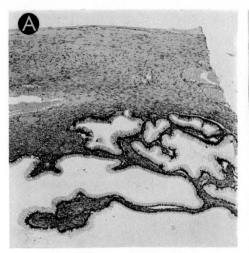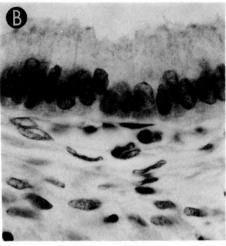

Fig. 7-15.—**A,** mucinous cystadenoma showing typical tall columnar epithelium lining the cyst. Note multiple daughter cysts in the connective tissue wall. (From Hertig, A. T., and Gore, H.: *Tumors of the Female Sex Organs: Part 3. Tumors of the Ovary and Fallopian Tube,* sec. IX, fasc. 33 of *Atlas of Tumor Pathology* [Washington, D.C.: Armed Forces Institute of Pathology, 1961].) **B,** the tall columnar picket cell of the mucinous cystoma resembles the secretory cells of the endocervix. This photomicrograph is of the endocervix. The intracytoplasmic mucin and the arrangement of nuclei at the base of the cell are characteristic features. (From McKay, D. G.: Clin. Obst. & Gynec. 5:1186, 1962.)

a rare complication but hydrothorax and ascites have been described. Hemorrhage may occur into a large cyst, or secondary infection and suppuration with rupture may occur. If penetration of the capsule occurs with subsequent implantation and growth of mucinous epithelium in the peritoneal cavity, the condition is known as pseudomyxoma peritonei. However, most authors feel that this is a malignant complication and occurs only in the malignant variety of tumor. Since these tumors reach extremely large size, the enlargement of the abdomen may be quite marked.

The accepted treatment for an obviously benign mucinous cystoma is unilateral oophorectomy, particularly in the younger patient. The opposite ovary should always be bisected and examined carefully for evidence of cystic disease. If the patient is over age 40 a bilateral oophorectomy should be done in conjunction with hysterectomy.

Although all papillary cystomas, both serous and mucinous, are considered potentially malignant, the precise diagnosis of carcinoma in a mucinous cystadenoma is somewhat difficult. Numerous sections should be selected from all portions of the neoplasm and particularly from the papillary or semisolid areas. The carcinomas tend to be well differentiated (Fig. 7-17) and in the series of Allan and Hertig 46 per cent were grade I, 48 per cent grade II and only 6 per cent were grade III. The majority of the tumors retain their multicystic nature when malignant and are papillary to a variable degree. In the study by Kent and McKay only 12 per cent of the 478 mucinous tumors at the Boston Hospital for Women were malignant. Malignant mucinous cystomas have a predilection to spread directly to the pelvic peritoneum and to adjacent pelvic organs, although the typical frozen pelvis is not common. These tumors do not metastasize by way of

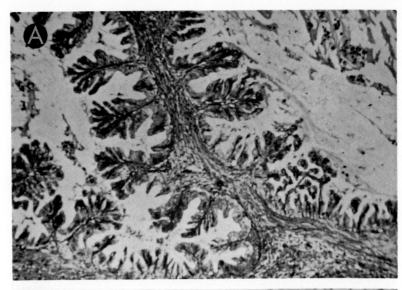

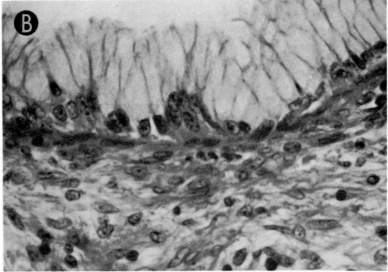

Fig. 7–16.—Mucinous cystoma. **A,** low power; **B,** higher power, to compare structure to that of endocervix seen in Figure 7–15. (From McKay, D. G.: Clin. Obst. & Gynec. 5:1190, 1962.)

the lymphatics as do the serous tumors. However, metastasis to the uterus is common.

Pseudomyxoma peritonei refers to the process of secondary implantation of mucinous tissue on the peritoneum, with subsequent local invasion and proliferation. It generally is accepted as a malignant type of mucinous tumor. Eventually there is a production of a thick, gelatinous, mucinous material which may entirely fill the pelvis and abdomen. Pseudomyxoma peritonei may also result from rupture of a mucocele of the appendix.

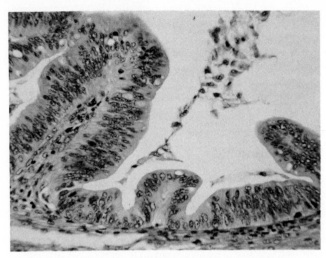

Fig. 7-17.—Mucinous cystadenocarcinoma. The epithelium is thrown into folds and, although a suggestion of mucinous character is present, the individual cells show anaplasia, increased mitotic activity, vacuolation and dyspolarity.

Clinically this condition causes a progressive enlargement of the abdomen with evidence of marked increase in abdominal pressure. Flank dullness is noted with anterior tympany but usually shifting dullness is not present as it is with ascites. Occasionally when the masses are rubbed together a typical grating sensation may be palpated.

The tumor consists of gray, jell-like masses, which are actually mucin in a colloid state surrounded by a pseudomembrane. Within this mucin, strips of epithelium are identified which show actively secreting columnar and low cuboidal cells. In certain areas, discharge of the secretion into connective tissue stroma may be noted. The peritoneum may show an aseptic foreign-body reaction. The condition is usually progressive and, although the histology may appear benign, the disease is clinically malignant since death frequently results from mechanical interference with vital structures. At surgery, the primary site and as much as possible of the mucinous material should be removed.

At the Boston Hospital for Women the optimum treatment for mucinous carcinomas is believed to be hysterectomy and bilateral salpingo-oophorectomy. This treatment is carried out even though the disease appears to be confined to one ovary since 15–25 per cent of these carcinomas are bilateral.

Cystadenofibroma, Benign and Malignant

This tumor may be regarded as a cystadenoma in which at least one-fourth of the tumor mass is solid and fibromatous. The epithelial component is derived from the surface epithelium and the connective tissue originates from the cortical stroma, the tunica albuginea or both. These tumors are more common than generally supposed since they are usually symptomless. It usually occurs in patients past the menopause and the majority are in patients over age 50. In 1942 Scott reviewed the literature and reported 31 cases, 14 of which were his own. Scott found that 93 per cent of the patients were over 40 years of age and 64 per cent were over 50. The tumor is usually a benign serous type although an occasional malignant variant has been reported. Other variations include a mucinous or endometrial epithelial component.

These tumors vary considerably in size; some are just barely visible microscopically, appearing as minute nodules on the surface of the ovary. The largest typical unilateral fibrous tumor is rare but may measure up to 20 cm. in greatest diameter and appear as irregularly lobulated masses. Tumors are bilateral in approximately 15 per cent of patients and vary considerably in the amount of cystic formation. The variety that is mainly solid, containing only small cystic areas, has been classified separately by some authors as serous adenofibromas (also so-called solid adenomas, fibroadenomas and fibromas with inclusion cyst). Other forms are largely cystic and hence papillations may occur within the cystic spaces. Grossly, a cystadenofibroma resembles a Brenner tumor or a thecoma. The cut surface is quite fibrous and yellow but numerous minute cysts and others as large as 10 cm. in diameter may occasionally be found. The fluid from these cysts is usually clear or straw color but thick, brown, viscid material is sometimes present. Papillary processes may be identified on the surface of the tumor or as papillary fibromas projecting from the lining of the larger cysts.

The basic histologic pattern of the cystadenofibromas is that of a dense connective tissue matrix in which are embedded innumerable small cystic spaces (Fig. 7-18). These cysts are lined by cuboidal to columnar epithelium which is often ciliated. The nuclei of this epithelium are centrally or basally placed, round or oval and relatively large. The fibromatous stroma is predominant and assumes a whorl-like arrangement of spindle cells with

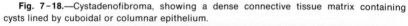

Fig. 7-18.—Cystadenofibroma, showing a dense connective tissue matrix containing cysts lined by cuboidal or columnar epithelium.

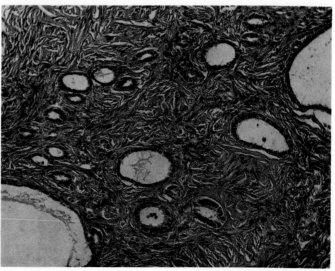

varying degrees of hyalinization. Papillae are usually composed of dense fibrous tissue covered by an epithelium similar to that which lines the cyst.

Carcinoma of the endometrium and hyperplasia have been associated findings. These endometrial lesions suggest that cystadenofibromas have an estrogenic effect which is consistent with the ovarian cortical derivation of their stroma. Hysterectomy and bilateral salpingo-oophorectomy are adequate treatment.

Endometrioid Carcinoma

In August, 1961, a conference of the Cancer Committee of the International Federation of Gynecology and Obstetrics was held in Stockholm for the purpose of standardizing both a histologic and a clinical classification for cancer of the ovary. Although only the common epithelial ovarian tumors were considered, it was proposed by Santesson of Sweden that a new group be added termed "endometrioid" because of the relatively frequent prevalence of this cell type. Although carcinomas arising in endometriosis had been recognized in the United States since Sampson's first description in 1925, this entity had been considered a rare phenomenon. Thompson reviewed the subject in 1957 and found only 30 previously reported cases including those reviewed by Kistner and Hertig in 1952. Thompson added 17 cases of his own and upon observing that all 47 were adenoacanthomas stated that all primary adenoacanthomas arose in endometriosis. Since that time, however, there have been a number of reports of endometrial-like cancers presumably arising in endometriosis but without squamous elements.

At the Stockholm Conference, according to Long and Taylor, Santesson presented 616 histologically reviewed primary ovarian cancers of which endometrioid tumors comprised 24.4 per cent. For inclusion in this category, Santesson did not require evidence of origin from endometriosis. Long and Taylor attribute the paucity of previously reported cases to a general adherence to Sampson's strict criteria of 1925 (see Chapter 9, endometriosis, pathology, p. 437).

Long and Taylor (following Dr. Taylor's participation in the Stockholm Conference) reviewed and reclassified 120 consecutive primary ovarian carcinomas at the Columbia Presbyterian and Francis Delafield Hospitals. After meticulously establishing histologic criteria for diagnosis, they found 20 cases of endometrioid carcinoma or 16.7 per cent. Forty per cent were classified as papillary serous cystadenocarcinomas, 10.8 per cent as mucinous carcinomas and 6.7 per cent were undifferentiated adenocarcinomas.

The histologic criteria used by Long and Taylor to differentiate these tumors from papillary serous cystadenocarcinomas are as follows: (1) glandular or acinar type of cellular arrangement with varying resemblance to primary endometrial carcinoma depending upon the differentiation of the tumor. (2) Papillae, when present, should be blunt in contrast to the finer branching papillae of serous tumors. (3) The growing border of the tumor should be even without the papillary projections of serous tumors. (4) Squamous metaplasia may be present. (5) With differential staining techniques glycoprotein and non-specific mucin can be distinguished in the apical regions of the epithelial cell and abundant extracellular mucin can be seen. Although most authors concur with these criteria for diagnosis,

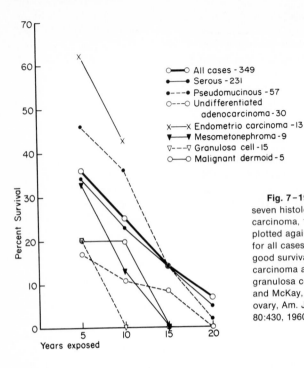

Fig. 7-19.—Survival curves for seven histologic types of ovarian carcinoma, 1904–1952, as plotted against the survival curve for all cases. Note the relatively good survival rate in endometrioid carcinoma and the low rate in granulosa cell carcinoma. (From Kent, S. W., and McKay, D. G.: Primary cancer of the ovary, Am. J. Obst. & Gynec. 80:430, 1960.)

Scully requires the absence of mucinous cells and the assurance that the ovarian tumor is not metastatic from the endometrium. Scully also includes those tumors which he believes arise from endometriosis, namely, clear-cell carcinomas (mesonephroma), squamous cell carcinomas, stromal sarcomas and carcinosarcomas.

Grossly, endometrioid carcinomas are cystic, ranging in size from 10 to 25 cm. in greatest diameter and contain a "chocolate" or mucoid fluid. They may be indistinguishable from the usual benign "chocolate" cyst. Although tumor masses may penetrate the cyst wall, the external papillary excrescences of serous cystadenocarcinomas are absent. About 30 per cent are bilateral.

Carcinomas arising in endometriosis have generally been associated with a favorable prognosis. Kistner and Hertig reported a 64 per cent five-year survival rate among their 14 cases of primary adenoacanthoma and Kent and McKay reported a 63 per cent five-year salvage for their 13 cases of endometriocarcinoma (Fig. 7–19). Although Long and Taylor's 20 cases of endometrioid cancer were not observed to arise in endometriosis, 14 or 70 per cent survived for five years compared to a 33.3 per cent survival rate for serous carcinomas during the same period. However, only 45 per cent of the patients with endometrioid cancer had primary extraovarian metastases while 75 per cent of the serous group had tumor dissemination to pelvic or abdominal structures. Also of significance is the relatively low histologic grade assigned the endometrioid tumors since fully 50 per cent were in the grade I category. Nevertheless, Long and Taylor showed an improved five-year survival rate for endometrioid carcinomas regardless of stage or grade.

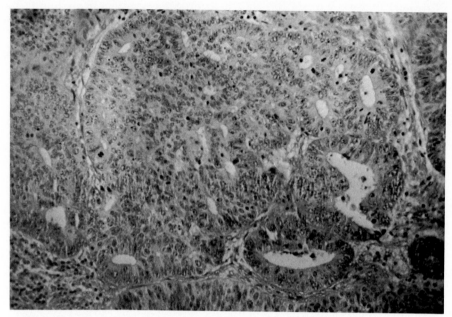

Fig. 7-20.—Endometrioid carcinoma of the ovary indistinguishable from a primary carcinoma of the endometrium. The tumor was unilateral and the uterine cavity was uninvolved.

Schueller and Kirol, in reviewing 302 cases of primary ovarian cancer classified 37 or 11.1 per cent as endometrioid. Although only 37.8 per cent survived five years (8.1 per cent followed for less than 5 years), the survival rate was twice that of patients with serous carcinomas observed concurrently.

In contrast to these reports, Gray and Barnes in reporting 25 endometrioid cancers not arising in endometriosis found only 4 surviving five years and an additional 3 living one to two years following diagnosis. For a point of reference, 250 endometrial carcinomas were histologically graded for comparison with the ovarian tumors. These authors found 19 of the 25 endometrioid carcinomas of high grade (III and IV) and that 17 had disseminated beyond the ovaries. They admittedly had difficulty in classifying these higher grade tumors as endometrioid.

It seems likely that although carcinomas arising in endometriotic cysts do have a favorable prognosis, the relatively good five-year survival rate associated with other endometrioid cancers is not independent of the stage and the grade of the tumor. To be *easily* recognized as endometrioid type, these tumors must necessarily be fairly well-differentiated and thus of low histologic grade. At the Boston Hospital for Women a definitive diagnosis of endometrioid cancer is still reserved for well differentiated tumors such as that illustrated in Figure 7-20.

Carcinoma of the Ovary

The subject of carcinoma of the ovary will be dealt with generally at this point since more than 90 per cent of ovarian malignancies fall into the "germinal" epithelial category.

Cancer of the ovary is the fourth leading cause of cancer deaths in American women, and ranks first in mortality among the gynecologic cancers. In contrast to the rapidly declining death rate from carcinoma of the cervix, the mortality rate from ovarian cancer has nearly tripled during the past four decades (from 3.2 to 8.9 per 100,000 per year).

The increase in ovarian cancer mortality is a result of an increasing incidence without concurrent improvement in the five-year survival rate above an average of 25 per cent. Although the greatest increase in incidence has occurred in the older age group where the relative five-year survival rate is the worst, the increased mortality is not simply the result of an aging population. Age adjusted rates show the same upward trend and compatible increases also are evident in specific age groups as well as in successive birth-date cohorts. Epidemiological studies have failed to uncover any environmental or other predisposing factors to explain the increase in incidence. Although single and nulliparous women appear to have a greater incidence, the significance of this observation has not been confirmed statistically. The incidence among Caucasians has been significantly greater than among non-whites although the gap has narrowed in recent years. Consistently higher death rates are found unexplainably in the Northeastern states.

Prevention.—Between 4 and 9 per cent of reported patients with cancer of the ovary, previously have undergone ablative pelvic surgery with conservation of one or both ovaries. These percentages have led many surgeons to advocate the prophylactic removal of normal ovaries at the time of hysterectomy. Proponents of ovarian salvage argue that the risk of developing cancer in a residual ovary is negligible and is outweighed by the evils of early castration. However, inimical sequelae to premenopausal castration have not been well defined particularly when exogenous estrogen is administered. There is no indication that the risk of ovarian cancer in women with residual ovaries differs from that of the general population or is reduced by removing only one ovary. If the 1962–1964 death rates prevail, more than one out of every one hundred women in the United States between the ages of 30 and 45 will eventually die from ovarian cancer. Only about 6 per cent of these deaths will be prevented by prophylactic ovariectomy at the time of hysterectomy, but the risk to the individual is reduced from 1 per cent to 0.

Detection and Diagnosis.—Recent reports indicate that treatment of cancers localized to one or both ovaries will result in a relative five-year survival rate near 75 per cent, while a 12 per cent five-year survival rate results if regional or distant spread has occurred. The distressingly poor survival rate for all cases is ascribed to the fact that fewer than 30 per cent of ovarian cancers are localized at the time of diagnosis. Obviously the detection of ovarian carcinoma during its localized or palpable stage is of the utmost importance. The infrequency of early diagnosis is attributed to the asymptomatic character of early cancer of the ovary. The presenting complaints as previously described usually include low abdominal pain, or pressure, or concern for a mass or abdominal enlargement. Unfortunately, these symptoms are related either to the accumulation of fluid, to the size and weight of the tumor, or to its adherence to surrounding structures with resultant traction or pressure. In other words, the usual symptoms are those of advanced growth. The fervent hope of many gynecologists that pelvic examinations attending the routine periodic Papanicolaou smears would uncover a greater number of early cancers of the ovary has not been realized. Neither the percentage of localized cases, nor the five-year survival rate has shown significant improvement in the past two decades. However, obstetrician-gynecologists tend to see women in the childbearing or menopausal ages. Elderly women without pelvic complaints, those more likely to have an *early* ovarian cancer, are also more likely to consult general practitioners or internists rather than gynecologists for their extra-pelvic complaints. Unfortunately, as late as 1958 a survey of Massachusetts internists suggested that less than 50 per cent performed routine pelvic examinations. Without question, greater emphasis should be placed on the importance of both the immediate examination of the patient with unexplained pelvic symptoms and the management of the patient with a pelvic mass.

Cytologic smears of the cervix and vagina occasionally are positive in patients known to have cancer of the ovary, but it is a rarity when a suspicious or positive smear is responsible for the detection of an early ovarian carcinoma. In 1964, Graham, Graham and Schueller reported on the pre-clinical detection of ovarian cancer by the cytologic examination of peritoneal fluid obtained from the transvaginal aspiration of the cul-de-sac. They obtained positive smears from 26 of 45 patients with known ovarian cancer and from 8 of 576 asymptomatic women. Of the seven patients subjected to laparotomy, metastatic breast cancer was found in one and suspicious atypical papillary lesions of the germinal epithelium, possibly pre-malignant, were found in 5. No lesion to account for the abnormal cells could be detected in the seventh patient. There were no complications from the technique, but adequate specimens could not be obtained from 20 per cent of the patients screened. McGowan, Stein and Miller screened 1,123 asymptomatic women over the age of 34 without obtaining a positive smear. However, mesothelial cells establishing the adequacy of the peritoneal sample were found in only 53 per cent of patients. There were no complications.

Although this technique appears promising, procurement of an adequate sample and interpretation of the cytologic findings seem to be major problems. Considerable refinement is needed before this technique can be accepted as a general screening measure. However, limited trials in the high risk age groups seem warranted.

Factors in Prognosis.—Survival curves for seven histologic types of ovarian cancer are illustrated in Figure 7–19. The survival curve for serous carcinomas which comprise 61 per cent of the total closely matches the survival curve for the whole group. Comparatively better five-year survival rates are found for the endometrioid and mucinous tumors, while poor rates are associated with undifferentiated adenocarcinomas and malignant teratomas.

The clinical stage of the disease, that is, the extent of tumor growth at the time of diagnosis, provides the best estimation of prognosis. A multiplicity of staging classifications has in the past prevented uniform reporting of the end results of therapy. The classification adopted by the International Federation of Gynecology and Obstetrics (FIGO) and approved by the American College of Obstetricians and Gynecologists should now be universally accepted.

Stage I   Growth limited to the ovaries
    Stage I-A Growth limited to one ovary; no ascites
    Stage I-B Growth limited to both ovaries; no ascites
    Stage I-C Growth limited to one or both ovaries; ascites present
        with malignant cells in the fluid
Stage II   Growth involving one or both ovaries with pelvic extension
    Stage II-A Extension and/or metastasis to the uterus and/or tubes only
    Stage II-B Extension to other pelvic tissues
Stage III   Growth involving one or both ovaries with widespread intraperitoneal metastasis to the abdomen (the omentum, the small intestine and its mesentery)
Stage IV   Growth involving one or both ovaries with distant metastasis outside the peritoneal cavity
Special Category   Unexplored cases which are thought to be ovarian carcinoma (surgery, explorative or therapeutic, not having been done)

The correlation between stage and five-year survival is demonstrated in Table 7-3 where Munnell's and Kent and McKay's series are combined and modified to fit the FIGO staging. Since older staging systems have not allowed for Stage I-C and II-A, the prognostic implications of these substages are as yet unclear. However, a few reported patients with uterine or tubal spread only (Stage II-A) have fared better than those with generalized pelvic dissemination (Stage II-B).

The histologic grade or degree of cellular differentiation of the epithelial cancers also correlates with five-year survival rates (Table 7-4).

The histologic grade apparently operates as an independent factor in determining prognosis and correlates with survival figures within a given stage. Thus, the five-year survival rate attending grade I tumors is three to four times that of grade III tumors regardless of stage. The microscopic grade correlates with prognosis only among the epithelial tumors and is of little value with granulosa cell tumors, arrhenoblastomas and dysgerminomas.

Although the histologic cell type appears to be important (Fig. 7-19), it probably has little influence on prognosis independent of stage and histologic grade. For example, the favorable prognosis generally ascribed to patients with mucinous carcinomas can be explained by the fact that 50 per cent or more are confined to one ovary (Stage I-A) and more than half are grade I tumors. By comparison only 25 per cent of serous carcinomas are either Stage I or grade I tumors. The favorable prognosis associated with endometrioid cancer has been discussed in this same regard. Undifferentiated adenocarcinomas by definition are of high histologic grade and therefore signify a poor prognosis.

TABLE 7-3.—RELATION OF STAGE TO PROGNOSIS
(Modified from Munnell and Kent and McKay)

STAGE	NO. OF CASES	5-YEAR SURVIVAL NO. OF PATIENTS	%
I-A	299	183	61.2
I-B	94	58	61.6
II	147	46	31.3
III	360	31	8.6
Totals	900	318	35.3

TABLE 7-4.—RELATION OF GRADE TO PROGNOSIS
(From Kent & McKay)

	No. of Cases	5-Year Survival No. of Patients	%
Grade I	83	54	65
Grade II	131	56	42.7
Grade III	115	12	10.4
Ungraded	20	5	25
Totals	349	127	36.4

The inadvertent rupture of malignant ovarian cysts with intra-abdominal spillage of the cyst contents during surgical removal has been considered an event of ominous portent. However, several large clinical studies including those of Munnell, Malloy, and Rubin failed to show an altered prognosis in this group. In a recent report from the Boston Hospital for Women, Grogan found that accidental cyst rupture had occurred in 16 of 124 patients (12.9 per cent) undergoing primary operation for ovarian cancer. There was no apparent compromise in survival among this group and early recurrence and death were associated only with advanced stage or high microscopic grade of the tumor.

The presence of ascites as an independent factor in determining prognosis of epithelial tumors has been debated. There is general agreement that this finding bears no influence once the tumor has disseminated (Stages II–IV). Some, however, feel that ascitic fluid containing malignant cells is an ominous sign in Stage I disease. For this reason the International Federation allocated Stage I-C for this group. There is little doubt that ascites signifies a poor prognosis when associated with cancers of germ cell origin.

In summary, the stage and grade of tumors of germinal epithelial origin are by far the most significant factors in prognosis, superseding the specific cell type in importance.

TREATMENT

The basic concept in the primary treatment of ovarian cancer is the extirpation of all gross tumor when feasible and when the patient's life is not thereby endangered. Hysterectomy and bilateral salpingo-oophorectomy, though adequate surgical treatment for patients with localized cancer, also are indicated when technically possible in patients with pelvic or abdominal dissemination. Even when extensive growth replaces both ovaries, lines of cleavage can usually be found between the tumor and adherent loops of bowel or other viscera. When spread to the pelvic peritoneum has occurred, a retroperitoneal approach along the iliac vessels and ureters will permit removal of the uterus, perimetrium, tumor and adjacent peritoneum *en bloc*. In such instances, plastic material, such as polyethylene or silastic, may be used to cover the denuded pelvic cavity, thus preventing prolapse of the small bowel. When localized involvement of the bladder or rectosigmoid occurs, these organs may be resected in contiguity with the primary mass. The common occurrence of tumor masses in the omentum makes omentectomy a frequent adjunct. Although the prophylactic removal of an uninvolved omentum is still advocated by some, this procedure has not improved end results and may predispose to later bowel obstruction.

Kottmeier, of Sweden, and Long, Johnson and Sala, in the United States, have advocated the use of radiotherapy prior to an extended surgical approach. However, the consensus at this time favors what Munnell has termed a "maximal surgical effort," at the time of initial operation. In reporting on 235 cases of primary ovarian cancer at the Columbia-Presbyterian Medical Center from 1952 to 1961, Munnell compared the results of treatment with those of two previously reported studies, covering the periods 1922–1943 and 1944–1951. The five-year survival rate of 40 per cent in the recent series represented a significant improvement over the 28 per cent survival rate observed in each of the two previous studies. Munnell concluded that the unexpected improvement was not the result of earlier diagnosis or a more favorable distribution of cases, but rather was due to a more aggressive surgical attack, as well as a more liberal use of postoperative irradiation. In considering 107 patients with upper abdominal spread, it was possible to remove most of the cancer in 36 with a 28 per cent five-year survival rate in this group. With only partial removal, the survival rate was 9 per cent while only 3 per cent survived five years if a biopsy alone was performed. In like manner, Hreshchyshyn observed a median survival time of 11.5 months in patients with Stage III (FIGO) disease, in whom more than 50 per cent of the tumor had been excised. The median survival time was only 3.5 months if less than half the tumor bulk had been removed.

Figure 7–21 shows survival curves according to stage and extent of surgical resection from a recent study by Griffiths at the Boston Hospital for Women. Surgical group A consists of those patients with abdominal dissemination in whom more than 75 per cent of the tumor bulk was excised and group B comprises the remainder. All patients with Stage II disease (pelvic dissemination) had maximal surgical procedures. The median survival time of the Stage II patients was 39 months with 7 of the 15 living without disease from 3 to 8 years following operation. Although the extent of disease was comparable in groups A and B, the group A survival curve more closely matches the Stage II curve up to 30 months. Despite the divergence at that point, four group A patients are living and well from 4 to 8 years after operation. No patient in group B survived 38 months.

Reoperation may have merit in patients with persistent or recurrent cancer following irradiation. Brunschwig performed radical operations excising as much tumor as possible in 65 patients. Significant palliation was achieved in 26 patients and an additional 5 patients were living and well from 5 to 10 years later. Dr. George V. Smith of the Boston Hospital for Women has reported four long-term survivors following radical surgery for recurrent seemingly hopeless ovarian cancer.

Despite an abundance of reports in the literature on the management of ovarian cancer, the role of postoperative radiotherapy remains an ill-defined subject. There is little question that irradiated tumor masses often regress in size or disappear entirely. However, the failure of postoperative irradiation to improve five-year survival rates in many reported series has led some authors to question its palliative value, much less its potential curability. The true value of postoperative x-ray has, in fact, been obscured

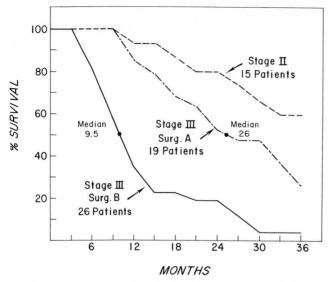

Fig. 7-21.—Survival curves by the life table method according to Stage and extent of surgical resection. Group A—75 per cent or more of tumor volume excised. Group B—less than 75 per cent excised.

by the lack of randomized series of patients. Thus, when radiotherapy is reserved for less favorable cases, as in many institutions, the irradiated group cannot fairly be compared with the prognostically more favorable, though non-irradiated, group. In addition, five-year survival rates cannot be used as a measure of palliation, since most patients with advanced disease succumb within three years, regardless of the treatment employed. However, increased survival in terms of months, during which time the patient returns to a normal or near normal existence, frequently has been observed following external irradiation. Palliation of this degree cannot be discounted.

A critical paper entitled, *Has Post-Operative Irradiation Proved Itself?*, was presented by Rubin, in 1961. In response to questionnaires on this subject sent by Rubin to major universities and cancer centers in the United States, most radiotherapists advocated the use of radiation, but expressed doubtful or negative opinions in regard to its curative value. After evaluating his own series and reviewing those published by others, Rubin concluded that a comparison of patients with Stage II disease with and without postoperative irradiation would provide the best assessment of radiocurability. Residual disease in the pelvis is certain postoperatively, but the tumor volume is relatively small and the area can reasonably be encompassed by a radiation field. Rubin found a 44 per cent, five-year survival in his own irradiated group (Stage II-B), with comparable rates being reported by others. Survival was consistently better than when surgery alone was used. Rubin considered these figures good evidence of the curative value of postoperative radiotherapy.

The effect of postoperative radiotherapy on five-year survival rates is presented by stage in Table 7-5. The significantly better survival rate of

TABLE 7-5.—FIVE-YEAR SURVIVAL RATES FOR STAGES I, II AND III
WITH AND WITHOUT POSTOPERATIVE IRRADIATION (COLLECTED SERIES)

STAGE	OPERATION ONLY		OPERATION PLUS IRRADIATION	
	NO. OF PATIENTS	%	NO. OF PATIENTS	%
I	274	62.4	281	58.4
II	110	19	190	42
III	312	3.5	298	11.4

irradiated Stage II patients is obvious. Even though irradiation has failed to improve survival among Stage III patients in individual series, a small difference is evident in this collected series.

For some years all patients at the Boston Hospital for Women with ovarian cancer, regardless of stage or the operation performed, have received postoperative radiotherapy. Dosage has been in the range of 3000r to 4000r to the lower abdomen and pelvis for all stages. Patients with extensive Stage II or Stage III disease have received an additional 2000r to 3000r to the upper abdomen with appropriate shielding of the kidneys. The advocacy of routine radiotherapy has stemmed primarily from the report of Kent and McKay in which significantly improved survival rates were observed among the irradiated patients with both Stage I and Stage II disease. The apparent benefit of radiotherapy for Stage I disease is in part the result of the unexpectedly low five-year survival rate of 49 per cent among the non-irradiated patients. Sixty-eight per cent of the irradiated patients survived five years. The latter figure is in keeping with survival figures for all Stage I patients (Table 7-3). Although the collected series (Table 7-5) fails to show improvement in Stage I survival by postoperative irradiation, it must be remembered that the poor risk patients, i.e., those irradiated, well may be benefited. Since the five-year survival rates of Stage I patients with poorly differentiated tumors (grades II and III) rarely exceed 50 per cent, postoperative irradiation seems indicated in this group.

Variation in the radioresponsiveness of specific cell types has been noted by a number of authors. Although radiotherapists have based their conclusions on the degree of observed tumor regression for a given radiation dose, gynecologists have noted an increase in survival with the irradiation of some cell types, but not with others. For example, with mucinous cancer Kent and McKay observed a five-year survival rate of 48.5 per cent with operation alone, and 50 per cent with operation plus x-ray. They thus concluded that mucinous tumors are relatively radioresistant. Rubin, after collating clinical experiences reported in the literature and responses to his questionnaires sent to radiotherapists, attempted to list ovarian cancers in order of radiosensitivity. He defines radiosensitivity as the dose required to produce tumor regression in relation to the tolerance of the surrounding normal structures. If the dose is low, the tumor is radiosensitive; as it approaches tolerance, it is radioresponsive and if it exceeds the tolerance of normal tissue, the tumor is considered radioresistant. The cell-types are listed below in order of decreasing radiosensitivity as modified from Rubin. Rubin feels that mucinous carcinomas are the least responsive of the epithelial group, but are not wholly radioresistant.

Dysgerminoma Granulosa Cell Tumor }	Sensitive
Serous Carcinoma Endometrioid Carcinoma Undifferentiated Carcinoma Mucinous Carcinoma }	Responsive
Mesometanephroma Teratoma }	Resistant

Chemotherapy

The observation in the early nineteen fifties that nitrogen mustard could produce a significant regression in the size of ovarian tumor masses has led to the widespread use of anti-cancer drugs for the palliation of advanced carcinoma.

The drugs most effective in inducing ovarian tumor regression are those classified as alkylating agents. This term refers to their ability to bind a highly reactive alkyl group to metabolically important sites within the cell rendering them incapable of functioning in their usual manner. The active component of the parent compound nitrogen mustard is the chloroethyl group which after being transformed into a cyclic ethyleneimine gives rise to a reactive center at the site of the ethyl moiety (Fig. 7–22). Since the mustards contain two chloroethyl groups, each capable of alkylation, they have been termed polyfunctional alkylating agents. Although they probably react indiscriminately with many cellular components, their primary anti-tumor action appears to be related to their ability to bind to the DNA of the cell nucleus. Recent studies indicate that the major site of alkylation is the 7-nitrogen of the guanine base in the DNA molecule. The exact mechanism by which the alkylating agents exert their cytotoxic effect is not known. However, cross linking may be an important reaction in which the two reactive groups of the mustard molecule join together two points, either in the same or different DNA chains in the manner of a grappling hook. This concept would account for the greatly enhanced activity of the bifunctional over the monofunctional mustards and might

Fig. 7–22.—Process of alkylation of an X receptor site by nitrogen mustard. The initial step is the release of chloride ion from one of the chloroethyl groups and the formation of a highly reactive cyclic ethyleneimine. This reactive center is capable of rapid binding to specific "X" receptor sites within the cell. Although not depicted, the second chloroethyl group undergoes the same process simultaneously. (From Hall, T. C.: New England J. Med. 266:129, 1962.)

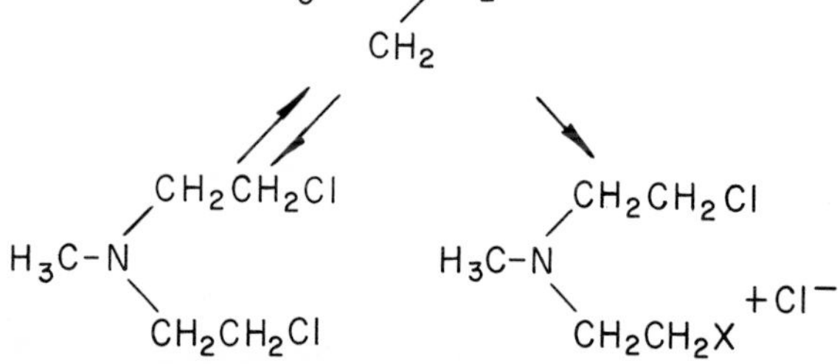

explain the apparent inability of these cells to undergo mitosis. Because of their direct attack on the DNA molecule, these compounds appear to be equally effective during any phase of the mitotic cycle and are thus relatively short acting. The effect of mustard on cells both in vitro and in vivo consists of nuclear enlargement or pyknosis with fragmentation or focal swelling of chromosomes. Although cytoplasmic growth may continue and bizarre early mitotic figures may be observed, cell division does not occur. Histologic similarities with irradiated cells have led some to refer to the alkylating agents as radiomimetic.

As with radiation therapy the anti-tumor action is dose related and the limiting factor in dosage is the tolerance of normal but susceptible tissue. None of the currently available chemotherapeutic agents are tumor specific. The rationale for their use is the exploitation of a differential in growth rate and metabolic activity between the cancer cell and the normal cell. Thus, rapidly proliferating normal cells such as those of the bone marrow and gastrointestinal mucosa are susceptible, though hopefully to a lesser degree. The toxic side-effects of nitrogen mustard therapy include leukopenia and thrombocytopenia reflecting bone marrow suppression. Because of the longer biologic life span of the red cell, anemia is uncommon even though reticulocytosis is inhibited. Hematopoietic depression usually becomes manifest seven to ten days following administration and may persist for several weeks. Vomiting is a frequent occurrence at the time of intravenous administration of nitrogen mustard but this effect is probably mediated through the central nervous system. Diarrhea is variable but is mild or absent when the dosage is within the recommended range. The extreme vesicant property of nitrogen mustard necessitates careful injection into a running IV infusion. Local thrombophlebitis at the injection site may occur.

Nitrogen mustard (mechlorethamine, mustargen, HN_2) is given intravenously in a dose of 0.4 mg./kg. divided over a two- to four-day period, followed in two weeks by a maintenance dose of 0.1 mg./kg. given at weekly intervals. It may also be given by intracavitary instillation in a dose of 0.4 mg./kg. for the control of pleural or peritoneal effusions. Should the white cell count (WBC) lie between 3,000 and 5,000 or the platelet count between 75,000 and 100,000 per cubic millimeter, only one-half the usual dose is given. The drug is omitted if the WBC falls below 3,000 or the platelet count below 75,000.

Various modifications of the mustard molecule have been made in attempts to reduce its toxicity and to promote a selective action against the cancer cell. Attempts to modify toxicity have included the substitution of the methyl group of nitrogen mustard with certain stable acid radicals to form mustard amides. The mustard is thus nonreactive until the amide is hydrolysed and the active dichlorethyl amine moiety is released.

Chlorambucil (Leukeran), a phenylbutyric acid substituted mustard (Fig. 7–23), can be administered orally and has a relatively slow onset of activity. It has the same degree of effectiveness against the same spectrum of tumors as nitrogen mustard. Although this drug has a wider margin of safety and minimal gastrointestinal side-effects, its prolonged use is associated with hematopoietic toxicity comparable to that of nitrogen mustard. Chlorambucil has been used extensively against ovarian cancer. The largest series has been reported by Masterson and Nelson from Kings

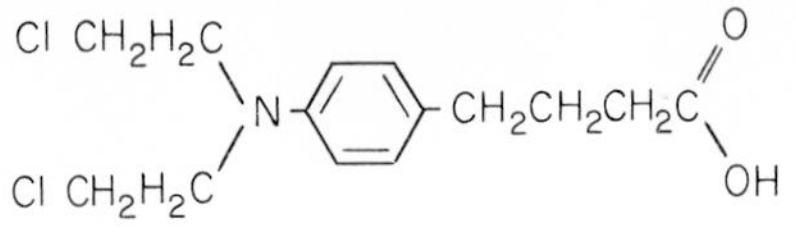

Cl CH₂H₂C
        \
         N—⟨benzene ring⟩—CH₂CH₂CH₂C
        /   \\O
Cl CH₂H₂C   OH

Fig. 7-23.—Structural formula for chlorambucil.

County Hospital who recommend an oral dose of 0.2 mg./kg. of body weight daily repeated in four-week courses. These authors found a 50 per cent objective response rate among 280 patients so treated. Their figures also suggest that a mild leukopenia should be maintained to insure optimal dosage.

The synthesis of cyclophosphamide (Cytoxan, Endoxan) is an example of an attempt to promote tumor selectivity as well as to reduce toxicity. Based on the studies of Gomorri and others which indicated that tumor tissue contained higher levels of phosphatases and phosphaminases, a cyclic phosphamide was combined with the mustard moiety (Fig. 7-24). It was hoped that this compound would be preferentially activated by the tumor cell. Unlike most other alkylating agents, cyclophosphamide is inactive in vitro and active in vivo only after breakage of the phosphamide ring. It now appears that this oxidative process takes place in the liver and is unrelated to phosphamidase hydrolysis. This drug seems to have a slightly wider spectrum of anti-tumor activity and greater tumor selectivity than the other mustards. Its toxicity is somewhat different in that thrombocytopenia is a rare occurrence. Countering the platelet sparing advantage is a 25 per cent incidence of alopecia and an occasional case of hemorrhagic cystitis. The latter is a result of the prolonged action on the bladder mucosa of active breakdown products which are excreted in the urine.

Cyclophosphamide may be administered orally at a daily dosage of 3 mg./kg. or intravenously in doses of 15 mg./kg. weekly. Previously irradiated patients usually require modification of this dosage but the white blood count is a reliable index to the optimal dose. This agent is the drug most used for advanced ovarian cancer at the Boston Hospital for Women both as an adjuvant to surgery and radiation in primary treatment or alone for recurrent disease. The dose is titrated against the white blood count to maintain a mild leukopenia (WBC 3,000-5,000) and during long-term therapy counts may be needed only every two to four weeks. In a collected series of 152 patients from seven institutions, objective remissions were observed in about 40 per cent regardless of prior therapy.

Another example of the "Trojan horse" approach is the phenylalanine substituted mustard, melphalan (Alkeran, L. phenylalanine mustard, sarcolysin) which was synthesized because of the avidity of certain tumors, particularly melanoma, for this amino acid (Fig. 7-25). Although this drug is activated prior to entering the cell as well as in vitro, it has a slow onset of action with toxicity comparable to that of chlorambucil. It has been used almost exclusively at the M. D. Anderson Hospital both alone and as an adjuvant to radiotherapy in the management of advanced ovarian carci-

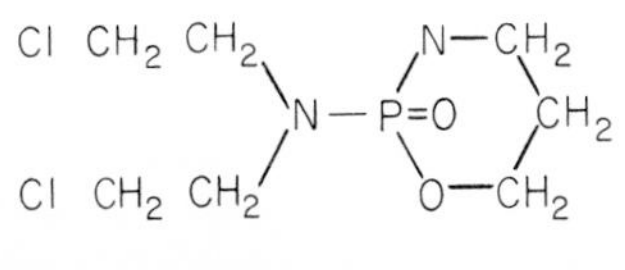

Cl CH₂ CH₂   N—CH₂
          \   /   \
           N — P=O   CH₂
          /   \   /
Cl CH₂ CH₂   O—CH₂

Fig. 7-24.—Structural formula for cyclophosphamide.

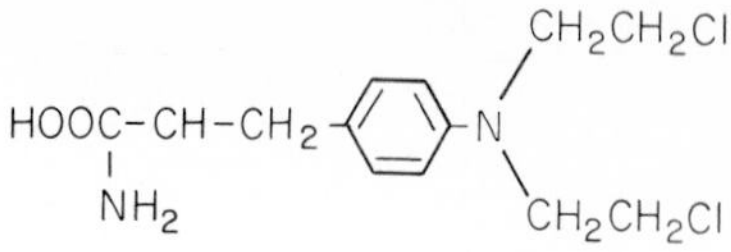

Fig. 7-25.—Structural formula for Melphalan. $HOOC-CH-CH_2-\langle\bigcirc\rangle-N\begin{smallmatrix}CH_2CH_2Cl\\ \\CH_2CH_2Cl\end{smallmatrix}$

$\underset{NH_2}{|}$

noma. Burns *et al.* from this institution have reported 116 objective responses among 185 patients treated. They have used the drug intravenously but currently recommend a course of oral administration at a dose of 1.0 mg./kg. divided over a five-day period which is repeated every four weeks.

The first alkylating agent used in a significant number of patients with ovarian cancer was triethylene thiophosphoramide (Thio-tepa). As can be seen on inspection of the structural formula (Fig. 7-26), this drug is not a mustard but contains three preformed ethyleneimine groups stabilized into a phosphoramide molecule. Although it is nonreactive, it acts somewhat faster than the substituted mustards. It is administered primarily by the intravenous route but is effective in reducing effusions when injected into serous cavities. Since it is not an irritant many physicians prefer it to nitrogen mustard for intracavitary instillation. The toxicity is similar to that of the substituted mustards. Hreshchyshyn has had wide experience with this drug in ovarian cancer and recommends an initial course of 0.4 mg./kg. on two successive days followed by a maintenance dose of 0.2 mg./kg. weekly. Using exceptionally strict criteria for objective response, he has reported twelve responses out of 68 patients treated.

At the present time the available evidence suggests that all of the alkylating agents have the same mechanism of cytotoxic action and with the possible exception of Cytoxan the same spectrum of anti-tumor activity. Certainly, none of these drugs has demonstrated therapeutic superiority over the others in the treatment of ovarian cancer. In addition, tumors with innate or acquired resistance to one alkylating agent will likely be resistant to other alkylating agents.

Table 7-6 lists the collected objective responses to each of the previously discussed agents obtained from a number of published reports. Differences in the ratio of objective responses to patients treated are related to variations in criteria for objective response and a variable selectivity of patients in the reported series. In regard to the latter, objective responses to an anticancer drug will be modified by the prior cancer therapy and, most important, by the patient's temporal relationship to the natural history of her disease.

In contrast to the alkylating agents which attack the DNA molecule directly, another class of chemotherapeutic agents, the antimetabolites, exert their antitumor effect by inhibiting the synthesis of DNA. Since they

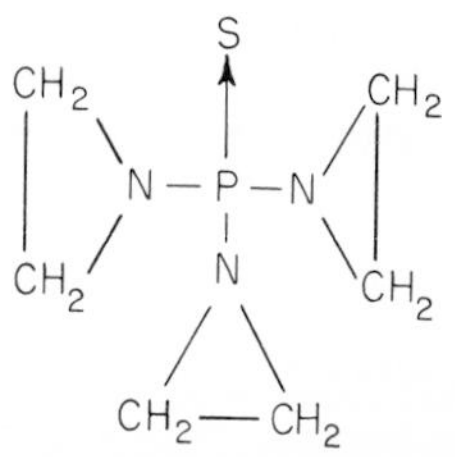

Fig. 7-26.—Structural formula for Thio-tepa.

TABLE 7-6.—COLLECTED RESPONSES OF OVARIAN
CARCINOMA TO ALKYLATING AGENTS

DRUG	COLLECTED RESPONSES	TOTAL NO. PATIENTS
Nitrogen Mustard	9	25
Thio-tepa	97	269
Chlorambucil	178	368
Cytoxan	60	152
Melphalan	122	208
Total	466	1022

act only during the phase of DNA synthesis (S phase) in the mitotic cycle, they must be given for prolonged periods. Gastrointestinal toxicity is more prominent than with the alkylating agents and may be manifested by oral ulceration, nausea and vomiting, and severe diarrhea. Moderate leukopenia and thrombocytopenia are common and are most severe 18 to 21 days after the initial dose. 5-Fluorouracil is the only antimetabolite that has been used to any extent for ovarian cancer and the results have been generally disappointing. Despite reports in the literature of objective responses in 15 per cent of patients, no favorable response to this drug has been observed at the Boston Hospital for Women.

The absence of tumor cross resistance to radiation and alkylating agents suggests that these two modalities act in different tumor cell populations. Nevertheless, the radiomimetic qualities of alkylating agents have led to their use as adjuvants to radiotherapy in the hope of increasing the radiosensitivity of ovarian carcinoma. In 1960 Miller and Brenner reported 16 of 19 objective responses among patients treated with x-ray and chlorambucil while only two of seven patients responded to x-ray alone. Hreshchyshyn found that the median survival time of 114 patients with advanced ovarian cancer treated by x-ray alone was only four months. A group of 23 similar patients simultaneously treated by irradiation and Thio-tepa had a median survival time of 13.5 months. This same survival time was obtained if the two agents were employed sequentially.

In reviewing the Stage II and III (FIGO) patients from the Boston Hospital for Women, Griffiths found a median survival time of 26 months in a group of 19 patients in which optimal surgery was followed by adequate irradiation. However, in a similar group of 13 patients in which Cytoxan or chlorambucil was given concurrently with the x-ray, a median survival time of 53 plus months was observed. In addition, the mean free interval (time till recurrence) was 10.5 months in the irradiation alone group and 18.3 months in the combined treatment group (p = .02). In the suboptimal surgical group irradiation induced the same proportion of objective responses as did the combined treatment. However, a greater number of complete responses was obtained in the combined treatment group than in the irradiation alone group and duration of response and median survival time of the responders were double those of the patients treated by x-ray alone.

In conclusion, radiation most likely is more effective than chemotherapy in the primary treatment of advanced cancer of the ovary but there is evidence that the combined or sequential use of these two modalities affords greater palliation and prolongation of life than does either one alone. As in the case of operative treatment, improved survival in terms of months appears to be inversely proportional to the volume of tumor treated by either agent. This suggests that a stepwise fractional reduction in tumor volume by the sequential use of surgery, x-ray and chemotherapy may in some instances reduce the number of surviving tumor cells to the point where normal host defenses will eliminate the residuum. This concept of "first order kinetics" currently being applied to the treatment of leukemia and choriocarcinoma thus may be applicable to the treatment of ovarian cancer as well.

Gonadal Stromal Tumors

The common origin of gonadal stromal tumors is adequate explanation for their marked histologic similarity and the difficulty with which pathologists distinguish one from the other. Therefore, all gonadal stromal tumors will be considered under this major heading whether they are derived from male-directed or female-directed gonadal stroma. The three major tumors under this classification are the granulosa-theca cell tumors, the arrhenoblastomas and the gynandroblastomas.

Granulosa-Theca Cell Tumors

Granulosa cell tumors may be considered a variant of the granulosa-theca cell neoplasms, sometimes called the feminizing mesenchymomas. These are tumors which are composed of elements of the wall of the graafian follicle. The histologic type and hormonal activity of the tumor will depend on the predominance of a particular cell type as well as its stage of maturity and ability to secrete sex steroids. Kottmeier has reported that combined granulosa-theca cell tumors constitute from 4 to 9 per cent of all ovarian neoplasms. Hertig and Gore found the incidence at the Boston Hospital for Women to be approximately 6 per cent. They also noted a distribution of the various types as follows: granulosa cell, 17.5 per cent; granulosa-theca cell, 15 per cent; theca cell, 67.5 per cent.

Tumors of this general variety may occur at any age from 1 to 90 years. However, most granulosa cell tumors occur during the postmenopausal years and only a few in the prepuberal era. In a study by Hodgson the average age was given as 52 years, with 61 per cent occurring postmenopausally, 37 per cent during the reproductive years and slightly less than 2 per cent before puberty.

The histogenesis of granulosa-theca cell tumors has not been clearly defined. It is generally accepted that normal granulosa cells and cells of the theca interna and externa arise from the ovarian cortical stroma if an ovum is present as a "cell organizer." Hertig and Gore believe that these tumors arise from the ovarian cortical stroma or its follicular wall derivatives. Other theories of histogenesis include that of Gilman, who suggested that the granulosa cells are derived from the germinal epithelium and the theca cells from the cortical stroma. Robert Meyer theorized that these tumors arose from "granulosa ballen" which he believed to be embryonic rests of granulosa cells in the ovarian cortex. Sternberg and Gaskill have traced the genesis of thecomas from cortical stromal hyperplasia, whereas Traut and Butterworth and McKay and associates have advanced the theory that these neoplasms originate from remnants of follicular epithelium in involuting follicles.

Animal experimentation lends support to the idea that granulosa-theca cell tumors may arise from residual cellular elements following death of the ovum and release of the follicles from their normal and cyclic gonadotropic stimulation. Thus, the experiments by Furth and Butterworth, in which irradiation of the ovaries of mice resulted in a high incidence of subsequent granulosa cell tumors, suggest that, following disappearance of the ovum, tumors develop as a result of constant gonadotropic stimulation. In other experiments, fragments of normal ovaries grafted into the spleens of gonadectomized mice also developed granulosa-theca cell tumors. The end-result of these experiments is to provide a constant stimulation of the follicular elements by gonadotropic hormones, since ovarian estrogen is actively removed from the general circulation by its shunt through the liver. The common denominator of the whole process is the loss of the ovum associated with aging of the follicular wall. Subsequent stimulation of residual cellular elements may then occur, as in menopause, when the level of gonadotropic-stimulating hormone is high and the level of estrogen is low.

The degree of hormonal activity in each tumor is variable. Further, the clinical characteristics which occur as a result of the secretion of estrogen will vary, depending on the patient's age. Thus, in the prepuberal child the syndrome of precocious pseudopuberty occurs. This is characterized by the development of adult feminine contour, breast growth, axillary and pubic hair, enlargement of the genitalia both internal and external, anovulatory bleeding, hyperplastic endometrium and an estrogenic vaginal smear (see Figs. 12–4 and 12–5). During the postpuberal period the clinical picture is not striking, but irregular menses are common if adequate estrogen is secreted. Ovulation is usually suppressed and a total secondary amenorrhea may be the presenting complaint. When the tumor occurs postmenopausally, the characteristic symptoms are irregular uterine bleeding and occasionally enlargement of the breasts. If the tumor is large, it may cause abdominal pain and pressure symptoms. Torsion of the pedicle with subsequent infarction occurs occasionally, and because of the soft, pultaceous characteristics of some varieties, rupture into the peritoneal cavity may cause a catastrophic incident. Ascites and hydrothorax have been noted rarely.

The granulosa cell tumor is generally regarded as having a low potential for malignancy (3–14 per cent) but the recurrence rate may be as high as 25 to 30 per cent. Certain of these tumors are histologically benign but are clinically malignant in that numerous local recurrences may be noted over a span of 10–15 years. There does occur, however, a definitely malignant type of granulosa cell tumor which has the characteristic histologic criteria of carcinoma. In these tumors the theca cells usually remain benign in appearance. Metastases from such a lesion may occur quickly via lymphatics and the blood stream.

Granulosa cell tumors are usually unilateral, only 12–18 per cent being reported as bilateral in some series. (Thecomas are almost always unilateral.) The tumor may vary in size from 0.4 to 40 cm. and may weigh as much as 35 lb. Grossly they appear as solid, mobile, oval or round encapsulated neoplasms with a smooth, lobulated, yellow-tan surface. Although the

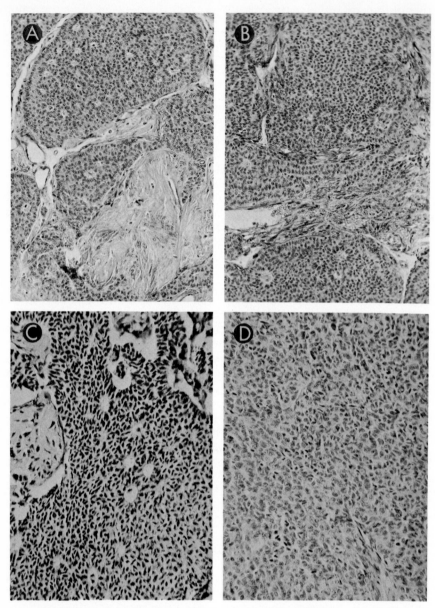

Fig. 7–27.—A, granulosa-theca cell tumor showing folliculoid pattern of granulosa cells and collagenous hyalinization of the thecal stroma. **B,** granulosa-theca cell tumor showing sarcomatoid pattern *(above)*, cylindroid pattern *(center)* and folliculoid pattern *(below)*. (A and B from Hertig, A. T., and Gore, H.: *Tumors of the Female Sex Organs: Part 3. Tumors of the Ovary and Fallopian Tube,* sec. IX, fasc. 33 of *Atlas of Tumor Pathology* [Washington, D.C.: Armed Forces Institute of Pathology, 1961].) **C,** granulosa-theca cell tumor showing typical Call-Exner bodies in a folliculoid pattern. **D,** granulosa-theca cell tumor showing pleomorphism and numerous mitoses in upper right. This is classified histologically as a malignant tumor, death occurring two years after surgery.

consistency is generally firm, if cystic degeneration or necrosis has occurred the tumor may be quite soft.

Cross-section of a typical tumor reveals it to be solid but partially cystic, quite cellular and slightly trabeculated. Areas of hemorrhage, necrosis or liquefaction are commonly identified. The consistency of the tumor will depend also on the relative proportion of epithelial to stromal elements. Thus, neoplasms which contain a small number of granulosa cells may have an extensive degree of collagen in the thecal elements and thus be a very firm tumor. The color seen on cross-section is a direct reflection of the degree of luteinization of the cellular elements.

The microscopic appearance of the granulosa cell tumor may be just as variable as the picture seen on cross-section. The characteristic cell is of course the granulosa cell. These cells are of uniform size, polygonal shape with poorly defined cytoplasmic borders. The cytoplasm is slightly granular and eosinophilic. The nuclei are large, round or oval, stain homogeneously but rarely show mitotic figures. The theca cells are easily differentiated since they are spindle shaped, have ovoid nuclei and resemble fibroblasts. Lipoid droplets in the theca cells may be accentuated by specific stains to differentiate these cells from fibroblasts. Theca cells may be differentiated from granulosa cells in some of the more anaplastic tumors by the use of a reticulum stain, since a supporting reticulum is always identified around theca cells but not around individual granulosa cells.

Numerous patterns of granulosa cell tumors have been identified histologically. These have been termed the folliculoid, adenomatoid, cylindroid, sarcomatoid and trabeculoid varieties (Fig. 7-27). The commonest pattern is the folliculoid, in which the cells are arranged in rosette fashion, with the nuclei placed at right angles to a central space. This arrangement resembles a developing follicle. If the pattern is exaggerated to the point of formation of glandular patterns, the form is called adenomatoid, whereas if the cells are arranged diffusely, it is called a sarcomatoid type. In the cylindroid pattern the granulosa cells are arranged in rather typical columns, with the theca cells arranged in diffuse sheets or whorls around these cell columns. When luteinization occurs, the cells increase in size, the outlines become more distinct and the cells may be vacuolated.

DIFFERENTIAL DIAGNOSIS.—In the differential diagnosis of granulosa cell tumors, consideration must be given to the age group in which they occur. In the prepuberal child, the precocious pseudopuberty induced as a pure estrogenic effect by this tumor must be differentiated from true precocious puberty. In the latter, there are normal ovarian cycles with ovulation, so that pregnancy may occur. This primary or "constitutional" precocious puberty accounts for 90 per cent of all premature female sex development. Usually it is due to a premature activation of the ovary by constitutional pituitary factors of unknown origin. Rarely, however, neoplasms or inflammatory lesions of the midbrain or choriocarcinomatous teratomas which produce gonadotropic hormone may cause a similar picture. Hormone excretion studies are frequently of diagnostic help. In true precocious puberty adult levels of pituitary gonadotropins as well as cyclic variations in urinary estrogen and pregnanediol will be found. In the pseudopuberty due to a granulosa cell tumor the estrogen levels in urine are considerably above the normal adult level and do not have cyclic variations. Furthermore, pregnanediol will not be found in amounts compatible with a luteal phase. In the absence of a palpable pelvic mass, laparotomy is rarely indicated; however, culdoscopy or laparoscopy may be of value. X-rays of the sella turcica together with funduscopic examination and visual field determinations should be done if a midbrain tumor is suspected.

During the reproductive period, the combination of menstrual irregularity and a solid adnexal mass should cause suspicion of the presence of a feminizing neoplasm. Following menopause any sign of increased estrogenic activity is important. If the vagina is well rugated and a vaginal smear is well cornified and particularly if endometrial hyperplasia is found in conjunction with a palpable solid adnexal mass, a granulosa-theca tumor is strongly suspected. These women frequently appear younger than their chronologic age and many will note the onset of menopausal symptoms, such as hot flushes and sweats, after removal of the tumor.

TREATMENT.—The treatment in the prepuberal group is unilateral excision. Removal of the feminizing tumor is followed by prompt and often dramatic regression of the precocious symptoms and signs. In women of childbearing age the minimum suggested therapy is a unilateral salpingo-oophorectomy. This pertains only if the lesion is nonadherent, unilateral, has an intact capsule and is not hemorrhagic on section. As previously mentioned, the malignant potential of these tumors was considered at one time to be quite low. However, as increasing numbers of patients are being followed for longer periods, it is becoming apparent that these neoplasms are frequently malignant. In a report by Henderson 60 per cent of the patients who had recurrence had been treated by simple oophorectomy only. A more radical approach may be in order, therefore, even in younger women. During the immediate premenopausal period as well as in younger women in whom there is evidence of extension, adhesions or metastases, hysterectomy and bilateral salpingo-oophorectomy should be performed.

There is no unanimity of opinion regarding the use of post-operative x-ray therapy in patients in whom there is evidence of extension or even in those treated by hysterectomy and bilateral salpingo-oophorectomy for confined disease. At the Boston Hospital for Women, 15 of 44 granulosa cell tumors were classified histologically as malignant. Of these 15 patients, 5 were treated by surgery alone, with 1 five-year survival (20 per cent) and 10 were treated by surgery plus x-ray, with 2 five-year survivals (20 per cent). None of the three patients surviving at five years was living at 10 years. These results are considerably at variance with the results noted at the Ovarian Tumor Registry, where 77 per cent of 96 patients who had granulosa cell tumors were living and well after five years.

There is another reason for performing a hysterectomy when a granulosa cell tumor is discovered. Endometrial hyperplasia or carcinoma of the endometrium may be a concomitant finding. Hertig and Gore, in a study of 75 feminizing mesenchymal tumors at the Boston Hospital for Women, reported that 60 per cent showed endometrial hyperplasia and one-fourth of these invasive carcinoma. Dockerty and Mussey found a 15 per cent incidence of endometrial carcinoma associated with granulosa cell tumors in their study. This finding has not been borne out in other reports, however, since Emge found endometrial carcinoma in only 3 per cent of feminizing mesenchymal tumors and Grady had a similar low incidence. Despite this fact the high incidence of leiomyomas as well as adenomyosis occurring in patients with granulosa-theca cell tumors is sufficient reason for performing a hysterectomy unless there are specific indications for preservation.

Thecoma.—As previously mentioned, the "thecoma" should not be considered a specific tumor made up of theca cells alone, since, if adequate sections are taken, a certain number of granulosa cells will be discovered. It is generally accepted that the hormone production of these tumors is from the active theca cell. Ketone-containing substances have been demonstrated in these cells by histochemical methods and it has therefore been assumed that the theca cells are the site of steroid synthesis. The exact type of hormone secreted—estrogen, progesterone or androgen—will depend on many factors, such as the availability of substrates and various co-factors as well as the kinetics of reaction in this particular synthetic pathway. It is generally accepted that the basic substrate cholesterol is converted into estrogens via Δ^5-pregnenolone, progesterone, 17-alpha-hydroxyprogesterone and Δ^4-androstenedione. Therefore these cells must be considered multipotential and able to produce and secrete progesterone, androstenedione and testosterone as well as estradiol.

The thecomas are not as common as the granulosa cell tumors, constituting only 1–2 per cent of all ovarian tumors and about 3–5 per cent of solid ovarian tumors. They have been reported in females from 1 to 90 years of age, but 70 per cent occur in the postmenopausal group. Thecomas are unilateral and usually benign. They vary in size from microscopic cellular aggregations of theca cells to ovarian masses measuring 15–20 cm. The larger tumors are frequently adherent to surrounding structures. The cut surface is either homogeneously yellow or has a somewhat fibrotic appearance that is diffusely mottled with yellow. Hyalinization or liquefaction may be present. Histologically, a thecoma resembles a fibroma with plump, fusiform cells arranged in a whorled pattern. In contradistinction

Fig. 7–28 (left).—Thecoma showing fibrillar appearance of cellular cytoplasm and interlacing bundles of fibrous connective tissue.

Fig. 7–29 (right).—Thecoma showing cluster of luteinized granulosa cells.

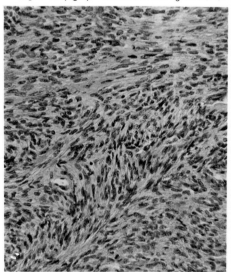
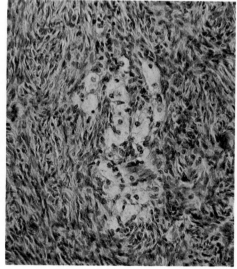

to fibromas, however, intracellular fat globules may be demonstrated with fat stains. Bundles of theca cells may be separated by interlacing bands of collagenous, fibrous connective tissue (Fig. 7–28). The cytoplasm of the theca cell is occasionally vacuolated but has a fibrillar appearance, with indistinct cell borders. Scattered throughout the tumor are clusters of luteinized granulosa cells (Fig. 7–29). Between the theca cells a reticulum may be identified by a silver staining method. In other areas of the ovary or in the opposite ovary, stromal hyperplasia or focal thecomatosis may be identified.

There is reason to believe that the histogenesis of thecomas differs from that of granulosa cell tumors. Woll *et al.* noted a change in the aging ovary which they designated as *cortical stromal hyperplasia* (Fig. 7–30). This consists of a diffuse or nodular thickening of the ovarian cortex which is unusually dense and often assumes the shape of spherical or scalloped masses. Usually there is a diminution in the number of ova and follicles, and the stromal cells are grouped into more than the usual number of whorls and fascicles. Intercellular collagen is scant, accounting for the fact that the cortex appears an unusually dark blue when the stained section is viewed by the unaided eye.

Such cortical thickening varies from patient to patient; in some ovaries it occurs only focally, producing nodular masses. These focal areas are often arranged in whorls and are identical with the histologic pattern of thecomas. The evidence, then, that theca cell tumors have their origin in cortical stromal hyperplasia is: (1) the histologic pattern of both tissues is identical, including the presence of hyaline plaques; (2) transitional stages between cortical stromal hyperplasias and thecomas are observed; (3) patients with theca cell tumors of one ovary almost invariably have cortical stromal hyperplasia of the opposite, uninvolved ovary, and (4) both conditions occur primarily in the postmenopausal age groups.

The clinical effects of thecomas are variable. Some patients may be asymptomatic, whereas others will have local discomfort or pressure effects which may be due to degeneration, hemorrhage, torsion or rupture of the cyst. Occasionally Meig's syndrome may be present with a thecoma. The clinical picture is not always clearly one of estrogen secretion. Although patients with thecomas often have anovulatory uterine bleeding, persistent flowing from secretory endometrium has been noted to accompany bilateral thecomas in women during the premenopause. The most characteristic clinical feature is atypical uterine bleeding similar to that found with granulosa cell tumors. Enlargement of the breasts is occasionally noted, together with microscopic evidence of fibrocystic disease. The uterus, even in the postmenopausal period, is found to be enlarged and softened and the endometrium is typically hyperplastic in nature. Leiomyomas of the uterus have been reported as occurring in 50 per cent of patients with thecoma, and a concomitant endometrial carcinoma may also be found.

Since the majority of thecomas are benign, conservative surgery is indicated. Less than 20 malignant thecomas have been reported in the world literature, and it may be that these tumors were actually granulosa cell tumors of the sarcomatoid variety. Histologically the malignant thecomas have shown a pleomorphic cell structure with excessive mitoses and ne-

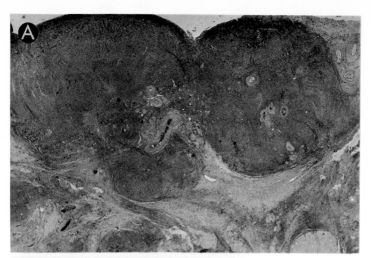

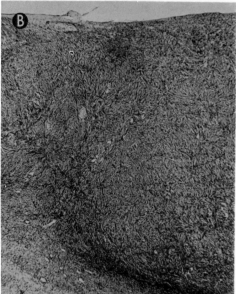

Fig. 7-30.—Cortical stromal hyperplasia. A, section of ovary of postmenopausal patient. The surface of the ovary is nodular, due to the proliferation of stromal cells into the periphery of the cortex. Occasionally the areas of stromal hyperplasia extend into the medulla and occupy almost the entire sectioned surface of the ovary. B, low-power view of ovarian surface, showing marked thickening of the cortex. Note the absence of ova and follicles and the fascicular arrangement of stromal cells. In left center are several foci of lutein cells. C, high-power view, showing characteristic large stromal cells with plump, blunted nuclei. In the central area is a focus of lutein cells arranged in clumps. These lutein cells are indistinguishable from those seen in some polycystic ovaries of patients with the masculinization syndrome. (Courtesy of Drs. Arthur T. Hertig and Hazel Gore.)

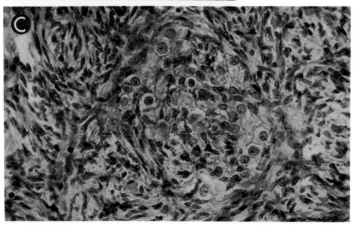

385

crosis. Invasion of the ovarian serosa has occurred together with metastases to omentum and bowel.

Treatment usually consists of unilateral oophorectomy and bisection of the opposite ovary in the young or middle-aged patient. This should always be accompanied, however, by a thorough curettage to rule out the presence of a simultaneously occurring carcinoma of the endometrium. If the endometrium is found to be hyperplastic at the time of laparotomy, subsequent ovulation and the secretion of progesterone will usually cause a reversion of this abnormal endometrium to the normal secretory type. If the patient is in the mid- or late forties or if she is postmenopausal, the usual treatment is hysterectomy and bilateral salpingo-oophorectomy. X-ray therapy is given only if malignant changes have been noted in the tumor.

Luteoma.—In certain classifications the term *luteoma* has been used to describe a specific ovarian tumor. Most observers contend that this neoplasm is actually a luteinized granulosa cell tumor since, in at least a small group of patients, the effects of progesterone on the endometrium have been demonstrated. The luteoma is a rare tumor and as such should be distinguished from the virilizing lipoid cell tumor (adrenal rest tumor) of the ovary. Luteomas are unilateral and benign, histologic examination revealing the cells to be rather large with pale-staining cytoplasm and well-defined cell boundaries. They may be difficult to distinguish histologically from the adrenal rest tumor but it is generally believed that "virilizing luteomas" are not true luteomas but are adrenal rest tumors. A sufficient number of patients having luteomas has not been reported to allow speculation concerning the incidence, the symptomatology or the malignant potential of the tumor. Simple surgical excision in most cases is deemed adequate therapy.

Hyperthecosis Syndrome.—Under the general heading of granulosa-theca cell tumors a consideration should be given to the hyperthecosis syndrome described by Shippel. He postulated the intriguing theory that the pure thecoma is in effect a masculinizing tumor. However, as a result of admixing with granulosa cells, the tumor may produce endometrial patterns ranging from cystic glandular hyperplasia to complete atrophy, together with menstrual abnormalities such as dysfunctional bleeding or amenorrhea. Shippel contended that the hyperthecosis syndrome comprised six pathologic phases, the first three being concerned with theca-granulosa synergism and the last three with thecal dominance. Thus, if untreated, patients who manifest various phases of irregular uterine bleeding will eventually progress to amenorrhea. Pathologically, the endometrium shows first crowding of glands, glandular intussusception, cystic glandular hyperplasia and finally atrophy. The female is transformed into a masculinized, hirsute, sterile, often frigid individual with temporal hair recession, atrophied uterus and endometrium, and occasionally enlargement of the clitoris and breast atrophy.

Although this is an attractive theory, the interruption of the pathologic process during the theca-granulosa synergistic state prevents adequate follow-up of the patient into the state of thecal dominance. As previously mentioned, subtle changes in the biosynthetic pathways of steroids in the theca cell may eventuate in an overproduction of estrogenic steroids followed later by incomplete synthesis and the production of androgen.

Arrhenoblastoma

The arrhenoblastoma is a rare ovarian tumor which characteristically causes amenorrhea, defeminization and virilization. It is the most common of the various masculinizing tumors of the ovary and occurs most often during the childbearing period, most cases having been reported in patients between ages 25 and 45 with an average age of approximately 32 years.

In 1960 Pedowitz *et al.* reported only 240 cases in the world literature. At the Boston Hospital for Women, Dr. Arthur T. Hertig has had the opportunity to study only 12 cases in consultation.

The arrhenoblastomas are unilateral in about 95 per cent of patients. Gross appearance is that of a smooth but occasionally lobulated tumor which may be solid or cystic. These tumors vary in size from 0.5 to 15 cm., although much larger neoplasms have been reported. The cut surface is firm and grayish yellow although necrosis, hemorrhage and cystic degeneration are common.

Histologically, three variants are recognized. (1) The *typical tubular* form (tubular adenoma of Pick) is a well-differentiated form in which round or oval tubules suggest a mature tubular adenoma (Fig. 7–31). (2) The *atypical* is a more solid or intermediate form which contains imperfect tubules and irregular columns of cells with nuclei at right angles to the long axis of the cell cords, sarcoma-like areas and clusters of typical Leydig cells. (3) The *undifferentiated* or *sarcomatoid* form has only suggestive cordlike or tubular patterns (Fig. 7–32).

Three major cell types are identified in arrhenoblastomas. The tubules or glands are made up of *cuboidal* or *columnar cells*, the sarcomatous

Fig. 7–31.—Arrhenoblastoma showing typical tubular adenoma form originally described by Pick (grade I). The tubules are well differentiated and the individual cells contain clear cytoplasm. Leydig (interstitial) cells are not seen. (From Hertig, A. T., and Gore, H.: *Tumors of the Female Sex Organs: Part 3. Tumors of the Ovary and Fallopian Tube*, sec. IX, fasc. 33 of *Atlas of Tumor Pathology* [Washington, D.C.: Armed Forces Institute of Pathology, 1961].)

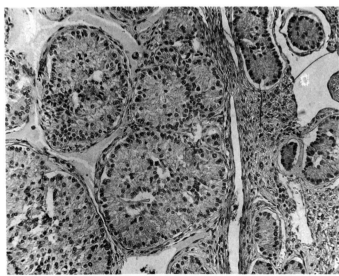

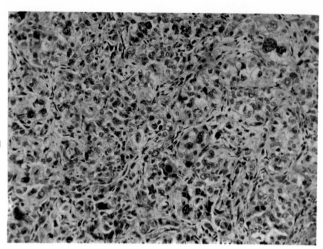

Fig. 7-32.—Arrhenoblastoma (grade III) of undifferentiated or sarcomatoid type. The cells are large, pleomorphic and show marked atypism with numerous mitotic figures.

areas are composed of *spindle-shaped* or *epithelioid cells,* and large polygonal cells with round, central nuclei and abundant cytoplasm represent the interstitial or Leydig cells. The Leydig cells are presumed to be the source of androgen secretion.

Arrhenoblastomas are thought to arise from ambivalent cellular elements in the ovary which tend to be of masculine cell type in their development, producing a hormone which activates both physical and latent psychic heterosexual characteristics. Although the precise histogenesis of the tumor has not been explained, Hughesdon and Frazier have indicated the following possibilities: (1) origin from an ovotestis; (2) origin from hilar "male-directed" cells; (3) origin from granulosa cell tumors; (4) origin from teratomas, and (5) direct origin from ovarian stroma resulting in a mixed mesodermal tumor with coelomic, testicular and müllerian derivatives.

Hertig and Gore feel that the embryonic gonadal stroma is fully capable of forming the nongerminal portion of the seminiferous tubule as well as its hormonally active stroma.

It should be emphasized that the presence of virilization is not necessary to make the diagnosis of arrhenoblastoma since the tumor may exist without external stigmata of androgen secretion. Thus, there is a gradual process of defeminization which is manifested originally by oligo-ovulation and then by total amenorrhea. This is followed by a regression of the female secondary sexual characteristics and in the full-grown syndrome there are usually marked hirsutism, partial alopecia, deepening of the voice and hypertrophy of the clitoris. Although virilizing signs diminish or disappear after removal of the ovarian tumor, hirsutism, may linger for a protracted time.

The diagnosis may be aided by certain laboratory studies but a definitive diagnosis can only be made by extirpation of the tumor. Virilization in the presence of an adnexal mass suggests arrhenoblastoma but the tumor is not palpable in 40 per cent of reported cases. The differential diagnosis includes adrenal cortical hyperplasia or tumor, basophilic pituitary adenoma, luteinized thecoma or luteoma, hilus cell ovarian tumor and gynandroblastoma.

Although the tumor usually produces excessive androgens, excessive estrogens may occasionally also be produced. The urinary 17-ketosteroid level may be normal or increased. However, direct analyses of tumor tissue have indicated the presence of progesterone, testosterone, androst-4-ene-3, 17-dione and androsterone. The finding of testosterone is of importance, since it explains the symptoms of virilism in the presence of normal or only slightly increased urinary 17-ketosteroids. (Moderate elevations of testosterone may produce virilism without significantly increasing the 17-ketosteroid level.) In reviewing the reports of steroid analyses of excised arrhenoblastomas, it seems likely that testosterone is the specific androgenic hormone causing the signs of virilization in most of these patients.

The presence of hypertension, diabetes, polycythemia and cutaneous striae suggests that the observed masculinizing signs are more likely due to adrenal cortical abnormalities and pituitary basophilic adenomas than to arrhenoblastoma. Similarly, masculinization occurring in the prepuberal girl is more likely to be due to adenomas of the adrenal cortex than to virilizing ovarian tumors. However, a few case reports indicate that both arrhenoblastoma and gynandroblastomas may occur in adolescence. When an adrenal cortical tumor is suspected, perirenal air insufflation and excretory urography may aid in the delineation of the tumor. In the congenital variety of adrenal cortical hyperplasia due to the inability of the adrenal cortex to synthesize hydrocortisone, the elevation of pregnanetriol levels in the urine is of diagnostic importance. Adrenal cortical hyperplasia may be differentiated from adrenal cortical tumor not only by the marked elevation in pregnanetriol, but also by a fall of the elevated 17-ketosteroid level in the patient with hyperplasia following intravenous administration of hydrocortisone.

It should be pointed out that most biologically active arrhenoblastomas are of the undifferentiated sarcomatoid type. However, the degree of differentiation cannot always be correlated with hormonal activity.

The malignant potential of an arrhenoblastoma is difficult to evaluate since five and 10 year follow-up studies are not available in most reported series. Javert and Finn reported malignancy in 22 per cent of 28 patients. Iverson stated that approximately 10 per cent of the tumors evidenced metastases and Henderson cited a 15 per cent recurrence rate. Metastases may occur to the periaortic and supraclavicular lymph nodes, lungs, liver, spleen, opposite ovary and bones.

The only method of treatment of an arrhenoblastoma is surgical excision. However, a unilateral oophorectomy should be performed only in the younger age group when conservatism is necessary for further childbearing. Of course, if local extension is present at the time of primary surgery, a complete hysterectomy and bilateral salpingo-oophorectomy should be performed. Similarly, in patients who have completed their family, complete extirpative surgery should be done. The value of radiation therapy as a postoperative adjunct is unknown. The signs and symptoms of virilization usually regress rapidly after extirpation, and menstruation may recur within one or two months.

GYNANDROBLASTOMA

The third tumor to be considered under the gonadal stromal tumors is known as the gynandroblastoma or Sertoli-Leydig cell tumor. This tumor is a mixture of various histologic elements which are compatible with both granulosa cell tumor and arrhenoblastoma. It was first described in 1930 by Robert Meyer, who theorized that it could arise from indifferent germinal epithelium surrounding the primordial germ cells. It is probable, however, that the gonadal stromal cells of common origin are differentiated into two major types. Thus, in some areas the tumor is rather typical of a granulosa-theca tumor, the theca cells showing varying degrees of luteinization. Presumably the biosynthesis of estrogen is carried to the usual end point in these cells. Similar routes of biosynthesis have been demonstrated in the human testis and the adrenal cortex. This unity in the biosynthetic process confers a potential for biologic heterofunction on all steroid-producing cells.

In other areas of the tumor a transition from folliculoid granulosa cell arrangement to tubular arrangement may be noted. Thus in areas around the epithelial cords or tubules are epithelial cells and interstitial (Leydig) cells which represent the prototype of ovarian theca interna and testicular interstitial cells. The interstitial cells in the gynandroblastoma demonstrate an eosinophilic cytoplasm with brown granular pigment. In one case at the Boston Hospital for Women described by Emig, Hertig and Rowe, areas were noted where typical granulosa cells were in immediate apposition to Sertoli-like cells and in between these areas were clusters of interstitial cells (Fig. 7–33). The latter cells have the potential for the secretion of either androstenedione, testosterone or estradiol.

Hertig has postulated that a gynandroblastoma simply represents a tumor of rather indifferent gonadal mesenchyme which retains the bisexual potential of the embryonic gonad. This is evidenced in both the epithelium and the stroma as well as in the variation in steroid synthesis in each stromal cell.

Less than 50 gynandroblastomas have been reported, but Hughesdon and Fraser, in a critical review, accepted only eight cases as being representative. Hertig has seen three additional cases, two from the Boston Hospital for Women and one in consultation.

The clinical observations on the reported cases indicate a dominant masculinizing effect of the tumor. However, the degree of virilism is variable and in some patients irregular uterine bleeding or hypermenorrhea may be the presenting complaint. In the one patient seen by the author at the Boston Hospital for Women, the presenting complaint was irregular and occasionally heavy uterine bleeding. At age 30 this patient had a right oophorectomy associated with a right salpingectomy for a tubal pregnancy. Following this she noted hirsutism which required daily shaving. Enlargement of the clitoris developed as did a male distribution of pubic hair. Menopause occurred at age 46 and at age 59 the patient was seen because of abnormal bleeding. The endometrium from the slightly enlarged uterus showed cystic and adenomatous hyperplasia with foci of carcinoma-in-situ. The circumscribed, gray, homogeneous tumor was identified in the hilar region of the left ovary and measured only about 1 cm. in greatest diameter.

The size of these tumors varies considerably from 1 to 20 cm. in greatest diameter. The microscopic picture has been described, but it should be mentioned that, because both granulosa cell tumors and arrhenoblastomas show marked variation in histologic pattern, caution should be exercised in making a final diagnosis of gynandroblastoma. The malignant

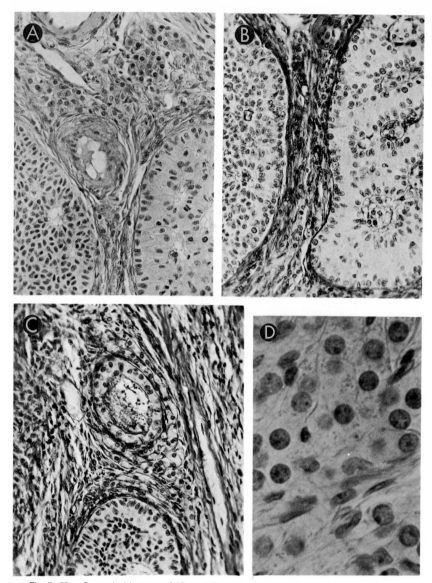

Fig. 7–33.—Gynandroblastoma. **A,** Sertoli-like epithelium is seen at lower right and granulosa cells at lower left. Multiple interstitial (Leydig) cells are scattered throughout the stroma but are clearly seen in the upper part of the photograph. **B,** high-power view shows an area of typical granulosa cells *(left)* and early tubule formation *(right)* in which the cells are of the Sertoli type. **C,** high-power view shows gradual transition between granulosa cells and Sertoli cells. The area below represents such a transitional area. The tubule above is surrounded by epithelial cells with stroma. The latter cells may be the prototype from which either theca interna or Leydig cells are derived. (A–C from Emig, O. R.; Hertig, A. T., and Rowe, F. J.: Obst. & Gynec. 13:135, 1959; Armed Forces Institute of Pathology photomicrographs.) **D,** higher power shows interstitial cells of Leydig. Pigment granules are seen in the clear cytoplasm.

potential of these tumors is unknown. The lesions reviewed by Hertig have not been morphologically malignant, but since granulosa cell tumors and arrhenoblastomas have a malignant potential one must assume that this tumor may behave similarly.

Germ Cell Tumors

DYSGERMINOMA

Several terms have been used for this tumor, such as small and large cell carcinoma and embryonal cell carcinoma, but the term *dysgerminoma,* first introduced by Robert Meyer in 1931, is most commonly used. The histologic morphology and clinical behavior of the dysgerminoma are identical to those of the male analogue, the testicular seminoma. The lesion appears morphologically malignant but has been considered in the past to be relatively benign.

The exact incidence of the dysgerminoma is difficult to determine. It has been estimated that these tumors constitute about 5 per cent of primary malignant ovarian tumors and about 1 per cent of all solid and cystic ovarian neoplasms. In a report by Kent and McKay only two cases were reported, both malignant, Pedowitz and Grayzel reported 17 cases in 1951, representing one of the largest individual series. Most patients are in the second or third decade of life although a 2-year-old patient has been reported. The oldest patient mentioned in the literature was 78. Pedowitz and Grayzel found an average age of 31 years in their 17 patients.

The histogenesis of dysgerminomas is obscure. The most acceptable theory suggests that the tumor arises from primordial germ cells before their differentiation into definitive sex cells. Pedowitz and Grayzel have suggested that the tumor arises from totipotential cells of the primitive gonadal mesenchyme. Since this tissue gives rise to the epithelial and non-epithelial components of the gonads in both male and female, the direction of differentiation of the cells will determine the nature of the specific tumor. Thus, in the female, male differentiation will result in an arrheno-blastoma while female differentiation will result in a granulosa-theca cell tumor. If the tumor arises from neuter cells, a dysgerminoma will result in the female and a seminoma in the male. Usually the cells of the dysgerminoma are neuter in regard to the production of male or female sex hormones. Occasionally the tumor secretes anterior pituitary-like hormone in the same manner as a seminoma of the testis. Numerous authors have reported mixed tumors composed of granulosa-theca cell tumors and dysgerminomas, further supporting the common origin from a totipotential mesenchymal cell. Similarly, teratomas and choriocarcinomas may be found occurring simultaneously since the totipotential cells also may give rise to these tumors.

DIAGNOSIS.—Although Meyer observed dysgerminomas in pseudohermaphrodites, most of the recently reported cases indicate that the tumor occurs in women of perfectly normal sexual development. Macmillan and Hertig have reported five cases of dysgerminoma removed during normal pregnancy. There are no characteristic symptoms but as the mass increases in size the patient may complain of vague abdominal pain, night sweats and fever. The abdominal pain and enlargement may be associated with recurrent attacks of nausea and vomiting. Leukocytosis is common since the dysgerminoma has a tendency to grow rapidly to a relatively large size, thus outgrowing its blood supply and predisposing to necrosis. Serosal involvement may produce an irritative peritonitis with associated pain, nausea and vomiting. Torsion of the cyst may occur, and Pedowitz and associates noted ascites in six of their 17 patients.

The only laboratory test of diagnostic value is one which determines the presence of chorionic gonadotropin. Thus, in a young individual with a solid ovarian tumor a positive pregnancy test is of diagnostic importance. After the removal of the tumor the pregnancy test becomes negative. The tumor should be examined carefully for presence of choriocarcinomatous tissue although the pregnancy test in a few cases has been positive without evidence of choriocarcinoma.

The simultaneous occurrence of choriocarcinomatous and dysgerminomatous elements within an ovarian tumor is exceedingly rare. Larson and co-workers reported a case in 1958 and cited four others in the literature. The signs and symptoms associated with this combined neoplasm are secondary to the secretion of chorionic gonadotropin. In the prepuberal female, there is usually early sexual maturation with an increased rate of growth and uterine bleeding. In the adult, changes similar to those noted during a normal pregnancy are seen; the breasts enlarge and colostrum may be expressed from the nipples. There is often an increased interval between the menstrual periods with subsequent hypomenorrhea followed by either amenorrhea or excessive flowing. Respiratory symptoms may be present if metastatic pulmonary lesions occur.

The dysgerminoma is usually a unilateral tumor which varies in size from 3 cm. to extremely large tumors which entirely fill the abdomen. The tumor is usually round or ovoid, and the surface may be smooth or covered by a fibrous capsule which disappears in the later stages of development.

Fig. 7-34.—Dysgerminoma showing solid groups of large, round or polyhedral cells with clear cytoplasm and a centrally placed nucleus. The fibrous connective tissue septa contain numerous lymphocytes. (From Hertig, A. T., and Gore, H.: *Tumors of the Female Sex Organs: Part 3. Tumors of the Ovary and Fallopian Tube,* sec. IX, fasc. 33 of *Atlas of Tumor Pathology* [Washington, D.C.: Armed Forces Institute of Pathology. 1961].)

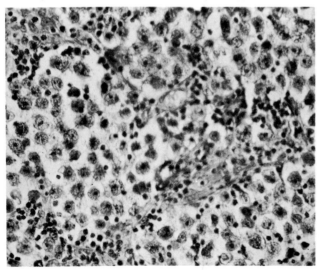

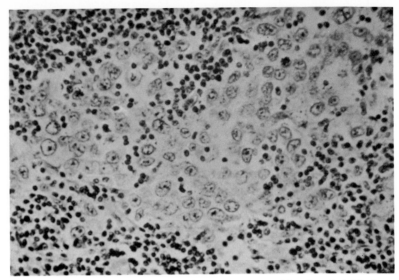

Fig. 7–35.—Dysgerminoma. High-power view shows typical lymphocytic infiltration.

Nodular excrescenses may be noted, and the tumor is rather rubbery in consistency unless extremely large, when it is quite soft and friable. On section the surface is grayish pink with foci of degeneration, necrosis and hemorrhage.

The microscopic appearance is characteristic. The cells which comprise the tumor are large, round or polygonal in shape with abundant clear cytoplasm and a large, centrally placed nucleus resembling the primordial germ cells of the indifferent embryonic gonad (Fig. 7–34). The cellular arrangement is alveolar and these alveoli are separated by strands of fibrous connective tissue which show hyalinization and infiltration with lymphocytes (Fig. 7–35). Mitotic figures in the epithelial cells may be numerous. In areas of degeneration large giant cells, similar to those seen in tuberculosis, may be identified. This was noted by Schiller to be fairly characteristic. This giant cell reaction has been confused with tuberculosis and when Mueller and associates reviewed the literature, they reported pulmonary tuberculosis in 176 of 427 patients with dysgerminoma. The dysgerminoma usually presents a uniform microscopic picture although, as previously mentioned, other malignant germ cell tumors may be associated. No apparent correlation exists between the histologic appearance of the tumor and its degree of malignancy.

Metastases may occur via the lymphatics or by direct contiguity. The organs involved are the omentum, liver, spleen, kidneys, gallbladder, pancreas, lungs, heart and even the thyroid gland and thymus. In four of the patients studied by Pedowitz, Felmus and Grayzel, hydroureter and hydronephrosis probably resulted from involvement of the periureteral nodes and paracervical area by the tumor.

Although only 6 per cent of patients have bilateral dysgerminomas at the time of primary operation, the contralateral ovary has a propensity for metastatic implantation. Pedowitz and associates noted that the residual ovary was the primary site of recurrence in 36 per cent of patients following conservative operations.

The prognosis attending a diagnosis of dysgerminoma has been an ill defined subject. Although this tumor has been considered a low grade malignancy in the past, Pedowitz, Felmus and Grayzel in 1955 reported a dismal 27.1 per cent five-year survival rate in a collected series of 102 cases. No patient with hemorrhagic ascites and only 12 per cent of patients with non-encapsulated tumors survived five years. Although these authors reported a 35.6 per cent survival rate with encapsulated tumors, the more recent studies of Malkasian and Symmonds and of Asadourian and Taylor suggest that an 85 per cent survival rate may be anticipated in this favorable group.

TREATMENT.—The optimal treatment of dysgerminomas is complete hysterectomy and bilateral salpingo-oophorectomy. At the time of operation all abdominal viscera as well as the para-aortic lymph nodes must be carefully palpated and biopsied when indicated to rule out the presence of metastatic disease. Since dysgerminomas are singularly radiosensitive, patients with metastatic disease including bilateral ovarian involvement, or with non-encapsulated tumors or ascites should undergo a course of radiotherapy. Postoperative irradiation has been effective both in preventing and treating recurrent tumor. Pedowitz and associates observed a 23.1 per cent five-year survival rate among patients with non-encapsulated tumors receiving postoperative radiotherapy. None in this group survived without irradiation. Malkasian and Symmonds at the Mayo Clinic have reported the survival of five of seven patients irradiated for recurrent disease. Metastatic sites included the abdomen, thorax and neck. Thoeny and Hunt from the same institution have advocated the use of prophylactic radiotherapy for all patients.

Since the majority of dysgerminomas occur in adolescence or young adulthood, there has been considerable interest in the preservation of childbearing function and the corresponding risk of conservative therapy. Malkasian and Symmonds found that the five-year survival rate of 27 patients with unilateral encapsulated dysgerminomas treated only by unilateral salpingo-oophorectomy was 80 per cent. The survival rate of 14 comparable patients treated by irradiation or more extensive surgery with and without irradiation was 87.5 per cent. Although 52.4 per cent of the conservatively treated patients developed recurrences, only 36.4 per cent of these died. The one patient in the radically treated group who developed recurrence was successfully irradiated. The recent report by Asadourian and Taylor is even more encouraging. Unilateral oophorectomy was the primary treatment in 46 of 71 patients with dysgerminomas confined to one ovary. The tumor recurred in ten of these (22 per cent) but was successfully controlled in six. The survival rate was 91 per cent. The same survival rate was observed among 21 patients undergoing bilateral oophorectomy with and without irradiation.

One must conclude that the preservation of childbearing potential in young patients with unilateral encapsulated dysgerminomas is possible but involves a calculated risk. Unfortunately fertility is apparently compromised in these patients since the subsequent conception rate in Malkasian and Symmonds' series was only 37.7 per cent. Candidates for the conservative approach should have resection of the opposite ovary as well as a unilateral salpingo-oophorectomy. The frequency of early recurrence in the opposite ovary suggests that occult metastases are common.

After all histologic sections have been examined, the surgeon must advise the patient and her family of her prognosis with and without further therapy. If the patient is reluctant to assume the calculated risk, reoperation should be performed.

BENIGN CYSTIC TERATOMA (DERMOID CYST)

The benign cystic teratoma is a unique neoplasm which is made up of anatomic structures derived from one, two or all three embryonic layers. Usually the structures are well differentiated and are predominantly of epidermal origin although some mesodermal and occasionally entodermal derivative may be found. Two forms of the neoplasm are recognized, one being a benign cystic growth which contains one or more nodules of well-differentiated structures in the wall. This is the common dermoid cyst. The other form is a more solid or microcystic tumor in which the histologic elements have a more embryonic structure, known as the malignant teratoma. The term "dermoid" is really a misnomer, since a tumor of the ovary which is composed of skin only is extremely rare. Usually two of the embryonic areas are represented and occasionally derivatives of all three layers may be identified, particularly if multiple sections are taken. A tumor which contains only one embryonic layer is called a monophyllom, whereas if two are present it is known as a biphyllom and if three layers are present, a triphyllom.

The benign cystic teratoma is a common ovarian tumor and in various reports the incidence ranges from 5 to 25 per cent of all ovarian neoplasms. At the Boston Hospital for Women 443 dermoid cysts have been recorded, an incidence of 17.5 per cent. Five were malignant. The majority of these tumors occur during the reproductive years but they have been reported in an infant of 7 weeks and in women in the eighth decade. A high incidence of dermoid cyst has been reported in the Japanese as well as in Negroes. There seems to be some familial tendency for development of this tumor, numerous reports indicating the existence in each of two or three sisters.

The histogenesis of benign cystic teratoma invokes three theories of origin: (1) parthenogenesis, (2) cellular rests and (3) blastomeric isolation. Dermoid cysts have been described as occurring in various areas in the body which have been traversed by the primordial germ cell, from the mesentery of the hindgut to the ovary. This observation favors the origin of the cyst by parthenogenetic development from the germ cell. Thus, dermoids in the bowel wall probably arise from an arrested germ cell during its migratory phase.

DIAGNOSIS.—Although many dermoid cysts are completely asymptomatic, Peterson and co-workers noted the presence of pain in 47 per cent of patients and of an abdominal mass or swelling in 15.4 per cent of 1,007 cases. In addition, abnormal uterine bleeding occurred in 15 per cent. A dermoid may frequently be discovered anterior to the uterus and freely mobile from that point (Küstner's sign). Since the tumor is commonly pedunculated, the cystic mass lends itself to ready palpation. A doughy, nontender, somewhat heavy adnexal mass is suggestive of this lesion.

The preoperative diagnosis may be aided by the roentgenogram. Frequently, calciferous shadows or teeth may be identified and occasionally there is a mottled central area (due to the sebaceous material and oil) surrounded by a more dense peripheral portion.

Since dermoids are so frequently pedunculated they may twist easily or may be completely separated from the pedicle and subsequently become parasitic. Adhesions and ascites do not commonly occur except in the presence of certain complications such as torsion or infection. Rupture of benign cystic teratomas is a rare and interesting gynecologic entity. Its exact incidence is unknown. Lippert noted rupture in 4.6 per cent of his cases, whereas in a review of the literature 38 years later, Van Orman and Mautner found only four cases. The discrepancy seems to stem from the fact that cystic teratomas more often rupture into hollow organs than into the peritoneal cavity. In a review of the literature in 1952, Kistner found 20 cases of intraperitoneal rupture and added two. Malignant degeneration, trauma, twisting with infarction and gangrene were etiologic factors in precipitating rupture of the cyst. Furthermore, the tumor size seemed to bear some relationship to the tendency to rupture. Dermoids in general do not exceed 20 cm. in diameter, and the average diameter of the cysts reviewed was 15 cm. Two of the cases of rupture occurred during pregnancy and one during the immediate puerperium. The intraperitoneal spill

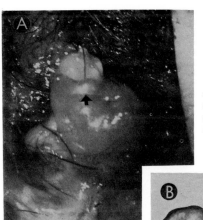

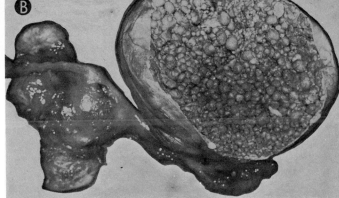

Fig. 7-36.—A, interior of cystic teratoma showing hair and a tooth *(arrow)* emerging from the dermoid process. **B,** large cystic teratoma (dermoid cyst) containing multiple pellets made up of lipids such as palmitin and stearic acid.

of dermoid contents sets up a granulomatous reaction in the peritoneum which, when viewed grossly, may be confused with tuberculosis or carcinomatosis. The peritonitis has been described as "chemical" and is due to deposition of neutral fat and fatty acid crystals, detritis, epidermal cells and crystals of cholesterol. In addition, tyrosine, leucine and xanthine have been identified, together with a yellowish, watery fluid, presumably a product of the sweat glands. Occasionally dermoids contain laminated pellets which are made up of lipoid, present as palmitin, stearic acid and other fatty acids (Fig. 7-36, B). Bilirubin, calcium and calcium soaps may also be found. The peritoneum may become excessively thickened and hardened and may simulate the rind of bacon. Microscopically, the granulomas are composed of lipoid-laden macrophages, lymphocytes, plasma cells and foreign-body giant cells. Dockerty has noted that similar granulomas may be caused by such exogenous factors as the tubercle bacillus, mineral oil, Lipiodol, beryllium, milk (as in plasma cell mastitis), colloid (as in granulomatous thyroiditis) or prostatic secretion (as in granulomatous prostatitis).

PATHOLOGY.—Dermoid cysts may vary in size from microscopic masses 4 mm. in diameter to extremely large masses weighing up to 40 lb. The majority measure less than 15 cm. in greatest diameter. They have been reported as being bilateral in from 8 to 15 per cent of cases. Multiple dermoid cysts may be present in one ovary, each containing a distinct dermoid plug separated from the others by ovarian tissue. As many as 10 separate dermoids have been reported in one ovary. The tumor is often spherical and occasionally has an hourglass appearance. The surface is usually smooth and glistening, without adhesions. The thick-walled cysts are usually white or yellowish, but when the wall is thin the yellow hue of the sebaceous material is more evident. When mixed with blood the cyst contents have a bluish or red color. On occasion a translucent amber color is due to a thin watery fluid. Hair or even the typical dermoid plug may occasionally be seen through a thin-walled cyst. Although the tumor is rather doughy in consistency, hard irregular masses which represent bone or cartilage may be palpated. The contents of the dermoid cyst are liquid at temperatures above 34 C. and therefore are fluctuant in situ. However these oils solidify below 25 C., as is frequently noted following extirpation of the cyst.

When a dermoid cyst is opened, a definite mound is noted which juts into the cyst cavity and which may be connected with the cyst wall by bridges of tissue. This nubbin is known as a dermoid process, dermoid plug or Rokitansky's protuberance. When bone and teeth are present they are usually found in this area, as is the hair so frequently seen (Fig. 7-36, A). In the cystic tumors the dermoid plug contains the well-differentiated structures that arise from the three embryonic layers. The surface of the plug is covered by skin, which grossly appears as the skin of a plucked chicken or even pigskin. Verrucae may be present on the skin surface and occasionally patches of mucosa are identified. On incising the skin, a layer of fat and connective tissue is exposed. Hair is found growing from the skin either as single or scattered tufts or as large diffuse patches. The cyst wall itself is smooth and there may be islands of skin or hair in some areas. Usually, however, the skin terminates abruptly at the base of the plug and the remainder of the cyst is lined by a glistening, reddish mucosal-like tissue.

The hair may be found free in the fatty contents or matted in an intertwined mass. Occasionally the cyst cavity may contain mucinous material if it is lined by gastrointestinal epithelium or mucinous fluid if respiratory epithelium lines the wall. All types of teeth may be found and in one report 108 teeth were identified in one large cyst. The teeth are usually of the second dentition, but milk teeth have been noted as well.

Complicated dermoids resembling dwarfed and distorted fetuses or fetal organs have been described. Thus, dermoids are seen with a rudimentary head, ear anlage, arm and forearm, cranium and brain, pelvis and cranial vault, ribs and studded vertebrae and even phalanges of a finger or foot.

Microscopically a wide variety of tissues has been found in dermoid cysts. The cyst wall is lined by a single layer of cuboidal or high cylindrical epithelium (Fig. 7–37). Occasionally an area made up of granulation tissue is present. Beneath the epithelium is a fasciculated connective tissue layer that merges into the fibrous cyst wall. The skin over the dermoid process is composed of stratified squamous epithelium without dermal papillae. Sebaceous glands, sweat glands and hair follicles are frequently found. The connective tissue resembles that of the skin. Although skin found in dermoids has been likened to circumanal or scrotal skin, there is considerable evidence that it represents the scalp. The cell nuclei of the stratified squamous epithelium are smaller than normal, and the stratum lucidum and stratum granulosum are occasionally absent. Cornification

Fig. 7–37.—Lining of cystic teratoma, showing desquamation of keratin, normal skin and sebaceous glands. (Fig. 7–37 to 7–40 and 7–42 from Hertig. A. T., and Gore, H.: *Tumors of the Female Sex Organs: Part 3. Tumors of the Ovary and Fallopian Tube*, sec. IX, fasc. 33 of *Atlas of Tumor Pathology* [Washington, D.C.: Armed Forces Institute of Pathology, 1961].)

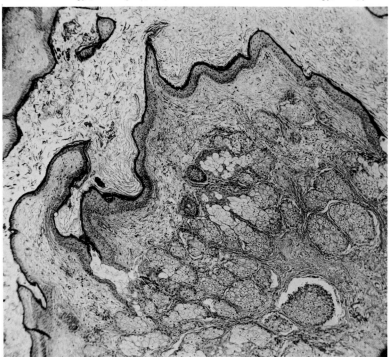

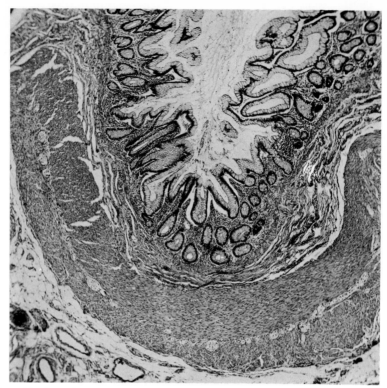

Fig. 7–38.—Large-bowel contents in a cystic teratoma. A mucinous cystoma may result from this portion of a dermoid cyst.

occurs to a greater degree than in the exposed skin and there is extensive maceration of the epithelium which is possibly caused by the contents of the cyst. Near the dermoid plug fat is a constant finding under the subepithelial connective tissue. In some instances the entire cone may consist only of skin, hair and fat. Although epidermal structures are most commonly found in the dermoid mound, mesodermal and endodermal derivatives are also found. Well differentiated glia, ganglion cells, nerve and brain tissue occur. Hyaline cartilage may be found, together with areas of calcification. All types of bones have been described, including long bones, flat bones, mandibular processes and teeth. Organs of special sense have been found occasionally, the structures related to the eye anlage being the commonest. All divisions of the respiratory tract have been identified and the presence of nasal mucosa has been reported by several authors. Gastrointestinal structures have been found in dermoids, sometimes only a few glands but occasionally complete organs (Fig. 7–38). Pelvis, vulva and urogenital sinus have been described and one report even mentions a penis. Gonads have never been found.

TREATMENT.—The optimum treatment of a dermoid cyst is surgical extirpation. Because of the possibility of a bilateral tumor, the opposite ovary should always be bisected and examined carefully. Every effort should be made to conserve ovarian tissue in the young patient since the prognosis is good except when there is a focus of carcinoma. If the dermoid has ruptured intraperitoneally, operative removal is the treatment of choice, with removal of the uterus and opposite ovary depending on the patient's age, parity and the presence of associated pathology. In these patients the intestinal tract should be closely inspected because of the tendency of the granulomatous process to form adhesions and omento-intestinal masses. Continuous intestinal suction and administration of antibiotics are suggested as prophylactic measures since postoperative ileus seems to have been a common complication in cases reported prior to 1930. Deaths in early reported cases were due to peritonitis but since 1924 this has not been a factor. In our study the previously generally accepted opinion that intraperitoneal rupture of dermoids causes fatal peritonitis was not borne out. The last seven patients in this series survived operation and were discharged from the hospital. If carcinomatous or sarcomatous changes have not occurred in the dermoid cyst and if intestinal obstruction does not occur postoperatively, the mortality associated with this condition need not be higher than that associated with any major laparotomy.

Struma ovarii.—This term has been used to describe a benign cystic teratoma composed entirely or largely of thyroid tissue (Fig. 7–39). The incidence of this finding has been 2.7–7 per cent in various reports of cystic teratomas. The average age of the patients with this unusual ovarian tumor was 42 years, and in a study of 139 patients 12 per cent showed evidence of thyrotoxicosis. In almost one-half improvement in the thyrotoxic state followed oophorectomy. The tumor is usually unilateral, measuring about 6–8 cm. in greatest diameter and having a smooth surface occasionally fixed by adhesions. Ascites has been found in 17 per cent of the cases

Fig. 7–39.—Cystic teratoma showing a focus of thyroid tissue in the wall (struma ovarii).

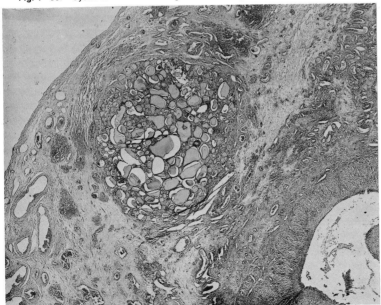

reported. On section the tumor has the glistening amber appearance of thyroid tissue, although variable amounts of hemorrhage and necrosis may also be evident. Microscopically the tissue is similar to that of the thyroid gland, with rounded follicles aligned with cubical or flattened epithelium. The colloid is homogeneous but tends to retract from the epithelial cells and is frequently vacuolated. Malignant change has been reported, with intravascular invasion. For benign tumors the treatment should be the same as that for a benign cystic teratoma, but if the tumor is malignant a hysterectomy and bilateral salpingo-oophorectomy should be performed, followed by x-ray therapy.

Primary Choriocarcinoma

This is a rare ovarian tumor which is composed of syncytiotrophoblast and cytotrophoblast usually occurring before puberty. Such tumors discovered during the childbearing period are usually secondary to choriocarcinoma originating in the uterus after a pregnancy (whether or not the pregnancy was recognized). It is important to differentiate a secondary from a metastatic choriocarcinoma. Secondary lesions include those resulting from neoplastic proliferation of chorionic tissue in a primary ovarian pregnancy as well as those lesions developing within teratoblastomas. Metastatic choriocarcinoma represents a spread from a primary lesion elsewhere, usually in the uterus. It has been suggested that choriocarcinoma of the ovary arising in a teratoblastoma not be regarded as a true primary choriocarcinoma but rather as a morphologic variant of another type of malignant neoplasm. Endocrine assays of the tumor as well as urinary excretory products may be of importance in deciding this important question.

The histogenesis of primary choriocarcinoma is believed to be from the primordial germ cell. The tumors are usually found in children and symptoms are due to massive ovarian enlargement. Pain and increase in abdominal girth, the latter due to ascites, are common. Premature puberty may occur, with development of secondary sexual characteristics. Recurrent vaginal bleeding and breast enlargement are due to secretion of estrogen. Occasionally, hemorrhage into the tumor mass results in rupture with intraperitoneal spill. This represents an acute surgical emergency, the symptoms and signs being similar to those seen in ruptured ectopic pregnancy.

These tumors may become quite large, reaching 15–18 cm. in greatest diameter, and may completely replace the ovary. The tumor surface is nodular and hemorrhagic beneath a thin capsule and is red or purplish in color. The tissue is extremely friable; on section it is a dark, reddish brown or purple. The mass consists of blood and infiltrated spongy tissue which resembles placenta. A hemorrhagic tumor is frequently traversed by firm, white or grayish, translucent bundles and plaques.

The microscopic appearance is similar to that seen in primary uterine choriocarcinoma. This tissue is composed of masses of cells with small, round, dark-staining nuclei arranged in a plexiform pattern, and light, homogeneous or vacuolated cytoplasm. These are the syncytiotrophoblastic cells. Boundaries between cells are indistinct or totally absent so that the neoplastic tissue appears as mass of cytoplasm containing numerous nuclei scattered in rows. Syncytiotrophoblastic masses may line blood-filled spaces similar to the intervillous spaces of the placenta or they may cover groups of cytotrophoblast. The latter are large polyhedral cells with distinct cell boundaries and granular or vacuolated cytoplasm. These cells resemble the typical Langhans cells of the placenta and contain well-defined nuclei with a conspicuous chromatin network.

Although the prognosis is practically hopeless, the optimum treatment is complete hysterectomy and bilateral salpingo-oophorectomy. Death usually occurs within one year as a result of extensive hematogenous metastases to lungs, brain and liver. The addition of x-ray therapy has not been of value, but the folic acid antimetabolite, Methotrexate, should be administered in full and complete dosage, since it is impossible to differentiate gestational from nongestational ovarian choriocarcinomas histologically. Gestational tumors arising in an ovarian pregnancy will respond to methotrexate or actinomycin-D, whereas those arising in a teratoblastoma will not. The usual dose schedule as recommended by Hertz for treatment of metastatic choriocarcinoma consists of successive five-day courses of intramuscularly administered Methotrexate in daily doses of 10–30 mg., the usual dose being 25 mg. Because of the marked toxic effects of this drug, caution must be exercised against irreversible changes by appropriate observations of hepatic, renal and bone marrow function both before and during therapy. Patients resistant to Methotrexate may be treated with vinblastine sulfate or actinomycin-D (see Chapter 11).

MALIGNANT TERATOMA

This is a rare tumor usually seen in childhood or early maturity. It tends to occur at a younger age than the benign cystic teratoma. Less than 1 per cent of all teratomatous growths have been classified as malignant, and at the Boston Hospital for Women only six cases have been encountered.

This lesion has also been termed a teratoblastoma or teratocarcinoma, the most widely accepted theory of histogenesis being that it develops from a primitive, unfertilized ovum. Usually the patient is asymptomatic until the tumor has reached rather large proportions and becomes sufficiently heavy to produce pressure symptoms. This period of growth may be quite rapid, so that abdominal enlargement with ascites may be the presenting complaint.

The lesion is usually unilateral and may present as a pedunculated or nodular mass with numerous adhesions. Section of the tumor reveals a soft, occasionally spongy or cystic tissue which may be multicolored, depending on the extent of hemorrhage into the cystic spaces. Microscopically the elements of the mesoderm are most abundant and there is a preponderance of connective tissue, elastic tissue, bone, hyaline cartilage and smooth and striated muscle. Mucus-secreting, anaplastic glandular epithelium may be identified, or well-differentiated canals lined by columnar or ciliated cells may be present as part of the endodermal constituents. Ectodermal elements are represented by masses of differentiated brain cortex, ocular structures, nerve trunks or ependyma. Three cases of malignant solid teratoma of the ovary, each of which showed well-differentiated tissues, have been reported by Benirschke and associates from the Boston Hospital for Women. In all three of the patients, aged 19, 22 and 40 years, the tissue elements were extremely well differentiated and this differentiation was maintained in the metastases. This is at variance with the usual malignant teratoma since there was no evidence of embryonic malignant mesenchyme. The tumor was fatal in two of the patients, both dying in less than nine months; one patient is alive three years after primary surgery.

The accepted method of therapy for malignant teratoma is a hysterectomy and bilateral salpingo-oophorectomy followed by supervoltage x-ray therapy. Recurrences are common and at the Boston Hospital for Women no patients have survived five years.

TERATOCARCINOMA

This is an undifferentiated carcinoma of the ovary made up of large, irregular cells which differ from those of müllerian carcinoma. It is a very rare tumor of children or adolescents and is uniformly fatal. The histogenesis is believed to be the same as that of malignant teratoma but in this particular tumor there is a striking overgrowth of the epithelial elements (Fig. 7–40). Grossly the lesion is similar to a malignant teratoma or a dysgerminoma. Microscopically the appearance is that of an undifferentiated carcinoma but precise diagnosis is extremely difficult and frequently is made on the basis of exclusion. Hertig has suggested that if a pattern of

Fig. 7–40.—Teratocarcinoma showing marked overgrowth of epithelial cells arranged in an adenomatous pattern.

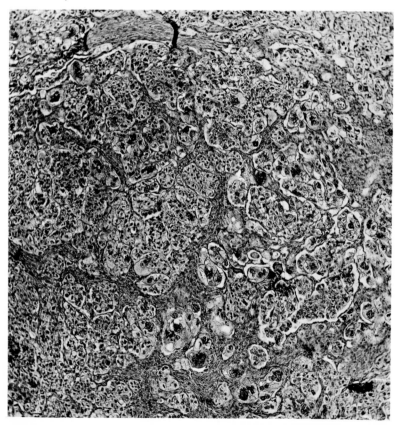

epithelial malignant cells does not fit that of any recognized histogenetic type of ovarian neoplasm, teratocarcinoma should be suspected.

Congenital Rest Tumors

Adrenal Rest Tumor

This is a rare, masculinizing ovarian tumor which grossly and histologically resembles the cortical tissue of the adrenal gland. It has been described in the literature under various headings such as hypernephroma, Leydig cell tumor, luteoma, masculinovoblastoma and virilizing lipoid cell tumor. Approximately 20 authentic cases have been reported and most of these lesions have been considered benign. The average age of the patients is 32 years, with a range of 15–61 years.

The histogenesis of the adrenal rest tumor is still theoretical. Since adrenal rests are commonly found in the ovary during childhood and aberrant tissue is frequently found along the course of the ovarian vessels, the most likely theory of origin suggests that the tumor arises from these adrenal cortical rests (Fig. 7–41). Hertig and Gore have suggested that the designation "adrenal rest" tumor be used for this specific group of virilizing tumors and that the less well-defined tumors interpreted as luteomas be regarded as a variety of arrhenoblastoma. They have also suggested that the nonvirilizing luteoma be grouped with the granulosa-theca cell tumors since the luteoma may be regarded as a luteinized granulosa cell tumor.

The symptomatology includes progressive defeminization, deepening of the voice, hirsutism, scanty uterine bleeding or amenorrhea and enlargement of the clitoris. Breast atrophy has been reported in about 50 per cent of the patients. Occasionally, twisting of the cyst results in emergency surgical extirpation before the symptoms are pronounced. The urinary excretion of 17-ketosteroids is usually elevated and FSH diminished. Fractionation studies of 17-ketosteroids may be of value in differential diagnosis since it has been found that in virilizing adrenal gland tumors (arising in the adrenal itself) the beta fraction of the elevated 17-ketosteroids is elevated. In patients with adrenal-like tumors arising in the ovary the beta fraction of 17-ketosteroids has not been elevated.

The findings of defeminization and progressive masculinization also are seen as a result of an arrhenoblastoma. However, in patients with adrenal rest tumors the additional findings of glycosuria, polycythemia and hypertension suggest the possibility of a disturbance in adrenocortical function or the possibility of a basophilic adenoma of the pituitary. The characteristic physical signs of Cushing's syndrome (osteoporosis, plethora, "buffalo humping," skin striae) do not occur in the adrenal rest tumor or arrhenoblastoma.

Adrenal rest tumors are usually well encapsulated, round or oval in shape and measure from 2 to 16 cm. in diameter. They are frequently buried within the substance of the ovary, are usually yellow and grossly resemble the adrenal cortex. The orange-yellow color which may be noted on cutting through the tumor is due to the presence of lipids within the cytoplasm of the large polyhedral cells. The histologic similarity of adrenal rest tumors, luteomas and luteinized granulosa-theca cell tumors is so striking that careful evaluation of the clinical signs is necessary for accurate classification.

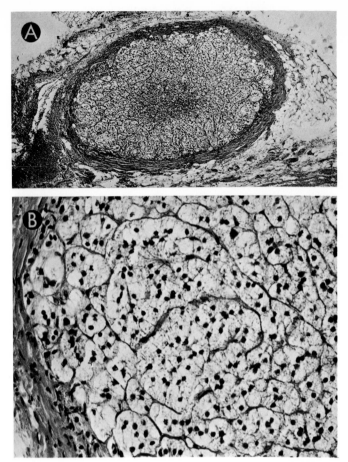

Fig. 7–41.—Adrenal cortex rest. **A,** adrenal cortex rest in the mesovarium. Note the capsule and structural similarity to the adrenal cortex proper. **B,** high-power view. The cells are large, rounded and spongy, being laden with lipoid. (From Morris, J. M., and Scully, R. E.: *Endocrine Pathology of the Ovary* [St. Louis: C. V. Mosby Company, 1958].)

Microscopically, the tumors consist of large polyhedral cells, suggestive of lipoid-containing cells or adrenal cortical cells, with deeply staining, granular nuclei (Fig. 7–42). The cells are arranged in strands or columns with a fine reticular stroma between the columns. An abundance of fat is noted when the tumors are subjected to Sudan-III stains. However, although the cells resemble the typical cells of the adrenal cortex, it should be remembered that the histologic appearance of the constituent cells is not an infallible criterion of their origin, especially since certain other cell types, such as lutein cells or the interstitial cells of Leydig, also closely resemble adrenal cells.

Treatment of these tumors is surgical, with unilateral oophorectomy usually being sufficient to bring about reversion to femininity. Enlargement of the clitoris and deepening of the voice are not always completely reversed.

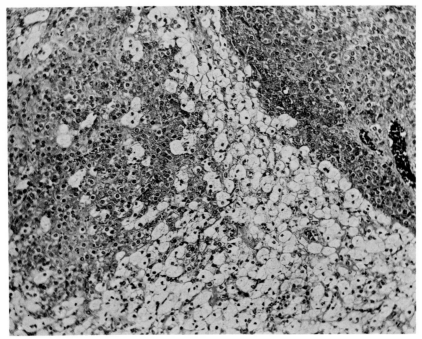

Fig. 7‑42.—Adrenal rest tumor removed from a patient with hirsutism and alopecia. The dark-staining cells resemble those found in the zona reticularis of the adrenal while the larger, vacuolated cells are similar to those seen in the zona fasciculata.

Mesometanephric Rest Tumor

These tumors, previously considered rare, are being reported with increasing frequency, although they have been variously termed mesonephroma, clear cell carcinoma, extra embryonic mesoblastoma, hypernephroma, endodermal sinus tumor, Grawitz tumor and Teilum tumor. Unfortunately the confusion and controversy involving terminology, histogenesis, and histologic appearance have surrounded these tumors with mystery and even cast doubt on their existence. Scully and Barlow recently have shed considerable light on the matter. In 1939 Schiller described a tumor consisting of a loose network of clear spaces lined by endothelial-like cells which projected into the spaces as small papillae (Fig. 7‑43, A). The resemblance to mesonephric glomeruli led Schiller to call this tumor mesonephroma ovarii and postulate an origin from mesonephric rests. Unfortunately, Schiller included in the same report a second tumor type which consisted of cystic or tubular structures lined by hobnail-like cells or large clear cells, the latter also forming solid masses (Fig. 7‑43, B). Although Schiller later denied a relationship of this second type to his mesonephroma ovarii, the tubular structures resembled renal tubules and the masses of clear cells suggested renal carcinoma (hypernephroma). Hertig termed these metanephromas and concurred with Novak's application of the word mesometanephroma to cover both varieties.

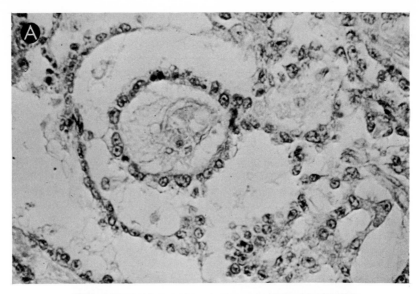

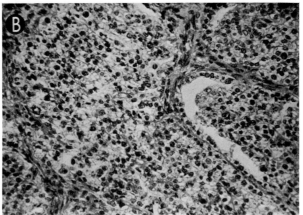

Fig. 7-43.—**A**, embryonic cell carcinoma classified as a germ cell tumor. Formerly it was termed "mesonephroma ovarii" of Schiller. Note the epithelial proliferation into a cystic space, which gives the appearance of a glomerulus. **B**, clear cell carcinoma—mesometanephroma. Solid masses of large clear cells resembling a hypernephroma; tubular structures *(right)* may be numerous, simulating renal tubules.

Meanwhile Teilum clarified Schiller's original paper by pointing out that two distinct unrelated tumors had been described. Teilum also demonstrated a resemblance between Schiller's "mesonephroma" and the endodermal sinuses of the rat placenta and suggested a germ cell origin for these tumors. Many authorities have agreed and the concept is supported by the occasional coexistence of these highly malignant tumors with dysgerminomas and malignant teratomas. Recently they have been termed embryonal carcinomas or Teilum tumors.

Most authorities, however, have continued to advocate a mesonephric origin for Schiller's second type, the clear cell tumor. Supporting evidence consists of their tubular architecture, the resemblance of clear cells to hypernephromas, and their extra ovarian occurrence at sites where meso-nephric remnants are often found. The mesonephric origin, however, has been challenged by Scully and Barlow who found that among 17 cases of mesonephroma four tumors arose from the lining of endometriotic cysts. Pelvic endometriosis separate from the tumor was found in five other cases. An additional eleven selected cases were presented showing a histologic relationship between mesonephromas and endometriosis. These authors conclude that mesonephromas are of müllerian, not mesonephric, origin and are closely related to endometrioid tumors.

The gross appearance of the mesometanephric tumor is not character-istic. The tumor may be quite large and may be densely adherent to sur-rounding structures. The cut surface reveals cystic areas with soft or solid stroma.

Since these tumors are malignant, the optimum therapy is hysterectomy and bilateral salpingo-oophorectomy followed by super-voltage x-ray ther-apy, even though they are relatively radioresistant. In the publication by Novak and Woodruff analyzing the 35 cases obtained from the files of the Ovarian Tumor Registry, the mortality approximated 50 per cent when the lesion was confined to the ovary irrespective of the extent of surgery or irradiation. Dissemination of tumor beyond the ovary resulted in a mortal-ity rate of 100 per cent. At the Boston Hospital for Women rapid lymphatic dissemination and death have been observed in all patients with extra ovarian spread.

Brenner Tumor

The Brenner tumor was originally described in 1907 and was designated *oophoroma folliculare.* Brenner used this term because he felt the tumor was related to the general group of granulosa cell tumors. Robert Meyer in 1932 distinguished the singular nature of this ovarian tumor and suggested that the origin of the tumor was from islands of indifferent cells known as Walthard's cell rests. In 1952 Greene offered evidence to support the fact that these tumors may originate in other constituents of the ovary, such as the stroma, rete ovarii and inclusions of surface epithelium via the process of metaplasia.

The Brenner tumor is relatively rare, the number of reported cases approximating 500. At the Mayo Clinic an incidence of 1.7 per cent was reported, whereas in the pathology laboratory of The Johns Hopkins Hos-pital only 19 cases were found in over 48,000 case specimens (.04 per cent). The Brenner tumor is most commonly found in women past the menopause, 50 per cent of the patients having been over age 50. If the incidental finding of a minute Brenner tumor is included as an entity, the ages of the patients will be diminished so that most will occur within the third or fourth decade.

The histogenesis of the Brenner tumor is presently unsettled but, as mentioned, it is generally accepted that many of these tumors have their origin from the peritoneal covering (coelomic epithelium) of the pelvis. The frequent occurrence of a mucinous cystadenoma with a Brenner tumor may thus be explained on the basis of common histogenesis. Hertig and Gore have suggested that Brenner tumors may arise from areas of squa-mous metaplasia in mucinous epithelium analogous to that seen in the endocervical mucosa. Schiller suggested that some of these tumors arose from the rete ovarii, and Greene has recently supported this contention.

Greene also suggested that the ovarian stroma itself may give rise to a Brenner tumor, and it has been shown that the fibrils between the epithelial cells are actually continuous with those of the surrounding connective tissue. A teratomatous origin has been suggested for Brenner tumors, supported chiefly by the fact that mucinous cystadenomas are also believed to differentiate from a teratoma.

These tumors do not produce characteristic symptoms since the growth rate is rather slow. Ascites is not common but hydrothorax may be an associated finding. The tumor is not hormonally active and therefore the menstrual history is usually not altered in patients who are in the childbearing age group. In postmenopausal patients there may be endometrial hyperplasia, and occasionally reports in the literature indicate that adenocarcinoma of the endometrium has been found in association with Brenner tumors. By and large, however, these tumors are looked on as being hormonally inactive though it is reasonable to assume that the stroma of certain tumors may become active and be converted into theca-lutein cells. In one series of 402 patients with Brenner tumors an estrogen effect was thought to exist in 7.5 per cent. The commonest symptom associated with development of a Brenner tumor is abdominal enlargement due to the tumor mass itself.

Many of these tumors are of microscopic size, whereas others may assume gigantic proportions. The largest recorded tumor weighed approximately 19 lb. Tumors usually measure between 10 and 15 cm. in greatest diameter and are usually unilateral. The consistency of the tumor in general is quite firm but cystic areas may occur. The serosal surface is smooth, occasionally slightly lobulated. When the tumor is sectioned it may appear similar to a fibroma, although occasionally a yellow tint may be scattered through the surface.

The microscopic picture is quite characteristic, the tumor being made up of nests of epithelial cells surrounded by a fibromatous connective tissue (Fig. 7-44). The nests, composed of cells which resemble squamous epithelium, are polyhedral with oval nuclei containing distinct nucleoli. Stratification of the cells occurs commonly but the morphology is characteristically uniform. A longitudinal groove has been described in the epithelial cells of the Brenner tumor similar to the groove found in the cells of the Walthard rest. Mitoses do not often occur and the cells in no way suggest malignancy. The epithelial nests may be arranged in ovoid forms and central degeneration of the epithelial islands is commonly noted. Calcification may be present, and differential staining has identified both glycogen and mucus in the epithelial cells. In the cystic cavities of the epithelial nests the cellular pattern may be typical of that seen in the usual type of mucinous cystoma. These "intraepithelial glands" have been described in approximately one-third of all Brenner tumors.

Although a few exceptions have been reported, Brenner tumors should be considered benign. A fine point in differential diagnosis may occur since there may be metastatic squamous cell carcinoma in the ovary which might appear to be a malignant Brenner tumor. Within the past decade approximately 15 malignant tumors have been reported. However, of the eight malignant Brenner tumors recorded in the Ovarian Tumor Registry, there is doubt as to the proper classification in six. Novak stated that in only two instances could the lesions be truly classified as examples of

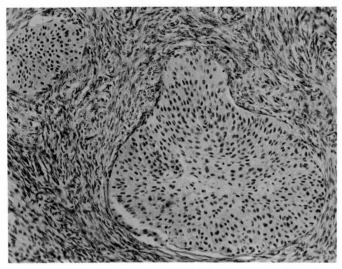

Fig. 7-44.—Brenner tumor. Nests of epithelial cells resembling squamous epithelium are surrounded by a fibromatous connective tissue matrix.

malignancy arising in a stratified epithelial structure. Only one malignant tumor has been seen in the material at the Boston Hospital for Women.

The treatment is usually unilateral oophorectomy but in postmenopausal women the procedure of choice is a hysterectomy and bilateral salpingo-oophorectomy. X-ray therapy should be administered only if malignancy is discovered in the excised material.

Hilus Cell Tumor

This is a rare masculinizing tumor of the ovary and arises from cells which are normally present in the ovarian hilus. These cells are usually associated with nonmyelinated nerve fibers and therefore the lesion is occasionally called a sympathicotropic cell tumor. The particular cells may be distinguished from adrenal cells in that they are darker, smaller and have a distinct nucleus. Usually they are arranged in an adenomatous pattern with a connective tissue matrix. The cells were originally described by Berger, who believed them to be identical with the Leydig cells of the testis. Novak and Mattingley reported 18 cases in 1960 in a comprehensive review.

Clinical virilism is a constant finding and this is frequently of rather long standing. The signs of masculinization include hirsutism, receding hairline, enlargement of the clitoris and deepening of the voice. The level of urinary ketosteroids has been slightly elevated in a few cases but otherwise has been normal. The causative agent responsible for masculinization is probably testosterone, since in the presence of a normal urinary 17-ketosteroid value one must assume that a very potent androgen, such as testosterone, is being formed by the tumor tissue. This explains the extensive virilism in hilus cell tumors as well as in arrhenoblastomas with normal urinary 17-ketosteroid assays.

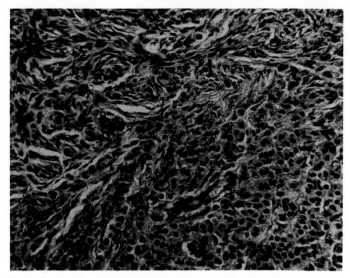

Fig. 7-45.—Hilus cell tumor. The cells are identical with the Leydig cells of the testis, being ovoid to polygonal with round nuclei and prominent nucleoli. There are fine connective tissue strands between the cells and several Reinke crystalloids near the center of the illustration. (Courtesy of Dr. Thomas Leavitt.)

Grossly the tumors are small, usually less than 5 cm. in diameter, and are generally unilateral. Although the tumor mass itself is usually found in the ovarian hilus, if it enlarges to 3 or 4 cm. it may replace most of the ovarian tissue. Grossly a hilus cell tumor is well demarcated from the surrounding tissue and is homogeneous and fleshy in appearance. The color may be yellow or yellow-brown, occasionally hemorrhagic. Microscopically the cells are identical to the Leydig cells of the testis. Both their nuclear and cytoplasmic structures are similar (Fig. 7-45). Both of these cells contain lipochrome pigment and albuminoid crystalloids of Reinke. An interesting observation made by Novak and Mattingley was that, despite the clinical virilism, the endometrium frequently showed hyperplasia or hyperplastic polyps. The cells making up a hilus cell tumor, although identical to the cells found normally in the ovarian hilus, are slightly larger and more pleomorphic. They have an eosinophilic cytoplasm with vesicular or round nuclei and one or more nucleoli.

In general these tumors have been thought to be uniformly benign but a case report by Stewart and Woodard described a definitely malignant hilus cell tumor. After surgical removal of the tumor the masculinizing features disappear rather quickly.

Nonintrinsic Connective Tissue Tumors
FIBROMA

Small fibromas of the ovary are seen commonly as tiny polypoid, wartlike structures on the surface or in the ovarian substance as firm, white, well-demarcated nodules. They are basically tumors of connective tissue and are composed principally of fibroblasts with varying amounts of collagen.

The incidence of these tumors varies considerably, depending on the care with which ovaries are studied pathologically. In the literature the incidence varies from 1.5 to 5 per cent, and in a study at the Mayo Clinic fibromas constituted a little more than 5 per cent of all ovarian tumors removed surgically. At the Boston Hospital for Women 740 fibromas occurred in 2,530 ovarian tumors, an incidence of 29.2 per cent. This high incidence is due to the inclusion of microscopic lesions in the total. This tumor is seen most commonly during the late childbearing period, the average age being 48 years.

Fibromas usually arise from the fibrous tissue elements of the ovarian cortex, although it has been suggested that the capsular connective tissue and perivascular connective tissue are common sites of origin. Some fibromas are secondary to Brenner tumors since in the latter a marked fibromatous reaction may occur which completely obliterates the characteristic cell islands.

The chief symptoms associated with ovarian fibromas are abdominal pain and pressure on the rectum or bladder. The large size of these tumors will produce gradual abdominal enlargement and this may be the only presenting complaint. Lesions have been reported which weighed as much as 50 lb. and, while this is unusual, the diagnosis of fibroma should be entertained when an extremely large firm mass fills the pelvis and abdomen.

Because of the weight of the tumor, elongation of the pedicle occurs. Twisting of this pedicle then may result in the formation of ascites or, if the blood supply is completely occluded, in massive infarction. Certain patients with a fibroma will have associated ascites and hydrothorax, the clinical picture known as Meigs's syndrome. The hydrothorax is probably due to the permeation of ascitic fluid through the lymphatics of the diaphragm. Meigs's syndrome is also seen in conjunction with other solid tumors of the ovary, such as Brenner tumors, granulosa cell tumors, thecomas and carcinoma.

A fibroma is a hard, homogeneous, fibrous tumor but on occasion it may appear edematous and even cystic. The average diameter approximates 6 cm., with about 5 per cent of the tumors exceeding 20 cm. The tumors are bilateral in about 10 per cent of cases, and multiple tumors are occasionally discovered within the same ovary. The cut surface is usually white with a yellow tinge, but if hemorrhage has occurred the tissue may appear multicolored with scattered areas of dark red, blue and green.

Microscopically the basic cell type is a connective tissue cell similar to the stromal cell of the ovarian cortex. There is a good deal of variation in the histologic appearance, some areas being made up of small fusiform or stellate cells with abundant intercellular substance. In areas that are more cellular, the typical spindle-shaped cells are closely approximated and arranged in individual bundles, giving a fasciculated appearance. In some tumors muscle bundles may be identified and such tumors are then designated as fibromyomas.

The fibroma may occasionally be confused with a thecoma and a fat stain is necessary for differentiation.

The usual, accepted treatment for a fibroma is simple excision. If the patient is postmenopausal a complete hysterectomy and bilateral salpingo-oophorectomy should be performed since the microscopic sections may reveal an ovarian sarcoma instead of a fibroma.

FIBROSARCOMA

This is a rare, malignant, connective tissue tumor of the ovary which usually occurs in postmenopausal women. It is associated with a poor prognosis because of its radioresistance and its propensity for spread by vascular channels.

The tumor is usually of moderate size and lobulated, the cut surface showing focal areas of necrosis and cystic degeneration. The microscopic picture is usually that of the spindle cell type. When a round cell sarcoma of the ovary is described, it is usually confused with a granulosa cell carcinoma, a dysgerminoma or a lymphosarcoma. In certain tumors myxomatous tissue is identified and the tumor is thus designated as a myxosarcoma.

Metastatic Tumors
KRUKENBERG'S TUMOR

This tumor is sometimes described under the term *fibrosarcoma ovarii mucocellulare carcinomatodes*. This is the term used by Krukenberg in his original description of this group of tumors in 1896. He believed this tumor to be a primary ovarian tumor, but subsequent authors have shown that such malignancies are usually, if not always, metastatic from the gastrointestinal tract, most often from the stomach. Although these tumors are usually firm, solid, bilateral growths of moderate size, they usually retain the shape of the ovary. On gross section they are quite hemorrhagic, spongy and mucinous. The average age of patients is about 48, and in a review of 530 cases Linnard found that the primary sites were the stomach in 70 per cent, the large bowel in 15 per cent and the breast in 6 per cent.

It is impossible to define exactly the criteria for diagnosis of a Krukenberg tumor, and Leffel has summarized the subject as follows: "There is as yet no agreement as to what constitutes a Krukenberg tumor; as to how metastasis occurs; as to whether a primary ovarian carcinoma may be impossible to distinguish from the Krukenberg tumor; as to whether the metastasis is in any way selective; or on how the lesion should be treated." The clinical picture may include symptoms associated with the primary lesion or the secondary ovarian lesion. Thus, the existence of breast carcinoma or carcinoma of the gastrointestinal tract would lead one to suspect secondary ovarian cancer should pelvic examination reveal ovarian enlargement. As previously mentioned, such tumors are usually firm, solid growths of moderate size, almost always bilateral. They may be kidney shaped or slightly lobulated, with a smooth surface and a well-developed capsule, but in general they do not tend to become adherent to surrounding structures.

Microscopically there is a great variation in histologic appearance. The stroma may be rich and cellular in certain areas while in others it is edematous or occasionally myxomatous. The epithelial elements may occur as clusters of small acini although, in a true Krukenberg tumor, these cells show varying degrees of mucoid epithelial change. It is true, however, that carcinoma which has metastasized from the gastrointestinal tract may simulate a carcinoma of germinal epithelial origin or one of mesometane-

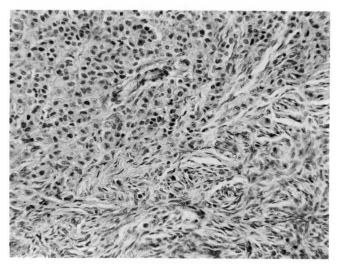

Fig. 7-46.—Carcinoma of the breast metastatic to the ovary. The upper part of this section shows cords of hyperpigmented mammary carcinoma cells which mimic a granulosa cell tumor.

phric origin. If the individual tumor cells are scattered through a loose stroma, they may simulate hilus cell tumors or even an arrhenoblastoma. The individual cells metastatic from a breast cancer which infiltrate ovarian stroma may closely mimic a granulosa-theca cell tumor (Fig. 7-46).

The pronounced variation that is possible in this tumor may thus give rise to large, rounded or polyhedral cells or very clear cells with a mucinous cytoplasm, the typical "signet ring" cell, in which the mucus compresses the nucleus against one side of the cell (Fig. 7-47). It is these signet-ring cells which have been stressed by most pathologists in the microscopic diagnosis of these tumors. However, they are not specific for designation as "Krukenberg" and may be found in any mucus-secreting tumor.

The route of dissemination of tumor cells from the various primary cancers to the ovary has not been definitely settled. Four possible routes have been suggested: (1) direct implantation on the ovarian surface transported by peritoneal fluid; (2) lymphatic metastases; (3) hematogenous transportation, and (4) direct continuity from adherent intestinal cancer. Hertig and Gore believe that the best explanation for the development of Krukenberg tumors from the stomach or bowel is via retrograde lymphatics. The fact is that, in many of these tumors, origin within the substance of the ovary seems definite. This favors the theory of lymphatic spread rather than that of peritoneal fluid sedimentation.

The treatment is essentially palliative. However, it is suggested that even though an ovarian tumor is thought to be metastatic a hysterectomy and bilateral salpingo-oophorectomy should be performed. A rare primary tumor may be mistakenly believed to be a Krukenberg tumor.

In summary, Krukenberg tumors are usually secondary lesions which are frequently metastatic from bowel carcinomas and are associated with a poor prognosis. However, in 1960 Woodruff and Novak reported a study of 48 cases, 10 of which appeared to be primary. All of these primary

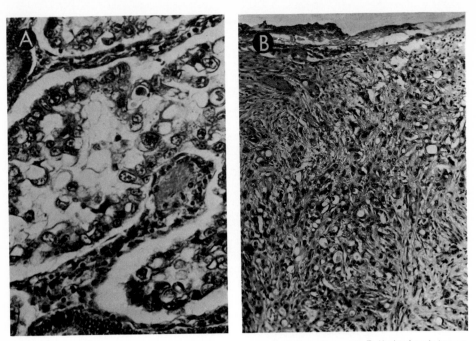

Fig. 7 –47.—A, carcinoma of the pancreas metastatic to the ovary. **B,** Krukenberg's tumor, showing rounded and polyhedral cells metastatic from a gastric cancer. Numerous "signet-ring" cells are seen.

tumors were obtained from reports of the Ovarian Tumor Registry and leave little doubt as to their validity. Four of the 10 patients with a seemingly primary tumor were alive and well five years after surgery.

SECONDARY OVARIAN CANCER FROM PELVIC ORGANS

Carcinoma of the corpus, cervix and oviduct may metastasize to the ovary, and occasionally even a benign carcinoid tumor of the appendix may show ovarian metastases. Adenocarcinoma of the uterine corpus metastasizes to the ovary in from 5 to 7 per cent of cases. In such cases the metastatic areas are usually found in close proximity to the hilus rather than on the ovarian surface. Carcinoma of the cervix metastasizes to the ovary in only about 1 per cent of cases. In a few of the reported cases of carcinoma of the oviduct metastases have also been identified.

The usual treatment is, of course, the treatment of the original primary tumor, usually a hysterectomy and bilateral salpingo-oophorectomy or in the case of cervical carcinoma a radical hysterectomy and pelvic lymph node dissection.

Sclerocystic Ovarian Disease (Stein-Leventhal)

In 1935 Stein and Leventhal called attention to a particular syndrome which has been considered by clinicians to be a singular disease process. As more basic research is accomplished, particularly in the field of steroid synthesis of the ovary, it is becoming apparent that this so-called disease syndrome may actually embrace many diseases of the endocrine system which result in persistent lack of ovulation.

As originally described, the syndrome was characterized by menstrual abnormalities, usually oligomenorrhea or amenorrhea, obesity, a tendency toward virilization with hirsutism in about one-half the patients, and infertility. The ovaries are large, frequently each ovary being larger than the uterus, and the surface of the ovary appears thickened, pale, and smooth (Fig. 7-48, A). They have been described as similar to large oysters in appearance. When the ovary is bisected (Fig. 7-48, B), numerous cystic follicles may be identified beneath the capsule. These measure 5-7 mm. in diameter and contain clear fluid. Microscopically there is fibrosis of the cortical stroma with areas of hyalinization (Fig. 7-49). Examination of the cystic follicles reveals an unusual activity of the theca interna cells with luteinization. Corpora albicantia and corpora lutea are usually absent, but on occasion one or more may be identified. Although at one time this microscopic picture was thought to be pathognomonic of Stein-Leventhal syndrome, recent studies have shown that it is merely representative of prolonged periods of anovulation from various causes. Scott and Wharton produced a similar appearance in the ovary by the administration of testosterone to monkeys in an attempt to eradicate areas of implanted endometriosis. A similar, though not identical, picture in the ovary has been described in association with abnormal adrenocortical function, adenomas of the pituitary, Cushing's disease and other syndromes in which amenorrhea is secondary. The uterus is usually of normal size in Stein-Leventhal syndrome and the endometrium shows varying degrees of proliferation, including hyperplasia. A few patients with concomitant endometrial carcinoma have been reported. Although research activity in this disease has yielded several significant findings, the precise etiology remains obscure and its pathogenesis is unknown.

Leventhal has reported observations of ovaries and adrenal glands in patients with Stein-Leventhal syndrome. Examination of the adrenal glands in two hirsute patients with typical Stein-Leventhal syndrome disclosed no histologic evidence of hyperfunction. Further, a study of

Fig. 7-48.—Ovaries of the Stein-Leventhal type. **A,** gross appearance, and **B,** on bisection. (*A* from Ingersoll, F. M.: Clin. Obst. & Gynec. 4:814, 1961.)

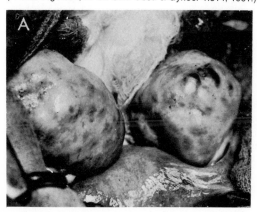
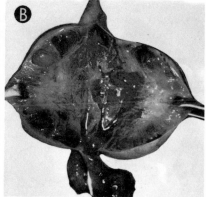

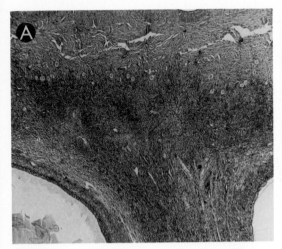

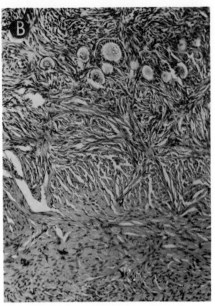

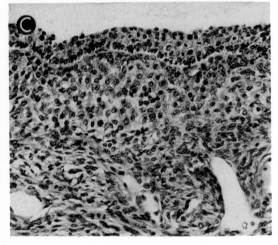

Fig. 7-49.—Ovary in Stein-Leventhal syndrome. **A,** low-power view. Note cystic follicles and collagenous character of the cortex. **B,** higher power. Numerous primordial follicles are seen in the zone between the normal cortex below and the hyperplastic fibrotic cortex above.

C, high-power view, showing the wall of a cystic follicle with a narrow layer of granulosa cells toward the lumen of the cyst and a wide layer of luteinized theca cells below.

ovarian tissue showed the hilus to be normal in each individual. The really significant anatomic finding was the unusual hyperplasia of the theca cells. This report agreed with the previous findings of Benedict as well as those of Sommers, both of whom described normal adrenal morphology in patients with Stein-Leventhal syndrome. Sommers described autopsy findings in 11 patients and, aside from the polycystic ovaries, the only endocrine pathology was a diffuse basophilia of the pituitary gland. Jones, however, in discussing the report of Leventhal contended that in approximately 25 per cent of cases there is an association between bilateral polycystic ovaries and adrenal function. Jones also felt that the primary site of pathology in this disease process might well be in the hypothalamus.

Wedge resection of the ovaries has resulted in the restoration of ovulation with subsequent menstruation in 80 per cent and pregnancy in 63 per cent of patients so treated. According to Goldzieher, this high success rate is obtained only with proper selection of the patient. It is obvious that wedge resection will not restore ovulation when the etiology of the anovulatory process lies in the pituitary, thyroid or adrenal gland.

In a few patients the menstrual history before the development of oligo-menorrhea or amenorrhea may have been perfectly normal. Usually, however, the menstrual history reveals a rather marked irregularity since the menarche. Breast development may be normal or may be slightly deficient in some patients.

ETIOLOGY

The basic etiology of the polycystic ovarian syndrome is unknown. Until 1956 it was theorized by many pathologists and clinicians that the cause of anovulation was the thickened cortex which trapped the ova beneath the hyalinized tunica, preventing their escape. This concept is no longer tenable. Greenblatt observed ovulation in a patient with Stein-Leventhal syndrome following simple extirpation of one ovary. Ovulation promptly occurred through the thickened cortex of the remaining ovary. Similarly, patients with borderline adrenocortical malfunction, in whom a moderate elevation of the urinary 17-ketosteroid level is found, will readily ovulate through the thickened cortex on the administration of small doses of cortisone. In these patients the lack of ovulation is thought to be due to abnormal adrenocortical function, with formation of excess adrenal androgens instead of cortisone. The elevated androgen level apparently prevents ovulation, but when this process is interrupted by the administration of cortisone, ovulation promptly ensues.

Other theories of etiology have included abnormalities of gonadotropic function. Thus, many of the ovaries appear pathologically similar to the ovary of the adolescent female except for the multiple cystic follicles. It has been suggested that these multiple follicle cysts and thickened cortex are the result of overproduction of FSH. However, a persistent elevation of FSH secretion has not been demonstrated in these patients.

Using the standard mouse uterine weight assay for "total" (FSH & LH) urinary gonadotropins, normal levels have been reported in numerous studies. Normal levels of FSH in urine have also been noted by the ovarian augmentation assay method. Another evidence in favor of the pituitary as an integral factor in the disease has been an irregular fluctuation of LH excretion as measured in urine using the ventral prostate assay method. Mishell has demonstrated this irregular, somewhat elevated LH activity in patients with this syndrome by the immunoassay method. In such a situation it might be possible that the burst of LH activity necessary to produce ovulation is lacking. Mishell, using immunoassay, has clearly shown a marked rise in LH, similar to that seen at the time of ovulation in the normal cycle, subsequent to the administration of clomiphene. This was followed by a rise in the basal body temperature and other indices of apparent ovulation.

Another theory of etiology suggests that the ovary in the polycystic syndrome is excessively sensitive to the stimulus of gonadotropic substances. Thus, the ovary responds by growth of numerous follicles which develop only partially and subsequently become cystic. Secondarily, hyperplasia of the stroma and luteinization of the theca develop as a result of the irregular but constant LH stimulation. An increased ovarian response to exogenous FSH has been demonstrated in patients with this syndrome and, as will be mentioned later, the response to clomiphene citrate seems equally labile.

Lloyd, Goldzieher and others have suggested that the basic derangement in the Stein-Leventhal syndrome lies in the hypothalamus. They postulate that the median eminence nuclei produce a *tonic* rather than a rhythmic discharge of releasing factors. This hypothesis of a constant, low-level gonadotropin discharge, chronically stimulated by estrogen, is consistent with the clinical findings. The polycystic ovary has the histologic and functional behavior of an overstimulated organ and persistent estrogen production has been documented.

STUDIES OF STEROID BIOSYNTHESIS

Prior to 1960, laboratory assays in patients with the sclerocystic ovarian syndrome were of no particular diagnostic value. The usual evaluation of the patient revealed normal values for total neutral 17-ketosteroids, FSH, protein-bound iodine and ketogenic steroids. The x-ray of the sella turcica was also normal. If all of these parameters were within normal range and the ovaries were thought to be enlarged, the most probable diagnosis, by exclusion, was a primary ovarian disorder of the Stein-Leventhal type. During the past several years, however, refinements in the techniques of laboratory assays for steroids in blood and urine have revealed the fallacy of this particular conclusion.

Two major ovarian steroidogenic abnormalities have been identified: (1) a deficiency in *aromatization,* i.e., in the conversion of 19-oxygenated androgens to estrogen with an accumulation of 19-oxoandrogens, and (2) a deficiency in 3-β-ol dehydrogenase, i.e., in the conversion of Δ^5-3-β-ol to Δ^4-3-keto compounds. These inadequacies are due to an insufficiency of specific enzymes as noted in Figure. 7–50.

Dorfman published the results of determinations of testosterone in human plasma obtained from normal men, normal women, hirsute women of the Stein-Leventhal type and hirsute women with diagnosis not established. The mean testosterone level in nine normal men was 0.56 μg./100 ml., whereas the mean level in 10 normal women was 0.12 μg./100 ml. Six hirsute women who had polycystic ovaries of the Stein-Leventhal type were studied and were found to have mean testosterone levels ranging from 0.25 to 0.42 μg./100 ml. The average for these individuals was 0.33 μg./100 ml. Four hirsute women with a diagnosis not established were studied in a similar manner, and the range was found to be 0.11–0.32 μg. of testosterone/ 100 ml., with a mean of 0.25. The total 17-ketosteroids excreted per day in urine in these two groups was, however, only 12.2 mg./24 hours in patients with Stein-Leventhal syndrome and 13.7 in hirsute women with unestablished diagnosis. Dorfman also reported studies on five virilized women with polycystic ovaries of the Stein-Leventhal type; the range for testosterone was 0.30–0.74 μg./100 ml., with a mean of 0.49. In the latter group the 17-ketosteroids ranged from 6.4 to 20 mg./24 hours, certainly not a high level in most laboratories. Bilateral ovarian wedge resection was performed in three hirsute women and reductions of plasma testosterone levels were seen in each patient. The mean testosterone levels before wedge resection in these three patients were 0.53, 0.77 and 0.58. All of these values ap-

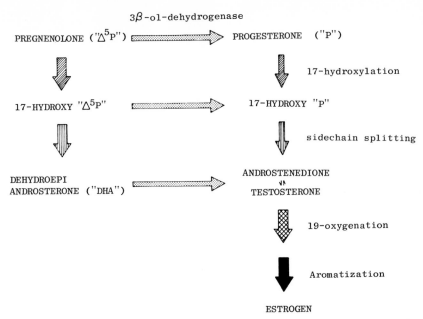

Fig. 7-50.—Enzymatic sequences in ovarian steroidogenesis. (From Goldzieher, J. W., in Behrman, S. J., and Kistner, R. W. (eds.): *Progress in Infertility* [Boston: Little, Brown & Company, 1968].)

proached that seen in the normal male. After wedge resection these values were 0.11, 0.34 and 0.22, respectively. Ovariectomy in five hirsute women with high mean testosterone values before surgery was followed by a mean value of 0.11.

In view of these most interesting studies of steroid biosynthesis in the ovary of the patient with Stein-Leventhal syndrome, it may be concluded that wedge resection causes a decrease in total hormone production which, in turn, permits pituitary-ovarian relationships to return to normal so that ovulation may be accomplished. Several other observations are also in keeping with the recent concept that polycystic ovarian disease is primarily an ovarian rather than a pituitary disturbance. Taymor and Barnard studied LH excretion levels in patients with typical Stein-Leventhal syndrome. They found elevated LH excretion levels in patients with normal-sized polycystic ovaries as well as in patients with typical, enlarged ovaries. Higher levels of LH in urine were noted when the polycystic ovaries were enlarged and suggested that the Stein-Leventhal syndrome was actually a later stage of a progressive endocrinopathy. They also found elevated LH excretion in four of nine patients with elevated 17-ketosteroid excretion, patients they believed to have adrenal hyperplasia. They concluded that LH excretion studies could not be utilized as a diagnostic tool for differentiating between ovarian and adrenal types of the polycystic ovary syndrome. They suggested that LH may stimulate both adrenal and ovarian androgens and, since androgens have been shown to be rather weak inhibitors of gonadotropin excretion, a stimulation-inhibition feed-back phenomenon may exist. Taymor and Barnard further theorized that the elevated LH excretion may be caused by the prolonged absence of progesterone and is not in itself an etiologic factor in this disease process. All of these observations are acceptable evidence in favor of the concept that the Stein-Leventhal syndrome is not in itself a specific entity but is merely a part of a progressive and probably polyglandular endocrinopathy.

DIAGNOSTIC MEASURES

In order to make an adequate diagnosis we feel that culdoscopy or laparoscopy should be performed in every patient. The process of gynecography may be used as an adjuvant diagnostic method.

At the time of admission to the hospital a complete endocrinologic survey is undertaken. This includes an x-ray of the sella turcica, examination of the ocular fundi, visual field determinations, protein-bound iodine and the basal metabolic rate. Urinary assays of 17-ketosteroids, 17-ketogenic steroids, FSH and LH are obtained. Since the finding of pregnanetriolone (11 ketopregnanetriol) is found only in patients with Stein-Leventhal syndrome or adrenal hyperplasia associated with adrenogenital or Cushing's syndrome, this assay is helpful in diagnosis. Ovarian and adrenal stimulation and suppression tests should be done.

ADRENOCORTICAL AND OVARIAN SUPPRESSION STUDIES

In 1951 Sohval and Soffer showed that administration of cortisone caused an immediate increase in gonadotropins in urine in a few patients with polycystic ovaries, and an increase in total gonadotropins in normal women after cortisone or dexamethasone has been reported by Barlow. Mahesh and Greenblatt showed a reduction in urinary dehydroepiandrosterone, androsterone and etiocholanolone after adrenal suppression in some patients with Stein-Leventhal syndrome but in others these metabolites remained elevated even after adrenal suppression. Subsequently, they were able to suppress the elevated 11-deoxy corticosteroids (after dexamethasone) by stilbestrol, suggesting an ovarian origin of these steroids.

Barlow noted an increase in urinary estrogens when dexamethasone was given to normal women during the follicular phase of the cycle but not during the luteal phase, and Netter noted an increase in urinary estrogens in patients with polycystic ovaries during dexamethasone suppression.

A further refinement in differential testing has been to superimpose stimulation of the ovaries by gonadotropin on the suppression of the adrenals with corticosteroids. On the basis of increased or decreased excretion of 17-ketosteroids after HCG stimulation, some observers felt that it was possible to differentiate adrenal and ovarian components. However, this interpretation depends on two assumptions: (1) that corticosteroids have a reproducible effect on the adrenal but none on the ovary and (2) that HCG affects the ovary but not the adrenal. There is substantial evidence that both of these assumptions are false. For example, corticosteroids increase the excretion of gonadotropins in urine and HCG evokes an adrenal response in certain patients. Thus it must be concluded that "adrenocortical" and "ovarian" suppression tests mean suppression of ACTH or gonadotropins but do not necessarily reflect a direct action of the suppressing agent on the target organ.

ADRENOCORTICAL AND OVARIAN STIMULATION TESTS

Lanthier showed an increased urinary excretion of androsterone and etiocholanolone after HCG but the degree of increase was no greater than that seen in normal subjects. HCG did not affect the excretion of pregnanediol or pregnanetriol in urine. Dignam showed an increase in plasma testosterone in some patients with polycystic ovaries after HCG administration.

The administration of homologous or heterologous FSH to women with polycystic ovaries results in gross ovarian enlargement but the steroid consequences of such stimulation are variable. Gemzell and Crooke noted a marked increase in estrogens in urine after such stimulation and Shearman noted a marked increase in estrogens plus urinary pregnanetriol and Δ^5-pregnenetriol. Mahesh and Greenblatt, however, noted an increase in urinary 17-ketosteroids, pregnanetriol and Δ^5-pregnenetriol but no increase in estrogens.

ACTH stimulation results in a greater increase in 17-ketosteroids, androsterone and etiocholanolone in women with polycystic ovaries than in controls. Mahesh also found an increase in pregnanetriol, Δ^5-pregnenetriol, tetrahydrocorticoids and 11-oxygenated 17-ketosteroids.

Although an exaggerated rise in 17-ketosteroids after ACTH stimulation is commonly found in hyperandrogenic states of adrenocortical origin, this response is not a consistently reliable test. An elevation of urinary pregnanetriol would suggest a biochemical adrenal defect similar to that found in congenital adrenal hyperplasia. A rise in 17-ketosteroids after ACTH in the Stein-Leventhal syndrome and suppression of the 17-ketosteroids by a corticosteroid would point to an important adrenocortical factor. Confusion regarding the pathogenesis of Stein-Leventhal syndrome is not likely to be dispelled in the near future, but a trial of corticosteroid suppression of a potential adrenal component has come to be an integral therapeutic preliminary before wedge resection of the ovary is performed.

TREATMENT

Stein and Leventhal suggested the original effective treatment of bilateral wedge resection in 1935. In their series, menstrual cycles returned to normal in about 95 per cent of the patients, and approximately 85 per cent of the infertile patients became pregnant within a short time after surgery. Since that time wedge resection has been extensively practiced and has been overused.

The use of wedge resection in treatment of this disease process should be the *last,* not the first, method employed. However, since curettage in some of these patients has revealed atypical endometrial hyperplasia, every avenue of therapy to produce ovulation should be explored.

The optimum therapy to be used initially, if the 17-ketosteroids in urine show elevations to 15 to 25 mg./24 hours, is that of cortisone or prednisone.

Forchielli and associates found a rather decided drop in mean testosterone levels after administration of 10 to 20 mg. of prednisone daily. Whereas the surgical procedure of bilateral wedge resection caused a net decrease of 0.41 μg./100 ml. of plasma (from a mean of 0.63 μg. to 0.22 μg.), prednisone effected a change from 0.34 to 0.07, a net decrease of 0.27 μg. of plasma testosterone. If the basal body temperature graph does not reveal apparent ovulation within six months of the initiation of cortisone therapy, a complete re-evaluation of the patient should be undertaken. We have employed doses of hydrocortisone of 30 mg. daily and if ovulation occurs therapy is continued for nine to 12 months. The medication is then withdrawn and the patient followed carefully to evaluate whether or not spontaneous ovulation occurs.

If the 17-ketosteroids in urine are normal, clomiphene citrate is given as primary therapy. In 1959 Dr. O. W. Smith and I reported induction of ovulation with a nonsteroidal estrogen antagonist, MER-25. Tyler reported similar results in 1962. Since this compound had certain toxic effects, a similar preparation known as clomiphene citrate, was substituted. The ovarian response to clomiphene was more striking but less physiologic than that demonstrated with MER-25. Clomiphene citrate seemed to be effective in the patient who had an arrest in the maturation of follicles but in whom adequate estrogen was present. This was particularly true of patients with Stein-Leventhal syndrome; in these patients the follicles seem ready to extrude their ova but a burst of LH activity was apparently lacking.

In a recent study 359 of 436 patients classified as having the Stein-Leventhal syndrome apparently ovulated after the first course of clomiphene, and an additional 58 did so after 2 or more courses of prolonged use. This incidence of effectiveness of 95 per cent is precisely equivalent to that reported by Stein and Leventhal as a result of ovarian wedge resection. The incidence of pregnancy subsequent to the use of clomiphene does not, however, approach the 85 per cent pregnancy rate reported for surgical intervention by Stein and Leventhal.

Effects of Clomiphene

The mechanism of action may be directly on the ovary or on the hypothalamus (Fig. 7-51). Greenblatt and co-workers found an initial rise in FSH excretion, followed by an increase in estrogen secretion and then a rise in LH. This LH peak was followed by a further rise in estrogen excretion and an increase in pregnanediol. The increase in estrogens was accompanied by a rise in urinary 17-ketosteroids and tetrahydrocorticoids. The changes in FSH and LH subsequent to clomiphene administration in women with polycystic ovaries have now been studied using immunoassay methods and, in general, parallel the pattern described above. In our original report only 38 per cent of patients became pregnant. There are numerous reasons which negate the validity of a direct comparison of results of surgery versus clomiphene:

1. Wedge resection is usually reserved for patients who are married and desirous of pregnancy, and usually is not performed until the male has demonstrated normal seminal fluid analyses; clomiphene, however, has been administered to numerous patients with the Stein-Leventhal syn-

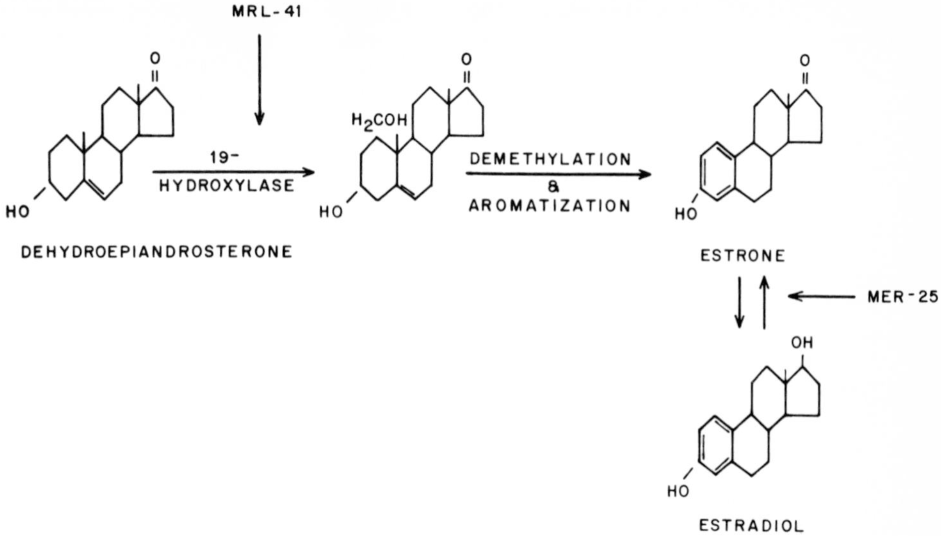

Fig. 7-51.—Graphic representation of possible sites of action of MRL-41 (Clomiphene citrate) and MER-25 on ovarian steroidogenesis.

drome who are unmarried, or married but not desirous of pregnancy, and without complete study of the male.

2. The length of follow-up of patients treated with clomiphene is not as long as surgically treated patients, since reports have frequently been submitted after 3 or 4 treatment cycles.

3. Many clomiphene-treated patients have not had a complete evaluation of tubal patency, whereas most of those treated surgically had tubal patency demonstrated either before or at the time of surgery.

Whereas clomiphene has been used in the Stein-Leventhal syndrome for the control of abnormal menses, wedge resection is usually reserved for infertility due to anovulation. If the permanency of ovulation following wedge resection approximated the 95 per cent reported by Stein and Leventhal, this certainly would be the procedure of choice. However, in numerous reports compiled by Goldzieher, a total of 1,079 patients, the incidence of ovulation approximated 80 per cent (range 6 –95) and a high rate of recurrence of oligo-ovulation was noted. The mean incidence of pregnancy was 63 per cent with a range of 13 to 89 per cent. Furthermore, we have recently been impressed with the number of patients referred to us because of recurrent amenorrhea or oligo-ovulation subsequent to wedge resection who have demonstrated extensive peritubal and periovarian adhesions by culdoscopy. Not only was the primary surgical procedure inadequate for the consistent regulation of ovulation, but it was responsible also for tubal adhesions of such severity that pregnancy was virtually impossible. None of these patients have become pregnant even though regular ovulatory cycles were established with clomiphene, and subsequent reparative tuboplasty undoubtedly will be necessary for restoration of normal tubal mobility and ovum pick-up.

In the young, unmarried patient with oligo-ovulation or secondary amenorrhea due to the Stein-Leventhal syndrome, it is obviously not necessary to secure recurrent ovulation with clomiphene, since prolonged treatment may be necessary for the restoration of normal cycles. But neither is it advisable to perform major surgery with the possibility of recurrent ovulatory insufficiency and tubal malfunction. Adequate, although temporary, therapy may be utilized in the form of cyclic estrogen-progestin combinations. These preparations will suppress the constant, irregular stimulation of the ovary by follicle-stimulating and luteinizing hormones. Since the histologic features of the ovary (hypertrophy, hyperplasia of the cortex, increased number and size of follicles) undoubtedly represent chronic stimulation by gonadotropic hormones, suppression of these stimuli should prevent the progressive changes noted in the ovary. The excessive androgen production will thus be reduced and hirsutism diminished. Finally, the tendency toward endometrial hyperplasia will be corrected by the progestin and regular withdrawal flow will occur.

There are a very small number of patients with Stein-Leventhal syndrome who apparently ovulate subsequent to the administration of clomiphene but in whom pregnancy does not occur. Leventhal has suggested that the ovarian cortex in these patients is excessively thickened and the indirect indices of ovulation, i.e., progesterone production, may be due to intra-ovarian ovulation without ovum release. In this small group of patients, wedge resection is advised. But this surgical approach should be the *last*, not the first therapeutic measure.

From the earlier discussion on pituitary-hypothalamic and ovarian factors in polycystic disease, an explanation for the empirically derived procedure of wedge resection seems to be at hand. It is most interesting that the wedging procedure should yield widely divergent results in different hands. The average success of wedge resection is high, with restoration of menstrual regularity in 80 per cent of patients and attainment of desired pregnancy in 63 per cent. However, in some series less than 10 per cent of subjects experienced regulation of menses.

The need for re-examination of the criteria used to decide upon surgery is apparent from the statistical facts given above, from the variability in surgical results, and from studies in anovulatory but otherwise endocrinologically normal women who do not present the alleged syndrome of Stein and Leventhal. Epstein *et al* reported on 19 such patients. In spite of the absence of the usual indications for surgery, wedge resection produced ovulatory menses in 74 per cent, and 8 of 14 patients achieved pregnancy. Numerous investigators have found no relationship between the response to surgery and the size of the ovaries, the 17-ketosteroid excretion, or any other laboratory parameter.

Why does wedge resection work? The following explanation has been suggested by Goldzieher. The fact that polycystic ovarian disease is usually associated with anovulatory menstrual function from menarche on strongly suggests that some disorder of hypothalamic-pituitary regulation of the ovary already exists at that time. One might speculate that the hypothalamic cycling center has failed to develop a proper rhythm to regulate the reproductive mechanism. With the absence or inadequacy of this regulation, there is an absence or infrequency of ovulatory cycles. The negative feedback effect of progesterone is missing, and estrogen production, acting continuously on the pituitary and hypothalamus, causes an outpouring and irregular release of gonadotropin. Thus, a vicious circle of noncyclic releasing-factor secretion, noncyclic and perhaps qualitatively abnormal gonadotropin secretion, and uninterrupted positive estrogen feedback exists. As a secondary result, the ovarian steroidogenic pathways become disorganized, with breakdown at the crucial aromatizing and 3β-ol-dehydrogenase systems. The existing estrogen production, at whatever level, is paid for with a disproportionately high production of androgens. Continuous abnormal gonadotropin stimulation causes the development and atresia of many follicles, producing the typical gross appearance and probably also the stromal hyperplasia.

The act of wedge resection inflicts a severe trauma on the ovary, particularly when the usual recommendations are followed and a generous portion of tissue, with incision well down into the hilus, is carried out. A transient but drastic reduction in ovarian hormone output, including the estrogens, has been shown to follow. As a consequence, there is an interruption of the vicious circle, of the positive feedback effect of estrogen. The pressure for continuous gonadotropin release is removed and gonadotropin may accumulate. The exhausted ovarian enzymes have an opportunity to reconstitute themselves. If the hypothalamic cycling center is able to resume a rhythm which the rest of the system can follow, cyclic menstrual activity ensues.

The fact that fertility is corrected less often than the menstrual rhythm may be the result of surgical factors, irreversible ovarian pathology such as capsular fibrosis, or other unknown influences. There is reason to believe that capsular fibrosis is a consequence of androgen overproduction. Administration or local implantation of testosterone to monkeys, for example, can produce ovarian capsular fibrosis. Clearly, the local concentration of androgens in polycystic disease would be much higher in the ovary itself than in the peripheral circulation.

The technique for wedge resection of the ovary used at the Boston Hospital for Women has been essentially that described by Stein and Leventhal in their original paper. A "generous" segment of ovarian tissue is excised from the antimesenteric border, the surface being about 3–5 mm. in width. We have not adopted medullary resection of the ovary since we did not wish to interfere with the ovarian blood supply and since, in view of the studies of Salhanick and Warren, the actual source of the androgenic hormone seemed conclusively to be in the cortex and not in the medulla. After the segment has been excised, the surfaces are approximated with a running suture of 000 chromic catgut. A single suture of inverted mattress type is then placed through the approximated edges in order to eliminate dead space and the accumulation of blood or fluid in this area. Meticulous hemostasis is imperative in order to prevent subsequent tubo-ovarian adhesions. Despite the importance and obvious success of ovarian wedge resection in patients with Stein-Leventhal syndrome, it now appears that the use of clomiphene citrate in this syndrome will relegate the surgical approach to a very minor position. Wedge resection is indicated in patients who apparently ovulate subsequent to the use of clomiphene but in whom pregnancy does not occur. At least six to eight courses of clomiphene should be given, however, before deciding that the patient is a "clomiphene pregnancy failure."

BIBLIOGRAPHY

Ovarian Tumors

Asadourian, L. A., and Taylor, H. B.: Dysgerminoma. An analysis of 105 cases, Obst. & Gynec. 33:370, 1969.

Burns, B. C., *et al.*: Management of ovarian carcinoma, Am. J. Obst. & Gynec. 98:374, 1967.

Brunschwig, A.: Attempted palliation by radical surgery for pelvic and abdominal carcinomatosis primary in the ovaries, Cancer 14:384, 1961.

Emig, O. R.; Hertig, A. T., and Rowe, F. G.: Gynandroblastoma of the ovary: Review and report of a case, Obst. & Gynec. 13:135, 1959.

Graham, J. B., *et al.*: Preclinical detection of ovarian cancer, Cancer 17:1414, 1964.

Gray, L. A., and Barnes, M. L.: Endometrioid carcinoma of the ovary, Obst. & Gynec. 29:694, 1962.

Griffiths, C. T.: Carcinoma of the ovary, in *Cancer—A Manual for Practitioners* (4th ed.: Boston: American Cancer Society, 1968).

————: X-ray, chemotherapy, and surgery in the management of advanced ovarian cancer, Proceedings of the American Society of Clinical Oncology, 1968.

Grogan, R. H.: Accidental rupture of malignant ovarian cysts during surgical removal, Obst. & Gynec. 30:716, 1967.

Hall, T. C.: Chemotherapy of cancer, New England J. Med. 266:129, 1962.

Henderson, D.: Malignancy of special ovarian tumors, Am. J. Obst. & Gynec. 62:816, 1951.

Hertig, A. T., and Gore, H. M.: Tumors of the Female Sex Organs: Part 3. Tumors of the Ovary and Fallopian Tube, sec. IX, fasc. 33, in *Atlas of Tumor Pathology* (*Washington, D.C.: Armed Forces Institute of Pathology, 1961*).

Hreshchyshyn, M. M.: Chemotherapy of Ovarian Cancer, in Lewis, Wentz and Jaffe (eds.): *New Concepts of Gynecological Cancer* (Philadelphia: F. A. Davis Company, 1966) p. 341.

Hughesdon, P. E.: Ovarian lipoid and theca cell tumors; their origins and interrelations, Obst. & Gynec. Surv. 21:245. 1966.

————, and Fraser, I. T.: Arrhenoblastoma of ovary: Case report and histological review, Acta obst. et gynec. scandinav. 32:supp. 4, 1953.

Idelson, M. G.: Malignancy in Brenner tumors of the ovary, with comments on histogenesis and possible estrogen production, Obst. & Gynec. Surv. 18:246, 1963.

Iverson, L.: Masculinizing tumors of the ovary: A clinicopathologic survey with discussion of histogenesis and report of 3 cases, Surg. Gynec. & Obst. 84:213, 1947.

Javert, C. T., and Finn, W. F.: Arrhenoblastoma: The incidence of malignancy and the relationship to pregnancy, to sterility and to treatment, Cancer 4:60, 1951.

Julian, C. G., and Woodruff, J. D.: The role of chemotherapy in the treatment of primary ovarian malignancy, Obst. & Gynec. Surv. 24:1307, 1969.

Kent, S. W., and McKay, D. G.: Primary cancer of the ovary, Am. J. Obst. & Gynec. 80:430, 1960.

Kistner, R. W.: Intraperitoneal rupture of benign cystic teratomas: A review of literature with report of 2 cases, Obst. & Gynec. Surv. 7:603, 1952.

————, and Hertig, A. T.: Primary adenoacanthoma of the ovary: A review of the literature with a report of 5 cases, Cancer 5:1134, 1952.

Kottmeier, H. L.: Modern trends in the treatment of patients with semimalignant and malignant ovarian tumors, in *Carcinoma of the Uterine Cervix, Endometrium and Ovary* (Chicago: Year Book Medical Publishers, Inc., 1962).

Long, M. E., and Taylor, H. C.: Endometrioid carcinoma of the ovary, Am J. Obst. & Gynec. 90: 936, 1964.

Long, R. T. L.; Johnson, R. E., and Sala, J. M.: Variations in survival among patients with carcinoma of the ovary, Cancer 20:1195, 1967.

Malkasian, G. D., and Symmonds, R. E.: Treatment of the unilateral encapsulated ovarian dysgerminoma, Am. J. Obst. & Gynec. 90:379, 1964.

Malloy, J. J., *et al.*: Papillary ovarian tumors, Am. J. Obst. & Gynec. 93:867, 1965.

Masterson, J. G., and Nelson, J. H.: The role of chemotherapy in the treatment of gynecologic malignancy, Am. J. Obst. & Gynec. 93:1102, 1965.

McGowan, L. L.; Stein, D. B., and Miller, W.: Cul de sac aspiration for diagnostic cytologic study, Am. J. Obst. & Gynec. 96:413, 1966.

McKay, D. G.; Hertig, A. T., and Hickey, W. F.: The histogenesis of granulosa and theca cell tumors of the human ovary, Obst. & Gynec. 1:125, 1953.

Meyer, R.: Pathology of some special ovarian tumors and their relation to sex characteristics, Am. J. Obst. & Gynec. 22:697, 1931.

Miller, S. P., and Brenner, S. M.: Combination therapy with cobalt-60 and chlorambucil in treatment of disseminated ovarian carcinomatosis, Cancer Chemotherap. Rep. 16:455, 1962.

Munnell, E. W.: The changing prognosis and treatment in cancer of the ovary, Am. J. Obst. & Gynec. 100:790, 1968.

Novak, E. R., and Mattingly, R. F.: Hilus cell tumor of the ovary, Obst. & Gynec. 15:425, 1960.

Novak, E. R., and Woodruff, J. D.: Mesonephroma of the ovary, Am. J. Obst. & Gynec. 77:632, 1959.

————; Woodruff, J. D., and Linthicum, J. M.: Evaluation of the unclassified tumors of the ovarian tumor registry (1942–1952), Am. J. Obst. & Gynec. 87:999, 1963.

Pedowitz, P.; Felmus, L. B., and Grayzel, D. M.: Dysgerminoma of the ovary: Prognosis and treatment, Am. J. Obst. & Gynec. 70:1284, 1955.
———, and Grayzel, D. M.: Dysgerminoma of the ovary: An analysis of 17 cases with special reference to histogenesis and therapy, Am. J. Obst. & Gynec. 61:1243, 1951.
Peterson, W. F., et al.: Benign cystic teratoma of the ovary: A clinicostatistical study of 1,007 cases with a review of the literature, Am. J. Obst. & Gynec. 70:368, 1955.
Robinson, D., and Hertig, A. T.: Histochemical observations on granulosa cell tumors, thecomas and fibromas of the ovary, Am. J. Obst. & Gynec. 1:125, 1953.
Rubin, P.: Has postoperative irradiation proved itself?, Am. J. Roentgenol. 88:849, 1962.
Sandberg, E. C.: The virilizing ovary. Part I—A histogenetic evaluation, Obst. & Gynec. Surv. 17:165, 1962.
Schiller, W.: Recent findings in solid ovarian tumors. J. Obst. & Gynaec. Brit. Emp. 43:1135, 1936.
Schueller, E. F., and Kirol, P. M.: Prognosis in endometrioid carcinoma of the ovary, Obst. & Gynec. 27:851, 1966.
Scully, R. E., and Barlow, J. F.: "Mesonephroma" of ovary, Cancer 20:1405, 1967.
———, Richardson, G. S., and Barlow, J. F.: The development of malignancy in endometriosis, Clin. Obst. & Gynec. 9:384, 1966.
Smith, G. V.: Ovarian tumors, Am. J. Surg. 95:336, 1958.
Teilum, G.: Gonocytoma, homologous ovarian and testicular tumors. I. With discussion of "Mesonephroma ovarii," Acta path. et microbiol. scandinav. 23:242, 1946.
Thompson, J. D.: Primary ovarian adenoacanthoma, Clin. Obst. & Gynec. 9:403, 1957.
Van Orman, F. L., and Mautner, L. S.: Intraperitoneal rupture of dermoid cysts, Am. J. Obst. & Gynec. 62:685, 1951.
Woodruff, J. D., and Novak, E. R.: The Kruckenberg tumor—study of 48 cases from The Ovarian Tumor Registry, Obst. & Gynec. 15:351, 1960.

Sclerocystic Ovarian Disease (Stein-Leventhal)

Andrews, W. C., and Andrews, M. C.: Stein-Leventhal syndrome with associated adenocarcinoma of the endometrium, Am. J. Obst. & Gynec. 80:632, 1960.
Benedict, P. H., et al.: Ovarian and adrenal morphology in cases of hirsutism or virilism and Stein-Leventhal syndrome, Fertil. & Steril. 13:380, 1962.
Charles, D.: MRL-41 in treatment of secondary amenorrhea and endometrial hyperplasia, Lancet 2:278, 1962.
Dorfman, R. I.: A review, steroid hormones in gynecology, Obst. & Gynec. Surv. 18:65, 1963.
Evans, T. N., and Riley, G. M.: Polycystic ovarian disease, a clinical and experimental study, Am. J. Obst. & Gynec. 80:873, 1960.
Forchielli, E., et al.: Testosterone in human plasma, Analyt. Biochem. 5:416, 1963.
Gold, J. J., and Frank, R.: The borderline adrenogenital syndrome: An intermediate entity, Am. J. Obst. & Gynec. 75:1034, 1958.
Goldzieher, J. W.: Polycystic Ovarian Disease, in Marcus, S. L., and Marcus, C. C. (eds.): Advances in Obstetrics and Gynecology (Baltimore: Williams and Wilkins Company, 1967) vol. 1.
———: Polycystic Ovarian Disease, in Behrman, S. J., and Kistner, R. W. (eds.): Progress in Infertility (Boston: Little Brown & Company, 1968).
———, and Axelrod, L. R.: The polycystic ovary. II. Urinary steroid excretion, J. Clin. Endocrinol. 22:425, 1962.
———, and Green, J. A.: The polycystic ovary. I. Clinical and histological features, J. Clin. Endocrinol. 22:325, 1962.
Greenblatt, R. B.: The syndrome of large, pale ovaries and its differentiation from adrenogenital syndrome and Cushing's disease, Postgrad. Med. 9:492, 1951.
———: The polycystic ovary syndrome, Maryland M. J., March 1961, p. 1.
———, and Baldwin, K. R.: The polycystic ovary syndrome (Stein-Leventhal syndrome), J. Clin. Endocrinol. 1:498, 1960.
———; Barfield, W. E., and Lampros, C. T.: Cortisone in the treatment of infertility, Fertil. & Steril. 7:203, 1956.
———, Roy, S., and Mahesh, V. B.: Induction of ovulation, Am. J. Obst. & Gynec. 84:900, 1962.
———, et al.: Induction of ovulation with MRL-41, J.A.M.A. 178:101, 1961.
Ingersoll, F. M., and McArthur, J. W.: Longitudinal studies of gonadotropin excretion in the Stein-Leventhal syndrome, Am. J. Obst. & Gynec. 77:795, 1959.
———, and McDermott, W. M., Jr.: Bilateral polycystic ovaries, Stein-Leventhal syndrome, Am. J. Obst. & Gynec. 60:117, 1960.
Jackson, R. L., and Dockerty, M. B.: The Stein-Leventhal syndrome. Analysis of 43 cases with special reference to association with endometrial carcinoma, Am. J. Obst. & Gynec. 73:161, 1957.
Jeffries, W. M.: Effect of small doses of cortisone upon urinary 17-ketosteroid fraction in patients with ovarian dysfunction, J. Clin. Endocrinol. 22:255, 1962.
Jones, H. W., and Jones G. S.: Editors note, Obst. & Gynec. Surv. 18:126, 1963.
Kase, N.: Steroid synthesis in abnormal ovaries. III. Polycystic ovaries, Am. J. Obst. & Gynec. 90:1268, 1964.

————, Forchielli, E., and Dorfman, R. I.: Biosynthesis of testosterone and androst-4-ene-3, 17-dione in patients with polycystic ovaries, Acta endocrinol. 44:8, 1963.

————; Kowal, J.; Perloff, W., and Soffer, L. J.: In vitro production of androgens by virilising adrenal adenoma and associated polycystic ovaries, Acta endocrinol. 44:15, 1963.

————, Kowal, J., and Soffer, L. J.: In vitro production of testosterone and androstenedione in normal and Stein-Leventhal ovaries, Acta endocrinol. 44:8, 1963.

Kaufman, R. M.; Abbott, J. P., and Wall, J. A.: The endometrium before and after wedge resection of the ovaries in the Stein-Leventhal syndrome, Am. J. Obst. & Gynec. 77:1271, 1959.

Keettel, W. C.; Bradbury, J. T., and Stoddard, F. J.: Observations on the polycystic ovary syndrome, Am. J. Obst. & Gynec. 73:954, 1957.

Kistner, R. W.: Induction of ovulation with clomiphene citrate (Clomid), South African J. Obst. and Gynaec. 5:25, 1967.

————: Induction of Ovulation with Clomiphene Citrate, in Behrman, S. J., and Kistner, R. W. (eds.): *Progress in Infertility* (Boston: Little, Brown & Company, 1968).

————, and Smith, O. W.: Observations on the use of a nonsteroidal estrogen antagonist: MER-25, S. Forum 10:725, 1959.

————, and Smith, O. W.: Observations on the use of a nonsteroidal estrogen antagonist: MER-25, Fertil. & Steril. 12:121, 1961.

Lanthier, A.: Urinary 17-ketosteroids in the syndrome of polycystic ovaries and hyperthecosis, J. Clin. Endocrinol. 20:1587, 1960.

————, and Sandor, T.: The urinary excretion of pregnanediol and pregnanetriol in the polycystic ovary (Stein-Leventhal) syndrome, Acta endocrinol. 46:245, 1964.

Leventhal, M. L.: Functional and morphologic studies of the ovaries and suprarenal glands in the Stein-Leventhal syndrome, Am. J. Obst. & Gynec. 84:154, 1962.

Lloyd, C. W., and Weisz, J.: Hypothalamus and Anterior Pituitary, in Behrman, S. J., and Kistner, R. W. (eds.): *Progress in Infertility* (Boston: Little, Brown & Company, 1968).

McArthur, J. W.; Ingersoll, F. M., and Worcester, J.: The urinary excretion of interstitial cell and follicle stimulating hormone activity by women with diseases of the reproductive system, J. Clin. Endocrinol. 18:1202, 1958.

Mahesh, V. B., and Greenblatt, R. B.: Isolation of dehydroepiandrosterone and 17-alpha-hydroxy-delta-5-pregnenolone from the polycystic ovaries of the Stein-Leventhal syndrome, J. Clin. Endocrinol. 22:441, 1962.

————, and Greenblatt, R. B.: Secretion of androgens by the polycystic ovary and its significance, Fertil. & Steril. 13:513, 1962.

————, and Greenblatt, R. B.: Steroid secretions of the normal and polycystic ovary, Recent Prog. Hormone Res. 20:341, 1964.

Mishell, D. R.: Daily immunoassay of luteinizing hormone excretion in patients receiving clomiphene citrate, Fertil. & Steril. 18:102, 1967.

Naville, A. H.; Kistner, R. W.; Wheatley, E. R., and Rock, J.: Induction of ovulation with clomiphene citrate, Fertil. & Steril. 15:290, 1964.

Roy, S.; Greenblatt, R. B.; Mahesh, V. B., and Jungck, E. C.: Clomiphene citrate: Further observations on its use in induction of ovulation in the human and on its mode of action, Fertil. & Steril. 14:575. 1963.

Ryan, K. J.: Biological aromatization of steroids, J. Biol. Chem. 234:268, 1959.

————, and Smith, O. W.: Biogenesis of estrogens by human ovary: I. Conversion of acetate-1-C-14 to estrone and estradiol, J. Biol. Chem. 236:705, 1961.

Scott, R. B., and Wharton, L. R.: Effect of testosterone on experimental endometriosis in Rhesus monkeys, Am. J. Obst. & Gynec. 78:1020, 1959.

Shearman, R. P.: The enigmatic polycystic ovary, Obst. & Gynec. Surv. 21:1, 1966.

————: Induction of ovulation, Australasian Ann. Med. 15:266, 1966.

Short, R. V.: Further observations on the defective synthesis of ovarian steroids in the Stein-Leventhal syndrome, J. Endocrinol. 24:359, 1962.

————, and London, D. R.: Defective biosynthesis of ovarian steroids in the Stein-Leventhal syndrome, Brit. M. J. 5241:1724, 1961.

Smith, O. W.: Chemical induction of ovulation (Letter to the Journal), J.A.M.A. 179:99, 1962.

————, and Day, C. F.: Effect of clomiphene on aromatization of steroids by the human placenta in vitro, Acta endocrinol. 44:519, 1963.

————, and Ryan, K. J.: Estrogen in the human ovary, Am. J. Obst. & Gynec. 84:141, 1962.

————: Smith, G. V., and Kistner, R. W.: Action of MER-25 and of clomiphene on the human ovary, J.A.M.A. 184:878, 1963.

Soffer, L. J., and Fogel, M.: Urinary concentration of gonadotropin (ICSH)-inhibiting substance in Stein-Leventhal syndrome, J. Clin. Endocrinol. 24:656, 1964.

Sohval, A. R., and Soffer, L. J.: The influence of cortisone and adrenocorticotropin on urinary gonadotropin excretion, J. Clin. Endocrinol. 11:677, 1951.

Sommers, S. C.: Pituitary cell relations to body states, Lab. Invest. 8:588, 1959.

————, and Meissner, W. A.: Endocrine abnormalities accompanying human endometrial cancer, Cancer 10:516, 1957.

————, and Wadman, P. J.: Pathogenesis of polycystic ovaries, Am. J. Obst. & Gynec. 72:160, 1956.

Southam, A. L., and Janowski, N. A.: Massive ovarian stimulation with clomiphene citrate, J.A.M.A. 181:443, 1962.

Stein, I. F.: The Stein-Leventhal syndrome: A curable form of sterility, New England J. Med. 259:420, 1958.

————, and Leventhal, M. L.: Amenorrhea associated with bilateral polycystic ovaries, Am. J. Obst. & Gynec. 29:181, 1935.

Taymor, M. L., and Barnard, R.: Luteinizing hormone excretion in polycystic ovary syndrome, Fertil. & Steril. 13:501, 1962.

————; Clark, B. J., and Sturgis, S. H.: The polycystic ovary. A clinical and laboratory study, Am. J. Obst. & Gynec. 86:188, 1963.

Townsend, S. L.; Brown, J. B.; Johnstone, J. W.; Adey, F. D.; Evans, J. H., and Taft, H. P.: Induction of ovulation, J. Obst. & Gynaec. Brit. Emp. 73:529, 1966.

Tyler, E. T.; Winer, J., Gotlib, M., Olson, H. J., and Nabkayashi, N.: Effects of MRL-41 in human male and female fertility studies, Clin. Res. 10:119, 1962.

Warren, J. C., and Salhanick, H. A.: Steroid biosynthesis in the human ovary, J. Clin. Endocrinol. 21:1218, 1961.

Chapter **8**

Endometriosis

ALTHOUGH ENDOMETRIOSIS WAS DESCRIBED in detail more than a century ago, it continues to be one of the unsolved, enigmatic diseases affecting the female. The first known report was written by Rokitansky in 1860, but following this only a few scattered reports appeared until about 1900 when Cullen and Meyer published extensive descriptions of their findings. Yet Cattell and Swinton were able to find less than 20 reports concerning endometriosis in the world literature prior to 1921.

In 1921 Sampson published the first of his series of reports, recording for posterity his theory of implantation as the causative factor in the disease. His papers awakened wide interest, even controversy, in the subject and today his theory kindles as much heated argument among physicians as it did after publication of his first papers.

Definitions.—*Endometriosis* may be defined as the presence of functioning endometrial tissue outside of its normal situation but usually confined to the pelvis in the region of the ovaries, uterosacral ligaments, cul-de-sac and uterovesical peritoneum. The development and extension of endometrial tissue into the myometrium is termed *adenomyosis*. This disease entity seems unrelated histogenetically and is characterized by an entirely different clinical situation. Furthermore, the pelvic examination presents none of the characteristics of endometriosis. It should be reiterated that the term endometriosis implies *proliferating growth and function* (usually bleeding) in an extrauterine site. An *endometrioma* may be defined as an area of endometriosis, usually in the ovary, which has enlarged sufficiently to be classified as a tumor. When the endometrioma is filled with old blood, resembling tarry or chocolate-colored sirupy fluid, it is commonly known as a "chocolate cyst." It should be remembered, however, that a corpus luteum hematoma may have an identical gross appearance, so that all chocolate cysts should not be considered due to endometriosis. Even in bona fide endometriomas the histology may be confusing, since endometrial glands and stroma may become compressed by the pressure of the trapped blood and the pathologist is unable to make a specific diagnosis. If the endometriosis is not completely "burned out," close examination of the wall usually reveals numerous hemosiderin-laden macrophages, lymphocytes and patches of condensed endometrial stroma without glands.

Histogenesis

The most popular theory of histogenesis is that **of** Sampson, who stated that viable fragments of endometrium are regurgitated with menstrual blood in a retrograde fashion through the oviducts with subsequent implantation on the ovaries or into the posterior cul-de-sac. Adequate evidence has now been accumulated to prove that at least some of the desquamated endometrium is viable and capable of growth. The experimental work of Geist demonstrated without question that clumps of endometrial cells could flow from the uterine cavity through the minute lumen of the interstitial portion of the oviduct. Subsequent work in Rhesus monkeys by Scott, Te Linde and Wharton proved that pelvic endometriosis could be produced artificially. They inverted the uterus so that menstruation occurred into the pelvis. Endometriosis developed in six of the first 10 monkeys so treated, although a rather prolonged period of time (75 to 963 days) was necessary to bring about the complete change. Recently Ridley and Edwards produced endometriosis in human subjects by injecting shed human endometrium into the site of a subsequent laparotomy incision.

One of the first ideas regarding pathogenesis was advanced by Russell in 1899. This author described glands in the ovary and suggested their growth from cell rests of the müllerian ducts. A similar theory was fostered by Robert Meyer. He suggested that the peritoneal mesothelium possessed totipotentiality so that recurring tubal reflux of menstrual detritus (blood, inflammatory cells and endometrium) stimulated this tissue to undergo metaplasia into functioning endometrium. There is no doubt that the serosa lining the coelomic cavity, including that investing the female genitalia, has not only a common origin but does not "use up" its developmental potential. Given proper stimulation, it may awaken to new activity and produce differentiated structures identical to those which it produced during the embryonic stage. Emil Novak tactfully embraced both theories, suggesting a metaplastic change in the ovaries as being primary with subsequent dissemination to surrounding peritoneal surfaces.

Areas of endometriosis have been described in the lungs, pleura, arms, thighs and pelvic lymph nodes. An explanation for these sites is given in the theory of Halban, who suggested that all heterotopic areas of endometriosis, wherever found, were metastatic growths originating in the endometrium and reaching their destination via the lymphatics. A common error is to assume that Sampson suggested that all endometriosis was due to reverse flow of menstrual blood through the oviducts. Sampson actually demonstrated endometrial tissue in both lymph and blood channels. He concluded that "we are warranted in stating that the invasion and dissemination of benign endometrial tissue employ the same channels as the invasion and dissemination of cancer." In all probability "more than one" avenue is available for the development and spread of this disease. Scott suggested that these various theories are not mutually exclusive. He states that the viability of endometrial fragments is definitely proved and that retrograde tubal passage of these fragments takes place, with secondary spread from functioning areas of endometriosis. He notes further that there is lymphatic and vascular spread to various areas and occasional transpulmonic passage to distant foci. Scott believes the coelomic metaplasia theory to be the least likely explanation for the pathogenesis of endometriosis.

Hertig has summarized the various theories of histogenesis as follows: "(1) The embryonic rest concept is no longer tenable in view of current reports. (2) The implantation theory is supported by findings such as reflux bleeding through the tubes, the viability of endometrium in tissue culture and in direct transplantation, plus the ingenious experiments in the monkey of diverting menstrual blood and detritus into the pelvic cavity. However, it has never been demonstrated whether the histologic sequence begins with implantation of endometrial fragments per se or arises from the inflammatory or inductive effect of menstrual blood on the pelvic peritoneum and its focal endometrial stroma. (3) The concept of lymphatic or vascular metastatic origin neglects or ignores the universally present endometrial stroma and the almost universally accepted concept of the müllerian potential of coelomic epithelium, in general, and germinal epithelium, in particular."

The probable sequence in the formation of endometriosis, as suggested by Hertig, is as follows: (1) formation of a fibrinopurulent exudate; (2) its organization by subperitoneal stroma, including endometrial stroma, and (3) formation of glandlike spaces lined by pelvic peritoneum. Thus Hertig considers ovarian endometriosis to be one of, or related to, the cystomas of germinal epithelial origin.

Certain mechanical, inflammatory and hormonal factors have been suggested as possible stimulating influences on the development of endometriosis. It is possible that each of these, or all of them, may act to incite the development of this unusual malady.

Mechanical transplantation of endometrial tissue during laparotomy, delivery or curettage is a possible etiologic factor. Blood is occasionally seen dripping from the fimbriated portions of the oviducts when laparotomy follows a thorough curettage performed during the late secretory or menstrual phase of the cycle. Tubal insufflation, especially if performed repeatedly during the luteal phase, has been mentioned as an inciting mechanism. Experiments in rabbits and guinea pigs in which air was forced through the oviducts on 10 consecutive days have resulted in the formation of endometrial cysts after a time lapse of four months. It has been suggested, therefore, that excessive tubal testing may actually initiate or potentiate the development of endometriosis. Uterine retroversion has been observed in from 15 to 50 per cent of patients with endometriosis. However, it is possible that retroversion in this disease is secondary to the scarring and fibrosis of the cul-de-sac. Numerous experiments have demonstrated, however, that a severe degree of uterine retrodisplacement may facilitate the flow of intrauterine fluid out through the oviducts, provided the subject remains in the supine position. Cervical obstruction, due either to stricture or to sharp flexion of the corpus on the cervix, has been mentioned as a factor which would tend to increase the possibility of retrograde flow through the tubes. However, studies of patients with congenital or acquired atresias of the lower genital tract, despite an increased frequency of hematocolpos, hematometra and hematosalpinx, do not show an increased incidence of endometriosis.

An inflammatory process of the pelvic peritoneum has been postulated as aiding the development of endometriosis. This is based on Sampson's original observation that regurgitated menstrual blood was irritating to pelvic peritoneum and on Frankl's description of an inflammatory reaction in areas of endometriosis. Most evidence now indicates that this cellular reaction is secondary and not a primary factor in etiology.

Hormonal factors are obviously associated with, but not necessarily the cause of, endometriosis. The disease occurs during the sexually active period of life, beginning after puberty and ceasing in most patients at the menopause. Ectopic endometrial tissue and normally situated endometrium respond, with minor variations, to ovarian hormones in a similar but not precise manner. However, the ability to stimulate already existing tissue to physiologic activity is not the same as the ability to initiate the development of new tissue. The relationship of endometriosis to infertility is a definite one but the question of precedence remains unanswered.

This review of the histogenesis is important because of its relationship to the following clinical observations in patients with endometriosis: (1) The disease occurs only after the female begins to menstruate and is of no serious consequence (except as it is related to ovarian cancer) after the menopause. (2) It is rarely seen in women with anovulatory cycles, but it is common in those who have uninterrupted cyclic menstruation for periods exceeding five years. (3) Endometriosis improves both subjectively and objectively during periods of physiologically induced (pregnancy) and artificially induced (hormones) anovulation. (4) Frequent pregnancies, if initiated early in menstrual life, seem to prevent the disease. (5) Endometriosis is commonly associated with infertility but it is not known whether endometriosis occurs because pregnancy is deferred or whether infertility is the eventual result of extensive endometriosis. There may be a combination of factors at work to prevent conception.

Pathology

The commonest site of endometriosis is the ovary, and in about 50 per cent of patients both ovaries are involved. Other areas and organs affected (in order of incidence) are: uterosacral ligaments and rectovaginal septum, sigmoid colon, lower genital tract (cervix, vulva and vagina), round ligaments, pelvic peritoneum, small intestine, umbilicus and laparotomy scars, bladder and ureter, breast, arm, leg, pleura and lung (Fig. 8–1). Early endometriosis may occur either as small, bluish, punctate or hemorrhagic areas on the surface of the ovary or uterosacral ligaments or as small cysts or foci of pink tissue lying beneath the surface epithelium or within the ovarian cortical stroma. The benign endometrial cyst of the ovary varies from microscopic size to a mass 8–10 cm. in diameter. The cysts may be multiple in the early stages but subsequently coalesce into a single large cyst. During the early stage of development, endometriotic cysts are usually free and have smooth surfaces. As growth progresses, however, and there is surface bleeding, the cyst becomes densely adherent to surrounding structures, particularly the serosa of the sigmoid colon. The convex border (lateral aspect) of the ovary is more often involved and may become adherent to the ileum or lateral pelvic peritoneum. Frequently the ovary shows multiple areas resembling "powder burns" as a result of changes in blood pigments. Minute red or blue cystic areas (raspberry or blueberry spots) with adjacent puckering may be identified on the ovarian surface but are noted more often on the uterosacral ligaments or pelvic peritoneum. The lining of the endometrial cyst varies from red to dark brown, depending on the extent and duration of bleeding. It may be thin and smooth or thick and velvety, depending on the preponderance of fibrous tissue or functioning endometrium. If discrete papillary or polypoid lesions are found in the cyst cavity, the possibility of malignancy should be con-

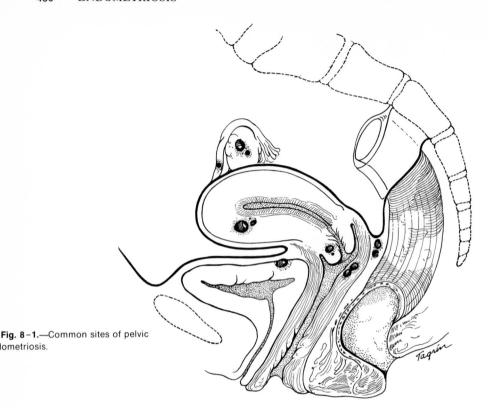

Fig. 8-1.—Common sites of pelvic endometriosis.

sidered. The contents of the cyst are usually thick, resembling chocolate sirup or tar.

The four basic structures seen microscopically in endometriosis are endometrial epithelium, glands or glandlike structures, stroma and hemorrhage (Fig. 8-2). Continuing function in areas of endometriosis tends to destroy its microscopic characteristics, thus Hertig's observation, "the more advanced the lesion clinically, the poorer the histologic detail" is the most descriptive. Early lesions, particularly those of the cul-de-sac, if excised in toto and properly oriented for the pathologist, usually demonstrate classic histology, whereas the large endometrial cyst of the ovary, obvious to the gynecologist at the operating table, may show only hemosiderin-laden macrophages with varying amounts of fibrous connective tissue and inflammatory cells. However, it is important to remember that it is the endometrial stroma which is responsible for bleeding in endometriosis, not the glands or epithelium. The presence of stroma alone is diagnostic of the disease and the experienced gynecologic pathologist usually makes the diagnosis of endometriosis without difficulty. The presence of a decidual reaction or a typical "naked-nuclei" cellular pattern surrounded by a delicate reticulum or spiral arterioles with adjacent predecidua, either with or without old or recent hemorrhage, is sufficient to permit the diagnosis to be made without glands.

Malignancy in endometriosis is rare and may be of the mixed variety, the so-called adenoacanthoma. These cysts tend to be larger than the

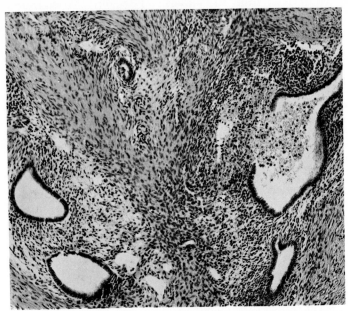

Fig. 8-2.—Endometriosis of uterosacral ligament. Typical endometrial glands and stroma are evident in the fibrous connective tissue of the ligament.

benign form, averaging 8-9 cm. When the tumor is sufficiently differentiated, the prognosis is considerably better than that associated with ovarian cancer in general. Kistner and Hertig described five primary ovarian adenoacanthomas which they believed originated in endometriosis. It is possible, of course, that many ovarian cancers originate in areas of endometriosis but are so undifferentiated at the time of laparotomy that exact diagnosis is not possible. Criteria for the diagnosis of carcinoma arising in endometriosis were outlined by Sampson in 1925 and are still acceptable. They are:

1. The ovary must be the site of benign endometriosis.
2. There must be a genuine adenocarcinoma.
3. A transition from benign to malignant areas must be demonstrable.

Only about 25 bona fide cases of carcinoma arising in ovarian endometriosis have been reported and a good number of these have been adenoacanthomas. These tumors rarely if ever metastasized widely, were rarely fatal, but were prone to local invasion.

Ectopic endometrium in endometriosis does not always respond to the stimulation of estrogen and progesterone in the same degree as does the normally situated endometrium. Frequently it exhibits only a proliferative or hyperplastic pattern during the luteal phase of the menstrual cycle. This refractory behavior to progesterone suggests that the displaced endometrium is immature or is incapable of complete differentiation—characteristics which argue against implantation of regurgitated portions of the "functionalis" layer. (It is not likely that the basalis is regurgitated.)

It has been suggested that endometriotic lesions which do not demonstrate cyclic activity in concert with the uterine endometrium are derived from the so-called "insensitive" basal layer, while the more active endometriotic lesions are derived from the superficial "reactive" two-thirds. However, Hartman excised the endometrium from monkeys as completely as possible, leaving behind only a few fragments of the basalis, and found completely regenerated, functional endometrium in these monkeys from 14 to 20 days after surgery. This procedure was repeated in the same animal as often as four times, yet many of these monkeys subsequently became pregnant and delivered normal fetuses. We produced typical secretory changes in the basalis of patients with endometrial hyperplasia by the administration of potent, synethetic progestins (norethynodrel and 17-alphahydroxyprogesterone caproate) for 40-60 days prior to hysterectomy. Thus, a valid conclusion seems to be that the basalis will respond if adequately stimulated.

Occasionally a full progestational response is seen in areas of endometriosis which cannot be distinguished from that of the uterine endometrium. The increasing levels of chorionic estrogen and progesterone during pregnancy usually bring about a rather typical decidual change in areas of endometriosis which mimics histologically the uterine decidua. In endometriosis of the cervix or vagina this change is frequently marked and is of a florid variety so that malignancy is frequently suspected. Biopsies reveal characteristic decidual stromal change with glandular regression. Decidual change in areas of endometriosis is not necessarily diagnostic of pregnancy, however, since "pseudodeciduosis" has been reported in nonpregnant women and is probably due to an exaggerated response to endogenous steroids. It may also be produced by the administration of potent synthetic progestational agents.

The uterosacral ligaments or rectovaginal peritoneum may be involved separately or there may be a fused mass incorporating both structures. (Fig. 8-3). The frequency of the disease in this area supports Sampson's theory since the force of gravity in the upright quadruped would permit "sprinkling of the soil" by viable endometrial fragments. The discovery of bluish red or brown nodules with surrounding areas of puckering on the uterosacral ligaments, adjacent cul-de-sac, peritoneum or serosa of the sigmoid is a characteristic finding, and if these reach adequate size, they may be palpated easily on rectovaginal examination. Eventually an intensive fibrous connective tissue reaction occurs, with fusion of the rectosigmoid to the back of the cervix and vagina. Masses of this type may become so firm that malignancy is suspected and unnecessary abdominoperineal reactions have been performed if biopsy is neglected. Since bilateral oophorectomy will almost always bring about permanent arrest of the disease, this procedure should be performed in preference to extensive bowel resection (see Treatment).

The bowel lumen may actually be invaded by endometriosis with resultant rectal bleeding, tenesmus and obstruction. Biopsy of the lesion either by proctosigmoidoscopy or at laparotomy is essential before start of therapy. A few cases have been reported in which endometrial stromal sarcoma of the sigmoid was believed to have originated in sigmoid endometriosis. In general, endometriosis attacks the bowel from the serosal surface and therefore the lesion is of an extrinsic nature, whereas colon cancer originates in the mucosa. Exceptions occur, however, so that precise diagnosis by gross inspection is not always possible.

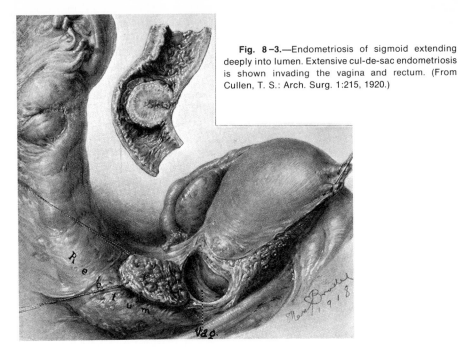

Fig. 8–3.—Endometriosis of sigmoid extending deeply into lumen. Extensive cul-de-sac endometriosis is shown invading the vagina and rectum. (From Cullen, T. S.: Arch. Surg. 1:215, 1920.)

The lower genital tract may occasionally be the site of endometriosis, lesions of the cervix, vagina and vulva having been reported. Usually there is a history of antecedent trauma, such as cervical cauterization or conization, vulvar surgery or episiotomy. Surface endometriosis of this variety is almost certainly derived from implantation of viable endometrium and, in general, responds actively to estrogen and progesterone. When endometriosis involves the portio vaginalis of the cervix, the gross examination is usually pathognomonic, with blue-black, elevated nodules, either discrete or confluent, being evident by speculum examination.

The round ligament is occasionally the site of endometriosis, and if the lesion exceeds 0.5 cm. in diameter, it can usually be palpated by examination of the inguinal areas. Subjective complaints in the region of the internal ring and/or canal of Nuck are frequently cyclic in nature and may be correlated with the menses.

Small bowel involvement is rare (about 0.1 to 0.2 per cent) but may lead to an erroneous preoperative diagnosis. There is usually twisting or coiling about the lesion with resultant symptoms of nausea and crampy midabdominal or periumbilical pain. Grossly the mucosal surface is usually smooth with subjacent fibrosis and scarring. In extensive pelvic endometriosis, several loops of ileum may be involved by contiguity so that resection of the areas is necessary. Similarly, the serosa of the appendix is often involved.

Endometriosis of the umbilicus and of laparotomy scars has been reported rather frequently. Although the theory of coelomic metaplasia is usually invoked to explain these lesions, Scott has suggested that various lymphatics situated along the obliterated hypogastric vessels might function as the route of transmission. Discomfort in the region of the umbilicus with cyclic nodularity and swelling or even gross bleeding serve to alert the clinician to the probability of endometriosis.

Urinary tract endometriosis is not common but probably occurs more often than is reported in the literature. The involvement of the serosal surface of the bladder is seen rather frequently but is usually asymptomatic. By the time the muscularis or mucosa is involved, the patient usually has noted cyclic hematuria and pain. Cystoscopy may show typical bluish "mulberry" lesions and endoscopic biopsy confirms the diagnosis. Ureteral involvement has been reported with increasing frequency during the past decade and probably explains many cases of idiopathic, unilateral hydronephrosis (Fig. 8–4). Cyclic flank pain, fever and pyuria may occur as a result of intermittent ureteral obstruction. The excretory urogram may show beginning ureteral dilatation if obtained at the optimum time in the cycle. A tentative diagnosis may be confirmed by noting cessation of symptoms and improvement in the urogram following prolonged periods of induced anovulation (see section on Treatment).

Several cases are now on record of biopsy-proved pleural and pulmonary endometriosis in which a hematogenous mode of dissemination must be postulated.

In summary, the pathologic process of endometriosis, although microscopically benign, produces extensive havoc in the pelvis as important structures are gradually involved. The process is unique in that it spreads in a cancer-like manner which is frequently terminated by fibrosis and scarring. The end result may be ovarian destruction, oviduct deformity, bladder dysfunction, large bowel obstruction and ureteral constriction

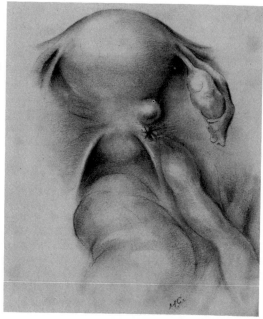

Fig. 8–4.—Endometriosis involving the right uterosacral ligament, with fibrosis producing marked right hydroureter. (Courtesy of Dr. Thomas Leavitt.)

Clinical Features

INCIDENCE

Endometriosis has been noted with increasing frequency during the past two decades and several reports have indicated that it is found in from 5 to 15 per cent of pelvic operations. It is not common in the Negro and seems to be found more among women of the higher socioeconomic groups. As such, it has been correlated with delayed or deferred motherhood. Meigs cited reports from the Masschusetts General Hospital which indicated that endometriosis was observed more often in private than in service patients. He even exhorted parents to subsidize young married couples so that early and frequent pregnancies could be undertaken. Cavanagh, however, in a study at the Sloan Hospital for Women in New York City, could find no evidence that endometriosis was related to voluntary delay of pregnancy or economic status.

The median age of patients at the time of diagnosis is about 37 years but about 15 per cent of patients are under age 30. It has been suggested that a specific body type and psychic demeanor are frequently found. The patient is said to be mesomorphic but underweight, overanxious, intelligent, egocentric and a perfectionist. These characteristics represent a personality pattern in which marriage and childbearing are likely to be deferred and therefore predispose to prolonged periods of uninterrupted ovulation. At the Boston Hospital for Women during the interval 1950–1965, endometriosis has been noted by microscope in specimens of about 18 per cent of all laparotomies performed for gynecologic disease.

SYMPTOMS

The characteristic symptoms associated with this disease are: (1) progressive, acquired, severe pain associated with or occurring just prior to menstruation, (2) dyspareunia, (3) painful defecation, (4) premenstrual staining and hypermenorrhea, (5) suprapubic pain, dysuria and hematuria and (6) infertility. Some patients do not have "acquired" dysmenorrhea but state that they have always had painful periods. Most will admit, however, to a recent increase in severity. In many patients the pain cannot be classified as dysmenorrhea but is actually premenstrual and varies from mild discomfort to severe pain that is characteristically in the lower abdomen, usually bilateral and associated with a sense of rectal pressure. A constant soreness in the lower abdomen or pelvis throughout the month that is aggravated just before the menses or during coitus may be the only complaint. The pain in endometriosis is of unknown cause but is probably related to the development of secretory changes, with subsequent miniature menstruation and bleeding in areas that are totally or partially encapsulated by fibrous tissue. That this is due to intermittent stimulation and withdrawal of progesterone is substantiated by the fact that dysmenorrhea is not evident if ovulation is prevented.

Pain is not always associated with endometriosis even when the disease is extensive. Bilateral, large ovarian endometriomas frequently are not symptomatic unless rupture occurs. On the other hand, incapacitating pelvic discomfort may be associated with minimal amounts of active endometriosis. Often there are only puckering and scarring of the posterior cul-de-sac with an adherent rectosigmoid to account for the multiplicity of symptoms. Since the factors causing pain are unknown, one must conclude that the amount of *evident* endometriosis bears no constant relationship to the degree of subjective discomfort.

The symptoms of peritoneal endometriosis, wherever located, are chiefly the result of attempted normal physiologic activity on the part of müllerian tissue in an abnormal location. Ectopic endometrium possesses the ability to menstruate, respond to the stimulus of pregnancy, retrogress at menopause, and at times even to become invasive, just as it does in the uterine cavity. It is the result of implantation, growth, invasion or surface spread, and most of all, the menstrual reaction of this tissue situated in or on the various pelvic structures. This produces the symptom complex of peritoneal endometriosis.

The disease, therefore, can manifest itself only during the period of menstrual activity, but sometimes discomfort will persist even after the menopause from some of the results of distortion and destruction. The symptoms, in the main, will bear a direct relationship to the menstrual period and will continue or increase as long as the menstrual function is maintained, although there is no uniformity in the time of the appearance, location, or duration of these symptoms.

In those patients who have had dysmenorrhea since puberty, it is impossible to tell when, if ever, the endometriosis became a factor. Unfortunately from a diagnostic standpoint, there is nothing absolutely characteristic about the pain of peritoneal endometriosis even when present, except in rare locations. It may vary in severity from mild discomfort to incapacitating pain and may be either localized or very diffuse, depending upon the distribution of the lesions, their nature, the degree of involvement of the organs affected, and the presence of complicating pathology.

Correlation with Infertility

There exists a definite correlation between infertility and endometriosis, and Rubin stated that the expectation of pregnancy when this disease is present is about half that in the general population. Thus, compared with a natural incidence of infertility approximating 15 per cent, in endometriosis the sterility incidence is 30–40 per cent. However, when operations are performed for the disease or when it is encountered during an abdominal operation, about one-third of the women will subsequently conceive if conservative procedures are carried out and if there is no other cause for infertility. Kelly and Rock reported endometriosis to be the causative factor of tubo-ovarian adhesions in 24 per cent of 143 women who had culdoscopy because of infertility, and Garcia stated that endometriosis is found in one-third of "infertility laparotomies." If studies of an infertile patient show ovulation to be occurring regularly, the oviducts to be patent, the endometrium to be normal and the postcoital test adequate, endometriosis should be considered and diagnostic procedures instituted.

The exact pathologic cause of the infertility is unknown. The oviducts are usually patent but perisalpingeal and perioophoritic adhesions are frequently found with an adherent, retroverted uterus. The endometrium is usually normal, and biopsies show secretory endometrium with progestational maturity. If other pathologic conditions such as submucous myomas and endometrial polyps are excluded, the author believes that the most important factor responsible for infertility in patients with endometriosis is an inadequacy of tubo-ovarian motility which is secondary to fibrosis and scarring. This results in imperfect ovum acceptance by the fimbria.

Diagnosis

The diagnosis may be suggested by the history, corroborated by the pelvic examination and verified by culdoscopy, biopsy and laparoscopy. On pelvic examination the finding of tender, nodular uterosacral ligaments in conjunction with a fixed uterine retroversion is almost pathognomonic. Biopsy of suspicious lesions in the vagina, perineum, umbilicus or cervix will prove the presence of endometriosis in those areas, and investigation of the cul-de-sac may be performed by culdoscopy or posterior colpotomy if the rectum is not too adherent. It should be recalled that small areas of suggestive endometriosis removed at laparotomy may show only stroma with hemorrhage and reaction to blood pigments. This should be sufficient for diagnosis in most cases but, in order to aid the pathologist, tiny blue spots or "powder burns" should be tagged with a suture for easy identification.

The nodularity of the cul-de-sac, so common in endometriosis, may be produced in rare instances by papillary lesions of ovarian carcinoma, metastatic bowel cancer or papillary mesotheliomas. A gastric carcinoma with ovarian metastases may occasionally present nodularity of the cul-de-sac which might be confusing diagnostically. Rarely, cul-de-sac irregularity may be produced by infestation with Oxyuris vermicularis.

Bidigital rectovaginal and bimanual abdominopelvic examination must always be performed in order adequately to palpate the uterosacral ligaments, the posterior surface of the uterus and the ovaries. The ovaries are so often fixed in or lateral to the cul-de-sac that they can only be palpated per rectum. The pelvic examination should be repeated during the first 24 hours of the next menstrual period or perhaps during the second or third day of flow. To facilitate the thoroughness of the examination, the bladder must be empty and the bowel cleansed by enemas.

Laboratory studies are not of particular value diagnostically but occasionally there are moderate leukocytosis and increase in the erythrocyte sedimentation rate.

Gross or microscopic blood in the urine or feces at the time of menstruation is highly suspicious of perforating endometriosis of the bladder mucosa or rectosigmoid. Cystoscopic and sigmoidoscopic examination may aid materially in establishing the diagnosis in certain patients and biopsy of bladder or sigmoid lesions is occasionally necessary. In specific instances upper and lower gastrointestinal x-rays may be of value in detecting lesions above the reach of the sigmoidoscope.

The differential diagnosis must include such diverse lesions as adenomyosis, pelvic inflammatory disease, nonspecific adhesions and ovarian carcinoma. Adenomyosis may produce similar symptomatology but usually occurs in an older age group and in multipara. The adenomyotic uterus may be symmetrically enlarged, nodular and tender but the cul-de-sac is usually normal. In pelvic inflammatory disease, the pelvic examination frequently reveals bilateral, tender, broad-ligament masses which are characteristically doughy or fluctuant. Objective and subjective improvement follows proper antibiotic and conservative therapy, and laboratory findings indicate the presence of an inflammatory process. Nonspecific adhesions may be diagnosed by culdoscopy and usually follow previous surgical intervention, especially appendectomy or incomplete surgery for pelvic infection. Ovarian carcinoma can only be excluded by laparotomy, and the presence of a persistent mass, especially if solid, in the adnexal area is an absolute indication for abdominal exploration.

Treatment

The crippling characteristics of this malady, occurring during the reproductive period of life, prevent the fulfillment of marital potential and too often terminate in hysterectomy or castration. An optimum method of treatment will secure pain relief, allow adequate coitus, prevent abnormal bleeding and preserve or increase the possibility of motherhood.

Therapy will be discussed under five headings: (1) prophylaxis, (2) observation and analgesia, (3) suppression of ovulation, (4) conservative operation and (5) extirpative operation.

Prophylaxis

If it is true that endometriosis develops as a result of the distribution by various routes of fragments of fully differentiated müllerian tissue primarily from the mucosa lining the uterus or tubes or that it can be produced in situ by the activation of the same tissue by trauma, it is evident that great care should be exercised in some of our diagnostic and operative procedures. The following observations are noteworthy:

1. During pelvic examination at or about the time of menstruation, forceful manipulation should be discouraged because of the danger of squeezing endometrial blood and detritus out into the tubes.

2. The Rubin inflation test or uterosalpingography should not be made too near the end of menstruation or immediately following curettage because of the danger of forcing bits of viable endometrium out through the tube. Experimentally, peritoneal implantations can be produced in rabbits and guinea pigs by insufflation.

3. Although it has been suggested that displacements of the uterus should be correlated to insure better drainage of menstrual blood, there is no conclusive evidence that women with simple third-degree retroversion of the uterus have an increased incidence of endometriosis.

4. Cervical obstruction should be corrected not only because of the possibility of increasing the tendency to retrograde tubal menstruation, but also to correct abnormalities of the endocervical epithelium and aid in sperm penetration.

5. If the patient is married, early pregnancy is suggested, and the patient is advised to have subsequent pregnancies as quickly as is economically sound. Meigs suggested pregnancy as the optimum prophylactic and therapeutic treatment for endometriosis, since the symptoms and signs regress during the period of gestation and for various periods of time thereafter.

This regression is probably due to a combination of anovulation and amenorrhea brought about by adenohypophyseal suppression. Kistner has suggested that the improvement may also be due, in part, to a transformation of functioning endometriotic tissue into decidua by the increasing levels of estrogen and progesterone secreted by the placenta. If pregnancy is not contemplated or is not desired, it is possible to secure anovulation by the administration of estrogens, androgens, progestins, or a combination of these. These therapeutic schemata are given in detail in the section on hormonal treatment.

There is suggestive evidence that women who have been taking oral contraceptives for prolonged periods of time, especially those with a potent progestin and minimal amounts of estrogen, may have a diminished chance of developing endometriosis. This is based on the observations that these agents produce endometrial atrophy and lessen menstrual flow, thus preventing tubal reflux of menstrual detritus into the peritoneal cavity. In patients subjected to hysterectomy and bilateral salpingo-oophorectomy at the time of withdrawal flow from oral contraceptives, step sections of the oviduct have not shown the usual intraluminal menstrual elements.

OBSERVATION AND ANALGESIA

Observation as a form of treatment is often rewarding, since many patients either "outgrow" their endometriosis or become pregnant and remain asymptomatic indefinitely.

Expectant treatment is worthwhile for the patients who have only minimal symptoms and pelvic findings, such as slight tenderness and nodularity of the cul-de-sac. Reassurance and mild analgesics are adequate for most patients. Some authors have suggested that the only treatment of endometriosis is surgical and that observation cannot be regarded as treatment. In this regard, the observations of Dr. Sampson made almost 40 years ago are still pertinent: "I would hesitate very much to suspend a retro-displaced uterus which was symptomless in order to prevent the possible incidence of endometriosis. I wouldn't operate on any patient with endometriosis in the absence of subjective symptoms." These admonitions are just as acceptable today if infertility is included as a subjective symptom.

If the patient is married, early pregnancy is suggested, and she is advised to have subsequent pregnancies as quickly as is economically sound. Should increased or irregular bleeding occur, a careful examination, with anesthesia, and thorough curettage are performed. Regular pelvic examinations should be scheduled at least every six months if endometriosis is suspected since, although the incidence of malignancy in endometriosis is low, rapid growth and the development of large endometriotic cysts may occur in a short time. At the time of pelvic examination, the ovaries should be carefully palpated and changes in their size and mobility noted. Progression of disease, as suggested by the obliteration of the cul-de-sac or the development of rectovaginal masses, necessitates specific therapy. If the patient is infertile, an adequate study of the husband should be made and endometrial biopsy, tubal insufflation and postcoital tests should be performed. If pregnancy does not occur after one year of study, including culdoscopy, observation and planned coitus, the methods of treatment outlined in the succeeding paragraphs are indicated.

SUPPRESSION OF OVULATION

Pregnancy has often been suggested as the optimum prophylactic and therapeutic treatment for endometriosis, since the symptoms and signs regress during the period of gestation and for varying periods thereafter. This regression is probably due to a combination of anovulation and amenorrhea brought about by adenohypophyseal suppression. The author has suggested that the improvement may also be due in part to a transformation of functioning endometriotic tissue into decidua by increasing levels of chorionic estrogen and progesterone. If pregnancy is not contemplated or is not desired, it is possible to secure anovulation by the administration of estrogens, androgens, progestins or a combination thereof.

Estrogens.—Beecham has stated that "physiological amenorrhea of pregnancy or the pregnancy equivalent induced by stilbestrol has produced regressive changes so remarkable that operative treatment once endorsed by all gynecologists is declining in popularity and usage." The author is in firm agreement with this statement. Some observers insist that the salutary effect of estrogen-progestin pseudopregnancy is due to the estrogen alone—that the progestin is converted to estrogen and has no specific progestational effect. This concept, however, completely ignores the extensive decidual effect in the stroma of endometriosis—similar to that seen during pregnancy—with subsequent necrobiosis and replacement by fibrous connective tissue. This conversion of stroma to decidua is not seen with estrogen alone.

Androgens.—The salutary effects of androgens are presumed to be due to direct action on areas of endometriosis. High doses will inhibit ovulation and cause involution and suppression of follicular growth, but amounts exceeding 300 mg. monthly frequently cause masculinizing symptoms.

Side effects, especially in sensitive individuals, include acne, hoarseness, edema, hirsutism, enlargement of the clitoris and occasionally hepatocellular jaundice. There is no doubt about the effectiveness of androgens in the relief of symptoms due to endometriosis. An anti-estrogenic effect of the androgen on endometriotic tissue may prevent the usual action of estrogen followed by estrogen-progesterone during the luteal phase of the ovarian cycle and thus prevent recurrent bleeding in foci of aberrant endometrium.

Progestins.—In 1956, the author began treatment of patients with endometriosis by means of a pseudopregnancy, giving combinations of estrogens and newer synthetic progestins for six to nine months. This concept of therapy was predicated on the fact that pregnancy usually brings about both objective and subjective improvement in patients with extensive pelvic endometriosis. Thus a state similar to pregnancy would seem of particular value when the patient was infertile, did not desire pregnancy or was unmarried. It was further suggested that the changes brought about in endometriosis by pregnancy were due to a combination of (1) anovulation and amenorrhea, (2) decidual transformation of functioning endometriotic tissue and (3) decidual necrosis and absorption. Figure 8–5 demonstrates the effects of endogenous estrogen and progesterone on a large rectovaginal mass which was biopsied during the fourteenth week of an apparently normal pregnancy.

A morphologically similar decidual reaction can be brought about both in the endometrium and in areas of endometriosis by the prolonged admin-

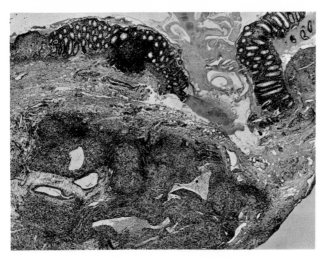

Fig. 8-5.—Biopsy of a mass in the rectovaginal septum during the fourteenth week of pregnancy. Rectal mucosa is seen at the top of the section. Approximately two-thirds of the rectal wall has been replaced by endometriotic tissue made up of inactive glands and decidua. The endometrial stroma (as decidua) is packed in whorl-like accumulations; ×40. (From Kistner, R. W.: Clin. Pharmacol. & Therap. 1:525, 1960.)

Fig. 8-6.—Endometrial biopsy after 15 weeks of increasing doses of norethynodrel with ethinyl estradiol. There is a variation in response in the separate levels of the endometrium. Note the pronounced edema and decidual necrosis under the surface epithelium. In the midzone there are moderate intercellular edema and minimal necrosis of decidual cells. The basalis is made up of compact, well-preserved decidual cells; ×50. (From Kistner, R. W.: Clin. Obst. & Gynec. 2:884, 1959.)

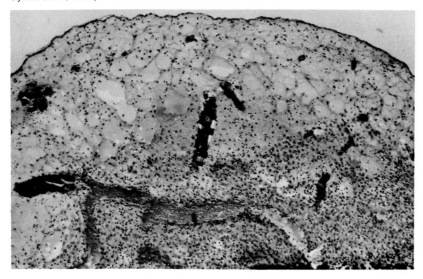

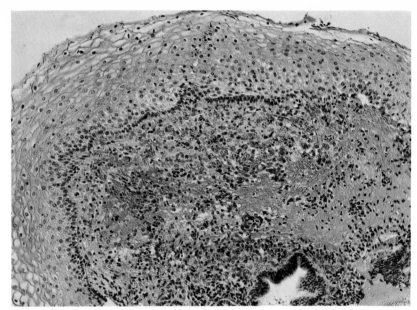

Fig. 8-7.—Biopsy of vaginal mucosa during stage of premenstrual staining. Typical endometriosis in a menstrual phase is evident. Note hemorrhage into stroma, inflammatory cells and an endometrial gland in the lower portion.
(Figures 8-7 and 8-8 from Kistner, R. W.: Fertil. & Steril. 10:547 and 549, 1959.)

istration of estrogens and progestins. Figure 8-6 demonstrates this change in an endometrial biopsy taken after 15 weeks of continuous estrogen-progestin therapy. There are marked edema at the surface, moderate decidual necrobiosis in the midzone and a well-maintained decidua in the basalis. It is suggested that the decidual cells undergo a gradual process of necrosis that is followed by liquefaction and absorption. Figure 8-7 illustrates endometriosis occurring in the vagina. The effects of Enovid given for 12 weeks are seen in Figure 8-8. The same process of decidual necrosis and edema is evident.

CHOICE OF HORMONE.—Numerous progestins are at present available for use in the treatment of endometriosis and they are illustrated in Table 8-1. The various regimens are shown in Table 8-2.

Each patient should be regarded as an individual problem. The specific agent and length of treatment should depend on the extent of the disease, the severity of the symptoms, the presence of infertility, and the response to pseudopregnancy.

USE OF HORMONAL THERAPY.—Hormonal therapy is contraindicated under the following conditions:

1. Unproved endometriosis or merely a suspicion of the disease by history with minimal palpable findings.

2. Obscure diagnosis of pelvic lesions, particularly when ovarian enlargement is of such degree that a neoplastic growth cannot be excluded.

3. Uterine leiomyomas of such size that stimulation of growth by estrogenic substances could initiate complications.

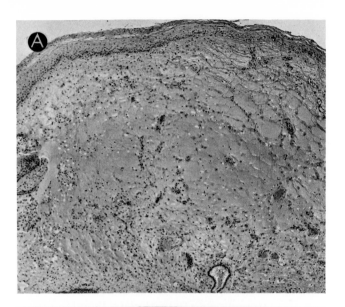

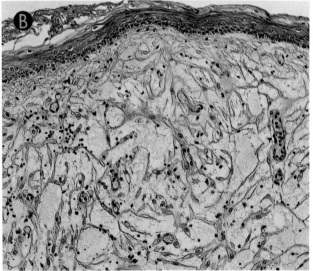

Fig. 8–8.—Biopsy of an area of vaginal endometriosis after 12 weeks of continuous norethy-nodrel with ethinyl estradiol therapy. **A,** there is evidence of a marked generalized edema throughout the endometriosis. Under the vaginal epithelium the decidua is well maintained but most of it is undergoing necrosis. **B,** high power of an area in *A.* An unusual pattern of decidual change is evident. Most decidual cells remain as "naked nuclei" or a cytoplasmic strand in an edematous stroma. A few lymphocytes and macrophages are present and suggest an absorptive process of the necrotic endometriosis.

TABLE 8-1.—COMMERCIAL PROGESTIN-ESTROGEN COMBINATIONS USED TO
INDUCE PSEUDOPREGNANCY FOR ENDOMETRIOSIS

DRUG	PROGESTIN	MG.	ESTROGEN	MG.
Enovid-5	norethynodrel	5.0	mestranol	0.075
Enovid-E	norethynodrel	2.5	mestranol	0.10
Ortho-Novum "2"	norethindrone	2.0	mestranol	0.10
Ortho-Novum "1"	norethindrone	1.0	mestranol	0.05
Norlestrin	norethindrone acetate	2.5	ethinyl estradiol	0.05
Norlestrin-1	norethindrone acetate	1.0	ethinyl estradiol	0.05
Norinyl	norethindrone	2.0	mestranol	0.10
Norinyl-1	norethindrone	1.0	mestranol	0.05
Ovulen	ethynodiol diacetate	1.0	mestranol	0.10
Lyndiol	lynestrenol	2.5	mestranol	0.075
Ovral	norgestrel	0.5	ethinyl estradiol	0.05

4. Excessive side effects such as nausea and vomiting, chloasma, extreme fluid retention, severe personality changes, or persistent breakthrough bleeding. Use of the newer agents has reduced markedly the incidence of these side effects.

5. Hepatic disease as manifested by abnormal liver function tests.

6. Previous mammary carcinoma.

7. Previous pulmonary embolism or phlebothrombosis.

Prolonged hormonal therapy is applicable in the following patients:

1. Unmarried patients with maximal symptoms and minimal palpable findings. Extension of the disease may be prevented and subsequent fertility preserved.

2. Patients with recurrent disease after a previous conservative operation. Pregnancies have been noted subsequent to treatment in patients to whom hysterectomy had been suggested.

Short-term hormonal therapy is indicated in the following situations:

1. Prior to conservative surgery. Areas of endometriosis will enlarge and appear hemorrhagic, making identification, excision and fulguration simpler and more complete. Six to eight weeks' therapy is adequate.

2. Subsequent to conservative therapy (in order to inhibit ovulation and prevent reactivation of remaining areas of endometriosis). Twelve to 24 weeks' therapy is adequate.

Results of treatment by various investigators have been uniform. About

TABLE 8-2.—SCHEDULE OF DOSAGE REGIMENS FOR TREATMENT OF ENDOMETRIOSIS

DRUG	DOSAGE
Enovid (or Enovid-E)	2.5 mg. daily for 1 week, 5.0 mg. daily for 1 week, 10.0 mg. daily for two weeks; increase by 2.5 mg. for breakthrough bleeding
Norlestrin (2.5 mg.)	1 tablet daily; increase by 1 tablet for breakthrough bleeding
Deluteval 2X	1 ml. IM weekly; increased by 0.5 ml. for breakthrough bleeding
Depo-Provera	2 ml. (100 mg.) IM every 2 weeks for four doses; then 2 ml. every 4 weeks; add oral estrogen or Delestrogen 30 mg. IM for breakthrough bleeding
Norinyl-1 Norinyl-2	Not marketed for endometriosis but may be given exactly as Norlestrin
Ortho-Novum-1 Ortho-Novum-2	Not marketed for endometriosis but may be given exactly as Norlestrin
Lyndiol	Not as yet marketed in the United States but may be given exactly as Norlestrin
Ovral	Not marketed for endometriosis but may be given exactly as Norlestrin

85 per cent of patients show improvement during the period of therapy and for varying times thereafter. In patients treated primarily with progestins, that is, without previous surgery, remissions have lasted as long as 6 years. In those patients who were not improved or whose symptoms were aggravated by hormones, it has been found that either adenomyosis or pelvic inflammatory disease coexisted with endometriosis. Patients who have recurrent endometriosis after preliminary surgery present a serious challenge to the gynecologist or surgeon. Prolonged pseudopregnancy has been of particular value in these patients, but therapy should be continued for 12–24 months to secure maximum results. It is also suggested that a period of anovulation be secured immediately after conservative surgery to obtain optimum benefit from the operation.

A summation of the results of prolonged administration of these steroids for endometriosis can be made here. (1) They are effective inhibitors of ovulation and produce a decidual reaction in areas of endometriosis. (2) About 85 per cent of the patients are improved during therapy and for varying periods thereafter. (3) No abnormalities of endometrial, ovarian or pituitary function have been observed during the post-treatment period, and subsequent pregnancies have occurred without incident in a high percentage of patients. Ulfelder, in a discussion of the various schemes presently available, stated: "At present it appears that hormone therapy for endometriosis will be the most widely applicable form of management in the future."

Surgical Treatment

In contemplating surgical treatment of endometriosis, one should always bear in mind that functioning ovarian tissue is necessary for the continued activity of the disease. Therefore, the successful treatment of endometriosis depends upon a knowledge of when it is reasonably safe or desirable to maintain ovarian function and when it is necessary to destroy it. It is quite obvious that ovarian function should be conserved in treating the very early and, perhaps, symptomless lesions and destroyed when the pelvic organs are hopelessly invaded by endometriosis. Unfortunately, from the standpoint of definite surgical indications, the majority of cases will fall between these two extremes and may present problems in surgical judgment seldom encountered in any other pelvic disease. As our knowledge of the life history of endometriosis has increased, there has been a definite tendency to become more conservative, particularly in the treatment of the early and borderline cases. In general it is believed that one should err on the side of conservatism; this belief is based on the fact that endometriosis (1) usually progresses slowly over a period of years; (2) is not, and rarely becomes, malignant; and (3) regresses at the menopause.

Early implantations on the surface of the peritoneum, wherever they are located, may be ignored, excised, or destroyed with a cautery. Small endometrial cysts on the ovary may be excised or a major portion of one or both ovaries may be resected. Small endometrial implants on the intestines should be excised. Conservative operations should also be accompanied by correction of uterine displacements, relief of cervical obstruction and removal of any other concomitant pelvic pathology to aid in the prevention of a recurrence of the condition. Endometriosis coexisting with uterine myomas, ovarian cysts or other pelvic pathology may be insignificant but, on the other hand, the extent or location may be such as to make conservative surgery hazardous.

Conservative Surgery Technique.—If childbearing function is to be preserved, operative procedures should be as conservative as possible. All surgical procedures should be preceded by a thorough curettage and every patient should have had vaginal cytology to exclude possible malignancy of the cervix.

The approach should usually be through a midline incision since, in almost all cases, a presacral neurectomy is performed; this is not facilitated if a transverse incision is used. Thorough exploration of the pelvic and abdominal organs should be performed routinely and the decision reached as to whether conservative or radical surgery is feasible. The uterus is frequently found to be adherent to the rectosigmoid. These adhesions are separated by either blunt or sharp dissection in the midline and the uterus is brought forward. Traction sutures of O chromic catgut are then placed around the round ligaments to lift the corpus forward and out of the cul-de-sac (Fig. 8—9A). With the uterus held forward, further adhesions may then be separated under direct vision. As previously mentioned, the use of progestational agents for 6 to 12 weeks preoperatively greatly softens the adhesions and makes the posterior dissection relatively easy. Endometrial implants in the uterosacral ligaments or cul-de-sac are excised. Care is taken not to dissect too far laterally or too deeply in order to bypass the uterine veins and the uterus. Similar excision of implants on the serosa of the rectosigmoid is then carried out (Fig. 8—9B). If the bowel lumen is entered, a layered closure of submucosa and seromuscular layers is done in the usual manner. After all areas of endometriosis have been removed, the edges of available peritoneum are closed with fine catgut. Occasionally the posterior aspect of the uterus may have to be approximated to the serosa of the rectosigmoid, thus obliterating the cul-de-sac, to secure adequate peritonization of the pelvis.

Endometrial cysts of the ovary are excised (Fig. 8–9C,D). These cysts are usually adherent and do not separate freely as do corpus luteum or follicular cysts. After as much of the cyst as possible has been removed, the walls of the ovary are approximated with several mattress sutures of fine catgut and the surface closed with a running, locked suture of 000 chromic catgut. Occasionally all ovarian tissue is destroyed and oophorectomy is necessary. However, it is remarkable how frequently an ovarian cyst can be enucleated and a fairly thick capsule of cortical tissue left in situ. We have had the experience of performing unilateral oophorectomy and resection of 90 per cent of the remaining ovary and of being rewarded by subsequent ovulation and pregnancy. However, this is not always the case; some patients have premature menopause following such surgery.

If reproduction is not a prime factor or if there is evidence of extensive involvement of other pelvic structures, such as bowel or ureter, a hysterectomy and bilateral oophorectomy should be done.

Since leiomyomas of the uterus are found in about 15 per cent of the patients with endometriosis, single or multiple myomectomy should be carried out as part of the conservative approach. It has been our practice to do a presacral neurectomy whenever the uterus is not removed. Even if the patient has not had dysmenorrhea or pelvic pain preceding surgery, these symptoms may develop postoperatively. The presacral procedure should be rather extensive, all nerve tissue between the right ureter and the superior hemorrhoidal vessels being excised. In addition, we usually remove a part of the uterosacral ligaments just at their insertion into the uterus, thus accomplishing a "pelvic denervation."

An appendectomy is performed at the time of surgery and we have been surprised to see functioning endometriosis of the appendiceal serosa in many patients. Endometriosis of the terminal ileum is seen only rarely and may be treated by superficial excision. If the muscularis and mucosa are involved, adequate resection and end-to-end anastomosis should be performed. A uterine suspension is performed routinely and the uterosacral ligaments are plicated in the midline. This accom-

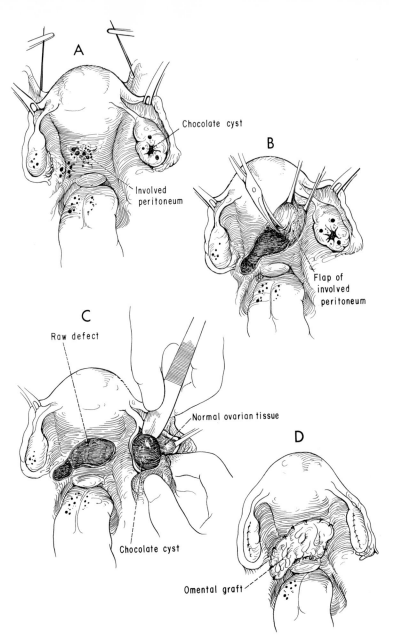

Fig. 8-9.—A, traction sutures placed around the round ligaments and the uterus is drawn forward; areas of endometriosis are shown on the ovaries, posterior aspect of the uterus and anterior surface of sigmoid colon. **B,** serosa of posterior aspect of uterus involved by endometriosis is excised. **C,** endometrioma of the right ovary is excised preserving as much normal ovarian cortex as possible. **D,** defects in both ovaries are corrected using fine catgut; a free omental graft is placed over the defect in the uterine serosa.

plishes forward fixation of the uterus and the shortened uterosacral ligaments produce a backward pull on the cervix effecting a more normal anatomic attitude. Pseudopregnancy is induced for a minimum of three months after operation, following which concerted efforts toward conception are made. About 30 per cent of women so treated will become pregnant if no other cause for infertility exists. Several authors have reported the incidence of pregnancy to be as high as 80 per cent following conservative operation, but this seems to be an exceptionally high success rate and may depend on patient selection.

Extirpative Surgery.—The treatment of choice for extensive endometriosis in women who no longer desire pregnancy is total hysterectomy and bilateral salpingo-oophorectomy. It has not seemed reasonable to us to leave the ovaries in situ if the uterus is removed for this disease, since ovulation continues in cyclic fashion and remaining areas of endometriosis may be stimulated to grow by endogenous estrogen and progesterone. In experimental endometriosis in monkeys, the most extensive growth has been obtained by the cyclic administration and withdrawal of estrogen and progesterone. This is exactly the situation that exists when functioning, ovulating ovaries are left in situ. When there is extensive bladder, bowel, or ureteral endometriosis, hysterectomy and bilateral oophorectomy will effect a cure.

Large bilateral ovarian endometrial cysts with extensive peritoneal endometriosis and numerous pelvic adhesions or with marked invasion of the rectosigmoid and rectovaginal space constitute the most urgent indications for radical removal of all the pelvic organs, regardless of the age of the patient. *Failure to castrate in the presence of marked endometriosis of the bowel is undoubtedly the most hazardous of all attempts at conservative surgery because of the dangers of subsequent intestinal obstruction.*

From the operative standpoint, early or moderately advanced endometriosis offers no unusual difficulties, but extensive endometriosis may present many technical problems. Endometriosis, in contrast to pelvic inflammatory disease (particularly that due to gonorrheal infection), produces an extremely dense type of pelvic adhesions with almost complete absence of planes of cleavage. Therefore, much of the dissection must be done with sharp instruments, and the dangers of damage to adherent structures are thereby increased. This hazard may be diminished by the use of preoperative pseudopregnancy.

A hysterectomy and bilateral salpingo-oophorectomy can usually be done on patients with large ovarian endometrial cysts and extensive pelvic adhesions and even on those with marked invasion of the rectovaginal septum. This may be facilitated by incising the posterior peritoneum above the insertion of the uterosacral ligaments. The endopelvic fascia and rectosigmoid may then be reflected and the danger of fistula is minimized. It may, at times, be necessary to leave a considerable portion of the growth attached to the bowel or other pelvic structures, but these remnants will regress along with other müllerian tissue in the pelvis following ablation of the ovaries, a fact of great importance in the treatment of this disease.

A few cases have been reported where this atrophy did not occur; however, one may suspect that all ovarian tissue was not completely removed in some of these cases.

It is frequently impossible to remove an adherent ovarian endometrial (chocolate) cyst without rupturing it and soiling the field of operation with its grumous contents. While this material is usually sterile, it is irritating to the peritoneum and it is good practice in these cases to insert a drain through the vaginal vault to prevent postoperative accumulations in the pelvis. Peritonization is often difficult following removal of extensive lesions, and areas which cannot be covered should be protected by some type of drainage, for it has been observed that postoperative ileus and partial intestinal obstruction are more common following operations on extensive endometriosis than on any other ordinary pelvic condition. Although the postoperative morbidity is high, the mortality has been very low, probably due to the age and generally good condition of the patients, the nature of the disease, and the absence of malignancy and infection.

There is no contraindication to the continuous administration of estrogen in small doses following hysterectomy and bilateral salpingo-oophorectomy. We have given Estinyl (0.05 mg.), Premarin (1.25 mg.) or Diethylstilbesterol (0.5 mg.) daily for indefinite periods to control untoward symptoms following surgical castration. Administration of these estrogens may gradually be diminished both in quantity and frequency over a period of years. In some patients a study of vaginal cytology will reveal the presence of adequate endogenous estrogen, presumably of adrenal origin, years after surgical castration. Exogenous estrogens need not be given to these patients. I have not seen endometriosis aggravated or "rekindled" by the use of estrogens after hysterectomy and bilateral salpingo-oophorectomy if the dose is as indicated above.

However, the use of estrogen-progestin combinations given in 20-day cycles or sequential estrogen-progestin preparations has been shown to reactivate endometriosis. These preparations should never be used in a patient who has had a hysterectomy and bilateral salpingo-oophorectomy for endometriosis. Similarly, they should not be given to postmenopausal women for relief of menstrual symptoms if the past history suggests that endometriosis might be present.

The use of x-ray or radium for nonmalignant pelvic conditions has been discontinued at the Boston Hospital for Women. This includes x-ray castration for endometriosis. Besides the possibility of a subsequent carcinoma of the cervix, endometrium or ovary, serious large and small bowel injuries may occur as late sequelae. Some gynecologists do employ x-ray castration to relieve intolerable pelvic pain in the immediately premenopausal woman who has already undergone one or more operations for the disease, but ovarian function may be markedly diminished in a far simpler fashion, e.g., by administering medroxyprogesterone acetate (Depo-Provera), 200 mg. every two weeks for four doses, then 400 mg. every month for one year. Measurements of ovarian steroids in urine have shown a diminution to postmenopausal levels within 10 days of the first injection. Furthermore, the action of this progestin is so prolonged that subsequent ovulation will not occur for at least one year subsequent to the conclusion of treatment.

Complications

Endometriosis, untreated, is rarely a fatal disease, and the complications arising from it are few except when the bowel or ureters are invaded or some accident occurs in an ovarian endometrial cyst.

Some degree of intestinal obstruction, usually in the large bowel, is perhaps the most frequent serious complication. In the small bowel it is most apt to be due to adhesions between loops of the intestine which may produce kinking and obstruction. In the large bowel the obstruction is nearly always located in the sigmoid at the level of the cul-de-sac and is most frequently produced by an invasion of the intestinal wall by peritoneal endometriosis.

An ovarian endometrial cyst is subject to many of the complications possible in any other type of ovarian cyst. It may become infected, it may rupture, and occasionally may become malignant. Twisting of the pedicle does not occur, as an endometrial cyst large enough to twist is almost invariably adherent.

The following are not considered, strictly speaking, complications but, rather, occasional manifestations of the disease: endometriosis in the groin, umbilicus, bladder, incisions, about the ureter, and in other unusual locations.

BIBLIOGRAPHY

Beecham, C. T.: Letter to editor, J.A.M.A. 163:678, 1957.
Cattell, R. B., and Swinton, N. W.: Endometriosis, New England J. Med. 214:341, 1936.
Cavanagh, W. V.: Fertility in the etiology of endometriosis, Am. J. Obst. & Gynec. 61:539, 1951.
Cullen, T. S.: Adenomyoma of the round ligament, Bull. Johns Hopkins Hosp. 7:112, 1896.
Frankl, O.: Adenomyosis uteri, Irish J. M. Sc. 7:303, 1932.
Garcia, C. R.: Personal communication to R. W. Kistner, 1959.
Gardner, H. L.: Cervical and vaginal endometriosis, Clin. Obst. & Gynec. 9:358, 1966.
Geist, S. H.: The viability of fragments of menstrual endometrium, Am. J. Obst. & Gynec. 25:751, 1933.
Gray, L. A.: The management of endometriosis involving the bowel, Clin. Obst. & Gynec. 9:309, 1966.
Green, T. H.: Conservative surgical treatment of endometriosis, Clin. Obst. & Gynec. 9:293, 1966.
Halban, J.: Hysteroadenosis metastica: Die lymphogene Genese der sog. Adenofibromatosis heterotopica, Wien, klin. Wchnschr. 37:1205, 1924.
Hartman, C. G.: Regeneration of the monkey uterus after surgical removal of the endometrium and accidental endometriosis, West J. Surg. 52:87, 1944.
Haskins, A. L., and Woolf, R. B.: Stilbestrol-induced hyperhormonal amenorrhea for the treatment of pelvic endometriosis, Obst. & Gynec. 5:113, 1955.
Hertig, A. T., and Gore, H.: *Tumors of the Female Sex Organs: Part 3. Tumors of the Ovary and Fallopian Tube,* sec. IX, fasc. 33 of *Atlas of Tumor Pathology* (Washington, D.C.: Armed Forces Institute of Pathology, 1961).
Karnaky, J. K.: Endometriosis, in Conn, H. F.: *Current Therapy* (Philadelphia: W. B. Saunders Company, 1957).
Kelly, J. V., and Rock, J.: Culdoscopy for diagnosis in infertility: Report of 492 cases, Am. J. Obst. & Gynec. 72:523, 1956.
Kerr, W. S.: Endometriosis involving the urinary tract, Clin. Obst. & Gynec. 9:331, 1966.
Kistner, R. W.: Observations on the effects of new synthetic progestogens on endometriosis in the human female, Fertil. & Steril., 16:61, 1965.
———: Current status of the hormonal treatment of endometriosis, Clin. Obst. & Gynec. 9:271, 1966.
———: Endometriosis and Infertility, in Behrman, S. J. and Kistner, R. W. (eds.): *Progress in Infertility* (Boston: Little, Brown and Company, 1968).
———:Endometriosis and adenomyosis, Davis' Gynec. & Obst., Vol. II, Chapt. 43:1-105, 1968.
———:The use of newer progestins in the treatment of endometriosis, Am. J. Obst. & Gynec. 75:264, 1958.
———: The treatment of endometriosis by inducing pseudopregnancy with ovarian hormones: A report of 58 cases, Fertil. & Steril. 10:539, 1959.
———: The use of steroidal substances in endometriosis, Clin. Pharmacol. & Therap. 1:525, 1960.
———, and Hertig, A. T.: Primary adenoacanthoma of the ovary: a review of the literature with a report of five cases, Cancer 5:1134, 1952.
Kourides, I. and Kistner, R. W.: Three new synthetic progestins in the treatment of endometriosis, Obst. & Gynec. 31:821, 1968.
Meigs, J. V.: The medical treatment of endometriosis and the significance of endometriosis, Surg. Gynec. & Obst. 89:317, 1949.

Meyer, R.: Anatomie und Histogenese der Myome und Fibrome, in Viet, J. (ed.): *Handbuch der Gynäkologie* (Wiesbaden: Verlag von J. F. Bergmann, 1907), vol. 1.

Novak, E.: *Gynecological and Obstetrical Pathology* (3d ed.; Philadelphia: W. B. Saunders Company, 1952), p. 490.

Ridley, J. H. and Edwards, I. K.: Experimental endometriosis in the human, Am. J. Obst. & Gynec. 76:783, 1958.

Rock, J.; Garcia, C. R., and Pincus, G.: Use of some progestational 19-norsteroids in gynecology, Am. J. Obst. & Gynec. 79:758, 1960.

Russell, W. W.: Aberrant portions of the müllerian duct in an ovary, Bull. Johns Hopkins Hosp. 10:8, 1899.

Sampson, J. A.: Intestinal adenomas of endometrial type: Their importance and their relation to ovarian hematomas of endometrial type, Arch. Surg. 5:217, 1922.

Scott, R. B.: External endometriosis: Mechanisms of origin, theoretical and experimental, Clin. Obst. & Gynec. 3:429, 1960.

Scully, R. E., Richardson, G. S. and Barlow, J. F.: The development of malignancy in endometriosis, Clin. Obst. & Gynec. 9:384, 1966.

Te Linde, R. W., and Wharton, L. R., Jr.: Further studies on experimental endometriosis, Am. J. Obst. & Gynec. 66:1082, 1953.

Ulfelder, H.: The treatment of endometriosis, M. Sc. 8:503, 1966.

CHAPTER 9

Infertility

General Considerations

INFORMATION NOW AVAILABLE indicates that for every 85 married couples producing one or more offspring there are still 15 couples in this country who are unable to conceive. As physicians, we must concern ourselves with the challenge of helping more than 3,000,000 involuntarily childless couples in the United States. Certain geographic and socioeconomic variations must be considered before broad statements are made regarding etiologic factors. Thus, in France there is a high incidence of oviduct closure; in Israel and in Scotland genital tuberculosis is a major cause of infertility in women. In this country, gynecologic clinics affiliated with large metropolitan hospitals are frequented by indigent patients or patients in the lower-income brackets. Pelvic inflammatory disease (gonococcal and enterococcal) and postabortal sepsis (streptococcal) are major causes of tubal closure in these patients; endometriosis and hormonal abnormalities are rarely seen. A review of recent literature dealing with the major causes of infertility reveals a gradient of this order: cervical factor, 20 per cent; tubal factor, 30–35 per cent; male factor, 30–35 per cent; hormonal factor, 15 per cent. In my patients the cervical factor is much lower and the hormonal factor much higher.

Current aspects of research in human reproduction do not, at the moment, hold the promise of immediate aid to the physician in his ultimate goal. Fortunately, the intricate processes involved do not demand meticulous control or perfected performance since in most people there is a helpful range of variation. There remain, however, a small number of apparently healthy, regularly copulating couples who fail to reproduce. In this specific failure group, a knowledge of reproductive physiology is necessary for success.

Certain demographic correlates pertaining to fecundability bear discussion. According to the United Nations Multilingual Demographic Dictionary, fecundity is the capacity of a man, a woman, or a couple to participate in the production of a live child. As we are interested in the probability of conception in the absence of contraception, the term *fecundability* is preferable. Generally speaking, then, four factors affecting the chances of fertility or fecundability emerge: (1) age of the wife, (2) age of the husband, (3) the rate of intercourse, and (4) the length of exposure.

Fecundability is maximal in the female around the age of 24 years, after which it gradually tapers down to the age of 30 and rapidly declines thereafter. Similarly, fecundability in the male is maximal around age 24 to 25, conceptions occurring in 75 per cent of couples in less than six months. In males over age 40, only 22 per cent of couples become pregnant.

MacLeod's 1953 study indicates that at almost any age level the proportion of conceptions achieved in less than six months rises with frequency of intercourse. He points out that the most important aspect of the semen in respect to ease of conception, i.e., the degree and quality of motility, is enhanced by frequent ejaculation. He states that from the single criterion of achievement of pregnancy the average of intercourse twice weekly reported by most married couples is by no means best, four times or more weekly being ideal to assure impregnation at all ages.

Observed and estimated studies on the number of months required for conception in the absence of use of contraception clearly indicate that 25 per cent of women will be pregnant within the first month, 63 per cent in six months, 75 per cent in nine months, 80 per cent in a year, and 90 per cent in 18 months. Thereafter, irrespective of the age of wife or husband or the frequency of coital exposure, the longer the couple have been married the greater the progressive decline in conception rate. Almost certainly, in these latter cases, other undiscovered medical factors exist.

The newly married couple thus has a predictable chance of conception depending on the age of the wife, the age of the husband, coital exposure, and duration of marriage, further modified by whatever other physical, physiological, or psychological medical factors pertain. These are the cases that will benefit from a complete investigation by the fertility specialist. It has been variously estimated that at least 10 per cent of them will be aided by such an evaluation, but with the advent of the newer ovulating agents (clomiphene and human menopausal gonadotropin, for example) management of hormonal deficiencies of the corpus luteum, improved surgical techniques for tubal reconstruction and uterine defects, therapy for immunological incompatibility, increased use of artificial insemination and improved diagnostic techniques such as culdoscopy and laparoscopy, it can be safely said that the eventual percentage of patients that can be helped is considerably higher.

Despite this apparent progress in infertility management, there remains an approximate 5-10 per cent of all married couples who are medically healthy and in whom no cause for barrenness can be determined. This group must be the focal point of future research and investigation and is, in fact, the background of the current tremendous interest in basic reproductive physiology as well as the raison d'etre for this chapter.

The so-called normal infertile couples obviously are *not* normal or they would not have an infertility problem, yet they are the most poorly managed patients. They must, then, *not be allowed to leave the office with the impression that they are normal.* Perhaps the significance of this problem has best been stated by Jones and Baramki: ". . . frequently unless a special effort is made to make them realize that they must have a factor which cannot be detected by current medical methods, such a couple is apt to leave your office with false impressions and unfounded high hopes. Actually, far from being a good prognosis, this factor offers a poor prognosis. In a group of 315 patients between the ages of 20 and 35 years, studied for infertility and completely investigated, and adequately treated we found a 46 per cent pregnancy rate, while in 15 patients in these series who were investigated with no factor found, only three pregnancies occurred."

Another serious and frustrating deterrent to an adequate diagnostic evaluation of the infertile couple is the indifference of the physician. Equally distressing is the lack of cooperation of the male partner. Too often the wife has accepted the responsibility for childlessness when, in fact, the husband may have been exposed to radiation or to heavy metal poisoning or is oligospermic as a result of chronic alcoholism or nicotine intoxication. It is therefore imperative that both marital partners share the responsibility in the planned investigation and subsequent treatment. Therapeutic nihilism and pessimistic abnegations are fruitless and, although the ultimate aim of the investigation is to enable the couple to bear a child, the ancillary purpose of prognosis is also served.

In summary, then, a thorough infertility investigation by an interested individual knowledgeable in the field of infertility has three important purposes: (1) It offers an explanation for the infertility; (2) it furnishes a prognosis which in itself is important to the psychological well-being of the couple; and (3) it may well afford a basis for therapy.

Clinical Management

An infertility study should have a definite plan with a predictable end point. Such a standardized regimen usually can be concluded in five or six office visits spaced at approximately one month intervals, and the couple should be so informed at the first visit. Today more and more infertile couples are seeking help in achieving conception and, perhaps because they are marrying early, they seem to be coming for help earlier. In this situation I believe that traditional injunctions to "wait and see" should give way to the concept that any couple who have cohabited normally and have not conceived within a year are entitled to a full infertility work-up. On the premise that infertility is often a syndrome of multiple origin, an adequate investigation therefore requires study of all reasonable etiologies in *both* husband and wife. Thus, the finding of a single causative factor—such as cervicitis in the wife—does not rule out the possibility of other causes as well—such as oligospermia in the husband. Nor does it rule out the possibility that more than one factor is operative in one or both partners. Although statistical data are only approximate, there is evidence that fully 35 per cent of all infertility problems are of multiple origin. The variety of possible causes (see Table 9–1) underscores the need for systematic investigation in both husband and wife, and only on this basis can therapy be undertaken with maximum expectation of success.

A well-organized program, in my opinion, can be best pursued by dividing the investigation into two phases, one involving the resources available to the physician in his office, and the other, those of the hospital. Hospital admission should be utilized to complete the work-up with a minimum of expense, inconvenience, and delay to the patients, for time is an important consideration. Generally, the patients have already spent at least a year in attempting to conceive. When they seek professional help, they hope their problem can be solved quickly. The physician's efforts should be, at the same time, both unhurried and unwasteful. With the proper balance be-

TABLE 9-1.—Etiological Interpretation of Cause of Infertility as Related to Husband, Wife, and the Couple as a Unit

Female Factors	Male Factors
General	General
Dietary disturbances	Fatigue
Severe anemias	Excess smoking, alcohol
Anxiety, fear, etc.	Excess coitus
(hypothalamus)	Fear, impotence, etc.
Developmental	Developmental
Uterine absence, hypoplasia	Undescended testis
Uterine anomalies	Testicular germinal aplasia
Gonadal dysgenesis	Hypospadias
	Klinefelter's syndrome
Endocrine	Endocrine
Pituitary failure	Pituitary failure
Thyroid disturbances	Thyroid deficiency
Adrenal hyperplasia	Adrenal hyperplasia
Ovarian failure, polycystic	
disease	
Genital Disease	Genital Disease
Pelvic inflammation, T.B.	Orchitis, mumps
Tubal obstructions	Venereal disease
Endometriosis	Prostatitis
Myomata and polyps	
Cervicitis	
Vaginitis	

Male-Female Factors
Marital maladjustments
Sex problems
Ignorance (timing, douching, sperm
    leakage, etc.)
Low fertility index
Immunologic incompatibility

tween the resources of his private office and of the hospital, a lead to the answers can often be obtained in short order. Since an expensive, time-consuming study of the woman serves no useful purpose if the male partner is azoospermic, the essentials necessary for adequate evaluation of the man will be outlined first.

Study of the Male Partner

If the husband is unwilling to co-operate fully, it is futile to study the wife unless her complaint is one of complete amenorrhea or it is known without doubt that tubal closure is present. An outline of minimal diagnostic procedures for the husband is given in Table 9-2; regardless of whether these procedures are performed by the so-called generalist or by the specialist, a systematic approach must be adopted.

The physician should question the patient specifically regarding certain illnesses (mumps, orchitis, childhood diabetes), occupational hazards (exposure to roentgen rays or to other radioactive substances), sexual habits (impotence, infrequent coitus), social habits (excessive smoking and alcoholism), and the use of precoital lubricants. The husband also should be questioned regarding coital positioning, premature ejaculation and his knowledge of vaginal entrance (we have seen several "infertility" patients with practically intact, rigid hymenal membranes in which, unknown to both partners, intromission had never occurred).

Occupations associated with the use of certain metals (lead, iron, zinc,

TABLE 9-2.—MINIMAL DIAGNOSTIC PROCEDURES — MALE PARTNER

1. History and physical examination
2. Laboratory studies
   Serology
   Blood count and sedimentation rate
   Urinalysis (including stained sediment)
   Prostatic secretion (fluid specimen and stained smear)
3. Protein-bound iodine
4. Semen examination

copper), such as painting, plumbing or printing, may affect the male fertility potential deleteriously. Prolonged periods spent behind the wheel of an overheated automobile with exposure to gasoline fumes and carbon monoxide may be undetected but important etiologic factors. The associated fact that heat affects spermatogenesis adversely is important, since most truck and taxi drivers may have excessive heat surrounding the scrotal area. Persons who lead sedentary, indoor lives, who are markedly obese, or who wear tight underclothing may have abnormal spermatogenesis due to interference with the thermoregulatory mechanism of the scrotum.

The family history and the couple's attitude toward parenthood should be reviewed. Details of surgical procedures, congenital defects and accidents should be obtained. The examiner should not overlook the importance of the effects of emotional and physical stress, dietary irregularities, weight loss or gain, and the availability of periods of rest, relaxation and diversion.

A complete physical examination of the male partner is mandatory, and particular attention should be given to certain secondary male characteristics and to evidence of endocrinopathy. Congenital abnormalities such as hypospadias, cryptorchism, absence of the vas deferens or penile-scrotal hypospadias are of obvious importance. Testicular atrophy, marked varicocele or prostatoseminal vesiculitis may indicate the need for subsequent definitive therapy. Excess or absence of hair, unusual fat deposits or evidence of malnutrition should be searched for. The examiner should gain a definite impression concerning the over-all habitus and general muscular development.

Table 9-2 lists the routine laboratory procedures that should be performed as part of the initial male survey. The most important procedure is the analysis of the semen. Any physician can do a preliminary semen analysis that is adequate to determine whether the aid of a specialist is indicated if he will observe the following simple rules. Before a final conclusion is made, at least three specimens obtained at intervals of two to four weeks should be examined.

1. The patient should observe approximately five days (or more) of sexual abstinence prior to examination.

2. The specimen should be collected in a clean, dry, glass container (not a condom or plastic jar; the alkaline pH of the semen should be preserved).

3. Examination for motility should be made within two hours.

4. An accurate sperm count should be made.

5. Sperm morphology by stained smear should be studied.

6. The semen study should be correlated with the past and recent history as well as with the physical examination of the husband (wide fluctuations in normal and abnormal spermatogenic behavior are common; a single specimen should never be interpreted as a true representation of total potential).

Certain normal variations in specific sperm characteristics should be recognized. Although normal semen is said to have a minimum volume of 3 cc. with 60 per cent motile spermatozoa after two hours, 60 million sperm/cc. and 60 per cent normal morphology, this "rule of the 60's" is not absolute. Furthermore, it has been suggested that too great a volume (over 6 cc.) is just as undesirable as too little (under 2.5 cc.). Clinical examination of sperm motility should include the character of motility and the number of motile sperm related to the time since ejaculation. Although a count of 60 million sperm/cc. is generally desirable, it has been shown that the count is frequently as low as 20 million in normally fertile men. It should be remembered that the sperm count is the result of spermatogenesis that occurred three weeks previously. Close attention to previous illnesses is imperative. A gram stain of the semen specimen may reveal leukocytes and bacteria, both of which may be regarded as potential contributing factors in male infertility. Certain bacteria may affect the fertilizing capacity of spermatozoa without affecting sperm count, morphology or motility. Also, the stained spermatozoa may show an increased number of abnormal forms (macrocephalic, microcephalic, tapered) which are incapable of fertilization.

If the semen specimen, examined according to the foregoing requirements, shows on more than one test a sperm count of less than 10 million/cc., other tests of endocrine function should be done. Since these procedures are usually under the direction of a urologist or an infertility specialist, they will merely be mentioned here. They include determinations of the urinary 17-ketosteroids and pituitary gonadotropins as well as serum protein-bound iodine level and basal metabolic rate. Testicular biopsies are suggested in azoospermia, in clinically demonstrable endocrine disorders and in severe oligospermia when the patients desire that every diagnostic procedure be completed. Occasionally, other diagnostic studies, such as a chest roentgenogram, intravenous urogram, catheterization of the ejaculatory ducts, seminal vesiculography and urethrography, may reveal a specific clinical entity responsible for the infertile state.

Therapy in male infertility remains controversial. With few exceptions, no specific treatment for oligospermia or azoospermia is currently available. The rebound phenomenon associated with the administration of testosterone has been found ineffective by most investigators, and this use of testosterone is not advised. The various vitamin compounds and mixtures of vitamins and hormones have also proved disappointing. The use of desiccated thyroid or L-triiodothyronine (Cytomel), even in euthyroid persons, has enjoyed widespread acceptance, but recent investigation reveals that the curative effects of thyroid hormones are much in doubt or are of limited value. Radiation therapy to the testes or pituitary gland has not effectively corrected abnormal spermatogenesis. Chorionic gonadotropin administered to normal men may cause hyalinization of tubules and must be used only for strictly defined indications.

What then can be offered to the husband in the way of positive therapy? Even if the semen analysis is normal, the following suggestions are frequently of value.

1. Avoidance of excesses of alcohol, tobacco, caffeine and coitus.

2. Regular hours of sleep, exercise and work.

3. A diet with adequate protein and vitamin constituents, and a weight-reduction diet for the obese patient.

4. Adequate vacations from business and social responsibility.

5. Adjustment of the local environment so that excessive and prolonged heat does not interfere with the thermoregulatory mechanism of the scrotum.

6. Correction of hypothyroidism by appropriate medication.

7. Administration of chorionic gonadotropin *only* to those patients who have a demonstrated deficiency in follicle-stimulating hormone and who have an immature testis revealed by biopsy.

8. Elimination of chronic sources of infection resulting in prostatitis and seminal vesiculitis.

9. Coitus at regular intervals—every two to three days. Prolonged continence may increase the total count but will diminish sperm motility.

Although surgical measures by themselves cannot correct abnormal spermatogenic activity, they are indicated when congenital abnormalities or obstruction prevents normal passage of spermatozoa. Correction of penile-scrotal hypospadias or epididymal obstruction by plastic procedures is associated with a high percentage of subsequent pregnancies. Varicocelectomy has been suggested as a wise prophylactic measure in prepuberal boys who have marked venous distortion, but it is doubtful that the operation will cure testicular atrophy. However, this should be an individual problem worked out with each patient with the realization that there may be a delay of one or two years after operation before maximum spermatogenesis or fertility appears. Recent evidence suggests that varicocelectomy may prove beneficial in elevating sperm count and increasing motility and I have found this to be of value in numerous patients. Testicular cooling has been suggested as a therapeutic measure but its value is yet to be determined. From the viewpoint of prophylaxis, the early correction of cryptorchism is of major importance. Recent evidence strongly favors orchiopexy before age 3 and certainly before age 5.

STUDY OF THE FEMALE PARTNER

The routine minimal diagnostic procedures for the evaluation of female infertility are given in Table 9–3. A detailed historical summary should in particular outline the menstrual pattern, including age of onset, duration and frequency of flow, amount of bleeding, presence or absence of pain and any gross irregularities. In addition, the physician should inquire about premarital and postmarital coitus, especially with relation to frequency and timing with ovulation. Other points of importance include use or disuse of contraceptives, present and past occupations, history of pelvic infections, use of cigarets and alcohol, past surgery, accidents or illnesses, and the use of intravaginal lubricants or douches.

When previous abdominal operations have been performed, I have found it advantageous to secure copies of the operative notes and the pathology reports. Surgery performed during childhood for a ruptured appendix suggests peritubal adhesions as a possible etiologic factor. Often an operation described by the patient as "conservative" has, in fact, been a bilateral salpingectomy. Extensive (and expensive) investigation is thus immediately avoided.

TABLE 9-3.—MINIMAL DIAGNOSTIC PROCEDURES — FEMALE PARTNER

1. History and physical examination
2. Laboratory studies
   Serology
   Blood count and sedimentation rate
   Urinalysis
3. Protein-bound iodine
4. Postcoital test
5. Endometrial biopsy
6. Tubal insufflation
7. Miscellaneous:
   Papanicolaou's stain
   Fern test — *spinnbarkeit*
   Schiller's test — cervical smear
   Hanging drop for candida, monilia and trichomonas
   Incompatibility test — cervical mucus and semen

During the physical examination the physician should pay particular attention to external body contour, hair distribution, fat deposits and breast development. The breasts should be thoroughly examined for nipple abnormality or dominant lumps (we have seen early breast carcinomas in two patients referred for endocrine infertility). Stigmata of hypothyroidism should be looked for. A thorough pelvic examination should be conducted, in which the size, shape and position of the internal and external genitalia are noted and particular search made for infections. Pronounced hypertrophy of the labia may be congenital but strongly suggests masturbation. An enlarged clitoris and male distribution of pubic hair should warn the examiner to look for other evidences of masculinization due to adrenal or ovarian tumors. If purulent material can be expressed from the urethral meatus or periurethral glands, it should be stained and cultured for gonococci. Specific vaginal infections, such as those caused by trichomonas and candida (monilia), may be important factors in infertility because the severe dyspareunia they cause may prevent normal frequency of coitus. The finding of a vaginal septum or double cervix demands that the uterus and oviducts be investigated radiologically for other congenital abnormalities.

Although the importance of the cervical factor will be considered separately, much can be gained at the first visit if (1) a cervical aspiration for cytologic examination is obtained (two slides may be made, one for Papanicolaou's stain to determine malignancy and one for the Harris-Shorr stain to determine estrogen effect), (2) Schiller's test is performed routinely and (3) biopsies are taken of all nonstaining areas and of obvious cervical erosions. Although the infertile patient statistically is less likely to have carcinoma in situ of the cervix than is her multiparous counterpart, she should not be denied a complete diagnostic survey.

The minimum laboratory procedures advocated are: (1) serologic test for syphilis, (2) complete blood count and erythrocyte sedimentation rate, (3) urinalysis, (4) chest x-ray, (5) serum protein-bound iodine and basal metabolic rate. The serum protein-bound iodine value should be obtained before performing Schiller's test. A false high value will be present for six to eight weeks after Schiller's solution (potassium iodide plus iodine) is applied to the cervix. If endocrine abnormalities are evident or if there is menstrual irregularity (especially amenorrhea), the following tests are ordered: (1) urinary 17-ketosteroids and 17-hydroxycorticoids, (2) urinary follicle-stimulating hormone, and (3) a roentgenogram of the sella turcica.

It has been mentioned that the various diagnostic procedures can be completed in approximately six visits, and prognostic advice may then be given the couple. (See Fig. 9–1.) The procedures require proper timing and interpretation, and each will now be discussed in some detail. Finally, certain specific factors causing infertility (cervical, uterine, tubal, ovarian) will be evaluated with particular reference to therapy.

The three most important office diagnostic procedures are the postcoital

Fig. 9–1.—Composite figure of major areas of investigation in cases of infertility. Large arrows indicate optimal day for each specific investigation. (From Behrman, S. J., and Kistner, R. W. (eds.): *Progress in Infertility* [Boston: Little, Brown & Company, 1968].)

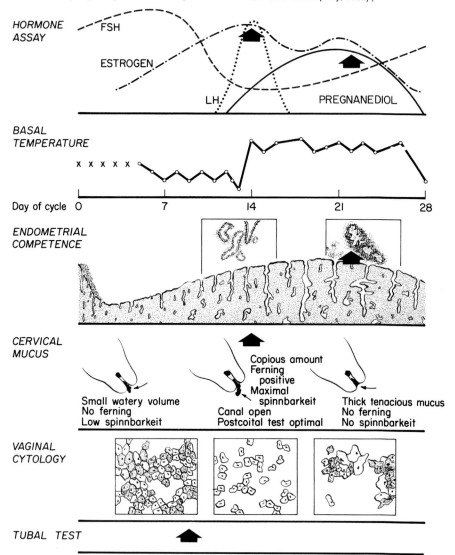

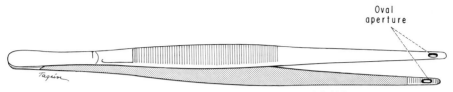

Fig. 9-2.—Long dressing forceps adapted for collection of seminal fluid from the endocervical canal.

examination of cervical mucus (Sims-Huhner test), the endometrial biopsy and tubal insufflation.

Postcoital Test.—This test is optimally performed at the time of ovulation, and, since experience with donor insemination has shown that conception occurs most frequently within the 48 hours just preceding the rise in basal body temperature, postcoital tests planned for 15 to 16 days before an expected menstrual period are often therapeutic. The interval between coitus and examination may vary, but a minimum of at least six hours (maximum, 16 hours) is desirable for the study of sperm survival. No douches or intravaginal medication should be used during the 48 hours preceding the test.

TECHNIQUE.—Figure 9-2 illustrates a long, narrow, dressing forceps with a small oval aperture at the tip. With this instrument a sample of mucus is easily obtained from high in the endocervical canal where sperm motility and survival are maximum. If the cervical os is too small to admit a metal instrument, a Silastic tubule may be inserted through the external os into the endocervix. A syringe may then be attached to the tubule and gentle suction will obtain an adequate specimen. If the mucus is clear, abundant and watery, with good elasticity, it is suitable for evaluation of sperm penetration. At the time of ovulation, the mucus forms a thin, continuous thread as it is pulled apart—a phenomenon called *spinnbarkeit* by the Germans. This physical characteristic is a function of increasing levels of estrogen and disappears after the appearance of progesterone. Such mucus, when allowed to dry on a slide, crystallizes into a fernlike pattern, the "arborization phenomenon" (see Chapter 4). This phenomenon also disappears after ovulation as a result of progesterone secretion. When the cervical mucus is examined under the high-dry magnification, the number of cellular elements (leukocytes) and spermatozoa per high-power field are noted. The motility and quality of progression of the spermatozoa are similarly observed.

INTERPRETATION.—No normal value may be assigned to this test, but in general the pregnancy rate is significantly higher if good mucus is associated with the finding of several actively motile spermatozoa per high-power field than if rare or inactive spermatozoa are observed. Spermatozoa are rarely seen in poor mucus, and therefore such a result on a *single* observation is of no prognostic value. The physician should remember that this test reflects not only the cervical environment of spermatozoa but also the ovarian function controlling it. As such, it is of extremely great value and, if numerous active spermatozoa are found, this test may be substituted for the laboratory analysis of semen. Furthermore, since the greatest number of conceptions in an infertile population occur within the menstrual cycle following the first consultation, a well-timed postcoital test is a most useful therapeutic contribution.

Endometrial Biopsy.—This is a convenient office procedure that causes only minor discomfort and does not require local or general anesthesia.

Although the test is usually employed as a test for ovulation, the finding of secretory changes in the endometrium is only *presumptive* evidence of ovulation (luteinized follicles may occasionally produce the same changes). Since the incidence of anovulatory cycles in infertile women is between 5 and 10 per cent, the significance of the test is obvious. The timing of the procedure is important, the optimum time being the first day of the menses. The bleeding may then be correctly interpreted as being menstrual or anovulatory in type, and the chances of disrupting a normal pregnancy are minimal. Some pathologists prefer the well-maintained late secretory endometrium of day 27-28 to the fragmented tissue obtained after menstruation has begun. In women with regular cycles this can be timed rather precisely but the patient is warned not to have coitus at the time of ovulation during that cycle. Biopsies at the time of menstruation have the added advantage of occasionally revealing tuberculous endometritis. Unfortunately, biopsy at this time is not always a practical arrangement, and an alternate method is to perform the biopsy on or before the sixth postovulatory day as estimated from the menstrual history. At this time the ovum is either in the oviduct or in the uterine fluid, since implantation does not occur until the fifth to eighth postovulatory day. If coitus is avoided

Fig. 9-3.—**A,** cutting edge of Duncan curet. This instrument can be introduced easily through an undilated, nulliparous cervical os without undue discomfort. **B,** proper technique of endometrial biopsy with the Duncan curet.

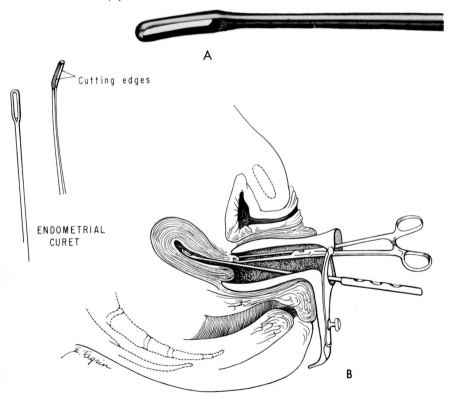

A

Cutting edges

ENDOMETRIAL
CURET

B

ENDOMETRIAL BIOPSY

during a given month, the biopsy specimen may be obtained at the theoretical apex of progesterone activity (i.e., day 22 or 23 of a 28-day cycle). This may be of particular importance in patients with an "insufficient luteal phase" when exacting studies of glandular and stromal changes in the endometrium are necessary.

TECHNIQUE.—A pelvic examination should precede the biopsy so that the position and size of the uterus can be ascertained. The cervix is exposed with a speculum and cleansed with Alkalol or Alevaire. Slight traction is placed on the cervix with a tenaculum. Although I prefer the Duncan curet (Fig. 9-3, A) because of its smaller size, any of the various types will give adequate samples. It has been my routine to obtain tissue from both the anterior and posterior surfaces of the endometrial cavity, using a firm but gentle stroke from the fundus to the cervix (Fig. 9-3, B). The most representative samples are obtained from high in the corpus. The tissue is immediately fixed in Bouin's fluid. Care should be taken not to traumatize the tissue in transferring it from the curet to the fixative.

INTERPRETATION.—Although exact dating of the endometrium during the secretory phase of the cycle is practiced by gynecologic pathologists, it is not absolutely necessary, and adequate interpretation or presumption of ovulation may be made in most patients. If the endometrial biopsy reveals abnormal tissue of any variety, a thorough curettage should be done for adequate diagnosis and to rule out malignancy.

Noyes has suggested certain essentials for obtaining and interpreting the endometrial biopsy. (1) Chart the basal body temperature and perform the biopsy during a BBT cycle. (2) Biopsy after two or three BBT cycles have been charted and biopsy at least during two cycles. (3) Biopsy on the sixth and ninth postovulatory days; be certain to get fundal surfaces. (4) Try to obtain superficial endometrium—don't go too deep. (5) Fix the tissue in Bouin's solution. (6) Date the endometrium, but date the most advanced area. (7) Look at your own slides.

Tubal Insufflation.—The most important single contribution to the promotion of fertility, with the exception of regular and completed coitus, is still the ingenious discovery of uterotubal insufflation by the late Dr. Isadore C. Rubin. Many gynecologists believe (and perhaps with good reason) that tubal insufflation and hysterosalpingography continue to be the outstanding measures in the treatment of infertility. One should realize, however, that functional occlusion of the oviducts is common and that a negative result, even if the technique is irreproachable, may still be indicative of tubal spasm and not of organic disease. Conversely, when the test gives a positive finding there may still be peritubal adhesions or endometriosis that causes tubo-ovarian malfunction.

TECHNIQUE.—A thorough pelvic examination should always precede the test since the presence of acute or subacute intrapelvic sepsis is a specific contraindication. The optimum time for this procedure is prior to ovulation and at least three to four days after the cessation of the menses. Selection of this time will avoid damage to a fertilized ovum or the possibility of a false-negative result from plugging of the internal tubal ostia with a ball-valve mass of secretory endometrium. Various instruments are now available for tubal insufflation (Fig. 9-4). Most employ (1) a constant source of carbon dioxide, (2) a flowmeter and (3) a pressure gauge and kymograph or some equivalent apparatus for reading the degree of peristaltic excursions that are presumably of tubal origin. *It should be emphasized that the use of room air or oxygen may be a likely source of fatal air embolism!* Since the most frequent error in the performance of the test is failure to obtain a leakproof applica-

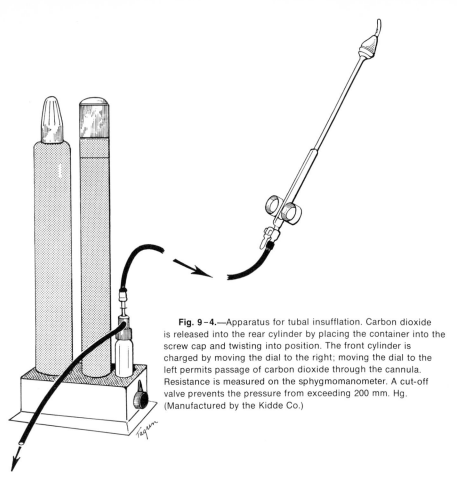

Fig. 9-4.—Apparatus for tubal insufflation. Carbon dioxide is released into the rear cylinder by placing the container into the screw cap and twisting into position. The front cylinder is charged by moving the dial to the right; moving the dial to the left permits passage of carbon dioxide through the cannula. Resistance is measured on the sphygmomanometer. A cut-off valve prevents the pressure from exceeding 200 mm. Hg. (Manufactured by the Kidde Co.)

To Sphygmomanometer

tion of the cervical obturator, the physician should have a supply of different-sized rubber acorns or should use the newer screw-type cannula. In patients with a patulous cervical os the use of a suction cup is invaluable. Leakage of gas at the cervical os may be checked by introducing fluid into the vaginal vault. In most cases it is not wise to exceed a pressure of 200 mm. Hg if the test is being performed for diagnosis only. (When insufflation is being performed to attempt to open closed tubes, the pressure has been allowed to rise to 300 mm. Hg.)

EVALUATION.—With normal tubal patency, the pressure rises to a variable height (usually 60-120 mm. Hg) and then falls to a relatively constant level. If blockage is present, the kymograph shows a steady rise until a pressure of 200 mm. Hg is reached; most units have cut-off valves at this level. The insufflation test indicates tubal patency only if gas is demonstrated under the diaphragm by the occurrence of shoulder pain or by roentgenography. Shoulder pain may be delayed in patients with extensive pelvic adhesions, marked obesity or old subdiaphragmatic pleurisy. The major principles in the evaluation of tubal function are the *necessity for more than one test* whenever the result of the initial test is abnormal and the utilization of other tests if the result remains doubtful. Further, if tubal function appears normal by one test (no other sterility factors being evident) and if pregnancy does not occur within a reasonable time, ancillary tests should be performed. The so-called triple tubal patency investigation embraces insufflation with carbon dioxide, hysterosalpingography and culdoscopy with injection of indigo carmine under visual control. The hysterosalpingogram aids in the diagnosis of lesions missed by insufflation and localizes areas of blockage. Abnormalities in the salpingogram are frequently clarified by culdoscopy and by tubal lavage with indigo carmine.

Hysterosalpingography.—Hysterosalpingography and insufflation by carbon dioxide should be regarded as complementary rather than antagonistic methods. Each serves specific purposes. Unfortunately, the ideal fluid for instillation is not as yet available. Theoretically, it should be water soluble, painless when injected and harmless and it should afford adequate contrast on roentgenograms and remain visible for a number of days after instillation. Figure 9-5 shows the normal findings obtained by tubograms

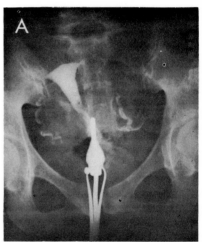

Fig. 9-5.—Hysterosalpingograms. **A,** visualization of uterus and both oviducts in a normal patient. **B,** second film, showing free passage of the dye from the oviduct into the peritoneal cavity. **C,** patient with chronic pelvic inflammatory disease and bilateral hydrosalpinges. Note the dilated and convoluted tube on the right and the accumulation of dye in sacculations at the tubal fimbria.

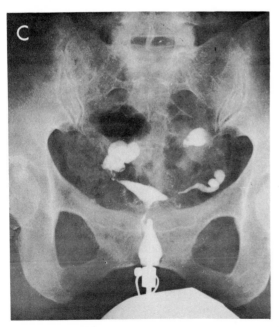

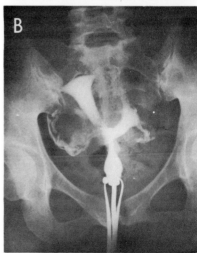

and the findings seen in chronic pelvic inflammatory disease. Viscous oils, such as iodized poppy-seed oil (Lipiodol), remain in the pelvic cavity for long periods and may cause oil granulomas. Iodine-oil preparations are no longer used in our clinic because of the high incidence of oil granulomas we have encountered. Nonviscous oils are quickly absorbed from the peritoneum but also remain in the pelvic cavity too long. Water-soluble media may cause abdominal cramps, and a 24-hour follow-up film is not possible because of rapid absorption. Many authorities still prefer the use of the opaque oils with a 24-hour film or special positioning of the patient after injection of 3–6 cc. of oil to fill the uterine cavity and oviducts. Thus the patient may be placed on the right side, the left side and then in lithotomy position so that spill through the pelvis can be demonstrated on the initial visit. Recently the procedure of cinefluoroscopy for evaluation of tubal motility and patency has been adopted in many clinics but its advantages over culdoscopy and indigo carmine lavage of the tubes remains to be proved. If oily media are not used, a substitute in the form of culdoscopy or culdotomy must be employed to diagnose adhesive processes.

Culdoscopy and Laparoscopy. —If tubal insufflations are unsatisfactory, if the hysterosalpingogram shows any abnormality, or if the patient does not become pregnant within a reasonable time, culdoscopy is suggested (Fig. 9–6). We prefer to perform this procedure in an operating room under local or hypobaric spinal anesthesia. A one-day admission to the hospital is necessary for this procedure; it is not recommended that it be performed in the office. Following routine inspection of the pelvic viscera, indigo carmine is injected through an intrauterine cannula. If the tubes are patent, the dye may be seen to efflux from the tubal fimbria and spill into the peritoneal cavity. Complications following culdoscopy are minimal, and much valuable information may be gained. In approximately three of four patients with abnormal salpingograms or unexplained infertility, some type of pelvic disorder, such as peritubal adhesions or endometriosis, is diagnosed by culdoscopy.

Obviously, additional tests are needed if no final diagnosis has been obtained up to this point. Among these tests are 24-hour urinalyses for 17-ketosteroids, total gonadotropins, estrogen, protein-bound iodine and T-3 and skull x-rays. To perform these on an outpatient basis is both cumbersome and costly, and they are frequently inaccurate because of the difficulty in collecting urine properly. Accordingly, I have arranged for my patients to be admitted to the Boston Hospital for Women for a 1- or 2-day stay so that these and other tests can be performed most expeditiously and at minimal cost. As a matter of fact, for the last five years I have not utilized carbon dioxide testing in my office and I use hysterosalpingography only to recheck a dubious finding at the time of culdoscopy. Obviously in a patient with habitual abortion a hysterogram is important in order to exclude various congenital abnormalities.

During this "rapid infertility workup" my patients have an x-ray of the chest and sella turcica, complete blood count and urinalysis and the endocrine studies noted above. These are initiated on the afternoon of admission and the next morning a culdoscopy (or laparoscopy), indigo carmine lavage of the tubes and dilatation and curettage are performed. The patient is then discharged the same evening. Prior to admission the patient is asked to chart her basal body temperature for 2 or 3 cycles and a post-

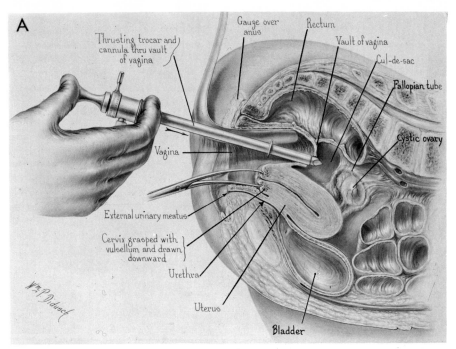

A

Thrusting trocar and cannula thru vault of vagina

Gauze over anus

Rectum

Vault of vagina

Cul-de-sac

Fallopian tube

Cystic ovary

Vagina

External urinary meatus

Cervix grasped with vulsellum and drawn downward

Urethra

Uterus

Bladder

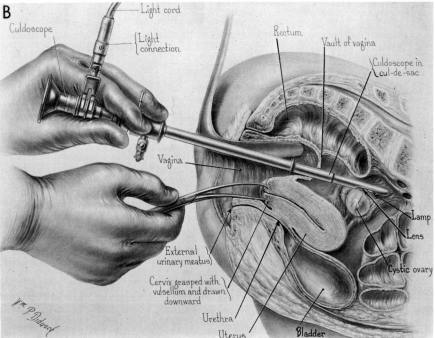

B

Culdoscope

Light cord

Light connection

Rectum

Vault of vagina

Culdoscope in cul-de-sac

Vagina

Lamp

Lens

Cystic ovary

External urinary meatus

Cervix grasped with vulsellum and drawn downward

Urethra

Uterus

Bladder

Fig. 9-6.—Technique of culdoscopy. **A,** the culdoscopy puncture is made with one thrust of the trocar through the vaginal septum. In the presence of cul-de-sac endometriosis or extensive adhesions, the index finger of the left hand is introduced into the rectum to "guide" the trocar below the rectum. **B,** the trocar has been removed and the culdoscope introduced through the cannula for visualization. (From Decker, A.: Clin. Obst. & Gynec. 1:610, 1958.)

coital test of cervical mucus is planned on the basis of apparent ovulation as indicated on the temperature chart. If the postcoital test is poor or inconclusive a complete seminal fluid analysis is obtained. It is surprising how many women will become pregnant during this 3-month period of initial observation, particularly those who have not had a previous infertility investigation. If the postcoital test and/or the seminal fluid analysis is adequate, the patient is then scheduled for admission. Obviously, those patients who have regular ovarian cycles and normal menstrual periods need not have determinations of gonadotropins, ketosteroids or estrogen. A protein-bound iodine and T-3 assay are done routinely, however. During this hospital stay multidisciplinary consultations can also be obtained.

Recently many gynecologists have been converted to performing laparoscopies due to several advantages. In the first place, the patient is in the lithotomy-Trendelenburg position, which is far less inconvenient for the operating staff and is most convenient in the event that surgery is to be performed immediately after the procedure. Visibility is far superior, and lysis of adhesions around the tube, biopsy of the ovary, and drainage of cysts are much more readily accomplished through the operating laparoscope. However, whether culdoscopy or laparoscopy is done, in our experience it has proved an extraordinarily useful method of investigation in problems of infertility—so useful that we feel it is essential to perform it sometime before any work-up is concluded. With its help we have found an incidence of undiagnosed pathology in the order of 12 per cent, including peritoneal adhesions separating tube and ovary, unsuspected endometriosis, pelvic tuberculosis, and even ovarian tumors.

It is clear, then, that only with this type of methodical and thorough investigation can one fulfill the criteria required to unearth the unsuspected and not so obvious etiological factors responsible for the infertility problem or give an intelligent prognosis for the future of the couple.

The Cervical Factor

The importance of the postcoital test has already been emphasized. The endocervical canal is lined by racemose glands composed of mucus-containing columnar cells. These cells produce a cervical mucus that contains a variety of sugars and amino acids and, although the effects of these substances on sperm metabolism and migration are not completely known, spermatozoa maintain motility longer in favorable cervical mucus than in seminal fluid.

Hormonal, anatomic and infectious aspects of the cervical factor are important. Stated simply, estrogen stimulates the secretory activity of the endocervical glands, and progesterone inhibits this activity. The estrogen effect may be assayed by microscopic examination of the mucus, which demonstrates the fern pattern, and by gross inspection, which reveals the formation of spinnbarkeit. Furthermore, estrogen produces specific anatomic changes in the isthmic canal. Two days before ovulation this area assumes a funnel shape due to relaxation of the sphincteric constriction, and it becomes shorter and wider. After ovulation the canal becomes longer and narrower. If estrogen deficiency is detected, exogenous estrogen may be administered, but care must be taken to keep the dose low enough so that ovulation is not inhibited. Ethinyl estradiol (Estinyl), 0.02 mg., or diethylstilbestrol, 0.25 mg., may be given daily for several months under these circumstances.

Anatomic variations in the position of the cervix do not seem to be as important as previously suggested by various observers. Spermatozoa seem to enter the anteriorly directed cervix associated with a third-degree retroversion as readily as they enter the cervix directed into the mythical seminal pool. The cervix that is prolapsed beyond the introitus, however, is poorly conditioned to accept the seminal fluid. Correction of the prolapse by pessaries, cervical cups or operation is frequently followed by pregnancy. Although the size and shape of the cervix may not be related to infertility, the hypoplastic cervix may be a predisposing factor because of scant mucus. Similarly, a small, tight endocervical canal and a tight internal os may be benefited by careful but not overzealous dilatation. As a matter of fact, in several recent articles the authors suggest that the passage of sounds or dilators through the cervix is attended by a large measure of success in overcoming infertility. Such success cannot be assigned to the process of dilatation alone, however, since one author recommended that this be followed by the orgiastic ritual of knee-chest coitus. Thus, hypothalamic and other stimuli might have had more effect than the cervical dilatation. If one chooses to follow this advice, care should be taken not to traumatize the endocervix by use of large dilators and perhaps predispose the patient to subsequent midtrimester abortion because of cervical incompetence.

Specific cervical lesions and infections demand careful and individual attention. If biopsy reveals invasive carcinoma, the indicated treatment immediately ends the reproductive potential. If carcinoma in situ is found, conservative therapy may allow further childbearing if the patient agrees to close follow-up supervision. Large endocervical polyps should be excised and the base lightly cauterized. Although cervical erosions and eversions are commonly found in infertile patients, their etiologic significance has been overemphasized. Nevertheless, erosions and eversions should be corrected by thorough electrocauterization or cryosurgery, but care should be taken not to destroy the endocervical mucosa. Gentle passage of a uterine sound should be performed after complete healing of the cauterized areas in order to prevent stenosis. Severely lacerated and distorted cervices occasionally may be improved by meticulous plastic surgery, comprising excision of the scar and restoration of as much of the normal anatomy of the portio vaginalis as possible. Conization (unless performed as a therapeutic measure in carcinoma in situ) is not advised as a procedure to increase the fertility potential.

Acute cervicitis should be treated by the antibiotics or sulfonamides indicated by cultures and the sensitivities of the responsible organism. At a later date, chronic foci of infection in the cervix should be obliterated by cauterization or by the use of topically or systemically administered antibiotics, or both. Recent evidence suggests that enzymatic debridement with fibrinogen-desoxyribonuclease preparations may be less traumatic to the cervix than cautery. In certain instances the anatomic or physiologic insufficiency of the cervix may be overcome by artificial insemination with the husband's semen. The use of polyethylene cups that can be trimmed to fit the contours of the grossly abnormal cervix has simplified the technique of this procedure.

Recent studies have shown that cervical secretions may contain ABO antibodies, thus suggesting an etiologic concept of infertility based on agglutination of the sperm by these secretions in incompatible ABO matings. Therefore, blood types should be checked in all patients who have infertility of apparently unknown cause. Research in the field of immunology will undoubtedly clarify many unsettled questions in the field of infertility, but at this time direct clinical application is not possible.

Various diagnostic tests have been designed to test the cervical factor in infertility. These are: (1) evaluation of cervical mucus for arborization and spinnbarkeit (described in Chapter 4), (2) the postcoital test, (3) an in vitro test of mucus penetration by spermatozoa, (4) pH of cervical mucus, (5) tests of cervical glucose, (6) test of cervical mucus chloride, (7) changes in cervical mucus proteins, and (8) cultures of the cervix.

The reader is referred to the chapter on The Cervical Factor in Infertility by Marcus and Marcus in *Progress in Infertility,* edited by Behrman and Kistner, for a complete review of the subject.

THE UTERINE FACTOR

The importance of an adequately developed, receptive endometrium was mentioned in the discussion of the endometrial biopsy. If luteal activity is believed to be deficient and if the endometrial biopsy reveals evidence of progestational insufficiency, improvement may be expected with the use of a progestational substance. A substituted progesterone is preferable to a 19-nor progestin for this purpose and therefore I have used Provera in a dose of 10 mg. daily from day 18 through day 25 of a 28-day cycle.

Therapy should not be started too soon after ovulation, nor should the dose be excessive, since glandular and stromal abnormalities occur that may affect implantation deleteriously. Noyes has suggested that the endometrium may be either "overdeveloped" or "underdeveloped." If the latter, he prefers to administer human chorionic gonadotropin (to stimulate the corpus luteum) than to give exogenous progesterone. If the endometrium is "overdeveloped," he gives ethinyl estradiol, 0.05 mg., from the low point on the BBT cycle for eight consecutive days. Infertility resulting from endocrine abnormalities affecting the endometrium will be discussed in the chapter on habitual abortion.

Certain infertile women with no detectable abnormality are found to have endometrial hypoplasia with associated malfunction of the uterus and oviducts. Several studies have suggested that stimulation of end-organs by progesterone and estrogen for several cycles may be associated with improved function and subsequent pregnancy. When therapy is administered in this manner, pituitary gonadotropins are inhibited, so that the results may be a combination of end-organ priming followed by so-called pituitary rebound. The suggested compound is one of the sequential oral contraceptives given from day 5 through day 25 for three consecutive cycles. In the first cycle after treatment, ovulation may be delayed for three to five days, occasionally longer; subsequent cycles ordinarily revert to the duration usual for the individual patient.

The presence of large submucous leiomyomas may be verified by diagnostic curettage and hysterography. Their importance in infertility and repetitive abortion has been established, and myomectomy (see Chapter

5) is indicated if tubal patency is assured and study of the male partner is adequate.

Uterine retroversions should be corrected by manual replacement and the insertion of a Smith-Hodge pessary (see Fig. 5–25). If pregnancy occurs, the pessary should be left in place until the twelfth week of gestation. Suspension of the retroverted uterus as a primary procedure for infertility is not warranted unless more conservative measures have failed. As previously mentioned, suspension is not necessary to place the cervix in a more favorable position for the reception of semen. In certain patients the uterus cannot be replaced manually even under anesthesia. In such cases, provided all other studies are normal and the patients have been observed during a 12-month period of involuntary sterility, culdoscopy is performed. Laparotomy and suspension are suggested if specific etiologic factors are discovered. Endometriosis or pelvic adhesions will be found to be the cause of uterine retroversion in most of these women. Congenital abnormalities of the uterus (bicornuate or septate uterus, etc.) may be diagnosed by hysterography and should be corrected surgically if they are associated with infertility or repetitive abortion.

Postpartum curettage will occasionally result in permanent intrauterine damage with destruction of the endometrium (Asherman's syndrome). The possibility of restoring fertility by surgery in these patients is small, although transplantation of endosalpingeal mucosa has been attempted. Spontaneous regeneration occurs but may take four to five years. Prognosis for subsequent pregnancy is poor. Louros has suggested the use of an intra-uterine device immediately following a curettage to break up the adhesions. The uterine walls are thus prevented from coapting and the patient is started on an estrogen-progestin pseudopregnancy. Preliminary results from this method of therapy seem encouraging and Comninos has reported pregnancies after the use of this method.

Inflammatory lesions of the endometrium are known causes of infertility. Moyer has suggested six general categories:

1. Endometrial infections may follow procedures that destroy or alter the usual protective role of the cervical secretions. Bacteria are normally present in the vagina and lower cervical fluids but are absent in the upper endocervical canal. When the normal secretion of the endocervical glands is altered, bacteria may find their way into the endometrial cavity. Procedures at fault include extensive biopsy, conization, and cauterization of the cervix.

2. Endometrial infections may result when the normally contaminated cervical mucus is pushed up into the endometrial cavity by instrumentation. Endometrial biopsy, hysterosalpingography, and tubal insufflation procedures, as well as criminal abortions, use of the stem pessary for dysmenorrhea, and insertion of gauze or radium into the uterine cavity may be the cause of infection.

3. Uterine infections are more likely to occur when the bacteriostatic environment of the endometrium is altered, as during the parturitional period when the endometrium is atrophic and quiescent. At this time the tissues are not stimulated by estrogen, so that marked changes in the secretion of uterine fluid and alteration of the phagocytic system take place.

4. Ascending infection of organisms having the ability to penetrate the usual bacteriostatic mechanisms of the cervix, such as *Neisseria gonorrhoeae,* may produce infections of the uterine lining.

5. Infections may be borne to the endometrium by the blood. For example, the tuberculosis organism is the etiological agent in chronic granulomatous endometritis.

6. Drainage of purulent material from chronically infected fallopian tubes may produce endometritis. This mechanism occurs rarely, and may take place early in the course of chronic salpingitis, because the longer the tubes remain infected, the greater the possibility of occlusion of the isthmus.

The Tubal Factor

The fact that blocked tubes can be opened—by time, sexual rest and antispasmodics—has been well documented. Some investigators have advocated repeated tubal insufflations with pressures as high as 300 mg. Hg together with pelvic heat and sexual abstinence as a method superior to tubal surgery. Unfortunately, the two methods utilized to evaluate tubal factors in infertility demonstrate only passage or nonpassage of the medium through the oviduct and are not significant in evaluating details of tubal anatomy, physiology or pathology. The clinician should remember that the fertilized ovum remains in the oviduct for three or four days before reaching the endometrial cavity. Research in tubal physiology is scant, but the data suggest that the oviduct is more than just a transporting organ (e.g., certain mammalian ova, transferred from the oviduct to the uterus within 20 hours of fertilization, do not implant). The effects of steroid hormones on tubal physiology and ovum transport are definite and measurable, but clinical application must await more extensive study.

Recent studies of patients with pelvic inflammatory disease have negated the generally accepted opinion that most salpingitis is due to the gonococcus. Cultures obtained from pyosalpinges frequently reveal that the etiologic organism is a gram-negative rod of the colon group. Therefore, therapy for the acute episodes should be initiated with one of the broad-spectrum antibiotics effective against Escherichia coli, Aerobacter aerogenes and Bacillus proteus in order to preserve the function of the endosalpinx.

Surgical treatment for a closed oviduct occasionally may be indicated when the husband is normal and all studies in the female indicate normal function except for nonpatency of the tubes on *repeated examinations* with both carbon dioxide and liquid media.

If the oviducts are apparently closed on the basis of both carbon dioxide insufflation and salpingography, I insist upon lavage of the oviducts either by culdoscopy or laparoscopy before proceeding to tuboplasty. Then, even before beginning the tubal surgery, I attempt transuterine lavage with indigo carmine dye. This is easily accomplished by occluding the cervix with a special clamp, then inserting an 18-gauge needle into the uterine cavity via the fundus. I have been pleasantly surprised on numerous occasions to see an easy efflux of dye from the fimbriated portions of the oviducts when previous testing by insufflation, x-ray and culdoscopy indicated bilateral closure. Undoubtedly the false impression had been due to tubal spasm or improper technique.

Many surgeons view the surgical treatment of tubal closure as being quite simple. Nothing could be further from the truth. While a radical hysterectomy may be more daring and may even thrill the observer, the judgment, skill and patience of the surgeon doing reconstructive work is usually less well appreciated. There is no doubt that the inexperience of the operator will lead to poor results and therefore analysis of published reports must be viewed critically. Shirodkar has suggested that the three basic reasons for poor results are: (1) inexperience of the surgeon, (2) improper selections of cases and (3) poor techniques. Garcia has suggested that consistently good results can be obtained only by meticulous handling of tissues, guided by the judgment which can be gained only with practice. Skill can be achieved by years of critical appraisal of many cases, or more effectively after individual tutelage by assisting someone with wide experience. But without a knowledge of reproductive physiology even the most skillful surgeon will fail.

Although all reconstructive surgery performed on the oviduct is referred to as a *tuboplasty,* this overall term is misleading since certain procedures have a fairly good prognosis for eventual pregnancy and others do not. A classification suggested by Margaret Moore-White is as follows: (1) Salpingolysis—the separation of peritubal adhesions usually secondary to an infectious perisalpingitis or endometriosis. (2) Salpingoplasty—opening of the totally occluded distal end of the tube, as in a hydrosalpinx, either by a linear salpingostomy, removal of a wedge of tissue producing a fishmouth eversion, or by the more popular distal resection creating a new ostium and fimbrial cuff. (3) Midsegment reconstruction—removal of a segment of occluded oviduct due either to previous salpingitis or surgical ligation. (4) Cornual or interstitial resection and reimplantation.

The physician should present all of the available data to the couple and permit them to decide if surgery is desirable. The major types of corrective

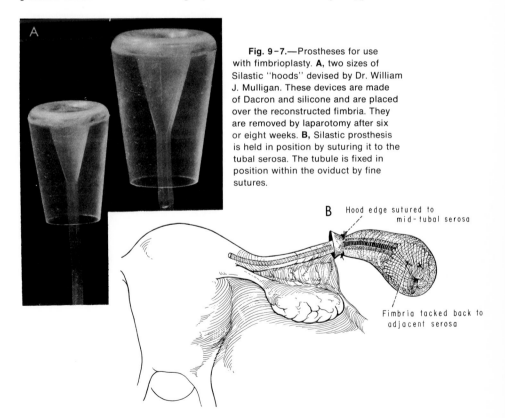

Fig. 9–7.—Prostheses for use with fimbrioplasty. **A,** two sizes of Silastic "hoods" devised by Dr. William J. Mulligan. These devices are made of Dacron and silicone and are placed over the reconstructed fimbria. They are removed by laparotomy after six or eight weeks. **B,** Silastic prosthesis is held in position by suturing it to the tubal serosa. The tubule is fixed in position within the oviduct by fine sutures.

Hood edge sutured to
mid-tubal serosa

Fimbria tacked back to
adjacent serosa

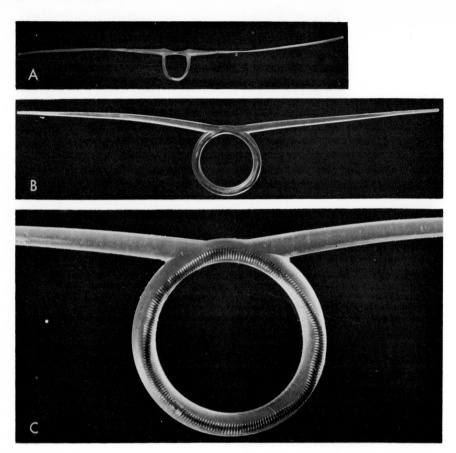

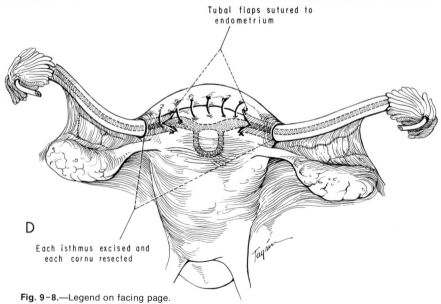

Tubal flaps sutured to
endometrium

Each isthmus excised and
each cornu resected

Fig. 9-8.—Legend on facing page.

operations on the oviduct are shown in Figures 9–7 and 9–8. Roland has devised a spiral Teflon stent to be used after salpingoplasty. It may be removed from its abdominal wall attachment without a second laparotomy. The reader is referred to an excellent review of these surgical techniques in the chapter on tubal reconstruction by Celso-Ramon Garcia in *Progress in Infertility.*

Since the physician is dealing with a malformed or diseased organ, the increased incidence of tubal ectopic pregnancy subsequent to operation is not surprising. Also, smoldering pelvic inflammatory disease may be reactivated at the time of salpingoplasty; this inflammatory reaction may be extensive enough to necessitate hysterectomy and bilateral salpingo-oophorectomy. The selection of patients for oviduct surgery and the choice of a surgeon to perform such an operation should be made on specific and stringent criteria.

The incidence of pregnancy after salpingolysis varies from 26 to 53 per cent and the overall salvage is 38 per cent. The number of pregnancies subsequent to fimbrioplasty varies from 4.8 to 53 per cent. In 868 cases the incidence of pregnancy was 18 per cent. The wide discrepancy obviously reflects patient selection, the degree of tubal destruction and, possibly, the use of protective hoods after the corrective procedure. Garcia has reported a gross pregnancy rate of 52.6 per cent in patients with bilateral hydrosalpinges whose tubes remained patent subsequent to surgery. The live birth rate corrected for ectopics and abortion was 36.8 per cent. In patients with bilateral hydrosalpinges of varying degree, it is sometimes advisable to perform a unilateral salpingo-oophorectomy on the most affected side combined with a fimbrioplasty and hood application on the better side. Grant reported a pregnancy rate of 32 per cent when tubal splints or hoods were used, whereas 35 per cent of women became pregnant without splints. He increased the latter figure to 43 per cent by the use of hydrocortisone transtubation every 3 days during the first 2 weeks after surgery, followed by chymotrypsin transtubation later.

The overall incidence of pregnancy in surgery for interstitial occlusion of the oviduct was 30 per cent in 583 patients reported by 17 authors. Unfortunately many reports give pregnancy results on the basis of patients with patent tubes after surgery, not on the overall number of patients treated. Most reports list the gross number of pregnancies that occurred without correcting for abortion, ectopic pregnancies and perinatal deaths. Ectopic pregnancies occur in from 5 to 10 per cent of women subjected to tubal surgery. Finally, many reports of tuboplasties do not indicate that they correct for patients in whom the contralateral tube was patent.

During the past two years we have cooperated in a study with Dr. Herbert W. Horne, Jr. utilizing dexamethasone (Decadron-Merck) and prometh-

---

Fig. 9–8.—Intrauterine prostheses for tubal implantation. **A**, plastic type devised by Shirodkar. **B**, Silastic type devised by Mulligan. **C**, a stainless steel ring is used in the Mulligan prosthesis to give resiliency and to aid in removal via the cervix. **D**, drawing showing prosthesis in position. A unilateral or bilateral resection of the diseased uterine portion of the oviduct is accomplished by incising the fundus transversely and dissecting out the oviduct. The prosthesis is then inserted into the uterine cavity and the oviducts threaded over the limbs of the prosthesis. The tubal flaps are bivalved, then sutured directly to the endometrium—in effect a "mucosa-to-mucosa" anastomosis. The uterine incision is then closed. The prosthesis is left in place for six months and is removed through the cervix with a tenaculum.

azine (Phenergan-Wyeth) in an effort to prevent postoperative adhesions in women undergoing surgery for infertility. There is no doubt that one of the major reasons for failure to accomplish pregnancy following tubo-plasty is the formation or reformation of adhesions with resultant tubo-ovarian malfunction. The rationale for using the combination of dexameth-asone and promethazine is based on the work of Replogle *et al* who showed that these compounds tended to minimize postoperative adhesions in dogs after deliberate abrasion of the bowel. The promethazine presumably acts to block the action of histamine and to enhance vascular integrity at the site of trauma and to minimize the early formation of a fibrinous exudate. The dexamethasone acts to inhibit local fibroblastic proliferation neces-sary for the formation of collagenous connective tissue.

The method utilized was as follows: dexamethasone, 20 mg. and pro-methazine, 25 mg. are given 2 hours prior to surgery and this dose is repeated intraperitoneally through a small catheter introduced into the cul-de-sac. The same amounts are then given intramuscularly at 4-hour intervals for a total of 12 doses.

Horne has reported the results of this method in 219 patients treated by 7 investigators. Ninety-nine (45 per cent) of the patients have become preg-nant and, of these, twenty-five have aborted and four have had ectopic gestations. Eight patients have had revisualization of the pelvis and in only one of these significant adhesions were present. Young and associates reported pregnancy in 32.5 per cent of 114 consecutive infertility laparot-omies at the Boston Hospital for Women during the interval 1961–67. These patients did not receive Decadron-Phenergan. If rugae were noted on the preoperative tubogram, the pregnancy rate was 60.7 per cent; if rugae were absent, only 2.5 per cent of women became pregnant.

THE OVARIAN FACTOR

The major abnormalities concerning the ovary are those involving the process of ovulation and the anatomic and functional changes following endometriosis. Several presumptive clinical methods for the determination of ovulation have already been given (endometrial biopsy, fern test). In addition, the patient may be asked to chart her basal body temperature for a period of three or four months so that some idea of the average point of ovulation and the thermogenic response to the secretion of progesterone may be gained. However, it is useless to indicate *a fertile day* to the patient, and prolonged observation of the basal body temperature probably does more harm than good. This soon becomes a fetish, and what should be an enjoyable communal act becomes stilted as a result of prearrangement. The best advice is to recommend coitus during days 11, 13 and 15 or days 12, 14 and 16 of a 28-day cycle. It is not necessary for the couple to abstain prior to these days in order to increase the sperm count since present evi-dence indicates that, although the count may be increased by this arrange-ment, sperm motility is diminished. Men who have intercourse four or more times weekly have somewhat lower sperm counts on each occasion, but it has been shown that the rate of conception is higher.

Induction of Ovulation.—A major difficulty confronting the clinician in the field of infertility is that of oligo-ovulation or anovulation. Not only is it difficult to evoke release of an ovum from a recalcitrant follicle, but the capricious occurrence of isolated spontaneous ovulation makes evaluation of specific therapeutic measures extremely difficult. Various investigations during the past decade have suggested a lack of specificity of most therapeutic schemes. Thus the effects of estrogens, alone or combined with synthetic progestins, of synthetic progestins alone, and of progesterone alone or preceded by follicle-stimulating-hormone priming have been critically observed and have been found inadequate. However, since lack of the ovulatory process may merely represent deficiencies in other endocrine organs, a systematized investigation is mandatory. An effort should be made to localize the cause as being of pituitary, thyroid, adrenal or ovarian origin.

CLOMIPHENE (CLOMID).—In 1960 Kistner and Smith reported successful induction of ovulation and pregnancies after administration of a nonsteroidal estrogen antagonist, MER-25, in four patients with Stein-Leventhal syndrome. MER-25 and Clomid are closely related compounds and their similarity in structural formulas is illustrated in Figure 9-9.

The clinical uses of clomiphene are based on several biologic actions in the anovulatory patients. If follicular maturation in the ovary is adequate, ovulation occurs as a result of release of increased amounts of follicle-stimulating and luteinizing hormones, the exact ratio of increase being unknown. Progesterone is subsequently secreted by the corpus luteum in amounts large enough to prepare the endometrium for nidation and to maintain the conceptus until chorionic estrogen and progesterone assume this role. In certain instances clomiphene may result in luteinization of cystic follicles, without ovulation, with subsequent secretion

Fig. 9-9.—Structural formulas for MER-25 and clomiphene.

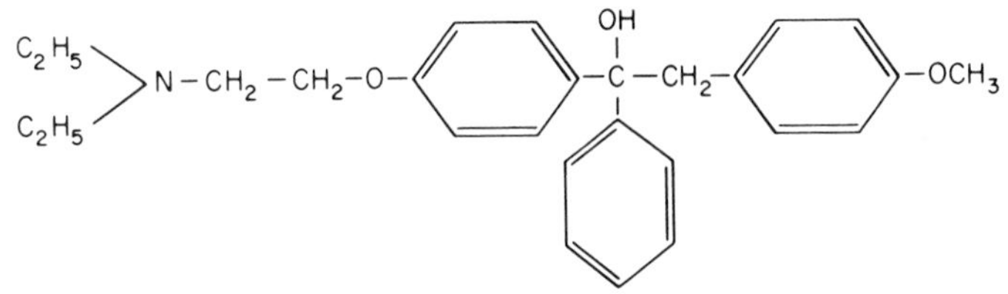

1-(p-2-Diethylaminoethoxy phenyl) -1-phenyl-2-p-anisylethanol

MER-25

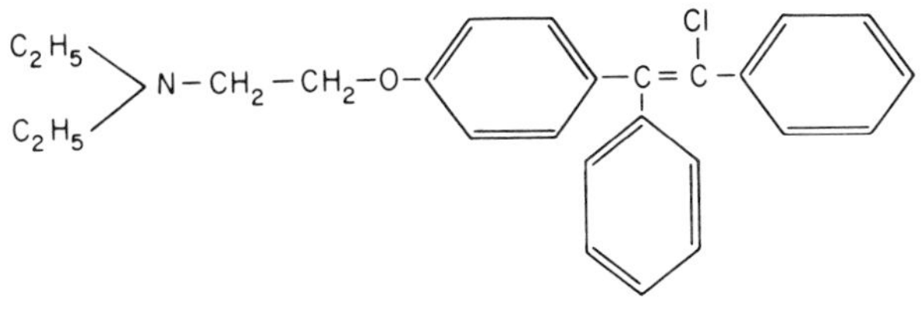

1 - [p-(β -diethylaminoethoxy) phenyl] 1,-2 -diphenyl-2-chloroethylene

Clomiphene

of progesterone from the luteinized cells. This will, of course, produce a sustained rise in the basal body temperature which might be mistaken for ovulation.

Clomiphene is indicated for the anovulatory patient with evidence of follicular function and adequate endogenous estrogen but lacking adequate and cyclic stimulation by pituitary gonadotropic function. The typical patient usually has normal or slightly elevated 17-ketosteroids, normal thyroid function and normal or slightly diminished pituitary gonadotropins. Evidence of adequate endogenous estrogen production by vaginal smear, endometrial biopsy, assay of urinary estrogen, or bleeding in response to progesterone gives a favorable prognosis for treatment. Although a reduced estrogen level affords a less favorably prognosis for subsequent ovulation, it does not always preclude successful therapy. Most patients with sclerocystic ovarian syndrome (Stein-Leventhal syndrome) exhibit an ovulatory response to clomiphene but only about 40 per cent have become pregnant (Fig. 9–10).

The numerous reasons which negate the validity of a direct comparison of results of surgery and clomiphene and instances where neither is advisable are discussed in Chapter 7.

Fig. 9–10.—Basal body temperature records of a 26-year-old patient with a history of three curettages for endometrial hyperplasia. The last endometrial tissue revealed carcinoma in situ and hysterectomy was advised. Ovulatory cycles with normal menses were obtained after the first two clomiphene cycles and the patient became pregnant about 12 days after the third clomiphene treatment.

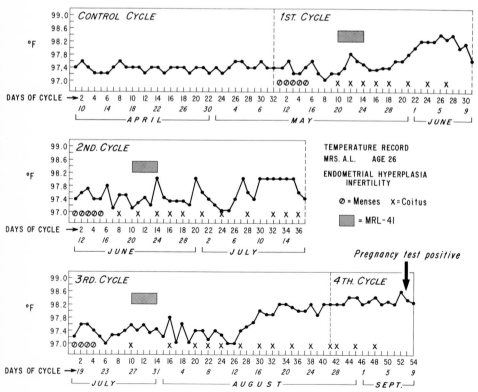

The precise dose of clomiphene citrate cannot be stated since it will depend upon the type of patient being treated and upon the sensitivity of the ovary. The usually recommended dose is 100 mg. daily (two 50 mg. tablets) for five days of the menstrual cycle. In patients with sclerocystic ovarian syndrome we have given 100 mg. for only one or two days. If natural or induced menstrual bleeding has occurred, we have reinitiated therapy on the eighth day of the subsequent cycle. If no response follows the first course of treatment, a second course should be initiated after 30 days. Since prolonged amenorrhea may render the endometrium less responsive, two or more cycles of therapy may be necessary before typical signs of ovulation with menstruation occur. We have recommended that at least six consecutive cycles of therapy be given before it is concluded that the patient is a "clomiphene failure". If there is no response to the usual dosage, we have given prolonged therapy in a dosage regimen of 100 mg. daily for 10 or 12 days. Some ovaries are so resistant that therapy of this length is occasionally necessary. In patients classified as having "hypothalamic amenorrhea" (low total gonadotropins, low estrogen in urine assays, and small, smooth ovaries evidenced by culdoscopy) we have secured ovulation by administering 100 mg. of clomiphene for 10 consecutive days followed by 10,000 International Units (IU) of human chorionic gonadotropin (HCG). The HCG is given in one dose, 4 days after the last dose of clomiphene.

If marked ovarian enlargement is noted with the usual 100 mg. daily for five days, the dose should be reduced during subsequent cycles. In general, we have recommended that the daily dose not exceed 100 mg. per day, that a given treatment course not be continued longer than five days, and that the total dose during a single course of treatment not exceed 500 mg. Slight variations of these cycles of treatment may be necessary in specific patients for hypothalamic amenorrhea and Chiari-Frommel syndrome.

Since the safety of long-term administration of clomiphene has not yet been conclusively demonstrated, this preparation cannot be recommended as "maintenance" therapy for the patient whose ovulatory defect recurs promptly when treatment is discontinued. Although we originally recommended estrogen-priming in patients whose endometrial biopsies were classified as atrophic, we no longer feel that this is a necessary part of treatment. We do feel, however, that the patient should not attempt to get pregnant during the first treatment cycle, since the incidence of abortion is increased, particularly if prolonged amenorrhea has existed. Careful pelvic examination should be performed before each course of clomiphene therapy, particular attention being paid to the size of the ovaries. Clomiphene should not be given if there is an ovarian cyst, but this contraindication does not apply to the moderate bilateral ovarian enlargement that occurs in patients with sclerocystic ovarian syndrome. However, as recommended above, the dose should be diminished in patients with this syndrome, particularly if moderate enlargement is noted following the initial course of therapy.

Ovulation may be expected to occur in approximately 70 per cent of women with secondary amenorrhea. The diagnosis of apparent ovulation is based on the finding of menstrual or secretory endometrium by biopsy, by basal body temperature graphs, or by increase in the assay of pregnanediol in urine.

Some patients respond regularly to each course of clomiphene therapy; others respond to some but not all courses of treatment. It should be pointed out that patients with severe panhypopituitarism (Sheehan's syndrome) have not responded even though other hormonal deficiencies have been completely corrected. Patients with complete ovarian insufficiency, such as ovarian dysgenesis (Turner's syndrome) or premature menopause, have not responded to clomiphene. About 50 per cent of patients with Chiari-Frommel syndrome have apparently ovulated and pregnancy has occurred in almost half of these.

Pregnancy has been reported in approximately 40 per cent of women who ovulate subsequent to the use of clomiphene. But this proportion is not a reflection of clomiphene failure since 10 per cent of women treated were single and other married patients were not immediately desirous of pregnancy. Furthermore, many patients were treated for only one or two cycles and in others tubal factors or male insufficiency predisposed to the infertility status.

There is an increased incidence of multiple pregnancy in patients conceiving immediately following clomiphene therapy, 1 in every 16. (The incidence of twins in the general population is 1 in 80.) The increased incidence of multiple pregnancy is undoubtedly due to fraternal twinning consistent with observation of superovulation after clomiphene therapy. The incidence of spontaneous abortion is not increased in pregnancies occurring after clomiphene if conception is avoided in the first treatment cycle.

The most striking side effect of clomiphene is ovarian enlargement due to the enlargement of cystic follicles, cystic corpora lutea, or other physiologic cystic structures. Such cystic enlargement is perhaps, the most convincing evidence that clomiphene is capable of stimulating ovarian secretory activity in the human female. Microscopic study of ovarian cysts and the associated endometrium has indicated that these structures are indeed of functional nature.

Experience has shown that these physiologic cysts regress spontaneously within 7 to 28 days following cessation of therapy. They should always be managed conservatively unless there is a specific indication for surgical intervention. Clomiphene therapy should be initiated subsequently only after the ovaries have returned to pretreatment size. If marked enlargement occurs during any course of therapy, the dose or duration of the subsequent course should be reduced. Careful pelvic examination should be performed before each course of clomiphene therapy, particular attention being given to the size and consistency of the ovaries. *Clomiphene should never be given in the presence of an ovarian cyst.*

Before initiating therapy with clomiphene, we have insisted upon a two-day admission to the hospital for certain endocrinological studies and culdoscopy. During this time assays of 17-ketosteroids, 17-ketogenic steroids, follicle-stimulating hormone, protein-bound iodine, T_3 and T_4 and x-ray of the sella turcica are performed. On the following day culdoscopy and uterine curettage are accomplished. In addition, vaginal cytology may be taken at the same time for determination of estrogen effect. A thorough evaluation of this type will materially reduce the incidence of patients who fail to respond to clomiphene. If the response, as measured by the basal body temperature or endometrial biopsy, is unfavorable, the various parameters previously evaluated must be rechecked. The patient may be amenorrheic because of premature menopause, and it is important that a repeat determination of total gonadotropins be obtained. Culdoscopy will permit making a diagnosis of ovarian agenesis and this may be aided by determination of nuclear sex as part of the original study. Every patient with primary amenorrhea should have a nuclear sex determination as well as an x-ray of the sella turcica and visual-field studies. Patients with secondary amenorrhea should be questioned carefully regarding the presence of headaches or visual abnormalities in order that a pituitary or extrasellar tumor will not be missed.

In patients having low levels of gonadotropins, both FSH and LH, low levels of estrogen, small ovaries by culdoscopy and atrophic endometrium, ovulation may be obtained by the administration of Clomid in a dose of 100 mg. daily for 10 days followed four days later by a single injection of 10,000 I.U. of chorionic gonadotropin. (See Fig. 9–11.)

Clomiphene is apparently more effective as a follicle-stimulating hormone than a luteinizing releasing hormone in such patients since it will not uniformly induce ovulation after follicular development has been produced with human menopausal gonadotropin HMG (Pergonal). Clomiphene acts in a similar fashion to HMG in effecting development of the follicle but the precise LH action of sequential HCG is necessary to rupture the mature follicle.

In order for clomiphene and HCG to be effective, a responsive pituitary and ovary must be present. Human pituitary FSH and HMG plus HCG will result in ovulation if total gonadotropins are absent (after hypophysectomy, e.g.) or are extremely low. In either case, however, the ovary must be capable of follicular development, maturation, and ovum release.

HUMAN MENOPAUSAL GONADOTROPIN.—In 1958 a new era in therapy for the infertile female was initiated by Gemzell in Sweden when he described the use of follicle stimulating hormone derived from human pituitary glands. When this substance was followed in sequence with human chorionic gonadotropin, basically luteotrophic in action, ovulation was induced in a large percentage of infertile and amenorrheic women. However, the supply of this substance is limited and therefore search for another source was begun. Lunenfeld, in Israel, and Rosemberg, in the United States, succeeded in isolating gonadotropic substances from the urine of postmenopausal females which, when followed sequentially with human chorionic gonadotropin, was capable of inducing ovulation.

At the present time there are two preparations of menopausal gonadotropins available for clinical investigation, Pergonal HMG* and Ortho HMG.** Pergonal has recently been approved by the Federal Food and Drug Administration for general use.

The FSH content of Pergonal has varied from 76 to 103 IU per ampule. At the present time each ampule contains 75 IU of FSH and 75 IU of LH plus 10 mg. lactose in the lyophilized form.

Infertility due to lack of ovulation is the chief indication for therapy with human menopausal gonadotropin. Patients having persistently low or

---

*Cutter Laboratories
**Ortho Research Foundation

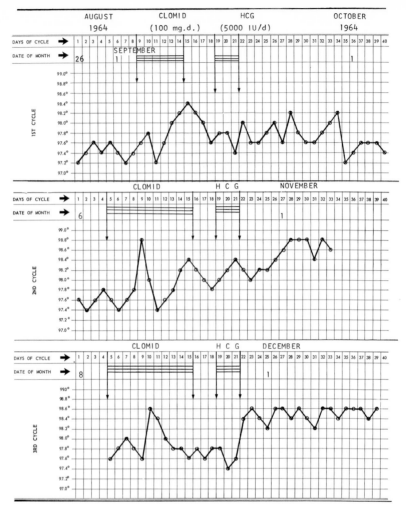

Fig. 9-11.—Basal body temperature graph of a 28-year-old female with secondary amenorrhea. The patient had been treated in 1963 with Clomid after a period of secondary amenorrhea lasting 4 years. Ovulation and pregnancy followed. However, following delivery, the patient again became amenorrheic, but did not respond to Clomid therapy. After 6 unsuccessful cycles with Clomid alone, sequential Clomid-HCG therapy was started. As noted above, ovulation and menstruation did not occur after 5 days of Clomid-HCG, but did after the length of Clomid administration was increased to 10 days. Normal menses ensued after both treatment sequences as shown.

absent gonadotropins may be treated if pituitary or hypothalamic tumors and cysts have been ruled out. Patients demonstrating primary gonadotropin insufficiency, hypothalamic amenorrhea, Sheehan's syndrome or an arrested pituitary tumor or cyst usually respond promptly to HMG-HCG therapy.

The etiologic factors causing many cases of secondary amenorrhea with normal gonadotropin levels remain obscure, yet ultimately many of these may respond to gonadotropin administration. All patients with normal gonadotropin levels should be given at least 6 courses of Clomid therapy before resorting to menopausal gonadotropin treatment. Certain patients who fail to ovulate with Clomid alone may do so with Clomid-HCG sequential therapy. (See Fig. 9–11.)

Patients with persistent anovulatory cycles who fail to respond to clomiphene or clomiphene-HCG will usually respond to gonadotropins if the ovary has not been depleted of follicles. Patients with marked elevation of endogenous gonadotropins will not respond to exogenous gonadotropins.

The combination of FSH and LH in menopausal gonadotropin stimulates the development of ovarian follicles and the subsequent secretion of estrogen. A direct chemical measurement of estrogen is the most accurate assessment of follicular activity. Following the administration of Pergonal, total estrogen levels have been noted to rise as high as 1,000 μg. per 24 hours. (normal 20–60 μg.). This marked rise undoubtedly represents follicular overstimulation. Elevated estrogen levels have been correlated with multiple pregnancies and with the occurrence of ovarian enlargement and ascites. It is important, therefore, to determine the extent of follicular activity in order to prevent excessive ovarian stimulation. The usual assay methods for estrogens in urine are complicated, time consuming and are not practical.

Most physicians rely on other evidences of follicular activity such as vaginal cytology or ferning of cervical mucus. In our clinic we have not found vaginal cytology to be more reliable than the fern test as an index of estrogen secretion and therefore prefer the latter test.

Before treatment with Pergonal is instituted, a thorough gynecologic and endocrinologic evaluation must be performed. This should include a hysterosalpingogram or culdoscopy and tubal lavage to exclude uterine and tubal pathology and documentation of anovulation by means of basal body temperature, serial vaginal smears, examination of cervical mucus, determination of urinary pregnanediol and endometrial biopsy. Evaluation of the husband's seminal fluid should be completed prior to Pergonal therapy. Primary ovarian failure should be excluded by the determination of urinary gonadotropin or a test dose of Pergonal. Careful examination should be made to rule out the presence of an early pregnancy. Since patients in late reproductive life have a greater predilection to endometrial carcinoma as well as a high incidence of anovulatory disorders, uterine curettage should always be done before starting Pergonal therapy. Finally, clomiphene citrate alone or followed by HCG should have been tried if the diagnosis indicates a possibility of response to these agents.

Dosage and Administration.—The dose of Pergonal to produce maturation of the follicle must be individualized for each patient. It is recommended that the initial dose should be 75 IU (one ampule) per day, administered intramuscularly for nine to twelve days followed by HCG, 10,000 IU one day after the last dose of Pergonal. The hyperstimulation syndrome has not occurred with administration of 75 IU per day for up to twelve days. Administration of Pergonal should be continued for at least nine days and should not exceed twelve days. If the ovaries are palpably enlarged on the last day of Pergonal therapy, HCG should *not* be administered. If there is evidence of ovulation but if pregnancy does not occur, this regimen should be repeated for at least two more courses before increasing the dose to 150 IU per day for nine to twelve days. Again, this higher dose should be followed by 10,000 IU of

HCG one day after the last dose of Pergonal. If evidence of ovulation occurs but pregnancy does not ensue, the same dose should be repeated for two more courses. Most pregnancies have occurred with 150 IU of Pergonal. Larger doses are not recommended.

During short course treatment with both Pergonal and HCG and during a two-week post-treatment period, patients should be examined at least every other day for signs of excessive ovarian stimulation. It is recommended that Pergonal administration be stopped if the ovaries become significantly enlarged or abdominal pain occurs. Ovarian hyperstimulation occurs after treatment has been discontinued and reaches its maximum at about 7–10 days postovulation. Patients should be followed for at least two weeks after HCG administration.

The couple should be encouraged to have intercourse daily, beginning on the day prior to the administration of HCG until ovulation becomes apparent from the usual indices. Care should be taken to insure insemination.

The contraindications for the use of Pergonal-HCG are:

1. A high level of endogenous gonadotropin indicating primary ovarian failure.

2. The presence of overt thyroid and adrenal dysfunction.

3. An organic intracranial lesion such as a pituitary tumor.

4. The presence of any cause of infertility other than anovulation.

5. In patients with abnormal bleeding of undetermined origin.

Pergonal is a potent gonadotropic substance capable of causing mild to severe adverse reactions. It must be used with caution.

Pergonal does not appear to influence the incidence of abortion in the subfertile individual. The abortion rate for the subfertile individual is reported to be approximately 20 per cent in patients with primary infertility and 30 per cent in secondary infertility. The abortion rate following Pergonal-HCG therapy has been 25 per cent.

Multiple births occur frequently following treatment with Pergonal-HCG, the incidence being approximately 20 per cent; four out of five multiple pregnancies being twins.

Taymor reached the following conclusions after extensive and detailed studies:

1. Human menopausal gonadotropin combined with or followed by human chorionic gonadotropin provides a potent method of ovulation stimulation.

2. This combination can be used as primary therapy in amenorrheic patients with absent gonadotropins. In patients with secondary amenorrhea associated with low or normal gonadotropin levels or with anovulatory cycles, its use should be postponed until other therapeutic measures have proven unsuccessful (e.g., clomiphene).

3. Each patient responds individually and close observation is mandatory. Patients who have secondary amenorrhea associated with normal gonadotropins as well as those with sclerocystic ovarian syndrome appear more sensitive. Thorough pretreatment work-up is necessary to avoid specific and known complications.

4. Therapy should be initiated with less than the maximum dose of HMG. A step-down pattern that continues 1 or 2 days after the first day of 3+ ferning should be utilized initially. Even this amount should be reduced if ovarian enlargement occurs.

5. The amount and duration of administration of HMG may be increased slowly in subsequent cycles.

6. HCG may be administered as 8–12,000 units in a single dose.

7. A pregnancy rate of 50 per cent within the first 2 treatment cycles may be expected to occur if no other causes for infertility exist.

8. Close adherence to precautionary measures will enable the physician to secure a reasonable conception rate in patients for whom no satisfactory treatment previously existed. Furthermore, most severe adverse reactions or multiple pregnancies beyond twins will be avoided. Undoubtedly complications will occur but they will be less frequent if slight under-treatment is utilized during the initial cycle.

Recently Cutter Laboratories has suggested that irregularly menstruating infertile women may be treated by giving 150 to 225 IU (2 to 3 ampules) of HMG on days 7, 8 and 9 followed by a single injection of 10,000 IU of HCG on day 11.

WEDGE RESECTION.—The Stein-Leventhal syndrome has been widely publicized as a specific ovarian defect associated with anovulation. Since ovarian cortical fibrosis and follicular cysts were described when biopsies of the ovary were obtained, it was assumed that ova were trapped by the pre-existing unyielding cortex and, under the persistent stimulation of adenohypophyseal hormones (perhaps luteinizing hormone), cystic luteinized follicles developed. Wedge resection of the ovaries resulted in subsequent ovulation and in pregnancy in a large percentage of patients. It has been impossible, however, for most pathologists to distinguish this "idiopathic cortical fibrosis" from that associated with adrenogenital syndrome or pituitary failure. Thus, if wedge resection does not result in subsequent ovulation, one may assume that the primary cause is not ovarian. Some doubt now exists as to whether the disease is ever of primary ovarian origin; but if it is, the problem is concerned more with an abnormal biosynthesis of estrogens by the ovary and less with the mechanical barrier of the cortex.

Aspiration of fluid from the cystic follicles of the Stein-Leventhal ovary (with the possible removal of large amounts of androstenedione) is said to have produced results as good as removal of large wedges from the ovary. Recent investigations by Dorfman and associates have shown an elevation of free testosterone in blood plasma in hirsute females with Stein-Leventhal disease and a return to normal after "generous" wedge resection of the ovaries. Ovulation subsequent to surgery is presumably due to a diminution in androgen and estrogen formation by the ovary and restoration of normal pituitary gonadotropin function.

Both the in vivo and in vitro studies reported to date provide unequivocal evidence of steroidal deviations in the Stein-Leventhal syndrome. No uniformly acceptable explanation has yet been advanced to account for these findings. As long as inadequate data prevent a solution to the enigma, the working hypotheses should be considered for what they are—theories to provide a basis for discussion and to stimulate further useful work. Among current hypotheses related to biochemical disturbances are: (1) impairment of ovarian enzymes resulting in alterations of steroid synthesis; (2) increased ovarian steroid output because of multiple active follicles; (3) mild adrenocortical disorders; (4) interglandular modulation of steroid synthesis between ovary and adrenal cortex; (5) alterations—either absolute or relative—in gonadotropin secretion; and (6) alterations in hypothalamic function.

Thus the delineation of a syndrome, together with the report of good results following wedge resection of ovaries, made sclerocystic ovarian disease a happy hunting ground for theorists, whose field of speculation was not encumbered by too many facts, and for surgeons, who were understandably delighted with a functional disorder that was amenable to such a simple and straightforward approach.

Little of significance occurred to alter this situation until the last decade, when a critical review by Goldzieher and his associates brought the disease into clear perspective–at least to those gynecologists who were not blinded by the reflected luminescence surrounding the surgical approach. In 1964 Goldzieher and Green reviewed all published cases of polycystic disease and found the following frequencies for the accepted clinical parameters: Amenorrhea was present in only about 50 per cent of the cases, sterility in 74 per cent, hirsutism in 69 per cent and obesity in only 41 per cent. These findings show that the key signs and symptoms are not found with sufficient consistency to justify the designation of a syndrome. Others have voiced similar conclusions: Netter and his associates in true Gallic style remarked that "the syndrome of Stein is a fugitive syndrome with limits less well defined than those of the Sahara or the Sudan"; in England similar sentiments were expressed in a paper, "Is There A Stein Syndrome?"

The pathophysiology and abnormal steroid patterns of sclerocystic ovarian syndrome are discussed in Chapter 7–The Ovary.

There is no doubt that wedge resection of the ovaries, in properly selected cases, results in a normal ovulatory process and pregnancy. Since the advent of clomiphene the number of patients needing this surgical procedure has markedly diminished. But there remain a few patients, possibly those whose ovaries have been subjected to abnormal gonadotropin stimulation for longer periods of time, who apparently ovulate after clomiphene but in whom pregnancy does not occur. Leventhal has suggested that "intra-ovarian" ovulation occurs in these patients and that ovum release from the thickened capsule is impossible. I have noted this in a few patients who apparently responded to clomiphene but in whom pregnancy did not occur after six or seven consecutive cycles of therapy. Subsequent wedge resection apparently was responsible for pregnancy. But I have seen many more patients of an opposite sequence, that is, failure to ovulate after wedge resection but early ovulation and pregnancy subsequent to clomiphene. In the latter group, however, it is impossible to say that this same result might not have occurred after clomiphene alone.

How does wedge resection work? Goldzieher suggests that the surgical procedure inflicts severe trauma on the ovary and that there follows a transient but drastic reduction in ovarian hormone output, both androgens and estrogens. The vicious cycle of constant positive estrogen feedback is eliminated, at least temporarily. The demand for constant gonadotropin release is removed and a process of pituitary regrouping and reorganization is permitted. Gonadotropins accumulate, exhausted ovarian enzymes are reconstituted, the hypothalamic cyclic center resumes its normal rhythm and cyclic menstrual activity follows.

But, unfortunately, the fact remains that fertility is corrected less often than the menstrual irregularity. This may be due to complications of the surgical procedure itself with production of peritubal and periovarian adhesions or to extensive capsular fibrosis. It is interesting to note the widely divergent results of wedge resection reported by different authors. The average rate of ovulation following wedge resection is high; approximately 82 per cent of patients will regain restoration of menstrual regularity and 63 per cent will attain pregnancy. But in reviewing all series, Goldzieher found that apparent ovulation varied from 6 per cent to 95 per cent and the incidence of pregnancy varied between 13 per cent and 89 per cent. This wide discrepancy must be meaningful.

If wedge resection is performed and ovulation is not forthcoming, the patient's ability to become pregnant subsequently is seriously diminished. These patients should have a complete endocrine evaluation, or re-evaluation if this was performed prior to surgery, combined with culdoscopy or laparoscopy and lavage of the oviducts. Certainly a wedge resection should never be done without prior evaluation of tubal patency since the ultimate goal of ovulatory success is pregnancy. If uterotubograms have not been done prior to surgery, the oviducts should be lavaged by the transuterine method at the time of wedge resection. I do not agree that wedge resection should be done in young, unmarried females to correct irregular bleeding, endometrial hyperplasia and hypertrichosis. Each of these entities may be successfully corrected or at least improved by the cyclic administration of estrogen-progestin combinations. Nor do I agree that the use of estrogen-progestin compounds will make it "more difficult or impossible" for these patients to ovulate after they have been discontinued. Such criticism evades the fact that these females are already in "ovulatory trouble." Quite the reverse seems to be true. I have treated numerous unmarried women for these undesired symptoms associated with, or due to, the sclerocystic ovary by administering estrogen-progestins for as long as two years. The administration of clomiphene immediately following cessation of treatment has been just as successful in inducing ovulation and pregnancy as in women whose ovaries had not been suppressed.

It is difficult to outline the precise indications for performing wedge resection. A rule of thumb is to try the simplest treatment first. The patient who is not desirous of pregnancy is treated by estrogen-progestin suppression. When pregnancy is desired, clomiphene citrate is given for at least six consecutive cycles. But I have had two patients who needed 9 cycles of therapy to accomplish pregnancy and Mishell has reported one patient who required twelve cycles of therapy. If the 17-ketosteroid assay is elevated, hydrocortisone or one of its derivatives is given. A few patients will ovulate and become pregnant only if hydrocortisone and clomiphene are given simultaneously. Others may need an injection of HCG subsequent to clomiphene–apparently clomiphene is capable of maturing one or more follicles in these patients but follicular rupture is effected only by the burst of LH activity brought about by HCG. I now perform wedge resection on patients who "apparently" ovulate following the use of the above regimens but in whom pregnancy does not occur. I think these patients are better treated by wedge resection than by prolonged (over 12 cycles) administration of clomiphene. In some of these patients ovarian enlargement and cortical thickening may progress during such therapy and the ovary may become more recalcitrant if hormonal treatment continues. One might say that prolonged medical management in such patients is more radical than wedge resection. I would caution, however, that wedge resection is of no value in patients in whom ovulation cannot be induced by clomiphene, clomiphene-HCG, or HMG-HCG. These patients have ovarian failure and surgical procedures are worthless.

Many of the time-worn criteria for wedge resection need to be re-evaluated. In the original paper by Stein and Leventhal the size of the ovary was emphasized as being an important criterion for selection. Gynecography was performed to demonstrate the marked bilateral enlargement deemed necessary to effect an ovulatory response. But Epstein and co-workers reported the induction of ovulatory menses in 74 per cent of patients who had normal size ovaries and who were otherwise endocrinologically normal except for their anovulatory status. Pregnancy occurred in 8 of these 14 patients. Numerous other investigators found no relationship between the response to surgery and the size of the ovaries, the 17-ketosteroid assays, or any other laboratory determination.

ENDOMETRIOSIS

Endometriosis has been definitely correlated with infertility, and it has been estimated that the expectation of pregnancy in this disease is about half that of the general population. Thus, with a natural incidence of infertility approximating 15 per cent, it is safe to say that in the presence of endometriosis the sterility incidence approaches 30-40 per cent. If the studies of the patient show that ovulation is occurring regularly, that the oviducts are patent, the endometrium normal and the postcoital test adequate, the presence of endometriosis should be considered. Diagnosis may be suggested by the history, corroborated by the pelvic examination and verified by culdoscopy, biopsy or laparoscopy. Treatment may be varied, utilizing analgesics and expectation, operation, hormones or combinations of these (see Chapter 8).

If childbearing function is to be preserved, operative procedures should be as conservative as possible. The optimum treatment for endometriosis is pregnancy. I have suggested the use of a pseudopregnancy in the infertile patient, utilizing increasing doses of estrogen and progestins for six to nine months. A decidual reaction is produced in the areas of endometriosis; these areas subsequently undergo degeneration and necrosis. Much of the endometriotic tissue may be absorbed so that subsequent fertility is improved. Therapeutic regimens are outlined in Chapter 8.

ADRENAL FACTORS

Certain disorders of the adrenal may lead to oligo-ovulation, anovulation, amenorrhea and infertility. Adrenal insufficiency, however, does not interfere with menstrual function. The most common type of disorder, congenital adrenogenital syndrome, is discussed in Chapter 12–Endocrine Disorders. Hyperfunction of the adrenal cortex associated with either Cushing's syndrome or adrenogenital syndrome, may produce irregular menses and infertility. Cushing's syndrome is characterized by an over-production of glucocorticoids and may be due to either bilateral adrenal hyperplasia, adenoma of the adrenal gland, adrenal carcinoma or a non-adrenal tumor. Cushing's syndrome is also discussed in Chapter 12.

But there are many patients who have an intermediate degree of adrenal abnormality who have neither Cushing's syndrome, a virilizing adrenal tumor, nor adrenogenital syndrome. They are neither virilized nor obese. As a matter of fact, they appear to be normal individuals. Some patients may have a variant of the Stein-Leventhal syndrome; others may have slight degrees of adrenal hyperplasia. But they are infertile and the infertility is usually due to irregular, or totally absent, ovulation. The endocrine survey reveals only two abnormalities: (1) a slight elevation in the 17-ketosteroids in the range of 15 to 30 mg., (2) a deficiency in the mid-cycle burst of LH. The precise mechanism by which the hypothalamus fails to elaborate LH releasing factor is unknown, but the disturbed physiological mechanism is corrected by the administration of hydrocortisone in a dose of 10 mg. three times daily. If the patient subsequently ovulates and becomes pregnant it is important that the hydrocortisone be continued until fetal organ development is complete. A recurrence of the elevated androgen levels could produce masculinization of the external genitalia of a female fetus.

The diagnosis of this "gray-zone" adrenal hyperactivity may be aided by testing with metyrapone, an 11-β-hydroxylase inhibitor, since this compound causes an excessive increase in 17-ketosteroids and pregnanetriol in urinary assays of patients with this disorder. A similar variation has been described in a few patients who noted irregular menses, slight virilization and infertility. Although the 17-hydroxysteroids and 17-ketosteroids are elevated, the patients do not have Cushing's syndrome. Chromatographic fractionation of the 17-hydroxysteroids showed that the elevation is due to desoxycortisol. This finding led to the diagnosis of an 11-β-hydroxylase deficiency producing this type of the adrenogenital syndrome.

THYROID FACTORS

Thyroid hormone has a narrow but specific application in the management of anovulation and subsequent infertility. Overt hypothyroidism may cause lack of ovulation and amenorrhea in the female and inadequate spermatogenesis in the male. Untreated thyrotoxicosis is associated with excessive fetal loss. These facts are well documented and therapy is available to restore normality to these processes. But the "thyroid myth" persists, perhaps because it was the first hormone to be used in the treatment of irregular menses and infertility. Because of its seniority, therefore, clinicians have been loathe to discard this old endocrinologic friend and I suppose that the indiscriminate use of thyroid extract won't die–it will just fade away.

Testimonials for the efficacy of thyroid extract in the management of every phase of reproductive behavior are quite easy to obtain–mostly on the basis of uncritical clinical experience, not from carefully controlled and properly designed experiments. Its magic has been extolled for the stimulation of sexual activity, improvement of fertility, prevention of habitual abortion and the reduction of pregnancy complications.

Both hypothyroidism and thyrotoxicosis may be associated with abnormalities in sexual interest and activity. In myxedema diminished sex interest and impotence have been noted. Undoubtedly this is related to the effect of thyroid dysfunction on the secretion, metabolism and end-organ responsiveness of gonadal steroids. But this should be evaluated in the light of the old cliche that 10 per cent of libido is derived from structures below the level of the sella turcica and 90 per cent arises above this area. Despite the extensive derangement in ovarian steroidal patterns in myxedema, the diminished sexual activity is probably more often due to lack of vigor, tiredness and apathy. A factor of more importance may be the complete disinterest of the husband, an expected result of the physical unattractiveness of his mate.

Sexual activity is altered more profoundly in thyrotoxicosis than in myxedema and while increased libido has been reported in this disease, the extreme degree of mental and physical exhaustion frequently causes complete sexual disinterest. From the therapeutic aspect, the clinician may assure the patient that those abnormalities in sexual behavior which are due to thyroid dysfunction will be corrected when a euthyroid state is effected. But those disturbances in sexual patterns which are brought about by emotional conflict will remain and will necessitate specific treatment.

Thyroid deficiency may be classified into three distinct syndromes: (1) myxedema, (2) hypothyroidism and, (3) pituitary myxedema. Impaired ovulation, irregular menstruation and infertility are frequently associated with both myxedema and hypothyroidism. In pituitary myxedema the absence of other trophic hormones regulating the adrenal and ovary accounts for total amenorrhea and infertility. The establishment and continuation of pregnancy in the myxedematous patient are rare and the reasons for the infertility are quite obvious. Only seventeen documented cases of pregnancy in myxedema have been reported, one woman bearing 6 children during 15 years. In mildly hypothyroid patients, however, the anovulatory process is frequently interrupted by spontaneous ovulation and an occasional pregnancy. Present evidence suggests that in myxedema there is adequate formation and secretion of FSH but diminished or ineffective LH. Most of these studies have utilized bio-assay methods and when these patients are re-studied using radioimmunoassay for gonadotropins, the basic inadequacy may be just the burst of LH needed at midcycle.

Hamolsky has summarized interrelationship as follows:

1. Thyroid hormone has a direct action upon gonadal function, either
   a. on specific biochemical mechanisms within the ovary or testis
   b. via a fundamental energy-controlling process in all tissues, or
   c. by indirect modulation of gonadal sensitivity to FSH, LH, LTH or prolactin.

2. Thyroid exercises an indirect effect on the gonads via a stimulatory or inhibitory effect on hypothalamic releasing factors.

3. Thyroid has an indirect effect on gonadal function by way of alterations produced in the adrenals.

4. The gonads have a primary role in determining thyroid function.

Feldman has explained the conflicting reports that (1) ovarian hormones depress thyroid function, (2) ovarian hormones increase thyroid activity, and (3) estrogens can both stimulate and depress thyroid function. Apparently estrogen has all of these functions, the ultimate effect depending on the dose of estrogen and its length of administration.

The controversial aspect of the thyroid problem, as it relates to infertility, centers on the diagnosis and treatment of an entity which may or may not exist. The syndrome is known as "subclinical hypothyroidism" and the diagnosis implies a mild but measurable degree of thyroid insufficiency which even protagonists are unable to demonstrate by objective criteria. If a patient is infertile or has irregular menses and all parameters of thyroid are normal, the clinician may still give a "small amount of thyroid" and even a "small amount of estrogen." Should pregnancy ensue, the conclusion is obvious. The patient had "subclinical hypothyroidism" and even "subclinical hypoestrinism." Such concepts persist and no amount of logical or scientific information will change them. Needless to say, I do not advise treatment of the euthyroid patient by small, large or intermediate doses of thyroid.

Therapy for thyroid dysfunction will be discussed in Chapter 10– Habitual Abortion. It should be remembered, however, that the normally functioning thyroid gland secretes daily the calorigenic equivalent of about 120 to 180 mg. of a potent preparation of desiccated thyroid. Therefore, in the absence of significant endogenous thyroid secretions, this is the usual maintenance dose. If this dosage does not correct fully all the signs and symptoms attributable to thyroid insufficiency, other causes of the symptoms should be sought. In patients with pituitary myxedema, it is imperative that the adrenal insufficiency be corrected before beginning thyroid extract. Not to do so might precipitate fatal adrenal insufficiency.

BIBLIOGRAPHY

Infertility

Behrman, S. J., et al.: ABO (H) blood incompatibility as a cause of infertility, Am. J. Obst. & Gynec. 79:847, 1960.

Bergman, P.: Treatment of sterility of intrauterine origin, Clin. Obst. & Gynec. 2:852, 1959.

Buxton, C. L., and Herrman, W.: Induction of ovulation in the human with human gonadotropins, Am. J. Obst. & Gynec. 81:584, 1961.

———, and Mastroianni, L.: Evaluation of tubal function, Fertil. & Steril. 8:561, 1957.

———, and Southam, A. L.: Human Infertility (New York: Paul B. Hoeber, Inc., 1958).

———; Kase, N., and Van Orden, D.: Effect of human FSH and HCG on the anovulatory ovary, Am. J. Obst. & Gynec. 87:773, 1963.

Charny, C. W., and Wolgin, W.: Cryptorchism (New York: Paul B. Hoeber, Inc., 1957), pp. 78, 124.

Getzoff, P. L.: Principles of management of the infertile male, Clin. Obst. & Gynec. 2:752, 1959.

Grant, A.: Evaluation of the tubal factor in infertility, Clin. Obst. & Gynec. 2:777, 1959.

———: The Fred A. Simmons memorial address: Experience, experiment and error in sterility, Fertil. & Steril. 11:1, 1960.

Greenblatt, R. B., et al.: Induction of ovulation with MRL-41, J.A.M.A. 178:101, 1961.

Hamolsky, M.: Thyroid Factors, in Behrman, S. J., and Kistner, R. W. (eds.): Progress in Infertility (Boston: Little, Brown & Company, 1968).

Jefferies, W. M.: Further experience with small doses of cortisone and related steroids in infertility associated with ovarian dysfunction, Fertil. & Steril. 11:100, 1960.

Jones, H. L., Jr., and Baramki, T. A.: Congenital Anomalies, in Behrman, S. J., and Kistner, R. W. (eds.): Progress in Infertility (Boston: Little Brown & Company, 1968).

Kelly, J. V., and Rock, J.: Culdoscopy for diagnosis in infertility, Am. J. Obst. & Gynec. 72:523, 1956.

Kistner, R. W.: Endometriosis and infertility, Clin. Obst. & Gynec. 2:877, 1959.

———: Infertility with endometriosis: A plan of therapy, Fertil. & Steril. 13:237, 1962.

———, and Smith, O. W.: Observations on the use of a non-steroidal estrogen antagonist: MER-25, S. Forum 10:725, 1959; Fertil. & Steril. 12:121, 1961.

Kupperman, H. S.: Treatment of endocrine causes of sterility in the female, Clin. Obst. & Gynec. 2:808, 1959.

McElin, T. W.; Danforth, D. N., and Young, I. J.: Study of infertility in the private practice of obstetrics and gynecology, Fertil. & Steril. 11:135, 1960.

MacLeod, J., and Gold, R. Z.: The male factor in fertility and infertility: VIII. A study of variation in semen quality, Fertil. & Steril. 7:387, 1956.

———, and Gold, R. Z.: An analysis of human male infertility, Internat. J. Fertil. 3:382, 1958.

Marcus, C. C., and Marcus, S. L.: The Cervical Factor, in Behrman, S. J., and Kistner, R. W. (eds.): Progress in Infertility (Boston: Little Brown & Company, 1968).

Moore-White, M.: Evaluation of tubal plastic operations, Internat. J. Fertil. 5:237, 1960.

Moyer, D. L.: Endometrial Diseases in Infertility, in Behrman, S. J., and Kistner, R. W. (eds): *Progress in Infertility* (Boston: Little Brown & Company, 1968).

Noyes, R. W.: Uniformity of secretory endometrium, Fertil, & Steril. 7:103, 1956.

———, Hertig, A. T., and Rock, J.: Dating the endometrial biopsy, Fertil. & Steril. 1:3, 1950.

O'Brien, J. R., and Arronet, G. H.: Operative treatment of fallopian tube pathology in human infertility, Am. J. Obst. & Gynec. 103:520, 1969.

Raymont, A.; Aronnet, G. H., and Arrata, W. S. M.: Review of 500 cases of infertility, Internat. J. Fertil. 14:141, 1969.

Riva, H. L.; Hatch, R. B., and Breen, J. L.: Culdoscopy for infertility: An analysis of 203 cases, Am. J. Obst. & Gynec. 78:1304, 1959.

Rubin, I. C., *Uterotubal Insufflation* (St. Louis: C. V. Mosby Company, 1947).

Schneeberg, N. G.: The thyroid gland and infertility, Clin. Obst. & Gynec. 2:826, 1959.

Siegler, A. M., and Hellman, L. M.: Tubal plastic surgery: Report of a survey, Fertil. & Steril. 7:170, 1956.

Southam, A. L.: Evaluation of cervical factors in infertility, Clin. Obst. & Gynec. 2:763, 1959.

———: What to do with the "normal" infertile couple, Fertil. & Steril. 11:543, 1960.

———, and Buxton, L.: Seventy postcoital tests made during the conception cycle, Fertil. & Steril. 7:133, 1956.

Stein, I. F.: The management of bilateral polycystic ovaries, Fertil. & Steril. 6:190, 1948.

———, and Leventhal, M. L.: Amenorrhea associated with bilateral polycystic ovaries, Am. J. Obst. & Gynec. 29:18, 1935.

Sweeney, W. J.: Pitfalls in present day methods of evaluating tubal function: I. Tubal insufflation, Fertil. & Steril. 13:113, 1962.

———: Pitfalls in present day methods of evaluating tubal function: II. Hysterosalpingography, Fertil. & Steril. 13:124, 1962.

Tyler, E. T.: The thyroid myth in infertility, Fertil. & Steril. 4:218, 1953.

———: *Sterility: Office Management of the Infertile Couple* (New York: McGraw-Hill Book Company, Inc., 1961).

Tubal Reconstruction

Garcia, C. R.: Surgical Reconstruction of the Oviduct in the Infertile Patient, in Behrman, S. J., and Kistner, R. W. (eds.): *Progress in Infertility* (Boston: Little Brown & Company, 1968).

Green-Armitage, V. B.: Tubouterine implantation, Brit. M. J. 1:1222, 1952, and J. Obst. Gynaec. Brit. Emp. 64:47, 1957.

Hanton, E. M.; Pratt, J. H., and Banner, E. A.: Tubal plastic surgery at the Mayo Clinic, Am. J. Obst. & Gynec. 89:934, 1964.

Hayashi, M.: Tubal factor in sterility, Proceedings of Third Asiatic Congress of Obstetrics and Gynecology, 1965, p. 361.

Horne, H. W.: Conservative laparotomy for infertility: A five year follow-up, Internat. J. Fertil. 9:391, 1964.

———, and Kosasa, T.: Prevention of postoperative adhesions by Decadron-Phenergan. Unpublished data.

Malkin, H. J.: Discussion on modern methods of salpingostomy, Proc. Roy. Soc. Med. 53:358, 1960.

Moore-White, M.: Techniques of tubal plastic operations, Ann. ostet. ginec. 81:90, 1959.

———: Evaluation of tubal plastic operations, Internat. J. Fertil. 5:237, 1960.

Mutch, M. G., Jr.: Sterility and tuboplasties: Critical analysis of 42 cases, Fertil. & Steril. 10:240, 1959.

Palmer, R.: Salpingostomy—A critical study of 396 personal cases operated upon without polythene tubing, Proc. Roy. Soc. Med. 53:357, 1960.

Replogle, R. L., *et al.*: Studies on the prevention of postoperative intestinal adhesions, Ann. Surg. 163:580, 1966.

Shirodkar, V. N.: *Contributions to Obstetrics and Gynecology* (Edinburgh: Livingstone, 1960), p. 65.

———: Plastic surgery of fallopian tubes, West. J. Surg. 69:253, 1961.

Siegler, A. M.: Tubal plastic surgery, the past, the present and the future, Obst. & Gynec. Surv. 15:680, 1960.

———: Tuboplasty, Clin. Obst. & Gynec. 5:820, 1962.

———, and Hellman, L. M.: Tubal plastic surgery: Report of a survey, Fertil. & Steril. 7:170, 1956.

Young, P. E.; Egan, J. E., Barlow, J. J., and Mulligan, W. J.: Reconstructive surgery for infertility at the Boston Hospital for Women, Am. J. Obst. & Gynec. 108:1092, 1970.

Induction of Ovulation

Charles, D.; Barr, W., and McEwan, H. P.: The use of clomiphene in dysfunctional bleeding due to endometrial hyperplasia, J. Obst. & Gynaec. Brit. Emp. 71:66, 1964.

Charles, D.; Loraine, J. A.; Bell, E. T., and Harkness, R. A.: The mechanism of action of clomiphene, in *Fertility and Sterility,* Proceedings of Fifth World Congress on Fertility and Sterility, Stockholm, 1966 (Amsterdam: Excerpta Medica Foundation, 1967) p. 92.

Gemzell, C. A.: Multiple births following treatment with human gonadotropins, in *Fertility and Sterility,* Proceedings of Fifth World Congress on Fertility and Sterility, Stockholm, 1966 (Amsterdam: Excerpta Medica Foundation, 1967) p. 92.

Goldzieher, J. W., and Axelrod, L. R.: Clinical and biochemical features of polycystic ovarian disease, Fertil. & Steril. 14:631, 1963.

———, and Axelrod, L. R.: The polycystic ovary, in Rashad, M. N., and Morton, W. R. M. (eds.): *The Genital System* (Springfield, Ill.: Charles C Thomas, Publisher, 1966).

———, and Green, J. A.: The polycystic ovary. I. Clinical and histological features, J. Clin. Endocrinol. 22:325, 1962.

Greenblatt, R. B.; Barfield, W. E.; Jungck, E. C., and Roy, A. W.: Induction of ovulation with MRL-41, J.A.M.A. 178:101, 1961.

Holtkamp, D. E.; Greslin, J. G.; Root, C. A., and Lerner, L. J.: Gonadotropin inhibiting and antifecundity effects of clomiphene, Proc. Soc. Exper. Biol. & Med. 105:197, 1960.

Johnson, J. E., Jr.: Outcome of pregnancies following clomiphene citrate therapy, in *Fertility and Sterility,* Proceedings of Fifth World Congress on Fertility and Sterility, Stockholm, 1966 (Amsterdam: Excerpta Medica Foundation, 1967) p. 101.

Kistner, R. W.: Use of clomiphene citrate, human chorionic gonadotropin, and human menopausal gonadotropin for induction of ovulation in the human female, Fertil. & Steril. 17:569, 1966.

———: Further observations on the effects of clomiphene citrate (Clomid) in anovulatory females, Am. J. Obst. & Gynec. 92:380, 1965.

———, Lewis, J. L., and Steiner, G. J.: Effects of clomiphene citrate on endometrial hyperplasia in the premenopausal female, Cancer 19:115, 1966.

———, and Smith, O. W.: Observations of use of non-steroidal estrogen antagonist: MER-25, Surg. forum 10:725, 1960.

———, and Smith, O. W.: Observations on use of non-steroidal estrogen antagonist: MER 25. II. Effects in endometrial hyperplasia and Stein-Leventhal syndrome, Fertil. & Steril. 12:121, 1961.

Lerner, L. J.; Holthaus, F. J., and Thomson, C. R.: A non-steroidal estrogen antagonist 1-(p-2-diethylaminoethoxy-phenyl)-1-phenyl-2-p-methoxy-phenyl ethanol, Endocrinology 63:295, 1958.

Mellinger, R. C.: Thompson, R. J., and Mansour, J. A.: Pituitary-gonadal stimulating effect of clomiphene, Clin. Res. 11:224, 1963.

Naville, A. H.; Kistner, R. W.; Wheatley, R. E., and Rock, J.: Induction of ovulation with clomiphene citrate, Fertil. & Steril. 15:290, 1964.

Paulsen, C. A.: Biologic Activities of Synthetic Progestins and a New Nonsteroidal Compound, in Goldfarb, A. F. (ed.): *Advances in the Treatment of Menstrual Dysfunction* (Philadelphia: Lea & Febiger, 1964), p. 55.

Riley, G. M., and Evans, T. N.: Effects of clomiphene citrate on anovulatory function, Am. J. Obst. & Gynec. 89:97, 1964.

Roy, S.; Greenblatt, R. B.; Mahesh, V. B., and Jungck, E. C.: Clomiphene citrate: Further observations on its use in the induction of ovulation in the human and on its mode of action, Fertil. & Steril. 14:575, 1963.

Shearman, R. P.: Induction of ovulation, Australasian Ann. Med. 15:266, 1966.

———, and Cox, R. I.: Clinical and chemical correlations in the Stein-Leventhal syndrome, Am. J. Obst. & Gynec. 92:747, 1965.

———, and Cox, R. I.: The enigmatic polycystic ovary, Obst. & Gynec. Surv. 21:1, 1966.

———, Cox, R. I., and Gannon, A.: Urinary pregnanetriolone in the diagnosis of Stein-Leventhal syndrome, Lancet 1:260, 1961.

Smith, O. W., and Day, C. F.: Effect of clomiphene on aromatization of steroids by the human placenta in vitro, Acta endocrinol. 44:519, 1963.

———, Smith, G. V., and Kistner, R. W.: Action of MER-25 and clomiphene on the human ovary, J.A.M.A. 184:878, 1963.

Southam, A. L., and Janovski, N. A.: Massive ovarian hyperstimulation with clomiphene citrate, J.A.M.A. 181:443, 1962.

Vorys, N.; Gantt, C. L.; Hamwi, G. J.; Copeland, W. E.; and Ullery, J. C.: Clinical utility of chemical induction of ovulation, Am. J. Obst. & Gynec. 88:425, 1964.

CHAPTER 10

Habitual Abortion

General Considerations and Management

HABITUAL ABORTION MAY be defined as a sequence of three or more consecutive failures of pregnancy before the end of the twenty-eighth week of gestation. The tendency for abortion to recur may be due to persistent factors in the maternal environment, to the permanent effects of a temporary environmental factor or to genes, maternal and fetal. It is probable that abortion involves many genetic factors, each interacting with the environment and with other genes. Habitual abortion occurs in approximately 0.2–0.4 per cent of all pregnancies.

A generally accepted estimate of the chance that abortion will occur in any given pregnancy is 15 per cent. Analysis of several recently reported series indicates that the chance of a second spontaneous abortion is about 20 per cent. There is a slight increase in this rate to approximately 25 per cent after three consecutive failures. These figures are at variance with previously reported, albeit pessimistic, statistics that indicated a risk of recurrence of about 84 per cent after three consecutive abortions. Caution must be exercised, therefore, in evaluating therapy since acceptance of the higher figure will lead to erroneous interpretations concerning the efficacy of various therapeutic schemes. This extensively quoted 84 per cent failure rate was merely a calculation based on a series of theoretic speculations and depended, in part, on a constant incidence of recurring factors (i.e., if the total incidence of spontaneous abortion is 10 per cent, accidental factors account for 9.6 per cent and constant recurring factors account for 0.4 per cent).

Etiologic Factors.—Two general concepts have been advanced in explanation of spontaneous abortion. One suggests that abortions are most often due to genetic abnormalities that result in pathologic ova, whereas the other holds that an abnormality of environment may result either in a pathologic ovum or in abnormal endomyometrial function. The importance of the first concept is emphasized by several independent observers who described pathologic ova in from 50 to 75 per cent of the specimens examined. However, it is conceivable that, after union of genetically normal male and female gametes, environmental conditions may be altered so as subsequently to produce an ovum that appears "pathologic."

It is obvious that treatment of any type could only affect the environment. Furthermore, it's a matter of record that such treatment usually starts during the second month of pregnancy. These observations were corroborated by Burge who showed that the proportion of malformed children in a group of salvaged threatened abortions was no higher than in a group of children who were products of uncomplicated pregnancies.

Carr and other workers have suggested that the underlying mechanism for anomalies in early pregnancy is located in lethal chromosomes. In a series of 400 abortuses weighing under 500 gm., he noted an incidence of 22 per cent of lethal chromosomes. However, to date no good evidence has been advanced to prove that repetitive abortions are due to chromosomal abnormalities. However, the volume of literature is growing which indicates that the male factor in the fertilized ovum may be of some significance in the etiology of repeated abortions. Joel studied the DNA of sperm by spectrophotometric methods and found the latter greatly diminished in 8 of 36 recurrent aborters. MacLeod and Gold state that there is perhaps a tendency for semen of poor quality to be associated with miscarriage. Although their study has not been validated statistically, it would tend to support the observations of Joel. To summarize, the possibility that defective germ cells play a role in a statistically valid percentage of recurrent abortions remains to be proved.

Although the precise incidence of abortions due to lethal chromosome is not as yet known, the association of these aberrations with abortion has been amply demonstrated and appears to be closest in the early stages of gestation. The abnormalities encompass trisomies of chromosomes of all groups (excluding Group F), triploidy, and the 45/XO condition.

Although the actual identification of the chromosomes involved in trisomies awaits further analysis, it is possible that trisomies of autosomes responsible for the established syndromes in extrauterine life are also responsible for intrauterine death before pregnancy becomes known. Szulman, long a student of the subject, feels that it is highly probable that such a relationship does exist. According to Szulman, trisomies of other chromosomes are evidently too lethal to permit survival to term, or even past the first trimester. The 45/XO condition of gonadal dysgenesis is the only one at present that has been unequivocally demonstrated to cause both abortions and a syndrome in extrauterine life; embryonic survival up to delivery is of the order of 1 in 60. (See Chap. 16.)

Szulman's figures suggest that a large proportion of abortions is inevitable and that they cannot be salvaged. The greatest number of karyotypically abnormal abortuses occurs in the first trimester and is roughly 60 per cent. The number falls precipitously after 14 weeks gestation. The results of cytogenetic study of abortions are in harmony with the pathologic findings and confirm the hypothesis of the embryo's intrinsic defect as an important cause of early demise.

Recent investigation into the possible causes of habitual abortion has suggested the importance of Mycoplasma hominis as an inciting factor. This organism is more frequently isolated in patients with cervicitis, urethritis and vaginitis although an etiologic role for M. hominis has not been established in these conditions. The organism has been isolated from the oropharynx of normal subjects and has been shown to produce pharyngitis when aerosolized into the nasopharynx of human volunteers. In 1965 Tully isolated M. hominis from blood cultures following the therapeutic abortion of a patient who was receiving immunosuppressive therapy for nephrotic syndrome. Jones has recently reported the isolation of M. hominis from the lungs of 5 aborted fetuses among 62 studied. He also noted antibody rises in the serum of a few women who harbored this organism in the vagina at the time of abortion. Harwick and associates have reported growth of M. hominis in cultures taken from the cervix of a patient who aborted during the third month of gestation. Maternal blood cultures and fetal liver cultures also showed growth of M. hominis. Although resistant to penicillin, most M. hominis isolates are sensitive to chloramphenicol and some are sensitive to tetracycline. Similar studies have indicted Listeria monocytogenes as a possible etiologic factor in spontaneous abortion. This organism is susceptible to penicillin, chloramphenicol, sulfonamides and erythromycin. Further inquiry is necessary into the pathophysiology of the process before it can be determined whether Mycoplasma or Listeria infections are the primary cause of the abortion or are simply the result.

Environmental factors, on the other hand, whether temporary or permanent, lend themselves to investigation, interpretation and correction. Recent advances in both medical and surgical therapy have engendered optimism about increased fetal salvage in this entity. The three most important aspects of the problem concern (1) a psychosomatic approach to the prevention of precipitating noxious stimuli; (2) the use of newer progestins and estrogens in the preconceptional period, and (3) the application of synthetic materials as temporary or permanent splints in the correction of anatomic defects such as the incompetent cervix.

Management of the Patient.—A plan of management in habitual abortion should include a comprehensive study of all factors that have potential etiologic significance. The approach to this intricate problem may be simplified by considering the etiologic processes involved—that is, psychic aspects, nutritional and chronic disease states, hematologic disorders, hormonal insufficiency and anatomic defects.

Psychosomatic Aspects

The intimate relation between mental processes and the causation of abortion has been emphasized in a recent study of over 160 women who habitually aborted. This analysis stresses the importance of the relationship between the physician and patient, since constant reassurance and encouragement are believed to be as important as vitamins or hormones.

This regimen, successful in over 80 per cent of patients, includes a program of frequent office visits with unlimited time for discussion. This is said to accomplish a type of psychotherapeusis that relieves stress and anxiety and permits the development of a "common understanding." If obvious serious emotional difficulties are present, psychiatric consultation is obtained. Regular attendance at mothers' classes augments the practical education of the patient and helps to dispel doubts, fears and worry. Preconceptional and prenatal interviews are unhurried and permit adequate time for evaluation of the patient's fears and problems, together with a sympathetic explanation of various symptoms. Over a period of weeks or months relief from tension and stress will result in a more complacent attitude toward pregnancy. The patient is repeatedly assured that the present pregnancy will terminate successfully.

This therapeutic program prohibits the use of many previously accepted measures. These include hot tub baths, heating pads, hot-water bottles, ice bags, bed rest, vitamin E, mineral oil, abdominal girdles, hormones and coitus. In order to prevent the development of decidual hemorrhage, however, vitamin C and vitamin K are administered throughout the period of the pregnancy. The efficacy of these preparations is doubtful, however, since no proof has been offered to indicate that a specific effect on decidual vessels occurs.

The problem of the relation of physical trauma to emotional shock and subsequent abortion has not been clearly delineated. Most studies have shown that the trauma incident to travel is not an important factor in abortion, and one may conclude that travel has no harmful effect on a *normal* pregnancy. Experimental evidence is available to support the idea that some tissue injury or "psychic shock" in the early stages of gestation may result in uterine contractions, owing to the liberation of epinephrine, and thus lead to abortion of an abnormal or normal embryo. It is known that the control of uterine contractile processes is dependent on, and varies with, the concentration of estrogen and progesterone. However, these hormones are effective through the mediation of specific ions (primarily potassium) in and around the myometrial cells. It may be concluded, then, that physical and emotional trauma may change the endocrine environment, the contractile substance of the myometrium or the ionic concentration of potassium and sodium sufficiently to cause uterine contraction, decidual hemorrhage and abortion.

Numerous authors have indicated the importance of psychological factors in the etiology of spontaneous, repetitive abortion. Deutsh outlined the following psychological mechanisms bearing on the expulsion of the fetus: (1) destructive tendencies directed against one's self or against others, (2) fear of the inability to become a mother, (3) fear of failure expressed in a tendency to abort. Dunbar and Squires describe patients who acquire the "abortion habit" in a similar fashion to certain individual's acquiring the "accident habit." They described two basically different personality profiles in their observations: (1) the predominantly immature woman who finds it impossible to accept the challenges of mature femininity and the responsibility of motherhood, and (2) the independent, frustrated woman who has adjusted to a man's world and whose main aspirations are beyond her feminine limits.

Psychotherapeutic successes in patients having the "abortion tendency" support the hypothesis that habitual abortion is indeed a psychophysiologic disorder. Tupper and Weil studied two groups of habitual aborters and demonstrated that supportive psychotherapy is capable of preventing pregnancy losses. James elaborated on the work of Tupper and Weil and proved statistically that psychotherapy was effective.

CHRONIC DISEASE AND NUTRITIONAL DISORDERS

Obvious deficiencies as well as evidence of chronic disease states are well-recognized causes of repeated abortion. Diabetes has been considered a possible predisposing factor but is mentioned only rarely in large series in which etiology is considered. Syphilis no longer seems to be an important cause of early, repeated incomplete pregnancy. Early and adequate treatment of both diabetes and syphilis has immeasurably increased fetal salvage in these illnesses.

Chronic renal and hypertensive vascular disease, unless severe, do not usually cause early abortion but may result in repeated premature labor or intrauterine death of the fetus. Some patients with these disorders, however, may have repetitive midtrimester pregnancy accidents some time between the twentieth and twenty-eighth weeks. Treatment in these conditions is based on the premise that, as a result of a generalized vasoconstrictive process, the blood supply to the placenta and the fetus is inadequate. Every effort is therefore made to prevent the development of superimposed toxemia by careful dietary restriction of sodium, prevention of weight gain and the use of vasodilating, hypotensive drugs. The patient should have a nutritious diet with adequate protein and vitamins but a minimum of fats. The daily intake of sodium chloride should not exceed 1 Gm. If weight gain due to edema exceeds 2 lb. per month, diuretic agents may be employed.

Visits should be scheduled at weekly or biweekly intervals, especially if there is elevation of the diastolic pressure. Protoveratrine or a combination of reserpine and protoveratrine should be administered as soon as the diastolic pressure exceeds the baseline normal for the patient. If treatment on an ambulatory basis does not control the increased blood pressure or if albuminuria develops, hospitalization is recommended. Although the outlook for fetal survival is not favorable in patients with chronic renal diseases, many babies can be salvaged in the chronic hypertensive group by meticulous management.

A careful review of the dietary habits of the patient should be made when the initial history is taken. Irregular eating habits and food fads should be eliminated and instruction given concerning the importance of proper nutrition. A multivitamin preparation is usually added even when there is no precise evidence of avitaminosis. It has been our practice to encourage this improved dietary regimen and increased vitamin intake together with moderation in the use of tobacco and alcohol during the preconceptional period. Should pregnancy occur, no great effort is then necessary to adopt these habits. The patient should be instructed in a diet containing generous amounts of calcium- and iron-containing foods, green vegetables, and fresh citrus fruits, as well as one quart of milk daily.

Improvement in the treatment of habitual abortion was originally ascribed to vitamins C, E and folic acid. Javert, however, showed the same salvage rate with placebos as with ascorbic acid. Tupper and associates were unable to demonstrate a significant difference in the vitamin C levels of women who were normally pregnant from those who subsequently aborted. These same investigators also were unable to demonstrate differences in the vitamin E concentration in these same groups. The latest "fad" suggests that levels of serum folic acid below a certain point are indicative of incipient abortion.

Immunologic Factors

Complete blood typing of the couple should be done to determine the presence of a major blood incompatibility or the presence of immune antibodies in the maternal serum. Evidence now exists that verifies the etiologic role of A-B-O incompatibility in early and recurrent abortion. It has been suggested that abortion occurs after an antigen-antibody reaction with histamine release causing vasodilatation, increased capillary fragility and uterine spasm. Methods of averting this specific problem are not presently available—except that general supportive measures including the use of vitamins C and P are advised.

Certain patients exhibit defects in clotting with increased capillary fragility; in such women the level of vitamin C in the blood should be ascertained. Administration of vitamins C and P has improved the vasculature of the decidua and may avert decidual hemorrhage.

Specific pathologic changes in the villi of the great majority of placentas of spontaneous and habitual aborters have been described by J. D. Gray. These changes consist of fibrinoid and hyalin degeneration. A correlation between these lesions and those found among certain collagen diseases has been suggested even to the point of including spontaneous abortion in the "collagen disease group." Such an assumption might be acceptable if the immunologic phenomena, similar to those found in rheumatoid arthritis, for example, could be demonstrated.

A simplified version of the hypothesis presented by Tupper and Weil to explain the pathologic and immunologic changes in spontaneous abortion is as follows: (1) placental metabolic products diffuse into the maternal blood stream and act there as a specific antigen, (2) this antigenic activity invites the production of an antibody, (3) a portion of this antibody is absorbed by antigen in the maternal tissues and serum, and the remaining free antibody reacts with the antigen-producing placental cells, thus leading to the specific pathologic changes.

Another approach to the immunological background of spontaneous abortion was initiated in Boston by the work of Bardawil and associates. They assumed that the placenta and the attached fetus was a hybrid parasite with maternal and paternal components. Disturbances in the "host-parasite" balance may occasionally be severe enough to cause expulsion of the fetus. Patients classified as habitual aborters had repetitive hypersensitivity to the paternal part of the placenta. Habitual aborters rejected skin grafts from their husbands earlier than those of unrelated male donors. The authors concluded that this observation confirmed the hypersensitivity of these women to their husbands' tissue. Attractive as this theory seems, the investigators have not been able to secure complete desensitization of the habitual aborter against the paternal portion of the placenta.

Rh sensitization in the Rh-negative woman is not usually a cause of habitual abortion, since most of these pregnancies proceed beyond the twenty-eighth week. However, in a few patients who have been sensitized by administration of Rh-positive blood and whose husbands are homozygous there may be repeated intrauterine fetal deaths between the twenty-fourth and twenty-eighth weeks of gestation. Fetal transfusions are a feasible method of salvaging infants who would otherwise die in utero. If spontaneous labor does not ensue within three to four weeks, determinations of serum fibrinogen and fibrinolytic activity should be made. If there is evidence of increasing fibrinolysin and diminishing fibrinogen, the pregnancy should be terminated. Serious cases of hypo- or afibrinogenemia may thus be averted. Rh immunoglobulin will prevent the development of antibodies normally occurring after delivery of an Rh-positive baby. In order to prevent the 20,000–40,000 new sensitizations that occur yearly in the United States, 400,000 doses need to be given.

HORMONAL ASPECTS

Hormonal studies in patients who have a history of habitual abortion frequently show multiple deficiency patterns. The serum chorionic gonadotropin and the urinary excretion of pregnanediol have been consistently lower in these patients than in women proceeding through a normal pregnancy. In addition, both the basal metabolic rate and the protein-bound iodine determination have shown subnormal values for thyroid function. These three findings provide a rational basis for the use of hormone therapy. In essence the treatment may be considered substitutional, in that the placental secretions are deemed inadequate for the maintenance of pregnancy.

Although endocrine therapy for the many variations of disturbed reproductive physiology has been regarded with skepticism, in the problem of habitual abortion its use seems justified. Progesterone is the key hormone, necessary for complete endometrial preparation before implantation and for adequate vascularization of the decidua during the early development of the placenta.

Chorionic Gonadotropin.—If deficiencies in the serum levels of this material can be correctly evaluated as representing the poor developmental status of the conceptus, the use of chorionic gonadotropin as replacement therapy is untenable. In addition, equine gonadotropin preparations have induced local and systemic reactions. However, since human chorionic gonadotropin is readily available, if such therapy constituted substitution but not replacement, it would seem that repeated small doses might be administered to certain patients *when indicated by low gonadotropin levels.*

Normal patterns for the excretion of HCG in urine during pregnancy are well documented. Figure 10-1 shows levels of HCG in serum and Figure 10-2 illustrates HCG levels in urine during normal pregnancy and treated and untreated threatened abortion. Other investigators have assayed FSH separately and found that the concentration of FSH in the serum did not vary during pregnancy. They found values to be in the high normal range for adult, non-pregnant, premenopausal women. In reviewing the problem of the relationship of HCG to abortion, Brody concluded that, although sub-

Fig. 10-1.—Concentration of human chorionic gonadotropin (HCG) in serum during pregnancy. Urinary excretion closely parallels this curve. (From Mishell, D. R., Jr., Wide, L., and Gemzell, C. A., J. Clin. Endocrinol. 23:125, 1963.)

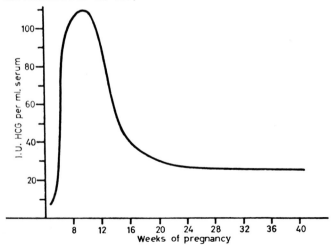

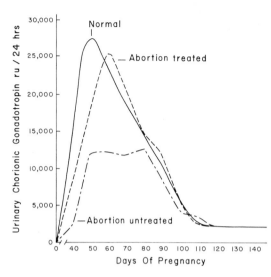

Fig. 10-2.—Urinary chorionic gonadotropin in normal gestation and treated and untreated abortion. Pregnancy may be maintained in some cases of threatening abortion due to hormonal insufficiency. Note that hormonal treatment may increase the level of urinary chorionic gonadotropin in cases of threatened abortion to comparable levels in normal gestation. The normal included 38 cases; the habitual abortion untreated, 24 cases; the habitual abortion treated, 68 cases. The statistical significance of the normal versus the untreated was $P = .01$; treated versus untreated, $P = .01$. (From A. W. Van Ness, New York J. Med. 55:3255, 1955.)

normal levels of HCG are usually associated with abortion, normal levels are occasionally found in unsuccessful pregnancy. I have used HCG in the correction of luteal phase insufficiency both prior to conception and during the cycle of conception. The therapeutic regimen is outlined in the discussion of inadequate luteal phase.

Thyroid.—Thyroid function may be measured by determinations of the blood cholesterol, basal metabolic rate, protein-bound iodine or the uptake of radioactive iodine. Desiccated thyroid has been used empirically either alone or as a supplement in the treatment of habitual abortion for many years. However, because several other medications were usually administered, interpretation of the results was not always possible. On the other hand, a recent study of women classified as habitual aborters revealed that inadequate thyroid function was the most conspicuous finding in 63 per cent.

We have utilized the protein-bound iodine method as an indicator of thyroid activity, levels of $4-8$ μg./100 cc. of serum being considered the normal range. This determination should be performed during the nonpregnant state; if the level is found to be subnormal, therapy may be instituted as a preconceptional measure and then carried through the first 28 weeks of pregnancy.

Crystalline thyroid preparations currently available offer the advantages of constancy of preparation and predictability of effect. Two such compounds now widely used are sodium L-thyroxine and L-triiodothyronine (Cytomel). Triiodothyronine offers the advantage of rapid establishment of therapeutic benefits as well as relatively rapid dissipation of effect. This is considered to be the effective hormone in cellular metabolism; it causes increase of the basal metabolic rate and protein-bound iodine value, decrease of elevated serum cholesterol levels, and normalization of glucose tolerance. The usual maintenance dosage is 100 μg. daily, full therapeutic effect being obtained in about two or three days.

An accepted regimen of treatment for mild hypothyroidism (PBI between 3.0 and 4.5 mcg.) is as follows: (1) 30 mg. desiccated thyroid or 0.1 mg.

sodium levothyroxine daily, (2) increase by increments of 15 mg. or 0.1 mg. at intervals of 30 days, (3) evaluate the patient at 30-day intervals and PBI levels should be used as guideposts until control is achieved, (4) final oral maintenance dosage is about 120 to 200 mg. of desiccated thyroid or 0.4 mg. of levothyroxine.

There is no definite evidence that triiodothyronine is more efficacious than desiccated thyroid or thyroxine for most patients. A disadvantage of triiodothyronine is that the PBI is not raised following treatment of hypothyroid patients and therefore this test cannot be used to follow the response to therapy. This is of particular importance in patients who have no clinical symptoms.

During normal pregnancy the range of the PBI is from 6.2 to 11.2 mcg. per cent, the average being 8.6 mcg. It increases about the third week and is back to normal within 2 weeks of delivery. In threatened and spontaneous abortions, levels between 2.8 and 5.8 mcg. have persisted throughout the first 16 weeks. The increase in the PBI during normal pregnancy is due to increased binding to globulin as a result of an increase in serum estrogens. The butanol extracted iodine test rises from 5.5 mcg. during the 8th week of pregnancy to 7.6 mcg. during the 10th week. Seventy per cent of women who demonstrate low butanol extracted iodine tests subsequently abort. The erythrocyte T-3 test falls during the fifth or sixth week of pregnancy as the amount of estrogen increases and the binding of T-3 to globulin is increased. The amount of thyroid available to be "taken-up" by the erythrocytes is therefore diminished. Failure of the T-3 test to drop during early pregnancy suggests inadequate estrogen production and abortion frequently occurs.

There is no evidence that exogenous thyroid medication is of benefit in habitual abortion when the protein-bound iodine level is truly normal. However, in patients in whom the PBI level is borderline, especially if only one determination has been made, the administration of triiodothyronine may have a beneficial effect.

Estrogen.—Therapy with estrogenic substances is based on the premise that these substances are capable of stimulating more normal secretion and metabolism of progesterone, but only if the trophoblast is able to respond to such stimulation. This theory is supported by the experimental evidence of Smith and Smith, who showed that diethylstilbestrol administered to pregnant women caused an increase in urinary excretion of pregnanediol, as measured by the Venning method. Other observers, however, using different methods for the determination of pregnanediol, were not able to confirm these findings. The dosage schedule advised by Smith and Smith is: 2.5 mg. daily when started at five weeks; 5 mg. at seven weeks; 10 mg. at nine weeks; 15 mg. at 11 weeks; 20 mg. at 13 weeks; 25 mg. at 15 weeks, and an increase of 5 mg. weekly thereafter until four weeks from term, when therapy is discontinued. With this treatment, viable infants were delivered by 74 per cent of 81 women who were habitual aborters. It should be remembered, however, that the chance for abortion to occur after three consecutive abortions is only 25 per cent.

The excretion of estrogens in the urine of pregnant women decreases rapidly in cases of inevitable abortion or fetal death. Although assays of urinary and serum estrogen have not been widely used in following the course of patients with threatened or habitual abortion, some observers

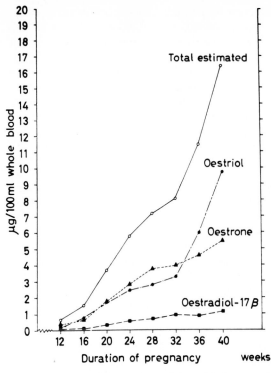

Total estimated

Oestriol

Oestrone

Oestradiol-17β

Duration of pregnancy   weeks

Fig. 10-3.—Blood estrogen concentrations during pregnancy showing the means for ten women. (From Roy, E. J., and MacKay, R. B.: J. Obst. & Gynaec. Brit. Comm. 69:15, 1962.)

believe that a demonstrated insufficiency of estrogenic substances in the urine is of greater prognostic value for the pregnancy than is the determination of pregnanediol.

Figure 10-3 illustrates the changes in blood estrogen concentrations during pregnancy. There is little reliable information about estrogen excretion in women who subsequently abort. What is available suggests that urinary estriol usually decreases before the abortion occurs.

During the first trimester of pregnancy, the corpus luteum and the maternal precursors (dehydroepiandrosterone sulfate and 16-hydroxy-dehydroepiandrosterone) are the main source of estrogens. During the second and third trimesters, the fetus has the predominant role. It has been shown that the placenta can synthesize estrogens by utilizing the circulating androgens in the blood of the fetus. Present evidence indicates that as early as the 15th week of gestation, and increasingly so thereafter, the bulk of estriol is derived from fetal sources, probably the fetal adrenals. For example, in pregnancies with anencephalic fetuses, the absence of the hypothalamic center and the anterior lobe the pituitary results in adrenal atrophy. Low levels of estrogens are characteristic in such pregnancies.

In order to state the precise correlation between abortion and estrogen insufficiency, it would be necessary to measure estrogen frequently, preferably in the serum, then determine whether a deficiency is correlated with an increased risk of abortion. This has not been accomplished.

Progesterone.—This hormone is excreted in the urine as pregnanediol, and the quantitative evaluation of urinary pregnanediol by serial studies has been advocated as a guide for therapy and prognosis in habitual abortion. Progesterone plays an important role in the very earliest stages of pregnancy, namely, at the time of implantation, since abortion may result from inadequate endometrial development or imperfect decidua at this critical period. Ovular loss is greatest during the preimplantation stage, the next greatest loss occurring during the week following implantation. The incidence of ovular loss after the first missed menstrual period may be as high as 28.6 per cent and is comparable to the abortion rate. Later, particularly toward the end of the first trimester, the progesterone-secreting function of the corpus luteum may be faulty or tardily transferred to the placenta, with a resultant transitory hormonal deficiency that may disrupt the physiologic mechanism for maintaining the uterus as the site of undisturbed gestation. It is logical, therefore, to correct endogenous progesterone deficiency by the administration of progesterone or progesterone-like substances.

Studies by Eton and Short who assayed plasma progesterone levels in patients with threatened abortion, were inconclusive and it was apparent that some women aborted in spite of perfectly normal progesterone levels. There is evidence, however, that many first trimester abortions are preceded by a fall in urinary pregnanediol excretion. Shearman has stated that "first trimester abortion is singularly rare with constantly normal pregnanediol levels." Although the patient with a low pregnanediol excretion is clearly a special risk of abortion, it is a mistake to assume that in this situation abortion is inevitable without treatment. Spontaneous restoration to normal levels occurs in 80 per cent of patients with continuation of the pregnancy. This is the crux of determining the effect of any therapy. In uncontrolled studies it is too readily believed that any improvement in pregnanediol excretion is due to the treatment given. The same criticism applies to uncontrolled studies using other and even less accurate parameters of progesterone secretion, such as vaginal cytology or cervical mucus.

The production rate of progesterone during pregnancy has been calculated at 92 mg./day at 15 weeks, 263 mg./day at 27–31 weeks, and 322 mg./day during the third trimester. Progesterone has been measured in serum at various stages of gestation, average values ranging from 5 mg./100 ml. of serum at 6 weeks to 20 mg./100 ml. at 37 weeks. These values may be compared with the average nonpregnancy luteal phase value of 1 mg./100 ml. Pregnanediol, the major metabolite of progesterone, shows rather wide daily variations during pregnancy. Furthermore, pregnanediol is not solely a metabolite of progesterone since it may be formed from other steroids. Thus its value in reflecting progesterone production is limited. The placenta is able to effect the biogenetic sequence of cholesterol—pregnenolone —progesterone, using either circulating precursors or those synthesized within the placenta itself.

What are the results of progesterone or progestin therapy in the treatment of habitual abortion? Uncontrolled studies of either preconceptual or postconceptual treatments, or both, have yielded a salvage rate of between 65 and 80 per cent. In many series the amount of hormone used was homeopathic in the light of current concepts of placental progesterone secretion rates, but this has not affected the results. Shearman has pointed out that equally good results have been obtained by methods as disparate as the administration of thyroid extract, estrogens, chorionic gonadotropin, psychotherapy, or the nonspecific use of antisyphilitic preparations.

A controlled study by Shearman and Garrett was reported in 1963 in which patients with two or more consecutive first trimester abortions were selected for study. The experiment was designed to assess the effect of progesterone or placebo of identical appearance in patients whose only observed abnormality was a low or falling pregnanediol. Those patients with evidence of uterine malformations were excluded. Urinary pregnanediol levels were assayed once weekly as soon as the diagnosis of pregnancy was made. Patients with persistently normal pregnanediol results were not treated. The final selection left 50 patients who were treated because of either a low or falling pregnanediol excretion. The progestine used was 17-α-hydroxyprogesterone caproate and the placebo was the vehicle only. Results in the treated and the placebo group were *not* significantly different.

Other double-blind studies in habitual abortion using different progestins have been published by Goldzieher, and by Klopper and MacNaughton. Each of these concluded that the rate of abortion was not affected by progestin therapy. There are no published reports of controlled studies of preconceptual treatment, utilizing chorionic gonadotropin or estrogen.

There is, without doubt, clear evidence of hormonal deficiency in the majority of spontaneous first trimester abortions: low or declining excretion of chorionic gonadotropin, estrogens and pregnanediol. No evidence can be adduced, however, to indicate that these deficiencies *cause* the abortion. Rather, the hormonal defects and the abortion are both due to a common factor: failure of placentation. When one examines a "blighted ovum" and notes the poverty of chorionic tissue, it is easy to visualize poor hormonal production. In an effort to correct the abnormalities of implantation, I have adopted a method of treatment for the habitual aborter which strives for the production of hormonal normalcy both prior to and during very early placentation. Therapy is administered before the diagnosis of pregnancy is possible. The optimum therapeutic benefit seems to be obtained in patients with "inadequate luteal phase."

Inadequate Luteal Phase.—This may be defined as a specific entity reflecting abnormal ovarian function with inadequate progesterone production and insufficient progestational effect on the glands and stroma of the endometrium. This finding, to be significant, in the etiology of infertility must be constant, not sporadic. The incidence of inadequate luteal phase has been given as 19 per cent of 406 infertile women in a single sample but only 3.5 per cent of 904 patients had a persistent luteal phase defect. The incidence is higher in secondary infertility, particularly when this is associated with repeated abortions.

The classic symptom of luteal phase defect is repeated abortion during the first trimester of pregnancy, usually prior to 8 weeks. The repetitive abortions may be due to an abnormal progesterone effect on: (1) the tube with too rapid transport of the ovum, (2) uterine motility—perhaps increased, or (3) the nidation site—inadequately prepared.

The basic and long reaching effect of inadequate luteal phase is identified in inadequate secretory endometrium. This finding implies: (1) inadequate progesterone, (2) inadequate estrogen preparation, (3) excessive estrogen in relation to the amount of progesterone (rare), or (4) the inability of the endometrium to respond to normal hormonal stimulation. In a study of endometrial biopsies from women with ovulation induced with exogenous human pituitary gonadotropins, it is evident that one of the causes of inadequate luteal phase is inadequate LH.

DIAGNOSIS.—The diagnosis of inadequate luteal phase is based on the repetitive finding of evidence of progesterone insufficiency. The simplest diagnostic approach, and the most accurate, is to combine endometrial biopsies with basal body temperature charts. The date of the endometrial biopsy should be timed according to the probable time of ovulation (low point or 24 hours prior to low point on the BBT) and the onset of subsequent menses. The endometrium should be fixed in Bouin's solution rather than formalin and is dated according to the criteria of Noyes, Hertig and Rock. The endometrial biopsy should be taken from the fundus of the uterus and should represent full thickness. Biopsies should be taken from the anterior and posterior surfaces. Endometrium taken from the lower uterine segment does not respond to hormonal stimulation. An intact surface epithelium is important for adequate histologic evaluation.

When should the endometrial biopsy be performed in the determination of luteal phase insufficiency? First of all, it is important that the patient chart several basal body temperatures graphs before taking the biopsy so that some idea of luteal phase sequence is obtained. Jones has advised taking the biopsy on day 26 of a typical 28 day cycle, that is, 2 days prior to the onset of bleeding. Although some investigators feel that the biopsy may be taken on the first day of bleeding, Jones feels that important morphologic criteria are lost in the occasionally confused "menstrual pattern."

If the patient is cautioned against coitus in a given cycle, the endometrial biopsy may be performed on the twenty-fourth day, at which time the effect of progesterone is at its peak. If the corpus luteum is poorly developed (or inadequately stimulated by adenohypophysial hormones), the secretion of estrogen and progesterone is deficient. Endometrial biopsies indicate a gross secretory appearance, but if analyzed histochemically they demonstrate a diminished storage of glucose, alkaline phosphatase and other enzymes presumably important at the time of implantation.

Assays of pregnanediol may be used to determine the presence of inadequate luteal phase but a single 24-hour urinary assay is not nearly as satisfactory as an endometrial biopsy. Although the diagnosis can be made very accurately by measuring the total pregnanediol excretion during the cycle, this is a nuisance for the patient and the expense is prohibitive. Furthermore, there is a wide variation in the normal day to day 24-hour pregnanediol excretion. However, if two or three 24-hour pregnanediol values are each below 2 mg. during the peak of the luteal phase, between day 19 and 25, the diagnosis of inadequate luteal phase is suspected.

Although the basal body temperature has been used to determine the presence of inadequate luteal phase, it is not a satisfactory diagnostic technique since it tends to show an all-or-none response. Its value lies in the fact that it may occasionally detect gross luteal defects and may alert the physician to the possibility of the condition. If repeatedly abnormal basal body temperatures are combined with endometrial biopsies showing inadequate progesterone response and deficient excretion of pregnanediol in the urine, the diagnosis of inadequate luteal phase may be accepted. Should specific treatment correct the deficiency and result in normal gestation, retrospective judgment as to the correct diagnosis would, of course, be corroborative.

Neither vaginal cytology nor cervical mucus changes can be used as a method for the quantification of progesterone production. Unfortunately, inflammatory changes, androgen, vitamins, digitalis and many other medications affect the total hormonal milieu exhibited by vaginal and cervical cells.

TREATMENT.—Several methods of therapy in this "luteal insufficiency" syndrome are available. A preconceptional plan may include estrogen, progesterone, triiodothyronine, ascorbic acid, nutritious diet and the avoidance of noxious stimuli.

The therapeutic approach to the luteal phase defect depends upon the specific etiology and the hormone deficiency involved. Every effort should be made to correct the primary cause of the condition, be it emotional tension, nutritional insufficiency, metabolic disease, or other forms of chronic illness or toxicity. If the cause is *idiopathic, hypothalamic,* or *pituitary insufficiency,* substitution hormone therapy is the only recourse. Clomiphene citrate has usually been unsatisfactory. One must know whether there is a simple progesterone insufficiency or an underlying estrogen dificiency. As previously discussed, this can be documented by an evaluation of the cervical mucus at ovulation in conjunction with vaginal cytology or with spot urinary estrogen assays throughout the cycle. Although the urinary estrogen assay is the most satisfactory method, the expense is often clinically prohibitive.

I have adopted the therapeutic measures advised by Dr. Georgianna Jones in the treatment of inadequate luteal phase and the regimens outlined are essentially hers. The reader is referred to the chapter on this entity by Dr. Jones in *Progress in Infertility.*

Estrogen Deficiency.—If an underlying estrogen deficiency is proved or suspected, the treatment of choice is continuous estrogen administration in low dosage; 0.1 mg. of stilbesterol daily or its equivalent is usually satisfactory. This amount of estrogen is ordinarily not enough to interfere with ovulation but sufficient to correct the inadequate cervical mucus at the time of ovulation and give a normal follicular phase endometrium in preparation for progestational stimulation. If the estrogen dose does delay ovulation, which it may do in approximately one-fourth of the patients, it can be stopped on day 10 of the cycle and resumed after ovulation.

If the cervical mucus remains scanty, e.g., if the picture is one of a "dry cervix" in the face of apparent sufficient estrogen stimulation as judged by vaginal cytology, the possibility of previous operative damage by cauterization or conization of the cervix should be considered.

Estrogen and Progesterone Deficiency.—If the estrogen deficiency seems to have been corrected but the endometrial pattern remains defective as judged by repeat biopsy during therapy, a progesterone deficiency may also be present. In this case both estrogen and progesterone should be administered in the latter half of the cycle.

Progesterone Deficiency.—If a simple progesterone deficiency exists, it can be corrected by progesterone substitution or by stimulation of the corpus luteum with chorionic gonadotropin. Progesterone per se is the treatment of choice rather than synthetic progestational drugs. Since the endometrial response is used to judge the adequacy of progesterone replacement, it is necessary to reproduce the normal physiologic-progestation-endometrium-pattern in both glands and stroma. Progesterone has been found to be the most efficient drug in this respect; synthetic progestational agents are prone to give unusual end-organ responses. The adjustment of dosage of long-acting progestational agents is often difficult from a practical clinical point of view because the absorption curve is such that in order to produce a proper concentration at the desired time it is almost necessary to give a sufficient amount to cause a pseudopregnancy reaction. The most convenient mode of progesterone administration is by vaginal suppositories; 50 mg. is given nightly after ovulation has occurred as judged by the shift in the basal body temperature chart or estimation of ovulation time from previously studied cycles. If the endometrial pattern has not been restored to a normal secretory one, as determined by a repeat biopsy during therapy, the mode of administration is changed to 12.5 mg. of progesterone in oil given intramuscularly daily. The aqueous suspensions of progesterone tend to produce a sterile abscess and hence should be avoided. For convenience of administration, the patient or her husband is taught to give the injections. The dosages described have been found to be sufficient to cause secretory changes in the properly prepared endometrium, but not enough to produce a pseudopregnancy reaction. Therefore, the progesterone administration is continued until menses begin, at which time it is discontinued and not resumed until after ovulation in the next cycle.

Although Jones still uses intravaginal progesterone suppositories, these are not available to most physicians. I have used an oral synthetic progestin, medroxy-progesterone acetate, since it is structurally similar to progesterone itself. This synthetic progestin is given in a dose of 10 mg. beginning 48 hours after the rise in the basal body temperature and continuing for 7 days. An alternative method is to continue the progestin for 21 consecutive days and then obtain a pregnancy test. This will obviate removal of the progestin at a most critical time in nidation.

If the expected menstrual period does not occur, pregnancy is to be suspected. Medication is then continued and a quantitative serum chorionic gonadotropin and urinary pregnanediol assays are performed. The serum gonadotropin will predict the normalcy of the embryonic development. If this assay result is poor and a repeat test taken ten days following the first is also abnormal, it is wise to discontinue progesterone, for the probability of producing a missed abortion from continuing treatment of a "blighted" ovum is to be anticipated. If the pregnanediol value is normal, progesterone can be gradually discontinued over a two-week period in the expectation that the trophoblastic hormone, HCG, has stimulated the corpus luteum to function normally. If the pregnanediol value is low, in spite of exogenous progesterone, it is necessary to continue with hormonal supplementation until the placental steroid function has been established. Under these circumstances, if the serum chorionic gonadotropin is normal, a long-acting progestational agent can be substituted, e.g., 17-α-hydroxyprogesterone caproate 125 mg. per week intramuscularly.

Chorionic gonadotropin can be used to stimulate endogenous progesterone secretion from the corpus luteum. A dosage of 2500 international units daily is adequate and usually unassociated with side effects. Although this is probably the most efficient way of replacing an inadequate corpus luteum function, certain considerations make such treatment impractical. The expense involved is a major point. Not only is the drug costly, but because it is a heat-labile hormone and a protein, which on disassociation can cause rather severe pyrogenic reactions, it is felt that administration should be by medical personnel, not patient or family. This precaution adds substantially to the cost and the inconvenience of the therapy. In addition to these rather practical considerations, it is sometimes difficult to preclude the possibility of a pseudopregnancy reaction and still be satisfied that a proper luteal stimulation has been maintained. Therefore, the patient must be cautioned that a delayed menses does not necessarily represent a pregnancy. Under these conditions, one cannot use the serum chorionic gonadotropin assay either as a pregnancy test or as an index for normalcy of trophoblastic development because the exogenous hormone administered will give a false biologic reading. This complication can sometimes be obviated by stopping the administration of the drug on day 26 of an ideal 28-day cycle, or two days prior to the anticipated menses.

I have varied the regimen of Jones slightly in that I have given a long acting progestin, 17-α-hydroxyprogesterone caproate in a dose of 500 mg. intramuscularly if the basal body temperature remains elevated over 18 consecutive days. This, of course, pertains only if the oral progestin is given for 7 or 8 days during the luteal phase and is not continued indefinitely. One week later a pregnancy test is obtained and, if positive, the intramuscular progestin is continued in the same dose, 500 mg. weekly, until the 16th week of gestation.

The advantage of such treatment is obvious since pregnancy may be assumed merely on the basis of the maintained elevation of the basal body temperature and progesterone may be administered at the most critical phase of gestation.

A few reports have appeared that suggest a correlation between the postconceptional administration of certain progestins and the masculinization of the external genitalia in newborn female infants. The changes have consisted in enlargement of the clitoris and fusion of the labioscrotal folds so that the infant is mistakenly considered a male. Wharton and Scott have produced similar changes in the fetuses of monkeys by the administration of norethindrone during pregnancy. Critical analysis of the data leads to the following conclusions:

1. The number of reported cases is small in comparison with the thousands of patients who have received progestogenic substances during early pregnancy.

2. Masculinization has occurred when certain progestins have been used early in pregnancy in *extremely* large dosage.

3. The preparations used in the reported cases are known to have some androgenic potential. These were anhydrohydroxyprogesterone (ethisterone, Pranone), crystalline progesterone and norethindrone (Norlutin). No cases have as yet been reported following the use of Delalutin or Provera. One equivocal case has been reported following the use of Enovid.

4. The fact that occasionally a female infant may demonstrate these superficial stigmata of virilization should not interdict the administration of progestogenic substances to women who might not be able to deliver a viable child without them. The defects, once recognized, are easily and permanently corrected surgically.

Use of Drugs in Early Pregnancy.—Certain drugs should not be given during the first trimester of pregnancy. As a matter of fact, a wide variety of agents would be contraindicated during early pregnancy if data from animal experiments were transferred to the human. Thus, depending on dosage and experimental circumstances, acetylsalicylic acid, caffeine, insulin, penicillin, streptomycin, thyroxin and vitamin A have produced malformations in the laboratory animal. Obviously, such data cannot be transferred. For example, cortisone given to a particular strain of pregnant mice will produce cleft palate in almost 100 per cent of the offspring. But its effect in pregnant women is questionable. Ultimately, only human experience is definitive.

In view of the international publicity given to the teratogenic effects of thalidomide, it is obvious that many of the newer drugs, hormonal and otherwise, should be restudied in pregnant animals, preferably in primates. Even then complete assurance could not be given that a specific substance might not cause congenital abnormalities, since the patient herself, because of intrinsic enzymatic abnormalities, may convert a "safe" compound into an "unsafe" one.

It is important, therefore, to administer drugs for specific indication only, and it is advisable that any drug or substance known to be teratogenic in animals be withheld during human pregnancy unless the life or health of the mother is endangered. The physician must select a preparation which has been proved safe by animal experimentation as well as by prolonged clinical investigation and widespread use.

Specifically, it would seem wise to limit medications during the period of organogenesis to the usual prenatal supplements of calcium, vitamins and iron. The judicious use of small doses of barbiturates for hyperemesis and insomnia seems acceptable on the basis of present evidence. If progesterone is indicated, the ideal steroid to use is progesterone itself. However, because of its rapid rate of metabolism and the fact that it is relatively ineffective orally, one of the synthetic progestogens may be substituted. The clinician should select a preparation which resembles the naturally occurring steroid most closely and which does not possess androgenic potency in animal assays. Both of these criteria are met by 17-alpha-hydroxyprogesterone caproate (Delalutin). Dihydrogesterone (Duphaston) is not androgenic in animal assays, but it has not been used as extensively as 17-alpha-hydroxyprogesterone caproate in this country and sufficient time has not elapsed to evaluate it fully. Although medroxyprogesterone (Provera) is structurally similar to progesterone, it has demonstrated androgenic potential in certain test animals. However, no virilized infants have been reported following its use in pregnant human females. Depomedroxyprogesterone has the disadvantage of producing prolonged anovulation and amenorrhea after being discontinued. Although there are probably a small number of patients who abort *only* because of inadequate endogenous progesterone, it is impossible for the clinician to determine precisely which patient to treat. The situation has not been clarified by two reports in which the fetal salvage rate in habitual aborters was not significantly increased in patients receiving synthetic progestagens. Both studies were done with "double-blind controls" and cast doubt on previously reported uncontrolled studies.

The physician should avoid the use of testosterone and testosterone-like substances during early pregnancy. These include ethynyl testosterone (Pranone), 19-nor-ethynyl testosterone (norethindrone, Norlutin) and certain protein anabolic agents such as 19-norethyl testosterone (Nilevar). All of the mothers whose infants showed enlargement of the clitoris and/or fusion of the labioscrotal groove received large doses (over 20 mg. daily) for prolonged periods. No masculinized female babies have been reported when these agents were employed as a three- or four-day pregnancy test or when the dose was below 10 mg. daily. Norethynodrel (the progestin in Enovid) does not demonstrate estrogen-antagonistic activity (as does norethindrone) and seems to have minimal androgenic potential. However, it should be noted that both norethynodrel (Enovid) and norethindrone (Norlutin) are rather poor progestational agents as measured by the McGinty test and both agents are ineffective in the maintenance of pregnancy in ovariectomized rats and rabbits.

Thalidomide and substances with a structural configuration similar to thalidomide should be avoided during the first trimester of pregnancy. Similarly, it would be wise to omit preparations having a basic phenothiazine ring. It is surprising how often an old-fashioned sedative such as phenobarbital, chloral hydrate or butabarbital is as effective or even superior in action to the newer, expensive tranquilizers for the relief of tension states or hyperemesis.

Cortisone or cortisone-like substances should be given only for strict medical indication even though a review of the literature in 1960 revealed only two instances of cleft palate in offspring of 260 pregnant women who had received corticoids during the first trimester. Thyroid extract has been used extensively during early pregnancy and has not been shown to cause congenital abnormalities. In most patients, however, the dose has been almost homeopathic.

Alkylating agents and antimetabolites ordinarily used in the management of carcinoma are obviously contraindicated, as are isotopically "tagged" preparations. Antibiotics and sulfonamides should be used only when specifically indicated for infection. Amphetamines and other preparations used as anorectics should be avoided, and diuretics are best withheld until the middle and last trimester. Drugs which interfere with cholesterol metabolism or disturb pituitary function should never be given to a pregnant woman.

ANATOMIC DEFECTS

Although the results of correction of anatomic defects which cause repetitive abortion are in general satisfactory, the total number of abortions due to these causes is relatively small. The most common abnormalities are infections, lacerations and incompetency of the cervix, bicornuate or double uteri, uterine malpositions and submucous leiomyomas.

The cervix should be thoroughly palpated and inspected at the time of the first examination. After adequate study by means of Schiller's test, cytologic examination and biopsy, lesions such as chronic cervicitis, endocervicitis and polyps should be treated by electrocauterization. Extensive lacerations, especially those of the "fish-mouth" variety, should be repaired surgically.

An "incompetent" cervix (Fig. 10–4) is suggested by a history of two or more midtrimester abortions, the pregnancies terminating painlessly and suddenly after spontaneous rupture of the membranes, usually without preliminary bleeding. In the nonpregnant state, a No. 18 Hanks cervical dilator may be passed through the internal cervical os without pressure, and hysterography will show dilatation rather than narrowing of the isthmus uteri. This condition may be corrected by a plastic operation as advised

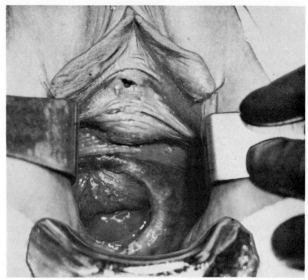

Fig. 10-4—Incompetent cervical os seen during the thirty-second week of gestation. The cervix is widely patulous and the membranes clearly visible. (From Easterday, C. L., and Reid, D. E.: The incompetent cervix in repetitive abortion and premature labor, New England J. Med. 260:687, 1959.)

by Lash or, as suggested, by the placement of polyethylene tubules or Dacron mesh (Mersilene) circumferentially around the internal os (Fig. 10-5). The latter procedures are performed during pregnancy and have resulted in a fairly high degree of fetal salvage when the patients were properly selected.

The following criteria for operability are rigid and should not be violated. (1) The patient should have had at least two, and preferably three, consecutive midtrimester abortions. (2) Repeated pelvic examinations should reveal progressive cervical dilatation. (3) The procedure should not be done before the fourteenth week of pregnancy to avoid "securing" an imperfect or blighted ovum. (4) In the presence of cervicitis, vaginal infection or rupture of the membranes, the operation is contraindicated, and (5) it is not usually advised after the thirtieth or thirty-second week of gestation.

The placement of the nonabsorbable mesh necessitates delivery by cesarean section even if the fetus is nonviable or if placental abruption occurs, whereas the polyethylene tubule has the advantage of being only a temporary splint that may be cut at the thirty-seventh or thirty-eighth week of gestation. The tubule may also be severed if labor occurs when the infant is nonviable, permitting pelvic delivery. It has also been suggested that the presence of nonabsorbable mesh may interfere with subsequent conception, especially if infection or local allergic manifestations occur. At present it is impossible to state which method is superior. The physician is cautioned, however, against the indiscriminate use of these procedures, since irreparable damage may simply convert the problem of habitual abortion into one of permanent sterility. Another disadvantage of the "permanent" band is its tendency to be extruded through the vaginal mucosa about eight or twelve weeks post partum. Since it must then be removed and replaced, it has no specific advantage over the "temporary" splint and will necessitate many unnecessary cesarean sections.

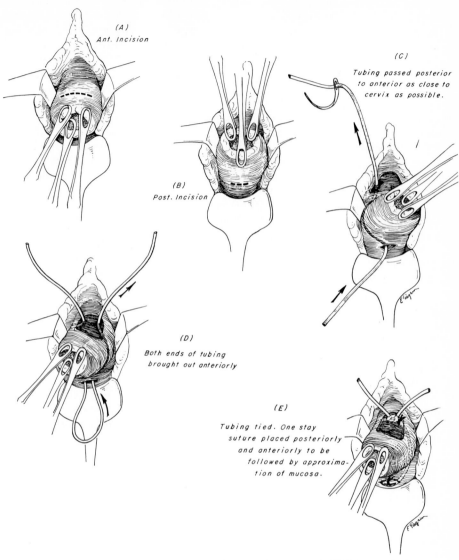

(A)
Ant. Incision

(B)
Post. Incision

(C)
*Tubing passed posterior
to anterior as close to
cervix as possible.*

(D)
*Both ends of tubing
brought out anteriorly*

(E)
*Tubing tied. One stay
suture placed posteriorly
and anteriorly to be
followed by approxima-
tion of mucosa.*

Fig. 10–5.—Repair of incompetent cervical os. **A,** the cervix is grasped with DeLee cervical forceps and an incision is made transversely on the anterior surface of the portio vaginalis. Bleeding is minimized by injecting epinephrine under the mucosa for a distance of 5–6 cm. The bladder is then advanced. **B,** a similar incision is made in the posterior fornix at the level of the insertion of the uterosacral ligaments. **C,** a polyethylene tubule containing silver wire is directed through the posterior incision close to the cervix and emerges anteriorly at the level of the upper end of the cervix. **D,** the other end of the tubule is passed around the opposite side of the cervix and emerges anteriorly. **E,** the suture is tied and is fixed anteriorly and posteriorly by silk sutures. (Since the usual tendency is to place the suture too low, another is placed above the first and tied in position). The vaginal mucosa is then closed with catgut sutures, and the ends of the polyethylene wire are secured with lead shot. They are thus available for easy removal if necessary. (From Easterday, C. L., and Reid, D. E.; in Reid, D. E.: *A Textbook of Obstetrics* [Philadelphia: W. B. Saunders Company, 1962].)

Submucous leiomyomas may disturb endometrial function or encroach on the cavity of the uterus to such a degree that implantation is prevented or its vitality jeopardized. Large intramural fibroids may rarely produce hyperirritability or dysfunction of the myometrium, resulting in abortion. The diagnosis may be made by palpation, curettage or hysterography. Surgical correction by myomectomy is indicated in the patient with repetitive abortion.

Uterine malpositions, especially third-degree retroversions, have been considered as predisposing to abortion. In most patients, however, the uterus gradually rises from its posterior position without incident. The use of a Smith-Hodge pessary may be of value in certain patients and is a simple office procedure. If other definitive intra-abdominal surgery is being carried out, suspension of the uterus should be performed. Primary suspension to correct habitual abortion is not recommended.

Incomplete fusion of the müllerian ducts may result in varying degrees of uterine duplication. The commonest congenital abnormalities are those of bicornuate, septate and double uteri. The diagnosis may be made by curettage or hysterography, and the treatment is surgical. The metroplasty (Fig. 10-6) advocated by Strassmann is the procedure of choice; a review of the world literature in 1955 reported that after 107 such operations 61 women became pregnant and 51 living children were delivered. Surgical intervention should be delayed until time and investigation have shown proper exposure in an infertile patient or until one or more abortions have occurred.

Howard Jones has classified maldevelopment of the vagina and uterus, depending on the degree of development of the müllerian duct, into a functional uterus as follows (see Fig. 10-7):

1. If the development of one müllerian duct is completely arrested, the uterus and fallopian tube may be formed entirely from the other duct. This so-called *uterus unicornis* or unicornuate uterus may not cause any problem at all or it may result in abortion or premature labor.

2. Most rudimentary horns are noncommunicating but in some cases the endometrium is nonfunctional so that no clinical symptoms are present. If the endometrium is functioning, a clinical situation may arise from the retention of menstrual blood. In other instances the endometrial cavity of the rudimentary horn may communicate through a narrow channel with the more normal opposite cavity. Under these circumstances, pain and very rarely pregnancy may occur. If a pregnancy does occur in a rudimentary horn under such a condition, the patient may present the classic picture of an ectopic pregnancy, including rupture. The communication is sometimes so narrow that it can be missed with the most careful scrutiny.

As with all examples of maldevelopment of the müllerian ducts, anomalies of the wolffian ducts may also be present, especially with a rudimentary horn. The anomaly of the uterine tract is invariably on the same side as the maldevelopment of the müllerian duct. Although the kidney may be malrotated, low lying, or actually within the bony pelvis, complete agenesis is not uncommon.

3. When the two müllerian ducts develop side by side without communicating with each other, a complete double uterus results. Each duct forms one cervix and one uterine body with a fallopian tube attached to each. The duplication may continue down into the vagina so that part of the vagina

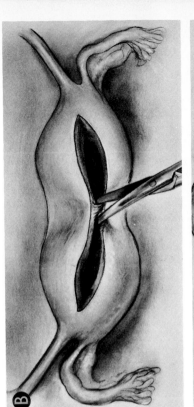

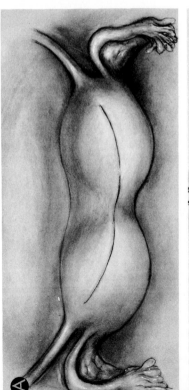

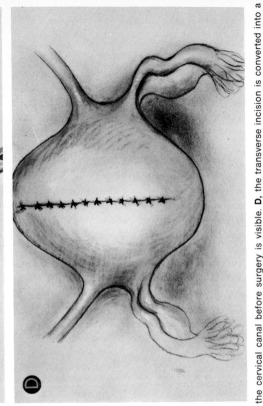

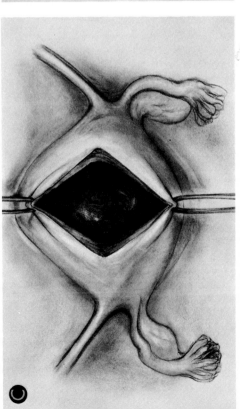

Fig. 10–6.—Operation for bicornuate uterus. **A,** a transverse incision is made over a uterine cornua and saddle, curving toward the round ligaments to avoid uterotubal junctions. **B,** uterine cavities are opened and the partition between them is split down the middle. **C** shows both cavities converted into a single cavity. Iodoform gauze pack inserted through the cervical canal before surgery is visible. **D,** the transverse incision is converted into a vertical suture line, preventing endometrial adhesions between anterior and posterior uterine walls. (From Strassmann, E. O.: Clin. Obst. & Gynec. 4:240, 1961.)

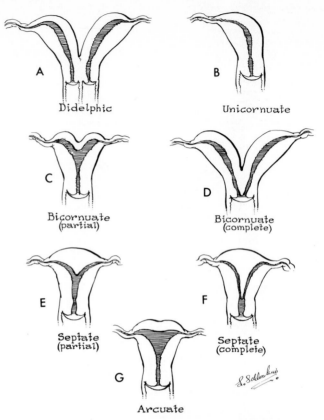

Fig. 10-7.—Nonobstructive maldevelopment of the uterus. **A,** uterus didelphys. **B,** unicornuate uterus. **C,** a partial bicornuate uterus as evidenced by the external configuration. **D,** a complete bicornuate uterus as evidenced by the external configuration and a double cervix. **E,** septate uterus as evidenced by a normal external configuration of the uterus and the septum which can be diagnosed only by radiographic means. **F,** arcuate uterus, which is the mildest form of malformation and seldom associated with reproductive difficulties. (From Jones, H. W., and Jones, G. S.: Am. J. Obst. & Gynec. 65:325, 1953.)

formed by the müllerian ducts is duplicated. Such complete duplication may be referred to as a *uterus didelphys.*

Most reduplicated uteri, however, are not so complete, and the fusion may involve only the upper portion so that the two uterine cavities communicate to a greater or lesser degree. Under this circumstance there is a single cervix and a single vagina. A rather simplified classification of such double uteri is convenient. If the two horns of a partially fused uterus are recognizable externally, the uterus may be designated as a bicornuate uterus. But sometimes the external configuration of the uterus is relatively normal so that it is almost impossible to recognize it from its external appearance; malfusion is represented only by a septum within the uterus. In this circumstance the uterus may be referred to as a septate uterus. If the condition is minimal, an arcuate uterus is said to occur.

The various degrees of reduplication of the uterus are usually associated with reproductive failure, especially repeated abortions. It should be emphasized, however, that an anomalous uterus may be compatible with a normal reproductive history. In our experience only about one-fourth of women with some form of this anomaly have reproductive problems. Miller gives an abortion rate among women with double uteri of 28.3 per cent; Smith a rate of 23.5 per cent; Schauffler a rate of 53 per cent; and Taylor a rate of 33 per cent.

The cause of the lowered fertility with a double uterus is not clear. The problem may be one of abnormal uterine contractions, inadequate stretching of the uterus, or improper implantation on the uterine septum.

Jones has stressed the fact that patients with reproductive failure and double uterus should be thoroughly investigated by all possible tests to eliminate other causes of reproductive failure. In essence, the diagnosis of reproductive failure associated with a double uterus is made by ruling out all other possible causes. Although any type of double uterus may be associated with reproductive failure, it is interesting that a septate uterus is much more likely to present a problem than a bicornuate one. This means that the operative procedure will be carried out on septate uteri most often. The procedure we have found most satisfactory varies in detail from the classic Strassmann procedure. In the latter operation no tissue is excised; the incision is made transversely from one cornu to the other across the uterine fundus, but the final suture line is in the anteroposterior axis of the uterus. The operative procedure of choice excises the septum and avoids the sensitive area of the cornu. This technique seems more applicable to the septate variety, for the bulky septum in many of these uteri does not lend itself to a convenient application of the Strassmann technique. It is to be recalled that the Strassmann technique was worked out in the days prior to the introduction of radiopaque material, when the diagnosis was always made by palpating two separate horns of the uterus. With the septate variety, one can seldom discern by bimanual examination a uterine abnormality but must depend rather on a hysterogram to reveal the details of the intrauterine pathology.

Technique of repair of septate uterus.—The description of the technique of repair is that of Dr. Howard W. Jones. The operation is begun by marking with brilliant green the lines of incision on the external surface of the uterus. It is also convenient to stain the endometrial cavity by the instillation of indigo carmine into the cavity so that during the course of the operation there is no difficulty in identifying the endometrium. Hemorrhage is usually not troublesome, but the local intramuscular injection of Pitressin (1 unit per cubic centimeter, maximum 20 cc.) renders the operation almost bloodless. After the excision of the septum the two halves of the uterus are sutured together from side to side in several layers. The deepest layer includes the endometrium, and 2-0 chromic catgut suture, either interrupted or continuous, is used. The second layer, which may be actually two rows of suture, approximates the myometrium. The third or outer layer includes the serosa (Fig. 10-8).

Depending upon the age of the patient, it is desirable to advise her to wait from 8 to 12 months following operation before attempting to get pregnant. Healing in the nonpregnant uterus is not to be compared with healing of cesarean section scars; there has been very little problem with the uterine incisions, and probably a good many of these patients could be delivered vaginally. However, in the average patient who has had considerable fetal wastage, we usually find ourselves dealing with a premium

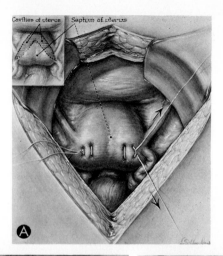
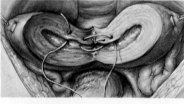
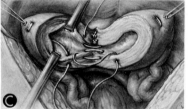
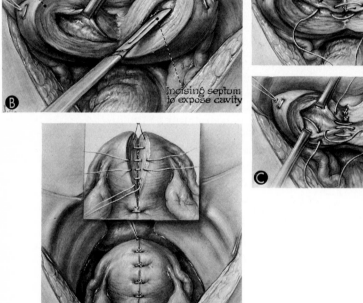

Fig. 10-8.—A, the appearance of a septate uterus at operation. Inset shows a thick muscular septum. **B,** excision procedure. After excision of a wedge-shaped segment of the uterus it is necessary to excise additional tissue to unroof each horn. **C,** unification of the two halves of the uterus. Two continuous sutures are used to approximate the endometrial cavities. **D,** further steps in the unification operation. Inset shows a second layer of sutures approximating the myometrium. The superficial layer includes serosa and myometrium. (From Jones, H. W., and Jones, G. S.: Am. J. Obst. & Gynec. 65:325, 1953.)

pregnancy. The patient may be in her late 30's, and there is always the possibility of a serious catastrophe with the uterine scar. For this reason we advise delivery by cesarean section.

In properly selected patients with repeated abortions, reconstruction of the uterus is a very satisfactory procedure and will result in a live birth in about three out of four patients.

BIBLIOGRAPHY

Chromosomal Abnormalities

Benirschke, K.: Cytogenetic Abnormalitites in Reproduction, in Behrman, S. J., and Kistner, R. W. (eds): *Progress in Infertility* (Boston: Little, Brown & Company, 1968).

Carr, D. H.: Chromosome studies in abortuses and stillborn infants, Lancet 2:603, l963.

————: Chromosome studies in spontaneous abortions, Obst. & Gynec. 26:308, 1965.

Hafez, E. S. E.: The Trophoblast and Its Relationship to Infertility, in Behrman, S. J., and Kistner, R. W. (eds.): *Progress in Infertility* (Boston: Little, Brown & Company, 1968).

Harwick, H. J.; Iuppa, J. B.; Purcell, R. H., and Fekety, F. R.: Mycoplasma hominis septicemia associated with abortion, Am. J. Obst. & Gynec. 99:725, 1967.

Jones, D. A.: Mycoplasma and abortion, Brit. M. J. 1:338, 1967.

Szulman, A. E.: Significance of Chromosomal Abnormalities in Spontaneous Abortion, in Behrman, S. J., and Kistner, R. W. (eds.): *Progress in Infertility* (Boston: Little, Brown & Company, 1968).

————: Chromosomal aberrations in spontaneous human abortions, New England J. Med. 272:811, 1965.

Thiede, H. A., and Salm, S. B.: Chromosome studies of human spontaneous abortions, Am. J. Obst. & Gynec. 90:205, 1964.

Tully, J. G., *et al.*: Septicemia due to Mycoplasma hominis type 1, New England J. Med. 273:648, 1965.

Inadequate Luteal Phase

Foss, B. A.; Horne, H. W., and Hertig, A. T.: The endometrium and sterility, Fertil. & Steril. 9:193, 1958.

Hughes, E. C.: Relationship of the endometrium to sterility and unsuccessful pregnancy, West. J. Surg. 67:166, 1959.

————: Jacobs, R. D.; and Rubilis, A.: Effect of treatment for sterility and abortion upon the carbohydrate pathways of the endometrium, Am. J. Obst. & Gynec. 89:59, 1964.

Jones, G. E. S., and Pourmand, K.: An evaluation of etiologic factors and therapy in 555 private patients with primary infertility, Fertil. & Steril. 13:398, 1962.

————: Inadequate Luteal Phase, in Behrman, S. J., and Kistner, R. W. (eds.): *Progress in Infertility* (Boston: Little, Brown & Company, 1968).

————, Woodruff, D. J., and Moszkowski, E.: The inadequate luteal phase, Am. J. Obst. & Gynec. 83:363, 1962.

Noyes, R. W.: Uniformity of secretory endometrium, Obst. & Gynec. 7:221, 1956.

————, Adams, C. E., and Walton, A.: The transport of ova in relation to the dosage of estrogen in ovariectomized rabbits, J. Endocrinol. 18:108, 1959.

————, Hertig, A., and Rock, J.: Dating the endometrial biopsy, Fertil. & Steril. 1:3, 1950.

Pathology

Hertig, A. T., and Sheldon, W. H.: Minimal criteria required to prove prima facie case of traumatic abortion or miscarriage: An analysis of 1,000 spontaneous abortions, Ann. Surg. 117:596, 1943.

Hughes, E. C., *et al.*: The Role of the Endometrium in Implantation and Fetal Growth, in Engle, E. T. (ed.): *Pregnancy Wastage* (Springfield, Ill.: Charles C. Thomas, Publisher, 1953).

Moyer, D. L.: Endometrial Diseases in Infertility, in Behrman, S. J., and Kistner, R. W. (eds): *Progress in Infertility* (Boston: Little Brown & Company, 1968).

Nesbitt, R. E. L., Jr.: *Perinatal Loss in Modern Obstetrics* (Philadelphia: F. A. Davis Company, 1957).

Wall, R. L., and Hertig, A. T.: Habitual abortion: A pathologic analysis of 100 cases, Am. J. Obst. & Gynec. 56:1127, 1948.

Thyroid Function

Buxton, C. L. and Herrmann, W. L.: Effect of thyroid therapy on menstrual disorders and sterility, J. A. M. A. 155:1035, 1954.

Comninos, A. C.: Thyroid function and therapy in reproductive disturbances, Obst. & Gynec. 7:260, 1956.

DeGroot, L. J.: Medical progress: Current views on formation of thyroid hormones, New England J. Med. 272:243, 1965.

Hamolsky, M. W.: Thyroid Factors, in Behrman, S. J., and Kistner, R. W. (eds.): *Progress in Infertility* (Boston: Little Brown & Company, 1968).

————, and Freedberg, A. S.: Medical progress: The thyroid gland, New England J. Med. 262:23, 1960.

Ingbar, S. H., and Freinkel, N.: Thyroid Hormones, in Antoniades, H. N. (ed.): *Hormones in Human Plasma* (Boston: Little Brown & Company, 1960).

Irizarry, S.; Paniagua, M.; Pincus, G.; Janer, J. L., and Frias, Z.: Effect of cyclic administration of certain progestin-estrogen combinations on the 24-hour radioiodine thyroid uptake, J. Clin. Endocrinol. 26:6, 1966.

Robertson, H. A., and Falconer, I. R.: Reproduction and thyroid activity, J. Endocrinol. 22:133, 1961.

Schneeberg, N. G.: The thyroid gland and infertility, Clin. Obst. & Gynec. 2:826, 1959.

Blood Incompatibility

Glass, B.: The relation of Rh incompatibility to abortion, Am. J. Obst. & Gynec. 57:323, 1949.

Grubb, R., and Sjostedt, S.: Blood groups in abortion and sterility, Ann. Human Genetics 19:183, 1955.

Hormonal Treatment

Brody, S.: Protein Hormones and Hormonal Peptides from the Placenta, in Klopper, A., and Diczfalusy, E. (eds.): *The Physiology of the Foeto-Placental Unit* (Oxford, England: Blackwell Scientific Publications, 1966).

————, and Carlstrom, G.: Immunoassay of human chorionic gonadotropin in normal and pathological pregnancy, J. Clin. Endocrinol. 22:564, 1962.

Brown, J. B.: Urinary excretion of oestrogens during pregnancy, lactation and the re-establishment of menstruation, Lancet 1:704, 1956.

Davis, M. E., *et al.*: Metabolism of progesterone and its related compounds in human pregnancy, Fertil. & Steril. 11:18, 1960.

Eton, B., and Short, R. V.: Blood progesterone levels in abnormal pregnancy, J. Obst. & Gynaec. Brit. Emp. 67:785, 1960.

Goldzieher, J. W.: Evaluation of Treatment of Abortion. A Problem in Experimental Design, in Barnes, A. C. (ed.): *Brook Lodge Symposium on Progesterone* (Kalamazoo, Mich.; Brook Lodge Press, 1961).

————: Double-blind trial of a progestin in habitual abortion, J.A.M.A. 188:651, 1964.

————, and Benigno, B. B.: The treatment of threatened and recurrent abortion: A critical review, Am. J. Obst. & Gynec. 75:1202, 1958.

Grumbach, M. M.; Ducharme, J. R., and Moloshok, R. E.: On the fetal masculinizing action of certain oral progestins, J. Clin. Endocrinol. 19:1369, 1959.

Guterman, H. S.: Progesterone metabolism in the human female. Its significance in relation to reproduction, Recent Prog. Hormone Res. 8:293, 1953.

Hughes, E. C.; Jacobs, R. D., and Rubulis, A.: Effect of treatment for sterility and abortion upon carbohydrate pathways in the endometrium, Am. J. Obst. & Gynec. 89:59, 1964.

Klopper, A., and MacNaughton, M.: Hormones in recurrent abortion, J. Obst. & Gynaec. Brit. Emp. 72:1022, 1965.

Kupperman, H. S.; Jeidl, J., and Epstein, J. A.: The use of progestins in habitual abortion. Notes on salvage and foetal abnormalities, Acta endocrinol. (Kobenhavn) Suppl. 51:673, 1960.

Rawlings, W. J., and Kreiger, V. I.: Studies in the prevention of recurrent abortion due to corpus luteum deficiency, M. J. Australia 2:561, 1958.

————, and Kreiger, V. I.: Long acting progesterone preparations and orally administered "Primolut N" in the treatment of habitual abortion, M. J. Australia 1:428, 1959.

Shearman, R. P.: Some aspects of the urinary excretion of prenanediol in pregnancy, J. Obst. & Gynaec. Brit. Emp. 66:1, 1959.

————: The urinary excretion of some steroidal metabolites applied to a study of ovarian and placental function, M.D. thesis, University of Sydney, 1965.

————; Hormonal Treatment of Habitual Abortion, in Behrman, S. J., and Kistner, R. W. (eds.): *Progress in Infertility* (Boston: Little, Brown & Company, 1968).

————, and Garrett, W. J.: Double-blind study of the effect of 17-hydroxyprogesterone caproate on abortion rate, Brit. M. J. 1:292, 1963.

Smith, O. W., and Smith, G. V.: The influence of diethylstilbestrol on the progress and outcome of pregnancy as based on a comparison of treated and untreated primagravidas, Am. J. Obst. & Gynec. 58:994, 1949.

Surgical Treatment

Barter, R. H.: Operations to preserve pregnancy, Clin. Obst. & Gynec. 1:963, 1958.

Danforth, D. N.: Cervical incompetency as a cause of spontaneous abortion, Clin. Obst. & Gynec. 2:45, 1959.

Israel, S. L., and Mutch, J. C.: Myomectomy, Clin. Obst. & Gynec. 1:455, 1958.

Jones, H. W., Jr., and Baramki, T. A.: Congenital Anomalies, in Behrman, S. J., and Kistner, R. W. (eds.): *Progress in Infertility* (Boston: Little, Brown & Company, 1968).

Lash, A. F.: Fertility and reproduction following repair of incompetent cervical os of cervix, Fertil. & Steril. 11:531, 1960.

Malone, L. J., and Ingersoll, F. M.: Myomectomy in Infertility, in Behrman, S. J., and Kistner, R. W. (eds): Progress in Infertility (Boston: Little, Brown & Company, 1968).

Strassmann, E. O.: Surgery for unification of double uterus, Am. J. Obst. & Gynec. 64:25, 1952.

CHAPTER 11

Hydatidiform Mole and Choriocarcinoma

Revised by Donald P. Goldstein

Approximately ten per cent of all pregnancies terminate in spontaneous abortions and about one-half of such abortuses are either pathologic or blighted ova. In two-thirds of these abnormal pregnancies the chorionic villi show early hydatidiform swelling. It may be concluded, therefore, that between 3 and 4 per cent of all pregnancies are potential hydatidiform moles but terminate in spontaneous abortion before full molar development has occurred. Hertig has stated that a true hydatidiform mole occurs only once in approximately 2,000 pregnancies, an incidence of 0.05 per cent (Fig. 11–1). In the Philippine Islands, however, the incidence has been described as 1 in every 173 pregnancies and on the island of Taiwan as 1 in 125 pregnancies. Although choriocarcinoma is said to occur in an approximate ratio of 1:40,000 pregnancies, the recent study from Taiwan revealed a much higher incidence of this malignant form of chorionic tumor. Thus, in a study of 172 trophoblastic tumors, 123 were classified as hydatidiform moles, 23 as invasive moles and 26 as choriocarcinomas. The reason for the high incidence in the Far East (and in Mexico) is unknown but is suspected to be correlated with low dietary protein.

Hydatidiform Mole

The pathogenesis of hydatidiform mole has been accurately described by Hertig and Gore. The molar tissue results from a progressive accumulation of fluid within the connective tissue spaces of the chorionic villi of the pathologic ovum (Fig. 11–2). The trophoblast is therefore still nourished by the maternal blood supply but is deprived of the fetal circulation. The immature villi, containing loose mesenchymal tissue, then begin to swell as a result of fluid inbibition and form multiple, isolated, grapelike cysts. Microscopic examination of these villi (Fig. 11–3) demonstrates that they exhibit varying degrees of trophoblastic activity, ranging from normal through hyperplastic, anaplastic and neoplastic degrees of undifferentiation (Fig. 11–4). Thus, the isolated villus tumor acquires the invasiveness of the early ovum.

Potential hydatidiform moles usually abort about the eleventh week of gestation, whereas true hydatidiform moles continue their development

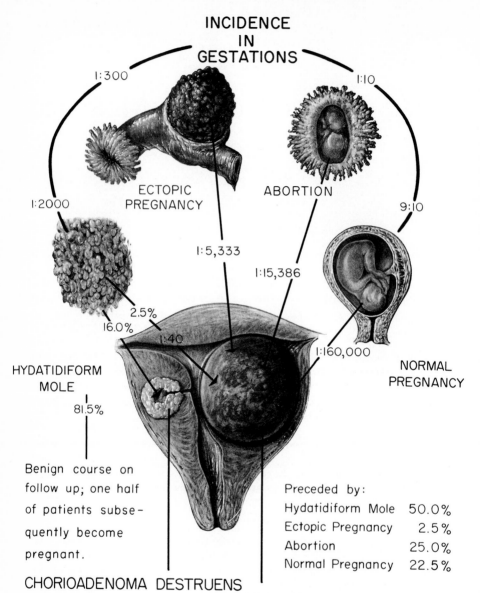

Fig. 11–1.—Schematic representation of the relation of various types of pregnancy to chorioadenoma destruens (invasive mole) and choriocarcinoma (true chorionepithelioma). Note that when pregnancies are followed by chorionic malignancy a hydatidiform mole can give rise to either variety of chorioma, although the other types of pregnancy appear to give rise only to choriocarcinoma. The more pathologic or abnormal the pregnancy, the more likely it is to give rise to a true choriocarcinoma. The tendency of any one type of pregnancy to become malignant is indicated by the ratios or percentages on the interconnecting lines. (From Hertig, A. T., and Gore, H. M.: *Tumors of the Female Sex Organs: Part 2. Tumors of the Vulva, Vagina and Uterus*, sec. IX, fasc. 33 of *Atlas of Tumor Pathology* [Washington, D.C.: Armed Forces Institute of Pathology, 1960].)

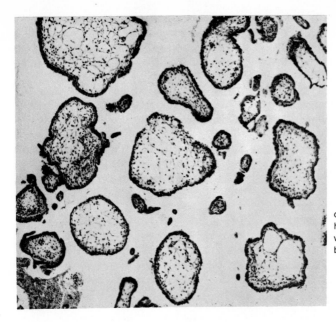

Fig. 11-2.—Pathologic ovum, showing villi with hydatid change. Edematous villi do not demonstrate fetal blood vessels.

Fig. 11-3.—Typical villi of hydatidiform mole. Note loose mesenchymal tissue, spaces due to edema and absence of fetal blood vessels.

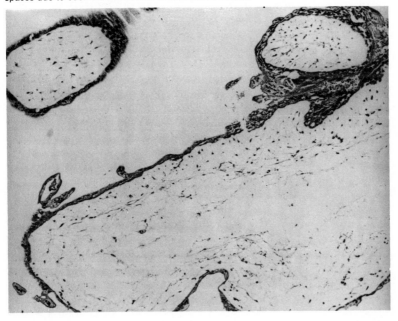

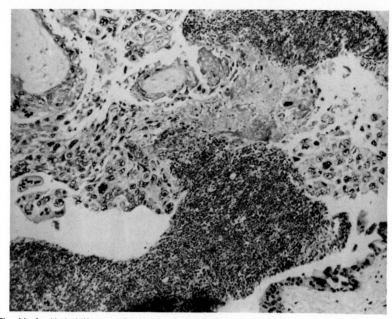

Fig. 11-4.—Hydatidiform mole showing hyperplasia and anaplasia of epithelial elements. Note syncytial border of villus at lower right and "tissue-culture" growth of pure trophoblast in center.

and are delivered somewhere near the sixteenth to eighteenth week of gestation. The classical description of a hydatidiform mole is "a missed abortion of a pathologic ovum."

The usual symptoms associated with an hydatidiform mole are summarized in Table 11-1. These data are based on the findings in a group of 107 patients with molar pregnancy treated at the Boston Hospital for Women under the auspices of the New England Trophoblastic Disease Center from July 1, 1965 through June 30, 1968. Irregular, painless bleeding occurs almost universally and ranges from dark brown or "prune-juice" type to bright red. The bleeding usually appears after the missed period and may be merely spotting or occasionally profuse hemorrhage. Uterine cramps occur only when molar tissue is being aborted. Owing to the rapid growth of molar tissue the uterus enlarges rapidly and in about half the cases is larger than would be anticipated for the duration of the pregnancy. Toxemia of pregnancy is noted in 22 per cent of patients and severe nausea and vomiting are seen more frequently than in normal pregnancy.

Pulmonary involvement manifested by diffuse rales is noted in 12 per cent of patients. When present the chest x-ray reveals varying degrees of infiltration. When lung involvement is extensive, patients exhibit shortness of breath, dyspnea on exertion, orthopnea, cyanosis and right heart failure. These signs resolve following evacuation and are not to be confused with the chest x-ray findings in the occasional patient who demonstrates the presence of a metastatic lesion of molar tissue or choriocarcinoma which persists following evacuation and requires further therapy.

Hyperthyroidism is manifested clinically by diffuse enlargement of the thyroid gland, tachycardia and warm skin. Muscle wasting and weight loss

TABLE 11-1.—CLINICAL SIGNS OF MOLAR PREGNANCY

	No. of Patients	%
Vaginal Bleeding	101	95
Uterine Enlargement	58	54
Hyperemesis	30	28
Toxemia	24	22
Trophoblastic emboli	13	12
Hyperthyroidism	11	10
Total	107	

is seen in 10 per cent of patients. Increased thyroid activity is documented by significant elevations of the protein bound iodine, red cell uptake, free thyroxine, thyroid-binding globulin, and radioactive iodine uptake tests. Exophthalmia has not been observed. This syndrome is limited almost exclusively to patients with marked elevation of chorionic gonadotropin levels (greater than 2 million International Units [I.U.] per 24 hours) and is thought to be due to the secretion by trophoblast cells of a thyrotropin-like factor.

Fetal movement is rarely noted and when reported must be questioned unless there is the coexistence of a normal fetus which is a rare event. Heart sounds likewise are absent and x-ray examination of the abdomen is advantageous only if the size of the uterus indicates the pregnancy to be beyond 18 weeks' duration. In normal pregnancy of this age the fetal skeleton is usually present. Pelvic examination may reveal bilaterally enlarged ovaries. These occur preoperatively in 15 per cent of patients with hydatidiform mole but are more common the later in gestation the mole is evacuated and the higher the level of chorionic gonadotropin.

Diagnosis.—Definitive diagnosis of molar pregnancy prior to evacuation can be obtained radiographically with injection of radio-opaque material into the uterine cavity. Patients are selected for this procedure who present one or more of the following signs: rapid uterine enlargement, borderline or elevated urinary or serum gonadotropin levels, first trimester vaginal bleeding, absent fetal heart tones, and absent fetal skeleton. Patients are prepared for the procedure by routine catheterization of the urinary bladder, by obtaining a preliminary radiograph of the abdomen, and by testing for sensitivity to the contrast medium to be used. The lower abdomen is surgically prepared and draped. A No. 18 spinal needle with stylet is introduced transabdominally into the uterine cavity at a point in the midline 3–5 cm. below the umbilicus. After aspiration to verify intrauterine location of the needle, 15–20 ml. of radio-opaque material (Renografin ®) are injected rapidly. The needle is then withdrawn and anterioposterior and lateral radiographs are taken within 5 minutes after injection.

A "moth eaten" or "honeycombed" pattern is consistent with a diagnosis of molar pregnancy (Fig. 11–5). Satisfactory radiographs have been obtained in 27 women with suspected molar pregnancy, twenty of whom had the condition. Of the remaining seven patients two had normal single fetuses, one had a twin gestation, one patient had quintuplets which aborted 6 weeks later, another had a benign cystic teratoma and co-existing normal intrauterine pregnancy, a sixth patient had a missed abortion, and the last patient had a large simple cyst of the ovary with a co-existing

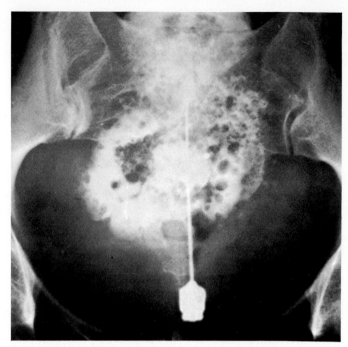

Fig. 11–5.—Intrauterine dye study showing the characteristic "moth eaten" or "honeycombed" pattern associated with a molar pregnancy.

pregnancy. To our knowledge there have been no reports of untoward effects on either mother or fetus from this procedure when properly executed.

The trophoblast cells of molar pregnancy produce human chorionic gonadotropin (HCG) which is identical to that produced by trophoblast cells of normal pregnancy so that the usual biologic and immunologic tests for pregnancy give positive results. Dilution tests on 12- or 24-hour urine volumes generally show titers of chorionic gonadotropin higher than that found in a single normal gestation. However, the titer associated with a twin pregnancy may be a confusing factor. Rarely, however, does the urinary chorionic gonadotropin level in patients with a normal single or multiple pregnancy reach levels in excess of 500,000 I.U. per 24 hours after the tenth or twelfth week of pregnancy. Molar pregnancy, in contrast, is associated with HCG titers above this level in approximately one half of the patients. In rare cases the tests for pregnancy are negative either because the chorionic tissue secretes very small amounts of HCG or because the method of assay is not adequate to test for low concentrations. In such instances HCG will be demonstrated if highly sensitive biologic or radioimmunologic tests are performed on serum or 24-hour urine concentrates (Table 11–2).

Studies of estrogens in the urine of patients with hydatidiform moles have indicated severe placental dysfunction as early as the tenth week of pregnancy. Individual levels of estrone, estradiol, and estriol, determined by gas-liquid chromatography and isotope dilution methods, were lower

TABLE 11-2.—Relative Potency of Commonly Used HCG Tests

Method	Index of Sensitivity
Bioassay	
Mouse Uterine Weight	1
Rat Ventral Prostate	2
Rat Ovary or Uterus	5
Mouse Ovary	7
Frog	40
Immunoassay	
Agglutination	20–40
Radioimmunoassay	0.01

than expected values for comparable periods in normal pregnancy. They actually approximated those of healthy menstruating non-pregnant women. The defect in estrogen biosynthesis may be assumed to be present in the trophoblastic cells of the molar villi. The main defect seems to be in the conversion of adrenal precursors to estriol which is the most abundant estrogenic fraction in normal pregnancy and which fails to rise in molar pregnancy. A similar defect has been demonstrated in women with invasive mole and choriocarcinoma (Table 11-3).

Similarly studies of human placental lactogen (HPL) in the serum of patients with hydatidiform moles have indicated severe impairment of the ability of trophoblastic cells to synthesize this interesting polypeptide hormone which normally can be detected in increasing amounts in normal pregnancy (Fig. 11-6). The detection of low values of HPL in the presence of normal or elevated levels of HCG is an excellent laboratory aid in the differential diagnosis of molar pregnancy from normal gestation or threatened abortion after the sixth to eighth week of gestation.

Recently there have been a number of interesting reports of genetic aberrations in molar pregnancy. Abnormal numbers of chromosomes have been found in the trophoblastic cells of molar villi as well as an overwhelming preponderance of chromatin positive (female) sex chromatin patterns. The significance of these genetic implications is still not well understood with respect to etiology and pathogenesis.

Clinically the differential diagnosis between an hydatidiform mole and a normal twin pregnancy or a threatened abortion is frequently difficult.

TABLE 11-3.—Estradiol/Estriol Production Rates

Subject	PR* E_2 ($\mu G/D$)	PR† E_3 ($\mu G/D$)	% Conversion E_2 to E_3
NL. Pregnancy (5 weeks)	842	214	7.9
NL. Pregnancy (9 weeks)	1519	374	8.6
NL. Pregnancy (14 weeks)	2913	2158	31.3
Hyd. Mole (16 weeks)	1335	152	5.1
Chorioca	1394	173	10.8

*PR-E_2 production rate of Estradiol
†PR-E_3 production rate of Estriol

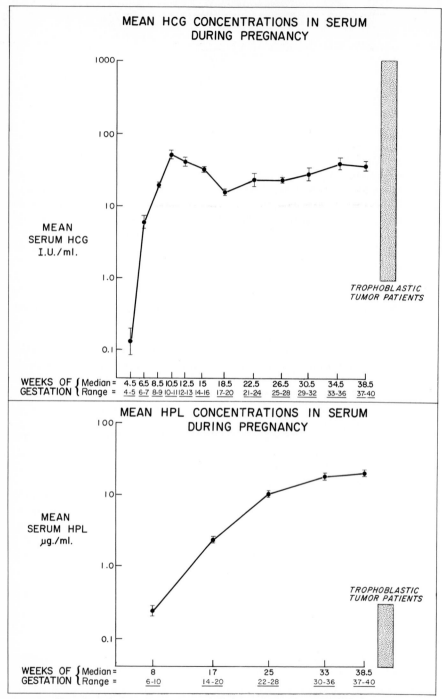

Fig. 11-6.—Graphs showing the characteristic pattern of serum HCG and HPL levels in normal pregnancy. Also illustrated is the range of serum HCG and HPL values in a series of patients with trophoblastic disease (invasive mole and choriocarcinoma).

However, if there is continuous or intermittent bleeding particularly of the "prune-juice" variety, a rapidly enlarging uterus in which fetal movement and heart sounds are absent, and x-ray evidence of intrauterine fetal death or absent fetal parts, the diagnosis should be strongly suspected on clinical grounds. While the association of toxemia is suggestive, the spontaneous expulsion of molar tissue is diagnostic. Studies of specific enzymes such as leucine aminopeptidase and alkaline phosphatase are most interesting and may, in the future, enable the clinician to make a more specific diagnosis.

Treatment.—The treatment of the disease process depends on the stage at which diagnosis is made. If diagnosis is made at the time of spontaneous expulsion of the mole, the approach should be vaginal. Most fragments of remaining molar tissue can be removed by finger curettage or an ovum forceps after the uterus has been made to contract with an intravenous infusion of oxytocin. Occasionally a large dull curet is needed to evacuate the uterine cavity completely. Suction evacuation offers an alternative and perhaps more expeditious method of uterine evacuation by the vaginal route with less chance of perforation and less blood loss. Regardless of the method utilized it is important that all curettings be sent to the pathologist for examination separately from the tissue spontaneously passed since the morphology of these specimens may be more representative of the extent of epithelial undifferentiation than that of the tissue expelled spontaneously.

Prior to the development of suction evacuation, if the uterus exceeded the size of a four-month gestation and molar tissue had not been passed, interruption of the pregnancy was best accomplished by abdominal hysterotomy. As with the vaginal route, blood should be available and oxytocic drugs should be given to effect rapid uterine contraction. This method offers the advantage of direct observation of the endometrium and myometrium to ascertain the extent of molar invasion. This advantage questionably outweighs that fact that the uterine scar may require repeat cesarean sections for delivery of future pregnancies. Of more importance, however, is the fact that endometrial curettage may be done under direct vision avoiding the possibility of uterine perforation.

If the diagnosis of hydatidiform mole is made after passage of the mole, treatment should include curettage after a 48- to 72-hour period of oxytocin infusion. The purpose of curettage in this instance is twofold: first, to ensure complete evacuation and thus diminish persistent vaginal bleeding and post abortal sepsis; and second, to obtain samples of endometrium and trophoblast for review by the pathologist.

Enlarged ovaries due to multiple theca lutein cysts return to normal size over a period of four to twelve weeks. Occasionally ovarian enlargement persists for longer periods even though the gonadotropin titer has returned to normal. Although ovarian twisting and infarction occur, rarely is it necessary to resect ovarian tissue at the time of hysterotomy.

In patients of advanced age or parity the treatment of choice is primary abdominal hysterectomy with the mole in situ. Well documented studies have demonstrated that, in the absence of pre-existing metastases, hysterectomy is generally curative.

Follow-up.—Following evacuation of a hydatidiform mole, regardless of the route, a chest x-ray should be obtained and assays of gonadotropins are done every two weeks. It is essential to obtain quantitative HCG levels of serum or urine using standard biologic or immunologic methods. When the assay of HCG drops below the level of sensitivity of these determinations (roughly 750–3000 I.U. per liter of urine), HCG determinations must be performed by more sensitive methods. This is necessary since it is impossible to distinguish between HCG produced by trophoblastic cells and gonadotropin of pituitary origin. The most widely used method involves bioassay of a kaolin-acetone concentration of a 24-hour urine specimen using the mouse uterine weight test. Involution of all molar tissue can only be ascertained by utilizing a system which is sufficiently sensitive to measure normal endogenous pituitary gonadotropin levels (Fig. 11–7). Other assay methods of similar sensitivity include the rat uterine and rat ovarian weight tests and the newer radioimmunoassay technique.

If these tests are unavailable it is essential to follow patients with semi-monthly chest x-rays, weekly quantitative pregnancy tests, and physical examinations. If normal menses ensue, uterine and ovarian involution

Fig. 11–7.—Graph compares the relative usefulness of routine pregnancy tests and the mouse uterine weight test for diagnosis, treatment, and follow-up in a patient with a hydatidiform mole who developed nonmetastatic trophoblastic disease after initial evacuation. Note that the routine pregnancy tests performed on unconcentrated urine (including bioassay and immunoassay methods) are unreliable when urinary gonadotropin levels are between 50 and 50,000 m.u.u. per 24 hours (equivalent to 5 and 5,000 I.U. per liter).

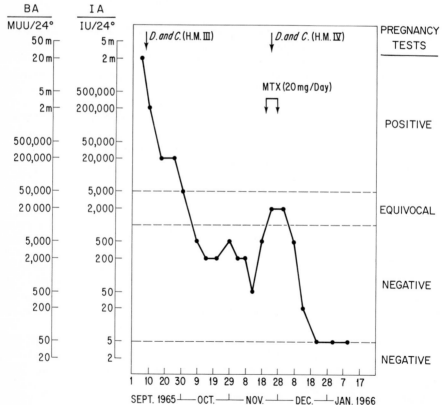

occur promptly, and lung fields remain clear, it is unlikely that trophoblastic tissue is present. This is particularly true if the original mole was of the benign type.

In almost 80 per cent of patients the gonadotropin assay reverts to normal pituitary levels within 30 to 60 days after evacuation. In these instances persistent trophoblastic tissue is absent. However, in patients whose gonadotropin titer remains elevated after 60 days or rises at any time after evacuation, at least 40 per cent will subsequently be found to have either invasive mole or a chorionic malignancy.

All patients who have passed a hydatidiform mole must remain under observation with regular physical examinations, x-rays of the chest, and assays of gonadotropin performed at monthly intervals for 6 months, then every other month until one year after obtaining the first normal gonadotropin level. Pregnancy should be avoided since an elevated level of gonadotropin due to the new pregnancy confuses hormonal evaluation. The oral contraceptive agents may be used since they do not affect the level of gonadotropin in serum or urine. An intrauterine device is not recommended.

PROPHYLACTIC CHEMOTHERAPY

The potential value of administering chemotherapy at the time of evacuation of a molar pregnancy has been suggested because of the success of these agents in patients with invasive mole and choriocarcinoma. A pilot study has been undertaken at the Boston Hospital for Women under the auspices of the New England Trophoblastic Disease Center to test the validity of this concept in a group of selected patients. Initially Methotrexate 0.3 mgm./kg. per day intramuscularly for 5 days was given either at the time of spontaneous delivery or two days prior to elective molar evacuation. Because of the frequency of abnormal liver function tests noted in patients receiving Methotrexate, actinomycin D was substituted in doses of 12 mcg./kg. per day given intravenously for 5 days. The results indicate a decrease in both metastatic and non-metastatic complications without severe morbidity (Table 11-4).

Adoption of this adjuvant technique in the management of molar disease awaits evidence from a larger series of patients.

TABLE 11-4.—PROPHYLACTIC CHEMOTHERAPY OF
HYDATIDIFORM MOLE

	TREATED*	UNTREATED†
Uncomplicated	29	52
Complicated		
Non-Metastatic‡	4 (14%)	16 (22%)
Metastatic	–	6 (8%)
Total	33	74

*Chemotherapy Administered at Time of Initial Evacuation
†Follow-Up Began <2 weeks following evacuation
‡HCG Level Elevated >8 weeks following evacuation

Invasive Mole (Chorioadenoma Destruens)

A diagnosis of invasive mole may be made in patients who have persistently high gonadotropin titers following passage of a mole. Pathologically the lesion is characterized by deep myometrial invasion of molar villi (Fig. 11–8). Metastases, though rare, have been observed and their presence should be excluded. The most common symptom is persistent and irregular vaginal bleeding associated with uterine enlargement and subinvolution. Ovarian enlargement is less frequent than in patients with uncomplicated molar pregnancy. Despite the presence of elevated gonadotropins and bleeding, a curettage may fail to disclose an intramyometrial lesion. The curettings indicate trophoblastic disease but usually are inadequate to make a precise diagnosis. Repeated curettage to obtain histologic confirmation of persistent trophoblastic tissue is unnecessary and hazardous. Uterine perforation, infection, and dissemination of metastases may occur subsequent to persistent invasion of the endometrial cavity.

In patients of advanced age and parity, hysterectomy is the procedure of choice when metastases are absent. The value of prophylactic chemotherapy at the time of operation is still under investigation.

An interesting approach to the non-surgical treatment of non-metastatic invasive mole has been described by Hertz and co-workers for patients who desire to preserve reproductive function. Therapy with Methotrexate (4-amino-n[10]-methyl pteroylglutamic acid) has eradicated hormonal and clinical evidence of disease in almost all treated patients in whom the histopathologic diagnosis was invasive mole. Subsequently many treated women have completed normal pregnancies and delivered normal infants. Hertz and co-workers suggest that the drug be given intramuscularly for five days in a daily dose of 15–20 mgm. The interval between courses ranges from seven to ten days. The frequency of subsequent therapy depends on the go-

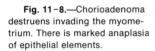

Fig. 11–8.—Chorioadenoma destruens invading the myometrium. There is marked anaplasia of epithelial elements.

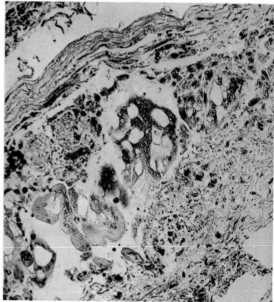

nadotropin response and the severity of toxic symptoms (Fig. 11–9). The hepatic and renal status must be determined before and during each course of treatment. Equally important is the determination of leukocytes and platelets daily during the first course and at least on alternate days during subsequent courses. The intervals between courses are dependent upon the severity of the resulting toxicity. Methotrexate is extremely toxic and therefore symptoms of stomatitis, intestinal irritation, or a cutaneous skin rash temporarily interdicts further therapy. The stomatitis may be detected early by giving the patient fruit juices daily. A burning or stinging of the tongue and mouth will be noted prior to actual stomatitis. The stomatitis usually precedes the leukopenia and other serious toxic reactions. To minimize life threatening toxicity, treatment should not be initiated or continued when any one of the following is encountered: (1) a white blood

Fig. 11–9.—Graph showing the gonadotropin response to chemotherapy in a patient with invasive mole treated with Methotrexate.

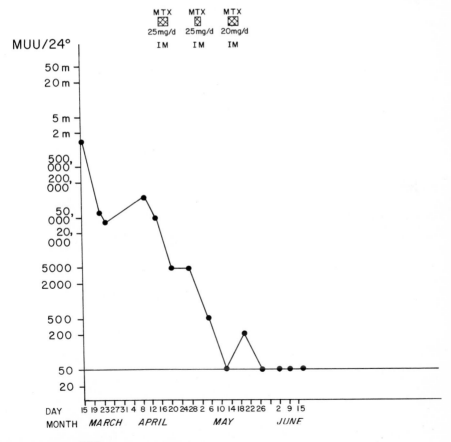

M.H.   AGE 23   G₁ P₀
Clinical Dx: Non – Met. T. D.
Operations: Hysterotomy   3 / 8 / 67   H M (Gp Ⅲ)

count less than 2500 per cu. mm., (2) a polymorphonuclear leukocyte count less than 1500 per cu. mm., (3) a platelet count less than 100,000 per cu. mm., (4) a significant rise in the serum transaminase levels.

Since toxic manifestations of drug therapy are largely predictable rather than idiosyncratic, clinical experience is essential in the proper appraisal

Fig. 11–10.—Graph summarizes the gonadotropin response in a patient with metastatic trophoblastic disease in whom remission was achieved with infusion of Methotrexate via the hypogastric arteries. Initial therapy with systemic Methotrexate and actinomycin D was followed by regression of the pulmonary lesion and an initial drop in the titer. Excessive hematologic toxicity prevented further systemic therapy despite persistence of gonadotropin titer. Pelvic arteriography revealed tumor in the left broad ligament adjacent to the lateral uterine wall. Catheters were inserted bilaterally via the inguinal route.

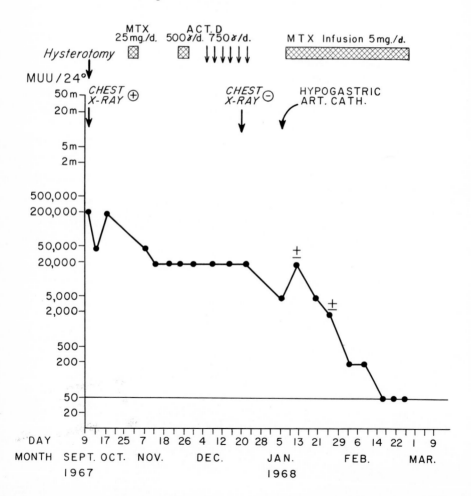

of severity. Therapy is continued until gonadotropin levels return to normal pituitary values. If resistence to drug therapy or excessive toxicity is encountered, hysterectomy should be performed even if the patient strongly desires subsequent pregnancy. In patients with resistant localized disease or excessive toxic reactions to systemic therapy, remission has been achieved by utilizing hypogastric artery infusion therapy. Catheters are inserted via the retroperitoneal route through bilateral inguinal incisions. One-fourth the usual dose of Methotrexate (0.1 mgm./kg.) is administered daily over a 4- to 8-hour period using an automatic constant infusion apparatus (Fig. 11–10).

After successful chemotherapy (or hysterectomy), gonadotropin assays should be continued for at least one year after which pregnancy may be permitted. If metastases are present, a similar therapeutic regimen should be instituted. Hysterectomy is not indicated regardless of the age or parity of the patient unless a surgical indication is present.

Choriocarcinoma

A choriocarcinoma is composed of pure malignant trophoblast in contrast to the locally invasive molar villi of chorioadenoma destruens and the benign molar villi of hydatidiform mole. This lesion may be localized anywhere within the uterus and usually shows a red, granular, hemorrhagic surface which may be discrete or diffuse throughout the cavity. Metastases occur early and generally are widespread. Chorionic villi are not seen grossly except in the rare case of simultaneously occurring choriocarcinoma and chorioadenoma destruens. Microscopically, the tissue recapitulates the pattern exhibited by the early villous ovum. There is a typical plexiform pattern of pure trophoblast with admixture of blood clot and fragments of necrotic decidua or myometrium (Fig. 11–11).

Fig. 11–11.—Typical plexiform arrangement of trophoblastic cells in choriocarcinoma.

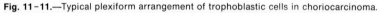
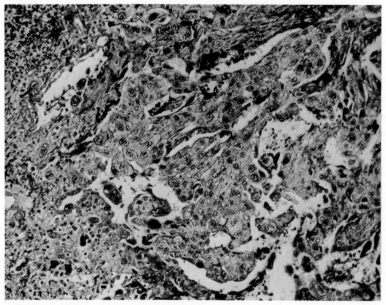

Choriocarcinoma may develop subsequent to an hydatidiform mole, an abortion, an ectopic or a full-term pregnancy. Hertig and Sheldon have indicated that about 2.5 per cent of hydatidiform moles progress to choriocarcinoma. The usual symptom is that of persistent abnormal uterine bleeding. However, if the chorionic malignancy is located deep in the myometrium, uterine bleeding may not be present. In certain patients the only symptoms may be due to the presence of metastases. The organs most commonly invaded are the lungs, vagina, brain, liver, and kidney.

A diagnosis of choriocarcinoma should be suspected in any patient in whom persistent bleeding occurs subsequent to the termination of a normal pregnancy, an hydatidiform mole, or an abortion. The presence of hemoptysis together with a positive result of a test for HCG is practically diagnostic of pulmonary metastases; usually the chest x-ray shows definite evidence of such lesions. In some patients metastases may be seen in the vagina or cervix. A diagnosis of choriocarcinoma is made most often by uterine curettage since large masses of endometrial tissue show anaplastic trophoblast in the absence of villi. Bilateral ovarian tumors due to theca lutein cysts may co-exist if the gonadotropin titer is markedly elevated. Liver lesions are generally silent unless capsular rupture occurs. Similarly brain lesions may go undiagnosed until hemiplegia or other neurologic abnormalities becomes manifest. Detection of metastases is possible by hepatic scan and arteriography and brain scan and electroencephalography. Since the histologic diagnosis of choriocarcinoma is frequently difficult or treacherous because of variations in the pathologic material, and because of the rarity of this condition, the general pathologist is advised to seek consultation.

When a presumptive diagnosis of choriocarcinoma is made by curettage and metastases are absent, therapy should be based on the patient's desire for subsequent pregnancy. Hysterectomy is suggested as primary therapy in most patients. Preoperative Methotrexate is advocated because of the poor prognosis associated with this disease. Without chemotherapy, only 42 per cent of patients with choriocarcinoma survive five years even if metastases are not present at the time of hysterectomy. If metastases are present and chemotherapy is not utilized, the five-year-survival rate is 19 per cent. Hertz has suggested that hysterectomy increases the possibility of embolization of malignant cells and diminishes survival time.

When the patient desires subsequent pregnancy, chemotherapy alone may be employed if the choriocarcinoma is apparently localized to the uterus. However, Hertz reported that even with intensive chemotherapy about one-third of patients will require hysterectomy because of persistently high levels of HCG due to the presence of a resistant choriocarcinoma in the myometrium.

In patients with metastatic choriocarcinoma the optimum treatment is chemotherapy alone. Hysterectomy does not influence the response to drug treatment or survival and is therefore unnecessary. The indications for surgery are limited to emergencies or the presence of a large pelvic mass. Hertz recently reported his results in the treatment of metastatic choriocarcinoma with Methotrexate, Vinblastine and actinomycin D. Of 75 patients with choriocarcinoma the remission rate was approximately 60 per cent, whereas of 34 patients with metastatic mole the remission rate following chemotherapy alone was 95 per cent. The over-all remission rate, as determined by hormonal assay, x-ray evaluation, and physical examination, was approximately 75 per cent. Hertz now suggests that sequential treatment with Methotrexate and actinomycin D affords optimum therapeutic results. If impaired hepatic function exists when the patient is first seen, Methotrexate is contraindicated and actinomycin D is substituted. Hertz estimates that a remission rate of approximately 50 per cent in patients with metastatic disease may be obtained with Methotrexate alone. If the disease recurs or fails to regress following Methotrexate therapy, treatment with actinomycin D is given and an additional remission may be expected in 50 per cent of these patients. Thus, an estimated over-all remission rate of 75 per cent has been obtained with this sequential method.

· BIBLIOGRAPHY

Acosta-Sison, H.: Chorioadenoma destruens: A report of 41 cases, Am. J. Obst. & Gynec. 80:176, 1960.

Bagshawe, K.: An Analysis of Tumor Growth Based on HCG Production by Trophoblastic Tumors, Fourth Rochester Trophoblast Conference, p. 305, 1967.

Bardawil, W. A.; Hertig, A. T., and Velardo, J. T.: Regression of trophoblast, Obst. & Gynec. 10:614, 1957.

Bonano, P., et al.: Estrogen levels in hydatidiform mole, Am. J. Obst. & Gynec. 87:210, 1963.

Brewer, J. I., et al.: Chemotherapy in trophoblastic diseases, Am. J. Obst. & Gynec. 90:566, 1964.

Brewer, J. I.; Rinehart, J. J., and Dunbar, R. W.: Choriocarcinoma: A report of the 5 or more years' survival from the Albert Mathieu Chorion Epithelioma Registry, Am. J. Obst. & Gynec. 81:574, 1961.

Coppleson, M.: Hydatidiform mole and its complications, J. Obst. & Gynaec. Brit. Emp. 65:238, 1958.

Douglas, G. W.: Diagnosis and management of hydatidiform mole, S. Clin. North America 37:379, 1957.

Douglas, G. W., et al.: Trophoblast in the circulating blood during pregnancy, Am. J. Obst. & Gynec. 78:960, 1959.

Goldstein, D. P., et al.: Radioimmunoassay of serum chorionic gonadotropin activity in normal pregnancy, Am. J. Obst. & Gynec. 102:110, 1968.

———, Couch, N., and Hall, T. C.: Infusion therapy in the treatment of patients with choriocarcinoma and related trophoblastic tumors, S. Forum 13:426, 1967.

———, Gore, H., and Reid, D. E.: Management of gestational trophoblastic disease, GP 35:114, 1967.

Gore, H., and Hertig, A. T.: Problems in the histologic interpretation of the trophoblast, Clin. Obst. & Gynec. 10:269, 1967.

Hertig, A. T.: Hydatidiform mole and chorion epithelioma, in Meigs, J. V., and Sturgis, S. H. (eds.): *Progress in Gynecology* (New York: Grune & Stratton, Inc., 1950), vol. 2.

———, and Mansell, H.: Tumors of the Female Sex Organs: Part 1. Hydatidiform Mole and Choriocarcinoma, sec. IX, fasc. 33 of *Atlas of Tumor Pathology* (Washington, D. C.: Armed Forces Inst. of Pathology, 1956).

———, and Sheldon, W. H.: Hydatidiform mole–a pathologico-clinical correlation of 200 cases, Am. J. Obst. & Gynec. 53:1, 1947.

Hertz, R.; Lewis, J., Jr., and Lipsett, M. B.: Five years' experience with the chemotherapy of metastatic choriocarcinoma and related trophoblastic tumors in women, Am. J. Obst. & Gynec. 82:631, 1961.

———, et al.: Chemotherapy of choriocarcinoma and related trophoblastic tumors in women, J.A.M.A. 168:845, 1958.

Hertz, R.; Ross, G. T., and Lipsett, M. B.: Primary chemotherapy of non-metastatic trophoblastic disease in women, Am. J. Obst. & Gynec. 86:808, 1963.

Hunt, W.; Dockerty, M. B., and Randall, L. M.: Hydatidiform mole, Obst. & Gynec. 1:593, 1953.

Klinefelter, H. F., Jr., Albright, F., and Griswold, G. C.: Experience with a quantitative test for normal or decreased amounts of follicle-stimulating hormone in urine in endocrinological diagnoses, J. Clin. Endocrinol. 3:529, 1943.

Lewis, J., Jr.; Gore, H., Hertig, A. T., and Goss, D. A.: Treatment of trophoblastic disease. With rationale for the use of adjunctive chemotherapy at the time of indicated operation, Am. J. Obst. & Gynec. 96:710, 1966.

Lewis, J., Jr.; Ketchum, A. S., and Hertz, R.: Surgical intervention during chemotherapy of gestational trophoblastic neoplasms, Cancer 19:1517, 1966.

Manahan, C. P.; Benitez, I., and Estrella, F.: Amethopterin in the treatment of trophoblastic tumors, Am. J. Obst. & Gynec. 82:641, 1961.

Novak, E.: Pathological aspects of hydatidiform mole and chorion epithelioma, Am. J. Obst. & Gynec. 59:1355, 1950.

———, and Seah, C. S.: Choriocarcinoma of the uterus: Study of 74 cases from the Mathieu Memorial Chorion Epithelioma Registry, Am. J. Obst. & Gynec. 67:933, 1954.

Park, W. W.: The occurrence of sex chromatin in chorion epitheliomas and hydatidiform moles, J. Path. & Bact. 74:197, 1957.
———, and Lees, J. C.: Choriocarcinoma: A general review, with an analysis of 516 cases, Arch. Path. 49:73, 1950.
Rock, J., and Hertig, A. T.: The human conceptus during the first 2 weeks of gestation, Am. J. Obst. & Gynec. 55:6, 1948.
Ross, G. T., *et al.*: Sequential use of Methotrexate and actinomycin D in the treatment of metastatic choriocarcinoma and related trophoblastic diseases in women, Am. J. Obst. & Gynec. 93:223, 1965.
———, Hammond, C. B., and Odell, W.: Chemotherapy for non-metastatic gestational trophoblastic neoplasms, Clin. Obst. & Gynec. 10:323, 1967.
Taymor, M. L.: Bioassay and immunoassay of human chorionic gonadotropin (HCG), Clin. Obst. & Gynec. 10:303, 1967.
Yen, S. S. C., Pearson, O. H., and Rankin, J. S.: Radioimmunoassay of serum chorionic gonadotropin and placental lactogen in trophoblastic disease, Obst. & Gynec. 32:86, 1968.

CHAPTER 12

Endocrine Disorders

DURING THE PAST decade the gynecologist has been called upon to diagnose and treat an increasing number of female disorders which involve abnormal function rather than disease processes affecting structure. Surgical therapy is still an important aspect of the specialty of gynecology but the most spectacular advances during the past decade have occurred in endocrine parameters, particularly the inter-relationship of the hypothalamus, pituitary, adrenal and ovary. For example, infertility may be caused by lack of ovulation which is corrected by the administration of hydrocortisone if the basic defect is due to acquired adrenal hyperplasia. Similarly, the persistent amenorrhea and galactorrhea which occur after pregnancy, the Chiari–Frommel syndrome, frequently respond to the administration of clomiphene citrate. Perhaps even more dramatic is the relief afforded the premenopausal female whose daily activities are severely limited by excessive and irregular uterine bleeding. Although these symptoms merely represent the inability of the aging ovary to secrete estrogen and progesterone in proper sequence, hysterectomy has been the only definitive therapeutic approach short of intra-cavitary radium or castration by x-ray. The administration of properly selected estrogen-progestin combinations to these patients results in regular and scanty bleeding which may be continued until the menopause. As a bonus, the patient is afforded conception control and amelioration of symptoms due to estrogen insufficiency.

This chapter considers the major abnormalities of endocrine function affecting "femaleness." It includes various disorders of menstruation which result from either inadequate or excessive secretion of pituitary, thyroid or adrenal glands. Specific endocrinopathies such as congenital adrenal hyperplasia, Cushing's syndrome, Sheehan's syndrome and Simmond's disease are discussed in a manner which permits diagnostic and therapeutic approaches by the practicing gynecologist, internist or general practitioner. The distressing and frequently perplexing problem of hirsutism is similarly treated. Although the precise cause of dysmenorrhea is not known, suppression of ovulation usually results in the occurrence of regular, painless menses.

Thus, in this chapter, an effort is made to outline the abnormal physiologic processes which produce gynecologic disorders and to suggest hormonal methods of control.

Premature Onset of the Menses

When uterine bleeding appears before the age of 10 years, it is generally considered to be abnormal and usually is associated with other symptoms and signs of so-called precocious sexual maturity. Although breast development (thelarche) and growth of pubic hair (pubarche) may normally occur in the female as early as the eighth or ninth year, the menarche usually occurs after age 10. Precocity may be due to either *constitutional* or *organic* causes. By and large, in most patients seen because of this symptom, subsequent classification will be that of constitutional etiology. However, it is important to distinguish these patients from those who may have menarche subsequent to lesions of the brain, ovary or adrenal.

While other factors undoubtedly are of importance, gonadal function depends primarily on the actions of the gonadotropins, which, in the absence of pregnancy, are secreted by the adenohypophysis. Without the pituitary, gonads atrophy and function drops to a low level. It is the present consensus that formation and release of the gonadotropins are regulated through the hypothalamus, which acts as the integrator of information from both the external and internal environment. The information reaches the hypothalamus over neuronal and humoral pathways. The channels of communication between the hypothalamus and the pituitary are vascular—the portal system of blood vessels. The means of communication are therefore limited to blood-borne chemical agents. Direct neuronal connections

Fig. 12–1.—Diagram showing method of production of amenorrhea and galactorrhea. At the left, luteotropic hormone is suppressed by hypothalamic-inhibiting factor. At the right, total blockade of hypothalamic-releasing factors produces amenorrhea whereas blockade of luteotropic-inhibiting factor permits release of constant luteotropin or prolactin. (Courtesy of Dr. Herbert Kupperman.)

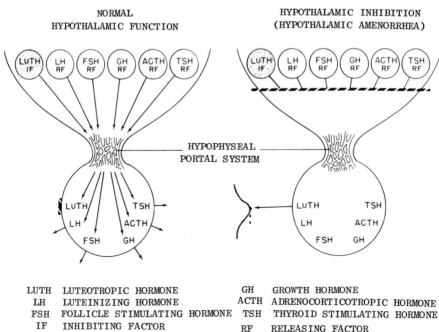

LUTH	LUTEOTROPIC HORMONE	GH GROWTH HORMONE
LH	LUTEINIZING HORMONE	ACTH ADRENOCORTICOTROPIC HORMONE
FSH	FOLLICLE STIMULATING HORMONE	TSH THYROID STIMULATING HORMONE
IF	INHIBITING FACTOR	RF RELEASING FACTOR

to the adenohypophysis appear to be restricted to fibers that are associated with blood vessels. (See Fig. 12–1.)

Just as gonadal function depends on gonadotropins elaborated by the pituitary, so does pituitary function depend on substances elaborated by the hypothalamus. When the vascular connections between the pituitary and the hypothalamus are severed, the synthesis of trophic hormone ceases. Only the production of prolactin is maintained—in fact, it increases. Electric stimulation of the hypothalamus or infusion of hypothalamic extracts into the pituitary has been found to induce ovulation. Recently, it has been shown that a pituitary transplanted under the kidney capsule and allowed to atrophy can be resuscitated when a hypothalamic extract is infused into the renal artery.

Szentágothai and co-workers have attempted to map out the areas of the hypothalamus where the regulatory factors originate. They implanted the pituitary into various sites in the hypothalamus of hypophysectomized animals. Only pituitaries that were located within a well-defined region in the median basal hypothalamus maintained their structure and function. This region of the hypothalamus has been termed the hypophysiotropic zone.

From this zone a series of fine axons has been traced to the region of the capillary network of the pituitary portal system in the stalk-median eminence region. Within these nerve fibers, fine granules perhaps representing neurosecretory products, have been observed. When the hypophysiotropic zone and pituitary are isolated from the rest of the brain, the structure of the pituitary and of its target organs is maintained. However, cyclic ovarian function is abolished. The ovaries contain either persistent follicles or, in some cases, persistent corpora lutea. Normal feedback relationships appear to have been abolished. Cyclic ovulation is possible only when the hypophysiotropic area remains connected to the rest of the brain anteriorly. These observations lend support to the postulate that the impulses responsible for the cyclic release of the ovulatory complex of hormones from the pituitary are mediated by a system of nerve fibers which arise from a wide area anteriorly in the septal region and converge toward the medial basal hypothalamus and median eminence. Electric stimulation of this system of neurons results in the release of LH and in ovulation.

Thus, tonic impulses for the maintenance of the gonads may originate in the hypophysiotropic area. For *cyclic* ovarian function, however, modulating influences from other regions of the brain are needed and the hypophysiotropic area may serve as the final common path.

A number of diseases of the endocrine system seem to be the result of interruptions of the hypothalamico-hypophyseal-ovarian circuit at any of a number of points. The region of the hypothalamus affected determines the defects that ensue. Damage of the region of the anterior hypothalamus causes gonadal failure. As lesions enlarge, they often involve the optic chiasm, producing visual disturbances, and may involve the ventromedial nuclei, producing obesity. Occasionally they extend more widely and cause emaciation. Changes in thyroid and adrenal function are less frequent and appear to be the result of more widespread damage. Lesions in the region of the median eminence also produce hypogonadism and, in addition, diabetes insipidus and varying degrees of thyroid and adrenal failure.

Generalized increase in ventricular pressure producing hydrocephalus is often associated with gonadal failure. Occasionally, hydrocephalus causes sexual precocity when other endocrine effects in the patient are minimal. Posterior hypothalamic lesions often produce sexual precocity. Sometimes released gonadotropins are sufficient to cause early maturation but not full gonadal function.

Sexual precocity with gametogenesis can result from posterior hypothalamic damage. In general, the area most frequently involved is the tuber cinereum and the mamillary region. This type of precocity is caused by stimulation of the gonads by pituitary gonadotropins. It is still not known whether the precocity results entirely from increased release of gonadotropin (perhaps through a lowered sensitivity of the hypothalamus to hormonal feedback such as is believed to occur at puberty), or whether the central nervous system lesions make the gonad excessively responsive to gonadotropin.

Even though gonadal function is stimulated to produce both gametes and sex steroids, not all of the children affected excrete detectable gonadotropin in the urine. The reason for this paradox has not been discovered. The demonstration of gonadotropin-inhibiting substances in urine of children and normal subjects has led to an interesting speculation that this type of precocity results from a deficit of the inhibitor.

The earliest cases of sexual precocity are the result of hamartomas. Constitutional precocity is the commonest form in girls, whereas this diagnosis is rarely warranted in boys. A much higher proportion of boys than girls have tumors in the region of the hypothalamus, producing precocity. Even in girls the diagnosis of constitutional precocity should be made with the reservation that a space-occupying lesion may eventually be discovered.

Constitutional Sexual Precocity

Constitutional sexual precocity may be described as a premature initiation of the normal physiologic and endocrinologic processes of adolescence characterized by breast development, appearance of pubic and axillary hair and menstruation. In some patients menstruation may occur prior to the development of the breasts. In 1944 Novak emphasized the frequency of this idiopathic cause of the menarche and showed that the number of patients with precocious puberty due to granulosa cell tumors of the ovary was relatively small.

The inciting factors in the process of constitutional sexual precocity are unknown. Obviously the signs are due to premature release of gonadotropic substances from the pituitary. It has been assumed that the hypothalamic inhibitory influence has been removed or diminished or that specific changes in ovarian estrogen metabolism may, in some unknown fashion, depress the hypothalamus or stimulate the pituitary.

Symptomatology and Diagnosis.—Uterine bleeding in constitutional sexual precocity has been reported in infants as young as 3 months. Most patients, however, are in the age group 5–8 years (Fig. 12–2), and usually an orderly and normal progression of development of the secondary sex organs takes place as estrogen is secreted from the ovary. However, this sequential pattern of development of breasts and appearance of pubic and axillary hair followed by menstruation is accelerated over the usual length

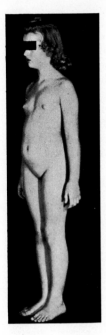

Fig. 12–2.—Constitutional sexual precocity in a girl, 7, who had just noted menarche. Vaginal smear showed evidence of estrogen stimulation. Height was above normal and bone age was 9 years. 17-ketosteroid level was 3 mg./24 hours and gonadotropins 8 m.u.u./24 hours. (From Lloyd, C. W.: The Ovaries, in Williams, R. H. (ed.): *Textbook of Endocrinology* [Philadelphia: W. B. Saunders Company, 1962].)

of time seen in the normal individual. When premature menarche occurs during infancy the bleeding may be the first abnormality noted. Premature breast development is not always due to or associated with constitutional sexual precocity. In a few patients premature thelarche and elevated levels of estrogens have been noted without uterine bleeding or growth of pubic hair. Similarly, the pubarche should not be diagnosed on the basis of vulvar hair growth. The latter is not indicative of sexual precocity.

The secretion of estrogen by the prematurely stimulated ovary results in an acceleration of linear growth and an advancement of bone age. The latter is not usually found when the excess estrogen originates in a neoplastic ovarian tumor, apparently because of the diminished interval between the initiation of estrogen secretion and the development of uterine bleeding in patients with, for example, a granulosa cell ovarian tumor. X-rays of the carpal bones as well as the epiphyses of the knees and elbows will reveal a pronounced developmental acceleration due to prolonged estrogen stimulation. Incidentally, from the viewpoint of differential diagnosis, an x-ray of the skull should also be obtained to exclude pituitary tumor or a site of calcification of the pineal gland. Girls aged 8 or 9 with constitutional sexual precocity usually are taller than their normal counterparts, but only for a two- or three-year period. Because of premature epiphyseal closure, the adult height is usually average or below average. In addition they may show rather excessive feminine hip contour and fat deposition in the buttocks. This appearance occasionally may be emphasized by the relative shortness of the lower extremities compared to the torso.

Certain assays of endocrinologic activity should be done to identify the precise cause of the premature menarche. Since patients with constitutional sexual precocity may or may not ovulate, the basal body temperature graph will not differentiate a granulosa cell ovarian tumor from the anovulatory pattern of the patient with constitutional disease. If the patient with constitutional precocity has cyclic catamenia associated with molimina, the basal body temperature graph will be biphasic, and cyclic changes may also be noted in the vaginal cytology. These findings would serve to differentiate constitutional precocity from that due to an adrenal or ovarian tumor. Actually adrenal tumors which secrete sufficient estrogen to produce precocious puberty in the female are extremely rare. Assays of gonadotropins in urine in females with precocious puberty have given results in the range usually seen in persons having normal menarche. These gonadotropic substances have demonstrated both follicle-stimulating and luteinizing activity. Usually, 17-ketosteroids are found to be within the normal range, whereas determinations of estrogen in urine give abnormally high values for this age group.

Diagnostic criteria in premature menstruation of constitutional etiology may be summarized as follows: a gradual development of the breasts and growth of pubic hair followed by uterine bleeding; an initial acceleration of linear growth and x-ray evidence of advanced bone age; an x-ray of the skull showing a normal sella turcica with possibly a calcified pineal gland; elevated levels of estrogens and pituitary gonadotropins in urine with normal 17-ketosteroids and 17-hydroxycorticoids. Kupperman has pointed out the value of a therapeutic response to progestational steroids in differentiating constitutional sexual precocity from bleeding due to granulosa cell ovarian tumors. As previously noted, the vaginal smear in constitutional precocious puberty will show cornification as a result of estrogen secretion, or secretory changes as a result of cyclic estrogen and progesterone if the patient happens to be ovulating. The vaginal smear in a patient with a granulosa cell ovarian tumor will show only proliferative, cornified cells. Kupperman found that norethindrone, norethynodrel or medroxyprogesterone given in adequate doses will suppress gonadotropic secretion, so that in sexual precocity of constitutional type, which is dependent on excess secretion of gonadotropins, there will subsequently be diminished gonadal estrogen. Thus, following administration of these agents, the vaginal smear will be made up mostly of basal cells (similar to that in the castrate). Since the progestins will not suppress the estrogen originating in a granulosa cell ovarian tumor, the vaginal smear following administration of these agents will show an atypical secretory effect. In diagnosis of precocious puberty due to adrenal neoplasm, intravenous pyelography, a flat plate of the abdomen and presacral air insufflation may be of help if sufficient enlargement of the adrenal gland has occurred.

Treatment.—The therapeutic approach in patients with premature bleeding due to constitutional sexual precocity is one of preventing the premature closure of epiphyses. To accomplish this, it is necessary to diminish or to negate the secretion of endogenous pituitary gonadotropins. Before the development of the newer progestational agents, therapy involved repeated injections of gonadotropic extracts from sheep, hogs or cattle. The extracts served as antigonadotropins, and titers of antigonadotropic substances could be determined. These extracts had to be given continuously to maintain an effective antigonadotropic level. After they were discontinued gonadal function resumed and normal development and menstruation occurred. With the advent of the progestational agents this therapy has become outmoded. Kupperman prefers depo-medroxypro-gesterone (Depo-Provera) to norethynodrel and norethindrone, since the latter are somewhat estrogenic and may be conducive to accelerating epi-physeal closure. This activity has not been noted with Depo-Provera which may be administered in a dose of 100–150 mg. intramuscularly every seven to 14 days. Such a dose will suppress the pituitary gonadotropins and will reduce the secretion of gonads to castration levels. A diminution in breast size will be noted, together with diminished estrogenic activity in the vagi-nal smear. Amenorrhea will usually follow. The bone age of the patient may be followed in order to determine the duration of therapy. After the patient has secured adequate stature, injections of this progestational agent should be discontinued.

The use of medroxyprogesterone acetate has occasionally been disap-pointing. Although menses and breast development have been suppressed, accelerated skeletal maturation has not been arrested. This may be due to delay in initiating treatment. When precocious puberty occurs at a very early age marked stunting of growth must be anticipated and unless epi-physeal closure is averted, the primary purpose of therapy is defeated.

Phenothiazine derivatives not only suppress ovarian function but also interfere with growth, perhaps by inhibition of growth hormone. Chlorpro-mazine, the most potent drug in this group, may negate premature release of FSH and LH. During puberty secretion of FSH and LH releasing factors by the hypothalamus is prevented by tonic inhibitory influences, probably neural in nature. Patients with idiopathic precocious puberty have been shown to have an increased incidence of abnormal electro-encephalo-grams which may revert to normal patterns after the administration of chlorpromazine. Lacey has reported two patients with constitutional pre-cocious puberty who responded to the administration of chlorpromazine in a dose of 25 mg. four times daily. The effect may be temporary and retreatment may be needed.

PREMATURE MENSTRUATION DUE TO ORGANIC CAUSES

Cerebral Lesions.—Animal experimentation has demonstrated that destructive lesions in the posterior hypothalamus cause premature pubes-cence. As a result of these observations and of clinical studies in patients with tumors of the hypothalamus, it has been suggested that the intrinsic posterior hypothalamic lesion interferes specifically with the hypophyseal portal circulation, resulting in excess secretion of pituitary gonadotropin (Fig. 12–3). The normal inhibitory influence of the hypothalamus on the pituitary is thereby removed, allowing for premature secretion of stored gonadotropins. Tumors of the pineal body may result in sexual precocity because of their proximity to and subsequent destruction of the posterior hypothalamus. Conclusive evidence that a hormonal secretion from a pineal tumor induces sexual precocity is lacking. Other cerebral lesions such as granulomas, hamartomas or hyperplasia of the tuber cinereum may also affect hypothalamic function, with precocious sexual develop-ment resulting. It is impossible to distinguish patients with sexual precocity on the basis of hypothalamic midbrain tumors from patients with constitu-tional sexual precocity unless x-ray examination reveals the presence of a pinealoma or other variety of space-occupying lesion. Occasionally neuro-

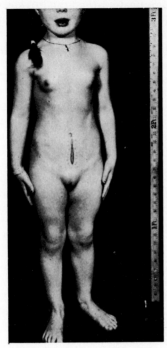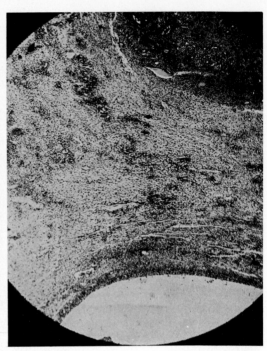

Fig. 12–3.—Sexual precocity due to hypothalamic lesion in 3½-year-old child with vaginal bleeding. Bone age was 4 years, the sella turcica normal. Gonadotropin excretion was 16 m.u.u./24 hours; 17-ketosteroid 2 mg./24 hours, and estrogens in urine 20 μg./24 hours. An electroencephalogram showed changes localizing the lesion in the hypothalamus; the pneumoencephalogram excluded tumor. Therapy with medroxyprogesterone resulted in complete disappearance of precocious maturation. The midline scar was due to an unwarranted exploration after the first episode of bleeding. Photomicrograph at right shows active ovarian stroma and a cystic graafian follicle obtained by biopsy at the time of laparotomy. (From Lloyd, C. W.: The Ovaries, in Williams, R. H. (ed.): *Textbook of Endocrinology* [Philadelphia: W. B. Saunders Company, 1962].)

logic symptoms due to the expanding intracranial lesion may be of value in differential diagnosis. However, in many patients with lesions of the hypothalamus the neurologic examination and roentgenograms of the skull are normal. An electroencephalogram may be of diagnostic aid in such patients. Mental retardation, grand mal or petit mal attacks may occur. Endocrine assays reveal elevation in the pituitary gonadotropin and estrogen levels, with normal range for 17-ketosteroids and 17-hydroxycorticoids. Thus it is impossible to distinguish this type of sexual precocity from the constitutional variety on the basis of the endocrinologic survey.

POSTENCEPHALITIC STATES.—Sexual maturation including menarche may follow a siege of encephalitis regardless of the cause of the infection. The precise mechanism for the initiation of precocity is unknown, but apparently hypothalamic suppression is removed, with subsequent release of pituitary gonadotropins.

MENINGITIS.—Precocious sexual maturity and the onset of menarche may rarely follow a severe case of meningitis, especially of tuberculous origin.

CRANIAL TRAUMA.—Occasionally a skull injury, with or without fracture, may precipitate precocious sexual development and menarche. Four to eight weeks is the average latent period.

The treatment of precocious sexual maturation following encephalitis, injury to the skull or meningitis is exactly the same. Suppression of pituitary gonadotropins is desirable until linear bone growth has been attained. Therapeutic measures utilizing depo-medroxyprogesterone as previously outlined are of value.

Adrenocortical Hyperfunction.—As noted in the classification of precocious puberty, premature menarche may be due to the production of estrogen in the young female by either the adrenal gland or the ovary. The premature menarche in these patients is part of the syndrome of precocious *pseudopuberty.* This differential classification is based on the fact that in true precocious puberty ovulation eventually appears if the patient is untreated, and normal ovulatory cycles and even pregnancy may occur. In pseudopuberty, the development of the target organs is due to the secretion of estrogen by a tumor of the adrenal gland or ovary and is not secondary to stimulation by pituitary gonadotropins.

Adrenal tumors.—Although adrenocortical hyperfunction may result in the development of axillary and pubic hair and an increased rate of skeletal growth, vaginal bleeding is rare. However, it must be included in this group for completion. In the report of Goldstein *et al.,* vaginal bleeding was found in only 2 of 44 cases associated with adrenal carcinoma. The development of adrenal hyperplasia, adenoma or malignancy usually delays the onset of normal menstruation in prepubescent females. The differential diagnosis should not be difficult because, even in the presence of vaginal bleeding, breast development is unusual but clitoral enlargement is common. Careful physical examination together with a determination of urinary 17-ketosteroids will suffice to differentiate the site of hormone production. The level of 17-ketosteroids in urine is elevated, the degree depending on whether adrenal hyperplasia, adenoma or neoplasm is present.

Ovarian tumors.—The isosexual type of precocious pseudopuberty is more often due to estrogen-producing tumors of the ovary. Although these lesions are quite rare, they are usually assumed to be the cause of precocious bleeding in most young females. Pedowitz, Felmus and Mackles reviewed the literature in 1955 and were able to find precocious pseudopuberty in only 85 patients. Sixty-five of these had granulosa-theca cell tumors, 3 had dysgerminomas, 12 teratomas, and 5 were reported as "follicular cysts." Thus it should be remembered that only about 5 per cent of granulosa cell tumors and only 1 per cent of thecomas occur before puberty. Pedowitz and associates reported two cases of precocious pseudopuberty, one in a 14-month-old infant with a thecoma and one in a 10-year-old girl with a granulosa cell tumor.

The youngest reported case of precocious puberty due to an ovarian tumor was in an infant, 14 weeks of age. Premature bleeding was most commonly seen in the granulosa-theca cell group, 56 patients having this symptom. In 74 patients of the total 85, vaginal bleeding was part of the symptomatology (Fig. 12–4).

Endocrine assays may be of extreme value in differential diagnosis. As previously mentioned, hormone levels corresponding to those of normal adults (cyclic estrogen-progesterone and normal gonadotropins) suggest

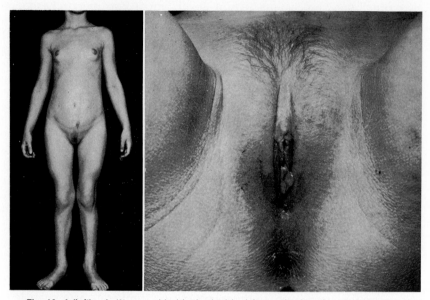

Fig. 12–4 (left).—A 4½-year-old girl who had had four episodes of vaginal bleeding in 5 months. She was tall and had a bone age of 6 years. Rectal examination: uterus, 4 cm. long; no ovarian enlargement. Vaginal smear showed marked estrogen effect. Gonadotropin excretion, negative at 4 m.u.u./24 hr.; pregnanediol excretion, 3.3 mg./24 hr. Diagnosis: luteinized granulosa cell tumor.

Fig. 12–5 (right).—Genitalia of patient shown in Figure 12–4. There is maturation of the structures but no clitoral enlargement.

(Lloyd, C. W., in Williams' *Textbook of Endocrinology* (3d ed.; Philadelphia: W. B. Saunders Company, 1962.)

true precocious puberty. Increased levels of estrogen with absence of cyclic variation strongly suggest a granulosa-theca cell tumor. Solid teratomas and dysgerminomas which contain chorionic elements may be associated with elevated levels of gonadotropins in urine, occasionally sufficient to give positive results in a test for pregnancy. The estrogen production by the theca cells of the granulosa-theca cell tumors is undoubtedly responsible for the premature menses, breast enlargement, increased bone age and acceleration of linear growth. In the vaginal smear there is a high percentage of cornified cells but without evidence of progesterone activity. The levels of gonadotropins and 17-ketosteroids in patients with feminizing granulosa-theca cell tumors are normal.

The diagnosis of an ovarian neoplasm as a cause for precocious pseudopuberty may be aided by the abdominal and rectovaginal examinations. Of the 85 patients in the study of Pedowitz and associates, 76 were found to have an abdominal mass and 65 a pelvic mass. In addition, 21 of these patients complained of pain and 12 had ascites.

Premature uterine bleeding may be one of the symptoms in solid teratoma of the ovary and, indeed, it was a presenting complaint in 10 of 12 cases reported by Pedowitz and associates. These tumors contained chorionic elements which secrete gonadotropic hormone. Therefore, the contralateral ovary may be stimulated by the chorionic gonadotropin to produce sufficient estrogen for endometrial proliferation and subsequent vaginal bleeding. Assays of chorionic gonadtropins in urine in patients with tera-tomas will frequently show elevated values. Chorionic tissue was identi-fied in eight of the 12 teratomas reported in the literature. The sexual precocity associated with lesions of this type is not accompanied by ovula-tion and therefore the vaginal smear will show evidence of estrogen effect only and the basal body temperature will be monophasic. Another diagnos-tic point is the absence of axillary hair in prepubescent females with ovarian teratomas. Thus the finding of premature bleeding with sexual precocity, breast development, absent axillary hair and high urinary go-nadotropin levels (which may give a positive pregnancy test result) is in-dicative of a solid teratoma of the ovary, particularly if a pelvis mass is palpable.

The mortality rate in patients with embryonic solid teratoma is almost 100 per cent. Despite the high degree of malignancy, complete hysterec-tomy and bilateral salpingo-oophorectomy should be performed. Neither Methotrexate nor other chemotherapeutic agents have been of value in nongestational chorionic tumors.

Precocious puberty due to dysgerminomas has also been associated with elevated gonadotropin levels in urine. Unsuspected choriomatous tissue was probably present, although not identified, in these patients. In the usual type of dysgerminoma occurring in the adult female, specific elabora-tion of chorionic gonadotropin has not been described except in one recently reported case. Occasionally granulosa-theca cell elements may be found in a dysgerminoma which, because of the elevated levels of estrogen secre-tion, may cause sexual precocity and uterine bleeding.

The removal of the ovarian neoplasm usually results in a rapid fall of the previously elevated levels of gonadotropin and estrogen. Reappearance of such hormonal entities, prior to the menarche, suggests a recurrence of the original tumor or the possibility of distant metastases.

Since in more than 90 per cent of patients precocious puberty will be found to be of constitutional or idiopathic type, exploratory laparotomy for patients with sexual precocity is not warranted unless ovarian enlarge-ment can be identified. Ovarian neoplasms which show surface or perito-neal extension and are nonencapsulated are preferably treated by complete hysterectomy and bilateral salpingo-oophorectomy. In the case of a neo-plasm of relatively low malignancy, such as an encapsulated granulosa-theca cell tumor, unilateral salpingo-oophorectomy is the treatment of choice. Most patients having the latter lesion were living and well without evidence of disease from three to five years following surgery in the series of Pedowitz and associates.

The treatment of encapsulated dysgerminomas has usually, in the past, been conservative because of the belief that this neoplasm was relatively benign. Recent evidence, however, by Pedowitz, Felmus and Grayzel in-dicates a five-year mortality rate of 73 per cent with a tendency toward early recurrence. In addition, involvement of the contralateral ovary has been reported in about 35 per cent of patients. In view of this high mortality rate and the bilaterality of the lesion complete extirpation of the pelvic organs seems warranted (see Chap. 7).

A unilateral cystic ovary has been described in several patients with premature menarche as well as other signs of premature pubescence. Such lesions may result from pituitary gonadotropic stimulation associated either with lesions of the hypothalamus or with true constitutional sexual precocity. In several instances, however, removal of the ovarian cyst was followed by regression of the signs of sexual precocity. Removal of such a cyst is adequate therapy; the ovary should be preserved.

Albright's Syndrome.—This syndrome consists of sexual precocity associated with disseminated bone lesions of cystic variety and patchy areas of increased skin pigmentation. Sometimes called polyostotic fibrous dysplasia, the disease is of unknown etiology although it was once thought to be related to involvement of the base of the skull by fibrous dysplasia. Sexual precocity has been noted, however, in patients without cranial lesions. Benedict reviewed the reported cases and concluded that the disease should be classified in the group of precocious pseudopuberty, since ovulation does not occur nor is there evidence of increased gonadotropin in the urine. In patients with Albright's syndrome ovulation subsequently occurs at the time of normal pubescence, and fertility is not impaired.

The various skin lesions have been described as café-au-lait macular spots of irregular size and shape. The cystic changes in the bones may lead to spontaneous fractures, and sclerotic overgrowth of the cranial bones may result in facial disfigurement. Occasionally pressure on the optic nerve may occur. There is no intrinsic abnormality of calcium or phosphorus metabolism, and there is no specific therapy for the bone abnormalities. Treatment is the same as that recommended for constitutional sexual precocity.

Miscellaneous Causes.—A report of Van Wyk and Grumbach has indicated that precocious menstruation, enlargement of the breasts and galactorrhea may be associated with or due to juvenile hypothyroidism. Pubic hair was not present in their patients, nor was there an advancement in bone age. These authors suggested that the pituitary gland responded to the thyroid deficiency by an increased secretion of gonadotropin as well as thyroid-stimulating hormone, with precocious sexual development and galactorrhea. Administration of thyroid extract resulted in cessation of galactorrhea and regression of the signs of sexual precocity.

Certain individuals with the XXX chromosome syndrome may note precocious puberty and premature onset of menstruation. (See Chapter 16.)

Pseudosexual precocity in a few instances has been the result of accidental administration of estrogens to prepubescent females. Diagnosis should be obvious from the history, although in certain cases the parents may be unaware of the hormone content of certain medications.

Delayed Menarche

This term is used here to describe the absence of menstruation in girls between ages 16 and 18 and further implies the presence of a functionally normal pituitary gland as well as the presence of normal reproductive organs which have not been adequately stimulated. The age at which the female secondary sex characteristics appear varies considerably. In any large series, approximately 5 per cent of girls will have their first menstrual period between 16 and 18 and almost 1 per cent will not have their first period until age 18–20. It has been noted that daughters tend to follow the pattern of menarche set by their mothers, indicating the importance of certain genetic factors in this regard. The menarche may also be delayed by marked obesity, malnutrition, anorexia nervosa or schizophrenia.

Delay of the menarche may be considered under three general classifications: constitutional, hypogonadotropism and hypogonadism.

Constitutional Delay in Menarche

The majority of patients with delayed adolescent development manifest no demonstrable organic pathology. The developmental retardation in these individuals represents a normal variation in endocrine function which will usually be rectified by time alone. For this reason, a most perplexing problem is *when* to commence a diagnostic program. The answer lies in the individualization of each case, taking into account the history, physical examination and the emotional attitudes of the patient and her family. However, the practice of initiating therapy to promote sexual development is to be deplored unless adequate diagnostic studies have been undertaken.

The endocrine defect in delayed adolescent development and delayed menarche is the lack of proper estrogenic stimulation necessary for maturation of the accessory sex organs and initiation of uterine bleeding. The secretion of estrogen is dependent on the elaboration of gonadotropic hormones from the adenohypophysis. The secretion of gonadotropins may be diminished or entirely lacking. In these individuals, for reasons unknown, it is assumed that both FSH and LH are held in abeyance. Perhaps the necessary stimulation from the anterior septal region of the brain to the basal hypothalamus is inadequate. Malnutrition due to starvation or chronic wasting diseases may be contributory. Similarly, emotional or psychosomatic factors are known causes of secondary amenorrhea and may act to delay the onset of the catamenia. Imbalances of other endocrine organs, such as the thyroid or adrenal glands, may also delay adolescent development and the menarche.

Clinical evaluation of the patients manifesting delayed adolescent development should begin with a complete and thorough history and physical examination. Careful scrutiny of the accessory sex organs and the genitalia is mandatory. The internal genitalia may be examined rectally; negligible mental trauma and physical discomfort ensue if the examiner is reassuring and careful. Roentgenographic study of the skull for evidence of intracranial lesions is imperative in all cases of retarded development and delayed menarche. Neurologic and ophthalmologic examinations are indicated if suspicious signs or symptoms such as headaches, scotomata or diplopia are manifested. The importance of a thorough rectovaginal examination is emphasized by the fact that delayed menarche may on occasion be due to a congenital mechanical obstruction in the vagina or cervix. Most commonly this is an imperforate hymen, and rectal examination reveals accumulated menstrual discharge in the vagina. Normal menses will immediately follow incision into the hymen and relief of the obstruction.

Assay of gonadotropins in urine will distinguish between hypophyseal and ovarian failure. An elevated gonadotropin titer suggests ovarian failure, whereas diminished titers focus attention on hypophyseal dysfunction. Both the total gonadotropin assay for FSH and LH by mouse uterine weight method and the more specific assays for FSH and LH by radio-immunologic methods indicate a marked deficiency in release of these hormones. Estrogens measured in urine or blood are in the range of the prepuberal or postmenopausal female. Yet the function of the endometrium is not altered since uterine bleeding may be induced by the administration of estrogens alone or estrogens followed by progesterone.

As previously stated, the majority of patients with delayed adolescent development manifest no discernible pathology. The prognosis for normal sexual development and reproductive function is excellent. In the absence of proved lesions or hormonal deficiencies, the use of endocrine preparations is deemed inadvisable. Reassurance, explanation and time comprise the desired therapeutic regimen. Systemic abnormalities such as obesity, cachexia, infection and hypothyroidism should be appropriately treated. Adequate psychiatric therapy, if indicated, should be initiated.

HYPOGONADOTROPISM

Lesions of the hypothalamus and pituitary are the most common causes of delayed menarche in this category. Occasionally there may be a specific gonadotropin deficiency associated with a craniopharyngioma (unitropic deficiency). These patients present clinically with signs of sexual infantilism but are not dwarfed. The specific gonadotropic deficit is probably correlated with involvement of the hypothalamus by tumor. Tumors of the third ventricle as well as internal hydrocephalus may be the etiologic factor in delayed menarche or primary amenorrhea.

The prognosis with proved hypothalamic and hypophyseal lesions is guarded, and the assurance of normal pituitary-ovarian function cannot be given. Maturation of the accessory sex organs and initiation of uterine bleeding in these patients are accomplished with substitutional estrogenic therapy after cranial tumors have been excluded. After linear skeletal growth has ceased, administration of estrogens, such as diethylstilbestrol in a dose of 1 mg. daily for 24 consecutive days, will not only result in cyclic withdrawal bleeding but also in appreciable growth and mature development of the breasts and vagina. Withdrawal bleeding usually occurs two to eight days after cessation of treatment, and these cycles may be kept up almost indefinitely. Estinyl may be substituted in a dose of 0.05 mg. daily. If bleeding becomes somewhat irregular this may be improved by the cyclic administration of one of the progestational agents with an estrogen, such as Enovid or Norlestrin. Once maturation of the secondary sex characteristics has been effected, the problem of continuing estrogen therapy to the age of menopause will undoubtedly arise. It is the opinion of the author that, as a result of recent studies on the beta-lipoproteins, the relationship of hypoestrogen states to atherosclerosis and coronary heart disease, it is prophylactically important to continue maintenance doses of estrogen indefinitely in these patients.

HYPOGONADISM

The menarche may be delayed also because of primary hypogonadism. The commonest cause of primary hypogonadism is an abnormality of chromosomal constitution, either an XO configuration (Turner's syndrome) or an XX chromosomal pattern with one of the X chromosomes being morphologically abnormal. Other patients with an XX chromosomal pattern have had congenital abnormalities, including polycystic or hypoplastic ovaries. The stature of the patient is quite helpful in differential diagnosis since it has been observed that most patients with primary amenorrhea due to chromosomal abnormalities were 58 in. or less in height, whereas the incidence of chromosomal abnormalities in young girls over 61 in. in height was rather small. (See Chapter 16.)

Scant or Absent Menstruation

OLIGOMENORRHEA

Oligomenorrhea (G., *oligos*, little; *men*, month; *rhoia*, flow) is the term used to describe a prolongation of the menstrual cycle to more than 35 days. In most patients with this abnormality the menstrual cycle lasts from 90 to 120 days, with menstruation occurring only three to four times yearly. Usually the menstrual flow is of normal duration and is not excessive, although some patients may note profuse flowing and clots on the second and third days of the menses. The term "oligomenorrhea" implies bleeding following ovulation. Therefore the prolonged interval is due to a lengthening of the preovulatory phase since the postovulatory phase is rather constant at 14–16 days.

Normal uterine bleeding occurring at longer than usual intervals is not infrequently encountered during the postmenarchal and premenopausal periods and represents fluctuations in ovarian activity. Although this situation need not represent a symptom of organic disease, lengthening of the menstrual cycle warrants investigation in sterility patients and in certain patients in whom this pattern represents a change from previously established menstrual patterns. Lengthening of the menstrual cycles may herald the approach of secondary amenorrhea. Although the precise pathogenesis remains obscure, relative ovarian failure is probably the causative factor in the vast majority of these patients. Systemic disease, malnutrition, obesity, dysfunction of other endocrine organs and psychic disturbances should also be considered. This variation of menstrual disorder may also be noted in patients with hyperthyroidism or pituitary tumors. It frequently is the presenting or earliest complaint in patients with Stein-Leventhal syndrome. Similarly, in patients with ovarian arrhenoblastomas defeminization occurs before the masculinization, and therefore oligomenorrhea usually precedes the amenorrhea.

The diagnostic and therapeutic procedures applicable to patients with prolonged cycles are similar to those discussed in the evaluation and management of secondary amenorrhea. One of the commonest etiologic factors is that of obesity. Complete restoration of normal cycles may be obtained by strict regulation of dietary intake. In another group of patients the oligomenorrhea may follow the puerperium. This is usually a temporary and self-limited endocrinologic derangement, but normal cycles may be brought about by progestin-induced, "artificial" cycles for three to six months. Thus, the administration of an estrogen-progestin in 20-day cycles will result in normal withdrawal flow and frequently will restore normal cyclic activity. Every effort should be made to determine the cause of anovulation since failure to do so may permit a pituitary, adrenal or ovarian tumor to go undiagnosed for a prolonged interval. In a small number of patients with oligomenorrhea the administration of cortisone in a dose of 10–30 mg. daily will increase the frequency of menstruation. The use of cortisone and clomiphene citrate for this particular indication is discussed under the Stein-Leventhal syndrome (Chapter 7).

PRIMARY AMENORRHEA

Amenorrhea denotes the absence or cessation of uterine bleeding and is a clinical symptom rather than a precise diagnosis. The expression *primary amenorrhea* usually designates failure of the menarche to occur by the eighteenth year of life.

Patients with primary amenorrhea may manifest normal secondary sex characteristics. In most instances, however, primary amenorrhea is associated with so-called hypogonadism, that is, underdevelopment of the breasts, sparse distribution of pubic and axillary hair and retarded maturation of the genitalia.

Etiologic factors are more easily determined if attention is focused on the various anatomic sites important to the initiation of the menstrual process or to the transport of menstrual fluid. These sites include the vaginal tract, uterus, ovaries, thyroid, adrenals, pituitary and hypothalamus.

Mechanical obstruction to the drainage of uterine secretions may occur in the vaginal tract or in the cervical canal. Stenosis in these areas is the result of congenital anomalies or infectious processes. An imperforate hymen is perhaps the most frequently encountered mechanical obstruction in patients with primary amenorrhea. In this condition, the absence of uterine bleeding is associated with intermittent attacks of vaginal, abdominal and lumbosacral pain. A palpable pelvic mass is often discernible. The condition, if unattended, leads progressively to hematocolpos and hematometra. Diagnosis of imperforate hymen is not difficult, and treatment consists in establishment of adequate drainage by hymenotomy. In young girls the diagnosis may be aided by a simple rectal examination which will reveal the accumulation of menstrual effluvium in the distended vaginal canal. The therapeutic procedure of hymenotomy should be carried out in the operating room under anesthesia and a thorough cruciate incision should be made. Patients with obstructive lesions of the vagina or cervix usually show normal ovarian and endometrial function. However, continued normality depends on correction of the mechanical impediment.

Agenesis of the vagina, resulting from aplasia of the vaginal segments of the müllerian ducts, is occasionally seen as the cause of primary amenorrhea. In most instances the uterus is also congenitally missing, but exceptions to this have been reported. Patients with congenital absence of the vagina usually possess normal secondary sex characteristics, indicating ovarian function and estrogenic stimulation. Diagnosis is not usually difficult and may be aided by the introduction of radiopaque substances into the introital orifice. Treatment is surgical correction of the anomalous condition. In most instances it is deemed advisable to postpone definitive surgery until the patient contemplates marriage. The prognosis for satisfactory marital relationships is excellent, provided careful attention is paid to surgical technique and postoperative care.

Congenital absence of the uterus, though not common, is occasionally found by the practicing physician or gynecologist. This anomaly results from abnormal development of those elements of the müllerian ducts destined to form the uterus. The vagina may be absent or may be normal.

Tuberculosis, sepsis or radiation may render the endometrium incapable of response to the stimulus of estrogens.

Primary amenorrhea is occasionally seen in association with a form of female pseudohermaphroditism in which the patients have ovaries, female ducts and varying degrees of masculinization of the external genitalia. The commonest is the so-called adrenogenital syndrome, occasionally called the compensated form of congenital adrenal hyperplasia.

The majority of patients manifesting primary amenorrhea as a complaint possess adequate ovarian tissue but, for one reason or another, lack adequate ovarian stimulation. Absent or diminished ovarian secretory activity results in most cases from an inherent ovarian defect or from abnormalities of the hypophysis or hypothalamus. The underlying cause of ovarian unresponsiveness in the presence of normal gonadotropic stimulation remains obscure. The complex metabolic derangement resulting from panhypopituitarism is a consequence of deficiencies of all the tropic hormones of the adenohypophysis. Panhypopituitarism in infants, or acquired at an early age, is characterized by defects in growth and development. The ovaries remain small, uterine bleeding is lacking and the secondary sex characteristics fail to develop due to the lack of gonadotropic stimulation. Panhypopituitarism may be congenital or may result from cysts, tumors, infection, infarction or malnutrition.

In the child the most common cause of failure of the pituitary to secrete gonadotropins is a tumor known as a craniopharyngioma. This tumor of embryonic origin is derived from Rathke's pouch and occupies a suprasellar position. If it is located in a relatively anterior position, defects of vision such as upper outer quadrant anopsia or hemianopsia may result from encroachment on the optic chiasm. Pressure of the tumor on the anterior hypothalamus may cause failure of the centers that stimulate gonadotropin release. If the tumor is located in a more posterior position, it may involve the median eminence and the tuber cinereum, in which case there may be failure of production of other pituitary tropic hormones as well as gonadotropin.

In rare instances, adenohypophyseal function is apparently normal except for a specific deficiency of the gonadotropic hormones. The precise pathogenesis of this condition remains to be elucidated. Gonadal dysfunction is often associated with hypothalamic lesions such as tumors or cysts. However, amenorrhea may result from abnormal hypothalamic function even in the absence of demonstrable pathology.

A rare type of primary amenorrhea is that due to a congenital anomaly known as "female with testes." Such patients have developmental anomalies of the genitalia with partial fusion of the müllerian ducts, a normal vagina and normal external genitalia. They are genetic males but the interstitial cells of the testes in these patients secrete estrogen and testosterone. The latter, however, is not effective at end-organ sites. The patients are externally feminized but do not menstruate because the ovaries and uteri are absent. (See Chapter 16.)

Either hypothyroidism or thyrotoxicosis may produce sufficient derangement of the pituitary-ovarian axis to delay sexual maturation.

Tumors of the pituitary gland may frequently be asymptomatic so that primary amenorrhea is the initial symptom. Amenorrhea was present in approximately one half of all female patients with chromophobe adenomas, according to several recent reports. Rogers has reported his experience in 15 patients, 10 of whom had chromophobe adenomas, three eosinophilic adenomas and two craniopharyngiomas, and noted that amenorrhea preceded the recognition of the pituitary tumor in all patients. It is important to remember that intracranial, extrasellar lesions may simulate primary pituitary malfunction and amenorrhea may be a presenting complaint. Aneurysm of the internal carotid artery, tumor of the third ventricle, obstruction of the aqueduct of Sylvius, glioma of the optic chiasm and meningioma of the floor of the anterior fossa may simulate pituitary tumors and cause amenorrhea.

Patients with primary amenorrhea due to pituitary or extrasellar tumors demonstrate abnormal growth and developmental features. Short stature is frequently observed but dwarfism is not a characteristic feature. Assays of gonadotropins in urine usually show normal or slightly diminished levels. Deficient adrenal or thyroid function is occasionally noted and estrogen secretion is greatly diminished.

One of the primary effects of a diminution in total caloric intake is an interference with gonadotropic function. In most patients there is a diminished excretion of follicle-stimulating hormone. Primary amenorrhea, therefore, may be directly correlated with and due to states of malnutrition. Experiments in animals have shown that chronic inanition did not diminish the content of gonadotropic hormone in the pituitary gland but *release* of these gonadotropins is prevented. Whether the amenorrhea is due to inadequate caloric intake or is secondary to a malabsorption syndrome, restoration of complete and normal pituitary-ovarian relationship occurs rather quickly after the deficiency is remedied.

Amenorrhea, usually secondary, has frequently been associated with the development of obesity. However, primary amenorrhea may also be associated with this state. It is not suggested that obesity is the cause of amenorrhea, since it is rather well established that the obesity may be the direct result of an emotional disorder. Therefore, the amenorrhea may be more definitely correlated with a psychogenic cause than with the obesity per se. There is no doubt, however, that as soon as these patients lose weight the menses begin rather readily. The rapid onset of menses suggests a rather expeditious output of stored gonadotropins that may be due to the establishment of a negative caloric balance but more likely is due to the correction of the psychosomatic factor.

Finally, primary amenorrhea as a specific symptom may result from emotional trauma. The psychogenic manifestations responsible for amenorrheic states vary from relatively superficial psychoneuroses to deep-seated psychopathic states. This type of amenorrhea, sometimes known as hypothalamic amenorrhea, is more common as a secondary development. However, it does occur as a primary situation, particularly in young girls who are tense or disturbed as a result of domineering parents. Excessive restriction or fear and concern regarding sexual matters may be etiologic factors. The general examination of patients with hypothalamic amenorrhea is usually within normal range. There is evidence of estrogen deficiency and the assay of gonadotropins is usually low. This is an important diagnostic laboratory test since primary amenorrhea of ovarian origin will be associated with elevated levels of pituitary gonadotropins whereas those of primary amenorrhea of pituitary origin will be characteristically low. It has been suggested that the relative state of hypoestrinism and lack of ovulation is related to the failure of release of LH. MacArthur noted a depression of LH excretion in two patients with psychogenic amenorrhea.

The diagnostic evaluation and clinical management of patients with either primary or secondary amenorrhea are similar. For this reason, the essential diagnostic procedures and therapeutic regimens applicable to patients with primary amenorrhea are included in the next section.

SECONDARY AMENORRHEA

Secondary amenorrhea designates the cessation of uterine bleeding in patients who have previously menstruated. The length of time which should elapse without external signs of uterine bleeding before consideration is given to secondary amenorrhea is difficult to define. In general, however, if a patient has not menstruated for a period equivalent to three or four of her normal menstrual cycles, investigation of the amenorrhea is indicated.

Certain physiologic states predispose to amenorrhea. The possibility of pregnancy must always be entertained, regardless of the negative history offered by the patient. Menstruation is held in abeyance for varying periods of time during the puerperium and during lactation.

Periods of amenorrhea, variable as to duration, are not uncommonly noted in the postmenarchal era and reflect normal fluctuations in ovarian activity. In most adolescent girls perfectly normal menstrual periods will resume in due time. Similarly, in patients in the premenopausal era amenorrhea is not uncommon in the form of skips and delays of flow as a reflection of waning ovarian activity.

Obstructive lesions involving the cervix may be responsible for states of secondary amenorrhea. Cervical stenosis that obstructs the drainage of uterine secretions may result from electrocauterization, conization, tracheloplasty, irradiation, chemical burns or infectious disease processes. The cessation of menstruation may follow the destruction of endometrial tissue. Asherman has described a syndrome of sclerosis of the endometrial cavity with multiple synechiae that results from overzealous curettage following spontaneous abortions or normal delivery. The patients usually have typical menstrual molimina and biphasic basal temperature curves but are totally amenorrheic. Use of radioactive substances or x-rays in the treatment of malignancies of the genital tract produces secondary amenorrhea. Destruction of the endometrium also has been reported following severe infection. In most instances, however, the consequence of irradiation and infection is twofold. In addition to the necrotizing effect on the endometrium, there is destruction of the more distant ovarian tissue. Another cause of secondary amenorrhea noted recently is the endometrial atrophy and ovarian inactivity that follow the use of long-acting progestational agents. Administration of depomedroxyprogesterone has resulted in periods of amenorrhea which may last 12–18 months. This amenorrhea is believed due to the protracted release of medroxyprogesterone from the injected site, with resultant depression of pituitary gonadotropins. Several patients with this iatrogenic amenorrhea have been successfully treated and ovulation induced by the administration of clomiphene citrate. The mechanism of action of this non-steroidal hormonal substance is discussed in the section on the Stein-Leventhal syndrome (Chapter 7).

Patients manifesting secondary amenorrhea on the basis of varying degrees of ovarian failure comprise by far the largest group in clinical practice. Hypo-ovarianism, in most instances, reflects either inadequate or improper stimulation by the adenohypophyseal gonadotropins or an inherent unresponsiveness of ovarian tissue to normal gonadotropic stimulation. The cause of ovarian failure in the presence of normal hypophyseal and hypothalamic function remains obscure. Patients with relative ovarian failure often have dysfunctional uterine bleeding before the inception of the secondary amenorrheic state. The underlying pathologic process is often one of gradual ovarian failure.

The average age at menopause has been stated to be 50 years, but a rather substantial number of women begin to have skips and delays of flow at age 40 and complete absence of menstruation by age 42 or 43. If the menses cease before age 40, particularly if there are associated symptoms of vasomotor instability such as hot flushes and sweats, it may be assumed that the cause is premature ovarian failure. Such a precocious menopause is characterized by diminished estrogen production and a rise in pituitary gonadotropins.

It is important that organic causes of amenorrhea be excluded before concluding that amenorrhea is due to ovarian failure. Once the diagnosis is made, however, the symptoms may be alleviated and premature athero-sclerosis and osteoporosis prevented, by the regular and cyclic administration of oral estrogenic preparations. If desirable, cyclic withdrawal bleeding may be effected by the use of estrogens alone or estrogens and synthetic progestins. There is no evidence that prolonged use of estrogenic substances in this fashion statistically increases the incidence of carcinoma of either the breast or endometrium in the human female.

Recent cytogenetic observations have demonstrated that precocious menopause may occur in patients with a XXX chromosome configuration. Such patients will usually show stigmata of sexual infantilism which is not evident in the usual patient with premature menopause.

Certain patients with hypogonadism demonstrate a variety of the Stein-Leventhal syndrome. The morphologic and physiologic variations of this condition are discussed in Chapter 7.

A variety of interesting endocrinopathies result from hypofunction or hyperfunction of the adenohypophysis. Despite the complex nature of the adenohypophyseal pattern of hormone secretion, a remarkably good accounting may be made of the symptomatology and metabolic aberrations of these endocrinopathies in terms of the known actions of the tropic hormones.

Extensive septic necrosis of the adenohypophysis following embolism leads to panhypopituitarism. This syndrome is known variously as Simmonds' disease or pituitary cachexia. Sheehan's syndrome is an interesting variation of this disease and has its onset in the puerperium as a result of postpartum hemorrhage and obstetric shock. (See p. 603.)

Amenorrhea of secondary type may result from functioning pituitary tumors such as eosinophilic and basophilic adenomas or from nonfunctioning tumors such as chromophobe adenomas or craniopharyngiomas (Fig. 12–6). Lesions involving structures immediately adjacent to the sella turcica may also be responsible for the development of secondary amenorrhea. Internal carotid artery aneurysms, tumors of the third ventricle, gliomas of the optic chiasm and meningiomas of the floor of the anterior fossa have been documented as etiologic lesions. These were discussed in the section on Primary Amenorrhea.

Hyperadrenocorticism in the human female is due to certain pathologic processes involving the pituitary gland or adrenal cortex (Cushing's disease and Cushing's syndrome, respectively). A state of hypercorticism may also be induced by the administration of the adrenocorticotropic hormone (ACTH) or certain adrenal steroids. In female patients with hyperadrenocorticism, regardless of etiology, dysfunctional bleeding and/or amenorrhea comprise part of the clinical syndrome. Inhibition of the adenohypophyseal release of the gonadotropic hormones by the elevated titer of adrenal steroids has been proposed as the mechanism responsible for the abnormal uterine bleeding and amenorrhea. However, recently reported data from animal experimentation suggest that the inhibition of gonadotropic activity which accompanies hyperadrenocorticism occurs at the ovarian rather than the adenohypophyseal level. (See pp. 588 and 598.)

Although amenorrhea is commonly found in association with variations

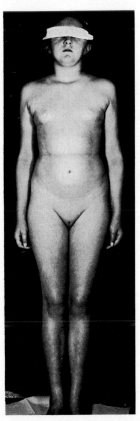

Fig. 12–6.—Secondary amenorrhea due to hypogonadotropic hypogonadism in girl, 16. Blindness developed from optic atrophy. A craniopharyngioma was partially removed at craniotomy. Postoperatively diabetes insipidus developed. Thyroid and adrenal function were normal. Growth had continued in prepuberal pattern. Estrogen excretion was low and gonadotropins negative at 4 m.u.u./24 hours. (From Lloyd, C. W.: The Ovaries, in Williams, R. H. (ed.): *Textbook of Endocrinology* [Philadelphia: W. B. Saunders Company, 1962].)

of excess adrenocortical function, it should also be remembered that amenorrhea may be a manifestation of adrenal hypocorticism or Addison's disease.

In certain patients, ovarian failure and amenorrhea result from a *specific deficiency* of the adenohypophyseal gonadotropins. The etiologic factors remain obscure. Inhibition of the adenohypophyseal release of the gonadotropins, resulting in the cessation of uterine bleeding, follows the administration of large doses of estrogen, progesterone or testosterone. The increased endogenous secretion of ovarian steroids that is caused by certain functioning tumors of the ovaries inhibits gonadotropic activity in a similar manner.

Malnutrition due to starvation or chronic wasting disease may result in hypofunction of the pituitary gland. Secondary amenorrhea following rigorous and severe reducing diets is not infrequently encountered and probably represents a state of relative hypopituitarism. The cessation of uterine bleeding is a clinical feature of anorexia nervosa, a specific syndrome seen in girls or young women who, on the basis of psychiatric etiologic factors, develop an aversion to food. These patients become extremely emaciated and occasionally cachectic. Anorexia nervosa is not a primary endocrine disorder and a state of hypopituitarism is not present. The gonadal insufficiency is due to inadequate release of gonadotropic hormones due specifically to the effect of starvation. The earlier stages of oligo-ovulation or anovulation may be due to inadequate release of LH. The patient with anorexia nervosa is alert and occasionally overactive, in definite contrast to the lassitude so characteristic of the patient with hypopituitarism. Body hair and skin pigmentation are normal in anorexia nervosa, the only finding of significance in the physical examination being extreme emaciation. Psychiatric therapy is indicated for such individuals and improvement in all parameters is noted following increased caloric intake.

Abnormal psychogenic states either cause or contribute to the development of secondary amenorrhea and other abnormalities of menstrual and reproductive function. The cessation of menstruation not uncommonly results from a fear of pregnancy, incompatible marital relationships, psychosexual conflicts, financial worry, intolerable family situations and other traumatic psychiatric states. Although the precise pathogenesis remains obscure, the *modus operandi* for the development of abnormal reproductive function in psychogenic states may be associated with hypothalamic dysfunction. For this reason, the so-called "emotional amenorrhea" has also been termed "hypothalamic amenorrhea." The absence of menstruation or the cessation of previously established menstruation does not, in the vast majority of patients, represent a serious threat to their well-being or longevity.

Amenorrhea as a specific symptom warrants evaluation in all patients. A concerted effort should be made to disclose underlying systemic disease, to uncover lesions of the various endocrine target organs and to investigate abnormalities of the midbrain and cerebral cortex. In the absence of proved organic lesions, amenorrhea warrants treatment only as it relates to infertility or to disturbed emotional states which not infrequently arise due to the absence or cessation of uterine bleeding. Treatment may occasionally be necessary because of an atypical hyperplasia of the endometrium which is considered to be premalignant.

Evaluation of the Patient with Amenorrhea

The evaluation of patients with either primary or secondary amenorrhea necessitates thorough testing of the functional integrity of each link in the chain of menstrual events, that is, the endometrium, the ovaries, the pituitary gland and the hypothalamus. Investigation of other endocrine systems such as the thyroid and adrenal glands and a search for underlying systemic disease should also be initiated. It would seem unnecessary to emphasize the importance of a complete history and physical examination, yet the number of patients in whom these simple procedures have been totally ignored by the physician is disturbing and appalling.

The author routinely obtains vaginal smears from all gynecologic patients. The cytologic characteristics of the desquamated cells reflect not only epithelial atypism, or occasionally even cancer, but also the degree and character of the endocrine stimulation of the genital tract. A drop of cervical mucus placed on a slide and allowed to dry will demonstrate the characteristic fern phenomenon diagnostic of adequate estrogen stimulation of the endocervical glands. Absence of the fern implies inadequate estrogen, the presence of progesterone or pregnancy.

Endometrial biopsies, obtained simply and easily in the physician's office, are valuable in determining the cause of a specific amenorrhea. Needless to say, the possibility of an intrauterine pregnancy should be entertained before undertaking this procedure. The investigation of an intrinsic endometrial defect as the cause of amenorrhea is not difficult. Endometrium, atrophied as a result of deficient ovarian secretion, maintains an inherent facility to respond to estrogenic stimulation regardless of the duration of the atrophy. If the basal glands of the endometrium have not been destroyed, withdrawal uterine bleeding will follow the administration of adequate amounts of estrogen. For this test diethylstilbestrol, 0.5 mg. daily by mouth for 20 days, or ethinyl estradiol 0.05 mg. twice daily by mouth for 20 days, is given. Withdrawal flow, if it is to occur, will usually be noted within four to five days after cessation of the medication. If uterine bleeding is not manifested after such therapy, diagnosis of an intrinsic endometrial defect, such as complete removal by curettage (Asherman's syndrome) or by x-ray or other caustic agents, is suggested.

The utilization of known endocrinologic relationships is helpful in differentiating between absolute and relative ovarian failure as the basis for amenorrhea. Withdrawal uterine bleeding follows the administration of adequate amounts of progesterone, provided the endometrium has been stimulated or "primed" with estrogen. If bleeding follows the administration of progesterone, or a synthetic progestin, estrogen is being elaborated to some degree by the ovary. If withdrawal bleeding does not occur, ovarian failure must be considered. For this test progesterone, 50 or 100 mg., is administered intramuscularly on two successive days. Withdrawal flow, if it is to occur, will be noted in from two to eight days after the second injection. Any of the oral synthetic progestins may be utilized in a similar fashion, giving 5–10 mg. daily for three days. Withdrawal bleeding will occur in from two to five days if the patient is not pregnant and if the endometrium has been adequately primed by estrogen.

The failure of withdrawal bleeding following administration of progesterone or synthetic progestins has been widely used as a test for pregnancy.

Careful examination of the internal genitalia and the use of a pregnancy test are helpful in establishing the diagnosis of an early gestation. The newer tests for pregnancy which are based on immunologic reactions to human chorionic gonadotropin appear to be superior to the older animal assay methods. Furthermore, these tests give positive reactions at a much lower level of sensitivity and therefore may be utilized after the first 21 days of gestation.

Reference is frequently made in the medical literature to persistence of the corpus luteum in a functional state as a distinct clinical entity. Existing evidence suggests that in the human subject the corpus luteum possesses an inherent life span, and considerable doubt has been cast on persistence of luteal function beyond this period. However, if one acknowledges the existence of persistent corpora lutea or corpus luteum cysts, inhibition of the adenohypophysis by continued ovarian steroidal elaboration can result in a state of amenorrhea. Quite obviously, withdrawal bleeding would not follow progesterone administration in this particular situation. Urinary pregnanediol assays would help differentiate this condition from absolute ovarian failure. We have routinely used culdoscopy to diagnose the presence of a corpus luteum of follicular cyst as the cause for amenorrhea. Cysts of this type will disappear if gonadotropins are suppressed with cyclic estrogens and progestins.

The concentration of estrogenic substances in urine and serum reflects the degree of ovarian activity. Determination of the estrogenic titer in body fluids is an invaluable aid in the diagnosis of certain of the endocrinopathies affecting the female reproductive system. Recent advances in the development of methods for the quantification of estrogenic steroids in body fluids have added another method for localization of the precise etiologic factor in amenorrhea.

Women manifesting ovarian failure secrete adenohypophyseal gonadotropins at a greater than normal rate and without cyclic fluctuations. The gonadotropin present in the urine of such patients is predominantly follicle stimulating in nature. Thus, the diagnosis of absolute ovarian failure can be established in a patient who (1) does not respond to progesterone administration with withdrawal bleeding and (2) demonstrates an elevated FSH titer.

Various abnormalities of the pituitary gland, as stated, may be responsible for amenorrheic states. Secretion of the adenohypophyseal gonadotropins is absent or significantly diminished in patients with abnormalities of the pituitary gland. The ovaries and hence the endometrium receive no hormonal stimulation and amenorrhea ensues. With lesions of the pituitary gland, (1) the concentration of FSH in the urine is low or absent, (2) withdrawal flow does not follow the administration of progesterone, but (3) the endometrium does respond to estrogenic stimulation by withdrawal bleeding.

Roentgenographic evaluation of the sella turcica is imperative in the clinical evaluation of all patients with amenorrhea. Neoplasms of the pituitary gland and adjacent structures give characteristic x-ray findings. Neurologic and ophthalmologic consultations are essential if pituitary or hypothalamic tumors are suspected. The association of headaches or blurred vision with amenorrhea should make the clinician suspicious of intracranial lesions. Parasellar tumors or arterial lesions may be diagnosed by specific angiograms or by the use of infra-red spectrophotometry.

Lesions of the hypothalamus are characterized by the failure of estrogenic elaboration in the presence of normal levels of FSH. The secretion of estrogenic substances depends on adequate ovarian stimulation by two of the gonadotropic hormones, FSH and LH. Convincing and substantial evidence has been accumulated to indicate that the adenohypophyseal release of LH is under the control of the hypothalamus. In conditions of hypothalamic dysfunction, (1) the endometrium is intact, as evidenced by withdrawal flow following estrogen treatment; (2) the ovaries are not active, as shown by the absence of uterine bleeding following administration of progesterone, and (3) the concentration of FSH in the urine is normal. However, radioimmunoassays of LH show low levels and inadequate "bursts" needed for ovulation.

Treatment of Amenorrhea

Two fundamental concepts, both equally important, should be stressed in the clinical management of patients with primary or secondary amenorrhea. First, the absence of menstruation or the cessation of previously established menstruation does not, in most patients, represent a serious threat to their well-being. Secondly, in the absence of proved organic lesions, amenorrhea as a specific symptom warrants treatment only as it relates to disturbed emotional states, to infertility or to abnormalities of the endometrium. Many physicians seem compelled to initiate cyclic uterine bleeding before they undertake an adequate investigation of the patient to determine the existence of serious organic lesions.

In order to obtain a complete endocrinologic survey within a short space of time the author follows the following plan. The patient is admitted to the hospital for a stay of 48–72 hours. During the first day a 24-hour urine collection is obtained for FSH determination. A lateral skull film is taken for visualization of the sella turcica, and a protein-bound iodine determination is made. (It should be noted that a Schiller test of the cervix or a previous uterotubogram will seriously alter the protein-bound iodine so that these tests should be avoided for six to eight weeks before this determination.) During the second day a 24-hour urine collection is obtained for determination of 17-ketosteroids and 17-ketogenic steroids. A vaginal smear is examined for estrogen effect and a fern test of the cervical mucus is performed. If the x-ray of the sella turcica is abnormal or if there are localizing cerebral symptoms, visual fields are plotted and a neurologic consultation obtained. A culdoscopy is then performed to assay the gross morphology of the ovaries adequately. A curettage follows, so that endometrium may be sampled and studied microscopically.

The procedures available to the physician for the clinical evaluation of patients with amenorrhea are simple and easily accomplished. However, in addition to investigating the functional integrity of the endometrium, the ovaries, the pituitary gland, the adrenal glands and the hypothalamus, attention should also be directed to the detection of systemic diseases, abnormalities of other endocrine organs and psychogenic factors. Appropriate treatment, when indicated, should be initiated if such pathologic states exist. In the absence of proved organic lesions, cyclic endocrine therapy may be indicated if the failure of uterine bleeding to occur emotionally disturbs the patient or if an abnormality of the endometrium is found. Under these circumstances, artificial cycles are initiated with combinations of estrogens and synthetic progestins as outlined for anovulatory uterine bleeding. Cyclic uterine bleeding resulting from withdrawal flow is easily accomplished in these patients provided inherent endometrial unresponsiveness does not exist.

The therapeutic management of sterility patients manifesting amenorrhea deserves special note. Relative ovarian failure is the most frequent cause of the amenorrhea and hence the infertility in the vast majority of these patients. Specific treatment for relative ovarian failure and the sterility which ensues is now available in the form of human FSH and human chorionic gonadotropin, concentrates of postmenopausal urine (Pergonal) and clomiphene citrate. (See Chapters 9 and 11.)

If the survey of the pituitary gland indicates the presence of a tumor, whether it be intra- or parasellar, consultation with a neurosurgeon is obtained. In the presence of a low or low-normal protein-bound iodine value, desiccated thyroid, 65 mg. daily by mouth, is administered. Desiccated thyroid gland U.S.P. is the oldest but still one of the best preparations available for hypothyroidism. It relieves all the known abnormalities of human thyroid deficiency. It contains levothyroxine and levotriiodothyronine in biologic proportions (0.2 per cent of iodine) as well as other iodinated thyronines, tyrosines and organic and inorganic iodides. The replacement dose for a patient with true hypothyroidism is generally between 100 and 120 mg. daily.

The diagnosis and management of the patient with adrenogenital syndrome is considered in detail later in this chapter. However, it must be realized that relative degrees of abnormal adrenocortical function also exist. This type of situation has been described as the postpuberal adrenogenital syndrome in the female. For completeness in the discussion of therapy for secondary amenorrhea, treatment of these patients will be considered here. The excretion of 17-ketosteroids in urine may be slightly or moderately elevated and the pregnanetriol level may be normal or only slightly elevated. A therapeutic test with corticoids may be used in these patients to establish whether or not there is an adrenogenital syndrome. If the borderline 17-ketosteroid value is depressed by the recommended doses of corticoids, such a patient must be considered as having some degree of hyperadrenocorticism and must be maintained on corticoid therapy until the anticipated therapeutic response is achieved. Therapy requires the use of glucocorticoids in doses sufficient to suppress the excessive ACTH secretion responsible for the elevated 17-ketosteroid excretion. The following preparations may be given orally three times daily at approximately eight-hour intervals: cortisone 12.5 mg.; hydrocortisone 10 mg.; prednisone or prednisolone 2.5 mg.; 6-methylprednisolone 2 mg.; triamcinolone 2–3 mg.; dexamethasone 0.375 mg.; paramethasone acetate 1 mg. There is usually no need for the parenteral use of corticoids in these patients. The doses advised are in the physiologic range so dietary restriction is not necessary, nor are potassium supplements needed. The patient may be permitted to take salt freely and the dangers of ulceration of gastric mucosa or activation of pulmonary tuberculosis are minimal. The dose of the corticoid should be one that will maintain the 17-ketosteroid excretion level at 10 mg. per 24 hours or below and/or keep the pregnanetriol level below 1.8 mg. per 24 hours. When corticoids are discontinued after three to six months of treatment in post-puberal adrenogenital syndrome, the patient's abnormal pattern of steroid excretion may not revert back to the pretreatment level. Hence, the postpuberal patient may not have to continue corticoid therapy indefinitely. This, of course, is not true in patients with congenital adreno-genital syndrome. The earliest response to the administration of corticoids is a decline in 17-ketosteroids in urine and a reversion of pregnanetriol levels to normal. Occasionally this may occur within 14 days following initiation of therapy. The next response to be noted is an increase in the secretion of FSH, and this is followed rather shortly by evidence of ovulation and subsequent menstruation.

In amenorrhea due to uterine causes, several etiologic factors may be responsible, and therapy will depend on the precise etiology. Congenital uterine agenesis or hypoplasia is a rare cause of primary amenorrhea. Such patients experience cyclic changes in the breasts as well as premenstrual molimina but have complete absence of catamenia. No specific therapy is available for this rare situation.

Primary or secondary amenorrhea may be due to a tuberculous infection of the endometrium, and specific therapy of the infection may result in subsequent menstruation. A suppurative endometritis may be of such extent that the entire endometrium is destroyed or is subsequently incapable of regeneration. Such a process may follow a septic, criminal abortion. In some patients the basalis of the endometrium is completely destroyed and subsequent exogenous hormonal therapy is of no value. Endometrial sclerosis (Asherman's syndrome) and the destruction of the endometrium by radiation therapy are other etiologic factors in secondary amenorrhea. Although results in the past have been discouraging in both of these processes, recent evidence has shown that large doses of estrogens given for prolonged periods may bring about growth of the basalis and subsequent normal menstrual patterns. The dose of the estrogenic substance should be three to four times as large as that given normally. In some patients we have given Premarin 2.5 mg. four times daily or Tace 24 mg. twice daily for six to 12 months. In certain patients no response was noted prior to the seventh or eighth month of continuous therapy. Attempts at transplantation of tubal mucosa or endometrium have not been successful.

The three major causes of ovarian amenorrhea are the precocious or premature menopause, the sclerocystic ovarian syndrome (Stein-Leventhal syndrome) and ovarian dysgenesis. The therapy for sclerocystic ovarian syndrome and gonadal dysgenesis are discussed in other chapters. As mentioned before, the only specific therapy for the patient with precocious menopause is substitutional estrogen therapy. Because of the extragenital effects of estrogen deprivation it is important that exogenous estrogens be provided in cyclic fashion ad infinitum. Therapy may be in the form of diethylstilbestrol 0.5 mg. twice daily, Estinyl 0.05 mg., Vallestril 3 mg., Premarin 1.25 mg. or Tace 12 mg. daily for 21 days of each month.

The treatment of amenorrhea due to hypopituitary states such as Sheehan's syndrome and Simmond's disease is discussed under these conditions later in this chapter. The therapy of patients exhibiting Chiari-Frommel disease is also given.

The therapy in hypothalamic amenorrhea is ideally administered by a psychiatrist. However, it is not unusual to see a patient who has had amenorrhea for years and, after initial interview and examination, reports spontaneous menstruation within a matter of months. It becomes obvious that hypothalamic or psychogenic amenorrhea is a delicately adjusted mechanism sustained by a relatively minor disorder of the hypothalamus and hypophysis, and occasionally minor adjustments in this important relationship will result in the spontaneous onset of menses. In other patients, however, psychotherapy is of no obvious value. If spontaneous menstruation does not recur despite all therapeutic and psychosomatic efforts, the case should be completely re-evaluated since some organic factor may have been overlooked.

In the patient who has associated obesity and amenorrhea, results may be obtained if a negative caloric balance is effected.

Endocrine preparations have been widely used both to inhibit and to stimulate pituitary gonadotropins in patients with both pituitary and ovarian amenorrhea. The rationale of treatment utilizes the observation that estrogenic substances, administered in large doses, block the adenohypophyseal release of gonadotropins. Existing evidence suggests that the gonadotropic hormones are accumulated or stored in higher concentrations in the pituitary gland during this period of endocrine therapy. Cessation of treatment, theoretically at least, releases the estrogenic blockage and a sudden burst of gonadotropic activity results. The desired effect of this so-called rebound phenomenon is to stimulate the ovaries sufficiently to promote ovulation and normal menstrual function. The use of cyclic estrogen and progesterone to promote ovulation and normal menstrual function in such patients has not met with uniform success.

In selected cases Kupperman has induced ovulation by the intravenous administration of an estrogen. It was previously shown that administration of estrogen to the menopausal patient will increase the luteinizing hormone excretion in the urine. The mode of action of the conjugated estrogens in inducing ovulation presumably is due to the effect these estrogens have on the center in the hypothalamus responsible for stimulating the release of LH. It is believed that this center lies in the area between the supraoptic and the paraventricular nuclei and that estrogen may induce a specific chemical change in this area. Animal experiments have indicated that deposition of an estrogen in this hypothalamic region will induce ovulation, apparently by a direct effect. The technique suggested by Kupperman consists in the intravenous administration of 20 mg. conjugated estrogens equine (Premarin) three or four weeks after the onset of an induced or spontaneous menstrual period. Rakoff suggests the use of dienestrol or diethylstilbestrol 0.1 mg. daily for 3 days, 0.2 mg. daily for 3 days, then 0.3 mg. daily for 3 days beginning immediately after an induced flow.

Gemzell reported on the use of a preparation of human pituitary follicle-stimulating hormone (HPFSH) and human chorionic gonadotropin (HCG). In one of his groups these preparations were given for the induction of ovulation in women who were sterile due to pituitary failure. The women chosen were treated for 10 days with daily injections of 250–500 units of HPFSH, followed on the eleventh to the thirteenth day by daily injections of 3,000 international units of HCG. Patients who had undeveloped secondary sex characteristics and infantile uteri were treated cyclically with estrogens for two to three months before administration of HPFSH. It is apparent from the work of Gemzell that preparations of human pituitary gonadotropin are highly effective in producing follicular growth and, when used with HCG, are effective in inducing ovulation. Superovulation may also occur, resulting in the birth of fraternal twins. A similar situation in regard to the increased incidence of twin pregnancy has been noted by us following the use of clomiphene citrate for the induction of ovulation. The use of human menopausal gonadotropin and clomiphene citrate is discussed in Chapter 9.

Dysfunctional Uterine Bleeding

Throughout this text the term *dysfunctional uterine bleeding* will be used to mean abnormal endometrial bleeding in which organic lesions cannot be demonstrated by ordinary means. The same process has been described as *functional uterine bleeding* or *metropathia hemorrhagica*, but the former implies the normal, cyclic discharge of blood and endometrial tissue which follows the cyclic *function* of ovulation, whereas the latter implies uterine pathology. Dysfunctional bleeding is extremely common and embraces a variety of apparently separate entities. These are: midmonth staining, premenstrual staining, normal uterine bleeding occurring at shorter than normal intervals, normal uterine bleeding occurring at longer than normal intervals, profuse or prolonged uterine bleeding at normal intervals, irregular endometrial shedding and constant or intermittent uterine bleeding.

The incidence of dysfunctional bleeding at the Boston Hospital for Women approximates 5 per cent of all admissions; in addition, this process accounts for about 60 per cent of all diagnostic curettages. It may be seen at any age, but the highest incidence is during the postmenarchal and premenopausal periods. Because derangements of function are common during the initiation and cessation of ovulation, bleeding during these times will in most cases prove to be of an anovulatory type.

The precise etiologic factors in dysfunctional bleeding are not known but most cases may be considered to originate in the cortex, the hypothalamus, the pituitary, the thyroid, the adrenal, the ovary or the endometrium. In contrast to normal menstrual cycles which are characterized by a regulated balance between gonadotropins and ovarian hormones resulting in ovulation and a *cyclic* efflux from the uterus, dysfunctional bleeding is characterized by anovulation and an *acyclic* pattern of bleeding. It probably results from an imbalance between adenohypophyseal and ovarian hormones rather than from a deficiency per se. Since the absence of ovulation is associated with *most* of the irregularities to be described, the ovary may be looked on as playing a dominant role. The anovulation may be due to intrinsic ovarian dysfunction or secondary to functional derangement of the hypothalamus or hypophysis.

The term *menstruation* is used to indicate a process of bleeding from secretory endometrium. Dysfunctional bleeding is most often associated with endometrial growth patterns in which the effects of progesterone are completely lacking or markedly deficient. One exception is the process known as "irregular shedding," in which the endometrial pattern is secretory. In other conditions of excessive or irregular uterine bleeding associated with secretory endometrium, the etiology is usually organic.

HISTORY AND PHYSICAL EXAMINATION

The diagnosis of this entity may be suspected by the history, corroborated by the pelvic examination and confirmed by the endometrial biopsy or curettage. Care must be given to minutiae in the details of the history, with exact dates of flowing, extent of flowing, number of perineal pads, the passage of clots, pain and associated moliminal symptoms. The bleeding of dysfunctional type may occur suddenly, may be slight or profuse, usually is associated with passage of clots but is often painless. Premenstrual moliminal symptoms of headache, backache, edema, acne and midline cramps are usually absent. If basal body temperatures are charted, the curve associated with anovulatory bleeding is monophasic whereas the curve associated with ovulation and menstruation is biphasic. A history of recent emotional stress or prolonged tension suggests a hypothalamic origin, as do outright psychoses, hysterias or depressions. Severe debilitating diseases such as tuberculosis or hepatic insufficiency or changes in dietary habits resulting in marked weight gain or loss are important etiologic factors and should be given due consideration. Frequently, episodes of dysfunctional flowing may occur after sudden changes of climate and may represent temporary adjustments of thyroid function. Specific endocrinopathies such as hyper- and hypothyroidism, adrenal hyperplasia and diabetes mellitus or insipidus may be elicited by careful history-taking. The presence of headaches, scotoma or blurred vision may suggest a pituitary tumor as the causative factor. Finally, the historian should inquire specifically about the use of medications. Patients are frequently given estrogens, progestins, androgens or adrenal corticoids without knowing their exact function or side-effects. Any of these may produce changes in the menstrual rhythm if not given in exact sequence and dosage. Similarly, certain drugs which affect the blood clotting mechanism may occasionally cause aberrations of endometrial bleeding. This history should, of course, include details of any radiation therapy or surgical procedure which might affect ovarian-endometrial interplay.

The general physical examination will delineate obvious endocrine problems such as gonadal dysgenesis (Turner's syndrome), myxedema, hyperthyroidism, dwarfism, gigantism, acromegaly, hypophyseal cachexia (Simmonds' disease), Cushing's disease, Cushing's syndrome and adrenal cortical insufficiency (Addison's disease). Obvious virilization and acquired hirsutism occurring in combination with oligomenorrhea or amenorrhea suggest adrenal cortical hyperfunction (tumor or hyperplasia, adrenogenital syndrome) or ovarian virilizing tumors (arrhenoblastoma, hilus cell tumors, masculinovoblastoma).

Pelvic examination and visualization of the cervix should be done on every patient who complains of any abnormality of the menses. This somewhat trite statement is italicized because it is so often omitted and therapy instituted without diagnosis. Pelvic examination will reveal, by inspection alone, such abnormalities as vaginitis, erosions, polyps or cancer of the cervix, prolapsed leiomyomas and foreign bodies which may be causing the abnormal bleeding. Similarly, enlargement of the clitoris and male-type pubic hair distribution suggest virilizing disorders. Inguinal or crural masses may be the testes of a true hermaphrodite. Bimanual examination will reveal the soft patulous cervix associated with an incomplete abortion, the small uterus and enlarged ovaries of the patient with Stein-Leventhal syndrome, and the cystic ovarian enlargement associated with a granulosa or theca cell tumor. In adolescents and unmarried young women with an intact hymen, the internal genitalia may be adequately evaluated by rectal examination.

Certain laboratory tests are of value in the diagnostic evaluation of a patient with dysfunctional bleeding. The most important of these is the endometrial biopsy. This may be done easily in the office or outpatient department without anesthesia and should be timed so as to obtain tissue *at the time of bleeding.* This will avoid invasion of the endometrial cavity when an unsuspected pregnancy exists and will usually provide an adequate sample for microscopic study. Care should be taken to gain access into the cavity of the corpus, thus preventing meaningless biopsies of the lower uterine segment. Thorough curettage of the entire cavity may be indicated, depending on circumstances which will be discussed in the sections on therapy. Basal body temperature charts are valuable if continued for three or four months so that they may be studied in relation to bleeding episodes. A basal metabolism test and protein-bound iodine determination are important adjunctive procedures, especially in patients with oligo- and amenorrhea. X-rays of the sella turcica are indicated in all patients with prolonged amenorrhea. Vaginal smears for quantification of estrogen effect are simple to obtain and interpret. Examination of cervical mucus is a simple office procedure; typical arborization with crystallization, if seen, is indicative of the presence of estrogen. A cellular pattern without arborization suggests either little or no estrogenic activity or suppression of this activity by progesterone. A minimum evaluation of the hematologic profile should include a platelet count and bleeding time. If thrombopenia is present, bone marrow aspiration should be done. If the bleeding time is abnormal, a diagnosis of pseudohemophilia or idiopathic bleeding-time defect may be made. The large majority of patients who have dysfunctional flowing as a result of hematologic disorders will have either idiopathic thrombopenic purpura (ITP) or idiopathic bleeding-time defect (IBTD).

Before we proceed to the specific manifestations of dysfunctional bleeding, a generalization regarding treatment may be made. Endocrine therapy, to be effective, must be based on an accurate diagnosis of the underlying hormonal defect. There is no place for trial or empirical therapy or for treatment without examination. Uterine curettage may prove to be therapeutic as well as diagnostic.

TECHNIQUE OF UTERINE CURETTAGE.—With the patient in the lithotomy position the vulva and vagina are prepared with aqueous and tincture of Zephiran. The bladder is emptied by catheterization and sterile drapes are applied. Careful examination should always precede dilatation and curettage in order to ascertain the correct size and position of the uterus as well as the presence of any adnexal masses. A previously unsuspected ectopic pregnancy or ovarian tumor may be discovered at this time, since complete muscular relaxation will now be afforded. In addition, the uterus may now be felt to be slightly soft and globular, indicating a previously undiagnosed intra-uterine pregnancy. The anterior lip of the cervix is grasped in the midportion by a pair of double tenacula and enough tissue included in the instruments to prevent tearing out and causing a cervical laceration. The tenacula originally devised by Cullen, with mouse-toothed hooks, are standard equipment at the Boston Hospital for Women since they obtain a firmer hold on tissues and cause less trauma than other instruments.

The cervix is drawn gently down toward the vaginal introitus; strong traction should be avoided. Dilatation of the nonpregnant cervix is most safely performed with Hanks's graduated dilators. Before passing the first dilator, a uterine sound should be gently inserted into the uterine cavity to determine the proper degree of angulation as well as the depth of the cavity. The first dilator should then be passed with extreme care since deviations or angulations of the canal or various obstructions may deflect the point of the instrument into and through the myometrium. When the uterus is atonic, as during intrauterine gestation or after menopause, a dilator may perforate the uterine wall with practically no resistance. If the direction of the endocervical canal is difficult to determine with the dilator, a fine uterine probe should be used.

After the proper direction has been established, dilators of graduated sizes are used until desirable dilatation is obtained. The necessary degree of dilatation will depend on the exact indication for the dilatation and curettage. Thus, in the treatment of primary dysmenorrhea dilatation is usually maximum, whereas in the infertile woman overdilatation may eventually result in cervical incompetence. We have not used Goodell's dilators because overzealous use may split the lateral fibers of the cervix, causing dangerous hemorrhage or subsequent incompetence. In a routine exploration or curettage of the endometrium, dilatation need not be carried beyond a no. 16 or 18 Hanks dilator. After the dilatation has been concluded, the uterine sound may be reinserted to ascertain the correct depth of the cavity. This instrument, which may be bent to the same angle as the dilators, should be inserted carefully since it may be pushed through the myometrium without undue pressure. A rule of thumb to avoid this complication is to exert no more pressure than is made by the friction of resting it on the forefinger.

Cervical dilatation is occasionally difficult, particularly in the hypoplastic anteflexed uterus in which there is a dense band of connective tissue at the internal os. Also in the atrophic uterus found in menopause and in the postirradiated uterus great care and perseverance are required to secure adequate dilatation. The best aid is good countertraction placed on the tenacula in an effort to straighten the endocervical angle. Frequently it will be necessary to locate the external cervical os with fine probes and then to proceed accordingly. Should a laceration of the cervix occur, repair should be undertaken immediately with fine catgut, since subsequent infection may produce a long-standing cervicitis.

In diagnostic curettage we begin with a large, sharp curet since this is less likely to perforate the uterus than the smaller variety. If a fractional curettage is being performed, the entire endocervix is curetted first, using the small curet or the endocervical curet devised by Kevorkian. The large curet is passed into the canal in the manner described for the uterine sound. It should not be bent at an angle sharper than that of the dilators unless it is being used to remove specific fragments of placental tissue. The entire uterine cavity is then thoroughly scraped in a systematic manner (Fig. 12–7) until the sharp scratch of the submucosa, the so-called *cri uterine*, can be heard. The curet should be passed into the uterine cavity lightly on the finger but may be drawn out vigorously and with considerable force. After the major portion of the uterine cavity has been treated, the small curet is used to explore the uterine cornua. Endometrial carcinoma may be localized in one of the uterine horns and will be missed if the smaller curet is not used. If the tissue removed is suggestive of malignancy, the curet is purposely carried somewhat deeper into the myometrium in order to determine by microscopic means whether or not the disease has invaded the subjacent tissue. Polypoid growths are usually soft and pliable and may be missed by routine curettage. Therefore it has been our routine to explore the uterine cavity thoroughly with a small placenta forceps or Kelly clamp at the conclusion of the procedure.

If the object of curettage is the removal of placental tissue and chorionic villi following an abortion, it is best to use a rather blunt curet. Frequently it is possible to perform a finger curettage to remove most of the products of conception, following which a continuous intravenous administration of dilute Pitocin solution will cause the uterus to contract and assume a relatively normal shape. A large, sharp curet may then be used if it is difficult to remove all the products of conception with the dull instrument. It is imperative, however, that the operator avoid being too thorough, since uterine perforation or dissemination of infection may result. It is not necessary to remove all of the decidua, and numerous cases have been reported of complete denudation of the endometrium by such overzealous curettage. Many patients with

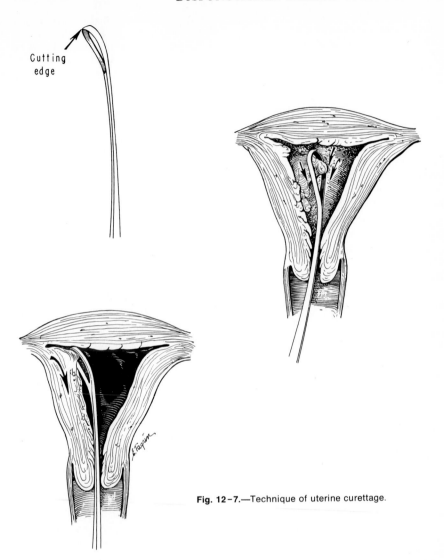

Cutting
edge

Fig. 12-7.—Technique of uterine curettage.

postabortal amenorrhea have been found to be ovulating normally but are amenorrheic because of scarification of the endometrium with subsequent adherence of the walls together with synechia formation. If it seems likely that small fragments of tissue have been left in the uterine cavity, these may be wiped out with a strip of gauze placed on a Kelly clamp or similar instrument.

No further treatment is usually necessary following a thorough curettage, and it is important to avoid douches and chemical applications for several days. If severe bleeding follows curettage, it is usually due to retained fragments of tissue rather than to vascular trauma. We do not pack the uterus following curettage although rarely a postabortal uterus may respond to this treatment. The small degree of venous oozing that occurs or the bleeding from the cervix due to the tenacula may be controlled by packing the vagina tightly for a few hours.

If patients are properly prepared and the operation done under antiseptic precautions, simple perforation of the uterus ordinarily does no harm and laparotomy is seldom necessary. The patient is watched carefully for hemorrhage although this is a rare complication except when there has been perforation with a large curet in a postabortal uterus. Larger wounds made by the placental forceps, especially in an attempt to remove fetal tissue, may permit the small intestine to prolapse into the uterine canal and vagina. In such cases immediate surgical intervention is obviously necessary.

Bleeding Associated with Ovulation

This abnormality is seen quite often in women during the latter half of their reproductive years and consists of bleeding or spotting for a two- or three-day period at the time of ovulation. The flow rarely is profuse but may linger until the onset of the next period. The term *pseudopolymenorrhea* has been adopted to describe this situation since the patient's usual complaint is that of a period "every two weeks." Premenstrual molimina are absent before this bleeding and a biopsy taken at the time of bleeding reveals late proliferative endometrium, occasionally with glandular changes suggesting ovulation. The bleeding probably results from endometrial breakdown and may be classified as a type of estrogen-withdrawal bleeding. As a result of follicular rupture and reorganization of the vascular integrity of the developing corpus luteum, a temporary decrease in the titer of estrogen occurs which apparently is sufficient to cause endometrial disintegration. A diagnosis may be made by a careful history supplemented by endometrial biopsy and a basal temperature chart. If this is the only abnormality of bleeding manifested by the patient, treatment consists principally of explanation and reassurance. When the bleeding is embarrassing or troublesome, the administration of small amounts of estrogenic substances (diethylstilbestrol 0.25 mg. or ethinyl estradiol 0.02 mg.) from day 10 through day 16 of a 28-day cycle will usually effect cure.

Premenstrual Staining

While premenstrual staining may often occur because of a submucous leiomyoma, the commonest cause is an endocrine imbalance. In the normal human female, menstruation occurs subsequent to a sharp decline in the elaboration of corpus luteum steroids. Teetering, fluctuation or gradual decline in the level of these hormones causes premature endometrial catabolism and results in bleeding before the onset of the expected period. The underlying pathology is usually an intrinsic, poorly understood corpus luteum failure. Histologically the endometrium shows varying degrees of progestational immaturity, and bleeding may occur from what is termed 24- or 25-day endometrium. Frequently there is a disparity between glandular and stromal development and, in particular, there is inadequate perivascular predecidual formation. Treatment is often unnecessary but if the problem is disconcerting to the patient it is simply obviated by giving an estrogen-progestin combination from day 20 through day 25 of a 28-day cycle. A long-acting progesterone (Delalutin) may be used with equal efficacy, 250 mg. given intramuscularly on day 14 of a 28-day cycle. Both methods are directed toward the support of a failing endometrium and should be repeated for a minimum of three or four cycles. If staining or bleeding occurs while the patient is receiving progesterone, underlying organic pathology is usually present; careful examination under anesthesia and curettage are indicated. Not infrequently patients with endometriosis will note premenstrual staining occurring simultaneously with pelvic pain.

Normal Bleeding at Less than Usual Intervals

Menstrual periods which occur every 18–21 days may be termed unusual or "not average" but must be considered normal if this is the established pattern of a given individual. Flowing which occurs at intervals of less than 18 days is abnormal and merits investigation. As previously mentioned, the postovulatory phase is a relatively constant 14 ± 2 days, with a preliminary three or four days being necessary for follicular maturation. If the bleeding is occurring as a deviation from the established pattern and the patient complains of periods "too close together," the condition known as *polymenorrhea* exists. This is not uncommon in postmenarchal girls because of fluctuations in ovarian activity. It may similarly be seen in premenopausal patients although skips and delays of periods are usually more common. Treatment in both instances is unnecessary if endometrial sampling is normal, since time will remedy the irregularity in the first instance by the establishment of normal ovulatory patterns and in the second by complete cessation of flow.

If normal, cyclic uterine bleeding occurs at intervals shorter than the established pattern for an individual or is associated with infertility, definitive therapy is warranted. Dilatation and curettage may be performed first to eliminate the possibilities of organic disease and to ascertain the functional status of the endometrium and ovaries. It should be performed in the late secretory or early menstrual phase. In almost all cases the endometrium will be found to be of normal secretory type, occasionally with "progestational immaturity" which may be evidenced as inadequate decidual reaction in the stroma or incomplete secretory glandular activity. Curettage alone does not usually effect reversion of the cycle back to its normal length so that hormonal treatment is necessary. Two methods are available. (1) If the shortened cycle is presumed to be due to premature maturation of the follicle, regulation may be accomplished by suppression of adenohypophyseal gonadotropins in the preovulatory phase. This is accomplished by the administration of estrogenic substances (diethylstilbestrol 0.5 mg. or ethinyl estradiol 0.05 mg. twice daily) from the third through the tenth day of the cycle. This may occasionally delay ovulation past the fourteenth day of the cycle, resulting in cycles of 30 or 32 days, but regulation of dosage and shortening of the treatment period will usually rectify this difficulty. (2) Induction of artificial cycles using estrogens and progestins in amounts sufficient to suppress ovulation completely is frequently effective in restoring cycles to normal length. Although the mechanism of this action is not well understood, it is believed due to a rebound phenomenon, with restoration of a normally balanced pituitary-ovarian endometrial axis. Artificial anovulatory cycles may be induced by diethylstilbestrol 0.5 mg. or ethinyl estradiol 0.05 mg. given twice daily from the fourth through the twenty-fourth day of the cycle with progesterone, 50 mg. intramuscularly, added on days 23 and 24. Withdrawal bleeding usually begins two to six days after cessation of therapy, and treatment is again instituted on the fourth day of flow and repeated for three such artificial cycles. Equally good results may be obtained with the use of one of the estrogen-progestin combinations which contain at least 100 mcg. of estrogen.

NORMAL BLEEDING AT MORE THAN USUAL INTERVALS

Because the length of the menstrual cycle is variable, an exact definition of prolonged cycles is difficult to establish. If menses occur at regular intervals of from 32 to 45 days, the cycles may be considered prolonged but not abnormal and may represent merely a prolongation of the follicular phase. It is not known whether this is due to insufficient gonadotropic stimulation or to follicular inadequacy. No therapy is indicated in such patients unless the prolongation of the cycle indicates a change from a previously established pattern or is associated with infertility. When the interval between menses exceeds 45 days and there is associated irregularity or diminution in the amount of flow, consideration must be given to the possibility of secondary amenorrhea developing.

Although the precise pathogenesis of this entity remains obscure, relative ovarian failure is probably the causative factor in most patients. This may be manifested as a premature menopause or may be associated with systemic disease and malnutrition. Hypothalamic influences, such as psychic disturbances, fright or obesity, may be etiologic in some cases.

The diagnostic and therapeutic procedures for patients with prolonged cycles are similar to those discussed in the evaluation and treatment of secondary amenorrhea.

PROFUSE OR PROLONGED BLEEDING AT NORMAL INTERVALS
(HYPERMENORRHEA)

The magnitude and the duration of uterine bleeding vary considerably among women and a precise definition of hypermenorrhea is difficult. Moreover, what seems to be excessive bleeding to one patient is considered perfectly normal by another. The problem is therefore relative, in that changes from an established norm must be considered. If a patient usually has a four-day flow and she uses three napkins a day, a change to a six-day flow with five napkins being necessary may properly be considered hypermenorrhea. Another patient may have always had a six-day flow necessitating six napkins a day and, for her, this is normal. If an average can be assumed, the length of the period will approximate four to six days with a change of napkins being necessary about three or four times daily during the height of flowing. Hematocrit and hemoglobin determinations frequently will aid in making a diagnosis of hypermenorrhea. If a patient considers the amount or duration of flow to be excessive, diagnostic and therapeutic steps should be initiated.

Before profuse or prolonged bleeding may be considered to be dysfunctional there should be a complete evaluation of the patient to eliminate organic causes. Leiomyomas, pelvic inflammatory disease, endometriosis, adenomyosis, polyps, blood dyscrasias, systemic diseases, carcinoma, constitutional defects and psychogenic disturbances must be considered in differential diagnosis. Examination of the endometrium by curettage or biopsy performed at the time of bleeding in cyclic dysfunctional hypermenorrhea usually discloses some degree of progestational activity, indicating prior ovulation. Frequently the pathologist will return a diagnosis of "progestational immaturity." This suggests that the corpus luteum has been inadequate or that the endometrial response to adequate progesterone is deficient. Knowledge of these fundamental hormonal interactions is meager at present and will remain so until accurate methods are devised for the isolation and quantification of pituitary and ovarian hormones in body fluids.

Treatment of cyclic hypermenorrhea associated with a secretory endometrium may actually be incorporated in the diagnostic procedure of curettage. Thus, in a high percentage of patients the periods subsequent to curettage will be normal and further therapy will be unnecessary. Such a curettage also affords the opportunity for a more complete pelvic examination to exclude organic disease. It is, therefore, recommended as an initial and integral procedure except in adolescents in the postmenarchal period or in certain young, unmarried women. Treatment in this younger group may be instituted with hormonal preparations after systemic and hematologic disorders have been eliminated. Occasionally, however, curettage is indicated if the bleeding is excessive or does not respond promptly to the usual regimens.

Hormonal therapy in this group is aimed at improving the progestational quality of the endometrium and accomplishing improved hemostasis. The simplest method is to give 50 or 100 mg. of progesterone intramuscularly on the twenty-fourth day of a 28-day cycle. Uterine bleeding of normal amount usually begins two to six days after the injection. This regimen should be repeated for three consecutive cycles. An alternative method is to have the patient take 10 mg. Enovid for one week during the luteal phase, that is, from day 17 to day 24 of a 28-day cycle. In some patients it may be desirable to produce hypophyseal suppression and inhibition of ovulation for periods of three to four months. This may be accomplished by giving one of the estrogen-progestin combinations from the fifth to the twenty-fourth day of the cycle. After the medication is stopped a withdrawal, albeit anovulatory, flow will occur in two to four days. The rationale for such treatment may be explained as follows: the progestins, administered as suggested, effectively inhibit the adenohypophyseal release of gonadotropins during the course of therapy. When treatment is halted, a more normal spectrum of gonadotropic elaboration often occurs. If intermenstrual or abnormal bleeding occurs while the patient is receiving progesterone therapy, or if hypermenorrhea recurs following treatment, intrauterine or intrapelvic pathology exists and curettage is mandatory.

If the patient is seen during the phase of profuse bleeding a degree of hemostasis may be secured by hormonal therapy. An endometrial biopsy is obtained to be sure the bleeding is truly from a secretory endometrium, and the patient is given 100 mg. progesterone intramuscularly. She should be cautioned that a rather profuse flow will occur in two to six days. Progesterone may then be given intramuscularly on the twenty-fourth day of the cycle as outlined previously and treatment repeated for at least three consecutive cycles. An alternative method is to give 20 or 30 mg. of any synthetic progestin daily for four or five days. This will usually control the hypermenorrhea in a matter of 24 hours. A withdrawal flow is permitted and a 10 mg. dose is then administered daily for 20 days, beginning on the fourth day of flow. This is repeated during three consecutive cycles. If satisfactory clinical results are not obtained, curettage is necessary.

The endometrial hemostasis produced by progesterone is dramatic but its exact mechanism is unknown. It may be the result of the ability of progesterone (and presumably other progestagens) to augment estrogen metabolism, converting estradiol to estrone and estriol and inhibiting their oxidation. It has been shown that estrone and estriol are proportionally greater during the luteal phase of the menstrual cycle, whereas oxidation products become much reduced.

The author no longer treats cyclic hypermenorrhea with estrogens or with estrogens and progestins in sequence since the results are equally good with progesterone (or synthetic progestins) when endogenous estrogen appears to be in adequate supply.

Irregular Shedding of the Endometrium

This term describes a form of dysfunctional uterine bleeding characterized by prolonged and profuse menstrual flow occurring at regular intervals from a secretory endometrium. The diagnosis is made by obtaining endometrial tissue by biopsy at least five days after the onset of flow. At this time in the normal cycle complete regeneration has occurred and the biopsy reveals early proliferative endometrium; in "irregular shedding," histologic characteristics of secretory endometrium plus incomplete regenerative changes are present. These findings suggest that menstruation has begun prematurely and has continued longer than usual because of the presence of progesterone. This idea has been supported by the finding of persistent urinary pregnanediol during the bleeding phase and suggests that the process is related to retarded regression of the corpus luteum. Dr. Arthur T. Hertig described this corpus luteum as "one that is dead but will not lie down."

Treatment of this condition is not specific or uniformly satisfactory. If it is suspected from the history or from a properly timed endometrial biopsy, curettage should be performed during the latter part of the bleeding episode. Curettage may prove to be therapeutic as well as diagnostic. In other patients, the use of estrogenic substances such as ethinyl estradiol, 0.05 mg. twice daily by mouth, beginning on the third or fourth day of bleeding will hasten endometrial regeneration and diminish the intensity of uterine bleeding. If this therapy is unsuccessful, artificial anovulatory cycles using progestins as previously described may be tried. In older patients surgical extirpation of the uterus may occasionally be advisable.

Constant or Intermittent Bleeding

This is the commonest type of irregularity found under the classification of dysfunctional uterine bleeding and is frequently seen during the postmenarchal and premenopausal periods when ovulation is infrequent or sporadic. If postovulatory menstruation may be described as *cyclic*, this variety of bleeding is typically *acyclic*, grossly unpredictable and characterized by profuse flow unassociated with the usual premenstrual molimina. Bleeding may be associated with the passage of large clots and may at times be almost exsanguinating. Determinations of hemoglobin, serum iron and hematocrit usually give low values and occasionally critical levels are reached.

Anovulatory dysfunctional bleeding seems more common in a specific body type, although exact correlations are not possible. The individual is frequently short, obese and appears hypothyroid. In most patients the onset of the menses is at the normal time but within two or three years prolonged intervals, up to four or five months, occur between periods. Weight gain is frequently excessive and may actually be an etiologic factor in perpetuating the abnormal hypophyseal-ovarian relation. Premenstrual molimina do not occur, and the patient may note an abrupt onset of profuse flow with the passage of clots after a prolonged interval of amenorrhea. The flow may continue to be heavy for 10–14 days and is frequently followed by another week or so of staining. This pattern becomes irregularly repetitious. Bleeding episodes of this type may follow full-term delivery or abortion but, in general, they are more common in the infertile group of patients.

Diagnosis may be suspected from the typical history and corroborated by basal body temperature graphs and properly timed endometrial biopsies. Since progesterone is not present, the temperature graph will be monophasic and the biopsy will show either proliferative or hyperplastic endometrium, depending on how long estrogen has been effectively stimulating endometrial growth. The optimum time for obtaining the endometrial biopsy is at the onset of bleeding. The diagnosis should be verified, in most cases, by a thorough, fractional uterine curettage under anesthesia. This will exclude the other major causes of constant or intermittent uterine bleeding, namely, malignancy and submucous leiomyomas. Elaborate diagnostic procedures such as urinary assays of estrogen and pregnanediol and hypophyseal hormones are expensive, time-consuming and, in most cases, unnecessary.

Treatment of this variety of dysfunctional bleeding is frequently difficult because of our inability to measure quantitative differences in the interplay of hormones. Curettage alone is not so often an effective therapeutic agent since it does nothing to re-establish a normal ovulatory pattern. In some patients a re-establishment of ovulation seems to be brought about by ancillary measures which are used after the diagnostic curettage. These include proper diet, weight reduction, vitamins, thyroid extract and simple reassurance. In other patients, however, therapy is substitutional in the form of pituitary or ovarian hormones. Pituitary hormones of animal derivation have been used in an attempt to simulate follicle-stimulating and luteinizing hormones. The results have been disappointing and occasionally these preparations have produced untoward reactions of systemic and local types. Follicular growth has been produced and, in some cases, the development of large follicular cysts has necessitated surgery. In most patients ovulation has not followed the use of the preparations.

Attempts have been made to secure ovulation in this group by the use of estrogens, progestins, androgens and various combinations of these steroids. No evidence is presently available to indicate that they "cause" ovulation in the oligo-ovulator any oftener than occurs by chance alone. Recent studies have indicated that in certain patients, not necessarily showing evidence of hyperadrenocorticism, the administration of small amounts of cortisone or hydrocortisone (10 mg. twice daily) will frequently be followed by ovulation.

Optimum results have been obtained in patients with the Stein-Leventhal syndrome by the use of clomiphene citrate. Wedge resection of the ovaries is rarely necessary. (See Chapter 9.)

Constant or intermittent uterine bleeding of anovulatory type is common during menarche and the climacteric. Curettage is not believed to be mandatory in the young patient (unless bleeding is exsanguinating) but is an integral part of the diagnostic regimen in the menopausal woman. If bleeding continues in the teen-aged girl, treatment may be instituted with cyclic use of an estrogen-progestin combination as previously described. A concerted effort should be made to find the cause of deficient ovulation in such patients, but bleeding may be converted to a cyclic process by the administration of these steroids. If these schemes do not control the irregularity, a thorough curettage should be done, since some organic lesion is probably present. Evidence now indicates that the prolonged use of the newer progestins, either cyclically or constantly, for four to six months, may convert many of the atypical endometrial hyperplasias into a less disturbing pattern and obviate hysterectomy in this young age group. The effect of these steroids is multiple, but a profound effect is seen on the growth pattern of endometrial glands.

In the premenopausal or menopausal woman a curettage is always done to eliminate the possibility of malignancy. If the bleeding is the result of progressive ovarian insufficiency, absent progesterone and teetering estrogen levels, nothing further need be done since the problem is usually self-limited. The management of recurrent bleeding in this age group after one diagnostic curettage has given negative findings is a difficult problem but is an adequate indication for hysterectomy since steroid therapy is not usually used in this age group. Occasionally, at hysterectomy, bleeding will be found to be due to a submucous fibroid, an undiscovered pedunculated adenomyoma or arteriosclerotic changes in the uterine vasculature. Curettage and cervical biopsy should always precede such hysterectomies, however, since malignancy may co-exist and this necessitates a more radical therapeutic approach. In certain patients in whom medical conditions contraindicate surgery, endometrial atrophy may be produced by the continuous administration of synthetic progestins.

Dysmenorrhea

Dysmenorrhea is the presence of abdominal and pelvic pain occurring just prior to or coincident with the onset of menstruation. It is one of the most common symptoms in gynecology and may be classified as primary (idiopathic, intrinsic) or secondary (acquired, organic).

Primary dysmenorrhea, the subject of extensive research and discussion, remains a disease of theories. To those affected by the malady, however, it is quite real and, despite the controversy over etiology, it remains a major problem wherever young women are employed. It has been estimated that approximately 140 million work hours are lost annually as a result of this entity. By definition, "primary" implies that the menstrual pain is observed in the absence of any discernible pelvic lesion and is due to hormonal derangement and an individual hypersensitivity of the target organ, the uterus.

The malady occurs most frequently in those under age 25 and is often seen in women under 20. McArthur noted that dysmenorrhea is the commonest of adolescent menstrual disturbances, 30–50 per cent of all puberal girls being subject to appreciable discomfort and 10 per cent being incapacitated for one to three days each month. It is more common in the nulliparous individual, parturition marking the endpoint of the disease in most patients. That this is not entirely due to cervical dilatation is evidenced by the fact that the cure rate seems just as high in patients undergoing abdominal delivery as in those who deliver pelvically.

Symptomatology.—Symptoms do not usually appear with the first few periods since these are almost always anovulatory. Suddenly, about a year or two after the menarche, pain is noted. Characteristically the discomfort begins a day or two before the onset of flow and lasts during the first and occasionally the second day of the period. Most patients describe the pain as being sharp and cramplike or as a severe aching in the midline just above the pubic symphysis. Generalized lassitude, backache, leg ache, headache, nervousness and nausea may be present in more severe cases. The psyche and morale may be adversely affected by uninterrupted monthly episodes of this variety, and anxiety neuroses may develop. Psychiatrists have suggested that this is reverse reasoning, since in certain patients dysmenorrhea is merely a signal of a deeper emotional disturbance. This is probable if the pain continues to be severe, persistent and resistant to the usual palliative procedures. While this may be true in fact, as well as fancy, it has been our observation that dysmenorrhea may be relieved completely or almost completely in both *adjusted* and *maladjusted* girls by the simple process of suppression of ovulation.

Secondary dysmenorrhea implies that the pain which occurs at the time of the menses is due to, or associated with, organic pelvic disease. The most common of these are (1) endometriosis, (2) inflammatory and infectious processes, (3) adenomyosis, (4) cervical strictures and (5) the pelvic congestion syndrome. The pain is usually located more laterally in the pelvis and seems to be of a deep, boring quality rather than being midline and crampy. Furthermore, especially in endometriosis and adenomyosis, onset of the pain antedates menstruation and is of reduced intensity after the flow starts although in certain patients it may persist throughout the cycle. The age incidence is usually higher in secondary dysmenorrhea, the average being the late twenties or early thirties. Adenomyosis seems to occur in multiparous patients in the late thirties and early forties and is frequently associated with hypermenorrhea. Each of these diseases producing secondary dysmenorrhea is discussed in detail elsewhere in this text.

Etiology.—Many factors have been suggested as being the major cause of primary dysmenorrhea. Some may be discarded without further discussion. These are cervical stenosis, uterine hypoplasia and uterine malpositions. One constant observation is of significance: primary dysmenorrhea is always associated with bleeding from a secretory endometrium. Suppression of ovulation by estrogenic substances, with subsequent cyclic withdrawal bleeding from a proliferative endometrium, is uniformly painless. If patients who are having induced anovulatory flows receive progesterone in the last half of the cycle, they experience dysmenorrhea. Whatever the cause of primary dysmenorrhea may be, its development depends on a progestational endometrium.

Considerable evidence has been presented to suggest that psychogenic factors are responsible for most of the dysmenorrhea seen today. Supporting this thought is the fact that a "recovery rate" may be obtained in approximately 70 per cent of patients by careful interview, explanation, reassurance, diet and attention to personal hygienic factors. This is about the same per cent of improvement noted in studies utilizing various analgesic and antispasmodic medications and is not much more than that obtained with placebos. However, in these same groups, complete relief may be obtained in almost 100 per cent of patients by suppression of ovulation. This would seem to indicate that, even in the presence of the factors necessary to cause pain, relief may be obtained in three patients out of four by various simple approaches.

Primary dysmenorrhea has been looked on by some as representing an abnormal hormonal balance. The typical patient is described as "asthenic with small breasts, a hypoplastic uterus and a congenitally eroded cervix." Although this suggests some degree of hypoestrinism, no evidence is available to verify this. Aberrations of hormonal interplay have been suggested also as the cause of spasm of both uterine muscle and vasculature, resulting in tissue anoxia and focal ischemia. Intrauterine balloon studies have demonstrated variations in amplitude and frequency of uterine contractions during different parts of the menstrual cycle. For example, during the postovulatory phase (when estrogen and progesterone are present), the contractions are less frequent but of greater amplitude than those which occur in the proliferative phase. This observation is somewhat at variance with the old theory that estrogen increased uterine tone and progesterone diminished it.

In summary, it may be concluded that primary dysmenorrhea is due to an unknown and probably varied etiology but is associated with the sloughing of a secretory endometrium. The latter process produces increased uterine motility with contractions of greater amplitude and, perhaps, with periods of arrhythmia and tetany. The effects might then be twofold: (1) vascular spasm with ischemia of the myometrium and (2) delayed expulsion of blood and endometrial fragments. Since there is a great difference in the threshold for pain in different patients and in the same patient from month to month or under difficult circumstances, this uterine "sensation" may be variously interpreted as heaviness, aching, discomfort or genuine pain.

Similarly, the milieu surrounding this process may be tempered by emotional, environmental and hormonal influences to a degree that a normal process takes on pathologic characteristics. Adjustment of the milieu may bring about as much pain relief as analgesic drugs or surgical denervation.

Treatment.—A complete physical and pelvic examination must precede any form of therapy. The physician should look for signs and symptoms of tuberculosis, chronic nephritis, rheumatic fever, avitaminosis and malnutrition, all of which may trigger menstrual pain. If a bimanual vaginal examination cannot be performed because of a virginal introitus, a gentle rectal examination may afford almost as much information. Congenital abnormalities and pathologic conditions of the pelvic viscera will become apparent if the pelvic examination is done thoroughly, although in certain overly tense individuals an examination under anesthesia is necessary. In most cases of dysmenorrhea the examination gives entirely negative results except for the presence of a congenital cervical erosion. If an adequate pelvic examination can be done, a uterine sound may be gently inserted through the cervical os (with experience this can be done with a finger in the rectum guiding the sound). In patients with primary dysmenorrhea this will duplicate the type of pain they have noted at the time of their periods. Presumably the sound produces uterine contractions and some degree of tetany. (The test is negative after adequate presacral neurectomy and in most multiparous patients with a patulous internal os.) During the vaginal and rectal examinations some idea may be obtained about the patient's pain threshold.

The optimum and simplest method of treatment is psychotherapy in the form of simple guidance, open discussion and instruction about the natural phenomenon of menstruation. The mystery and intrigue surrounding the process should be unveiled and a program of physical activity suggested. Warm tub baths are an effective therapeutic measure but usually have been prohibited by the parents or by tradition. Medications are limited to mild analgesics and antispasmodics. A particularly good preparation in our hands has been the combination of aspirin, phenacetin and Benzedrine (Edrisal) given for two to three days before the onset of flow as well as during the period. There is some evidence from animal experiments that amphetamine (Benzedrine) may prevent sustained, tetanic uterine contractions and its mood-elevating property is particularly desirable. Morphine and codeine are not advised because of the possibility of addiction. Many patients secure adequate relief by eliminating sodium chloride from the diet and others benefit from a diuretic such as chlorothiazide given four to five days before onset of flow.

Hormonal treatment may be utilized if the methods just outlined are not successful. The basis for their use is to secure adenohypophyseal suppression and inhibition of ovulation. The following estrogenic substances are effective: (1) diethylstilbestrol, 1 mg. daily for 21 days beginning on the fourth day of the cycle; (2) Premarin, 2.5 mg. daily for 21 days, or (3) Estinyl, 0.05 mg. twice daily for 21 days. A painless flow will usually occur three to five days after stopping medication, and the estrogen is then restarted so that three or four such cycles may be given. This treatment is temporary since dysmenorrhea usually recurs within one or two months. It is uniformly effective and, by alternating treatment periods, relief may be given for six to ten months of each year. No evidence exists to prove that such therapy permanently disturbs subsequent ovulation or menstruation. Androgens are not suggested for the treatment of primary dysmenorrhea since large doses must be given to inhibit ovulation, with the definite risk of hirsutism, acne and deepening of the voice. Progesterone has not been uniformly successful in providing pain relief. As a matter of fact, it may actually induce painful bleeding episodes in anovulatory women who have always had painless flowing. However, recent work with the newer progestogens and nor-testosterones has indicated that these preparations may be of considerable value if given from day 5 through day 24, thus inhibiting ovulation.

Surgical treatment of primary dysmenorrhea is best reserved for patients who do not secure adequate relief from psychotherapy or other conservative measures. An adequate trial period should be allowed, including several courses of adenohypophyseal suppression. If the patient has pain relief during these intervals but has no immediate possibility of marriage and motherhood, a presacral neurectomy may be considered. Before this is done, however, a simple cervical dilatation under anesthesia may be attempted. Whether this is effective because of temporary alteration in uterine innervation or because of improvement in endometrial drainage is not known. In any event, it produces pain relief in about 25 per cent of patients. Unfortunately, the improvement is not permanent and after five or six months the problem must be reconsidered. Presacral neurectomy, or resection of the superior and middle hypogastric plexuses, is a major operation requiring laparotomy and should be done only after all other measures have failed. There are certain complications associated with this procedure, mostly due to the anatomic situation of the nerve plexus. Ureters have been ligated, iliac veins have been entered, and large retroperitoneal hematomas have occurred. Postoperative persistent constipation and bladder atony have been reported, as have intestinal obstruction and peritonitis. The "cure" rate approximates 80 per cent and depends on proper selection of patients as well as adequate resection. Failures have been due to regeneration of nerve fibers, anatomic peculiarities of the plexus preventing adequate removal, inadequate tissue resection and selection of patients who might have fared better with psychotherapy. Orgasm is not affected by presacral neurectomy, and pregnancy occurs at a normally expected rate following the operation. The first stage of labor will be "completely painless" in about a third and "relatively comfortable" in another third of patients having had adequate resections. Such patients should be forewarned of this fact when pregnancy occurs.

Adrenogenital Syndrome

The adrenogenital syndrome in the female is a disorder due to an inherent defect in normal biogenesis within the adrenal gland and is recognized as an inherited error of metabolism. The clinical features in both the male and female are brought about by an excessive secretion of adrenal androgens. In patients who survive infancy and who are deprived of specific hormonal therapy, virilization and rapid somatic advance occur (Fig. 12–8). Adrenocortical activity begins in the fetus about the third month of gestation, before development and completion of certain genital structures. Thus, the female fetus is exposed to excessive androgenic stimulation from her own disordered adrenal cortex during the remainder of the pregnancy. The external genitalia are altered as a result of this stimulation. The urogenital sinus (which remains open as the introitus in the female) and the growth of the genital tubercles are diverted toward a male developmental pattern. The characteristic findings are (1) clitoral hypertrophy with some degree of ventral adhesion and (2) fusion of the labioscrotal folds. The external appearance is similar to that of a male with complete hypospadias and bilateral cryptorchism. The internal ducts and the gonads are unaltered in the human female fetus exposed to androgens from any source.

Similar alterations in the human fetus may be produced by administration of androgenic substances to the mother during the first trimester of pregnancy. For the most part, these abnormalities have been produced by the administration of the more androgenic progestins, ethynyl-testosterone (Pranone) and 19-norethynyl testosterone (Norlutin). Androgen-secreting

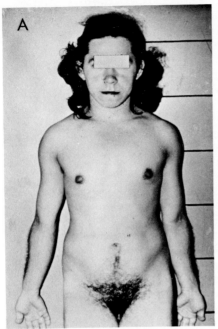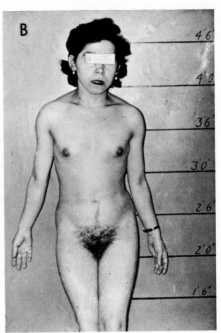

Fig. 12-8.—Classic adrenogenital syndrome in 19-year-old female. The 17-ketosteroid level was over 80 mg./24 hours and pregnanetriol was 48 mg./24 hours. **A,** before therapy. Note the masculinized female showing no evidence of feminization. **B,** after corticoid therapy there is a tendency for some loss of masculinizing musculature and beginning breast development plus female fat deposition. (From Kupperman, H. S.: *Human Endocrinology* [Philadelphia: F. A. Davis Company, 1963].)

tumors in the pregnant female, such as arrhenoblastoma, may also produce virilization of the female fetus, at least involving the external genitalia.

In some cases the degree of virilization is so pronounced that the urethra traverses the entire length of the genital tubercle (clitoris). The labioscrotal folds may become bulbous, rugated and deeply pigmented, resembling the skin of the scrotum.

Rarely the external genitalia of the newborn female infant are normal and virilization becomes evident during infancy, adolescence or adulthood. Studies on these individuals have revealed biochemical findings consistent with the diagnosis of adrenal hyperplasia of the inherited type. These cases have been regarded as acquired adrenocortical hyperplasia but the presence of an adrenal tumor must be considered. It has been suggested in these cases that, although the adrenal glands have a congenital defect of biogenesis, excessive androgens were not secreted until after the fifth fetal month and the external genitalia thus were normal.

If the female infant does not receive treatment, typical signs of complete virilization follow rapidly. There are deepening of the voice, appearance of pubic hair, enlargement of the clitoris, excess of facial hair and temporal baldness. Breast development and onset of the menses do not occur at adolescence. There is acceleration of linear bone growth, so that by the fifth or sixth year of life the height age may be the equivalent of that for 12 or 13 years and the bone age equivalent to that at age 15 or older. Premature fusion of the epiphyses then occurs, with the subsequent production of a dwarfed adult in a previously excessively tall female child. Muscular development is excessive and a masculine habitus appears.

In certain cases of congenital adrenal hyperplasia, symptoms resembling addisonian crisis develop shortly after birth, with excessive vomiting and subsequent dehydration. Death may occur rapidly in these patients. The condition is occasionally confused with hypertrophic pyloric stenosis because of the recurrent emesis, weight loss and rapid dehydration. These cases have been described as the "salt-losing" type of the disease and necessitate early recognition and rapid therapy. Certain complications have been described in the adult with adrenogenital syndrome, including vascular hypertension, hypoglycemia and recurrent fever.

The pathology of the adrenal cortex in patients with congenital adrenal hyperplasia reveals a hyperplasia of the reticular zone, and it is believed that these cells are the source of increased androgen production. Blackman has described irregularly arranged but compact, pigmented, eosinophilic cells with small basophilic nuclei in this region. The zona fasciculata is usually normal but the zona glomerulosa may be poorly developed. It has been suggested that the salt-losing form of congenital adrenal hyperplasia is due to the inadequacy of the zona glomerulosa. It has been postulated that the hyperplasia of the zona reticularis is due to excessive stimulation of the adrenal cortex by ACTH. Symington demonstrated that ACTH stimulation causes the "clear" cells of the zona fasciculata to become indistinguishable from the "compact" cells of the zona reticularis.

Abnormal pathologic findings have been described in the ovary, testis and pituitary gland of patients with congenital adrenal hyperplasia. Before puberty the ovarian histology is normal but in the postpuberal female the ovaries become cystic and have a thickened cortex with fibrosis, resembling ovaries in the Stein-Leventhal syndrome. Hyperplasia of the ovarian hilar cells has also been described.

The basic enzymatic defect in the adrenogenital syndrome is in the biosynthesis of cortisol. There follows a compensatory endogenous ACTH stimulation with enlargement of the target organ and overproduction of other adrenal secretory products, some of which are androgenic. A rise in circulating ACTH has been demonstrated. The levels of cortisol in the blood and the urinary metabolites thereof are either normal or within the lower range of normal. Many subjects with adrenocortical hyperplasia achieve compensation, so far as the secretion of cortisol is concerned, at the expense of adrenal enlargement with excessive production of androgens. The precise enzymatic defect was not appreciated until suitable methods for the routine estimation of pregnanetriol in urine became available. This substance has been found regularly and in large amounts in the urine of practically all patients with adrenogenital syndrome. Before age 2 pregnanetriol is barely present in normal urine; after age 15 it rises to an average of 1.5 mg./day. The precursors of pregnanetriol are 17-hydroxypregnenolone and 17-hydroxyprogesterone. The biogenesis of adrenal steroids is shown in Figure 12–9. The various enzymes of the adrenal cortex together with the urinary metabolites are shown diagrammatically in Figure 12–10. Several enzymes are necessary for the completion of this process. Pregnenolone is derived in great measure from the degradation of cholesterol. Pregnenolone is then converted into progesterone through the

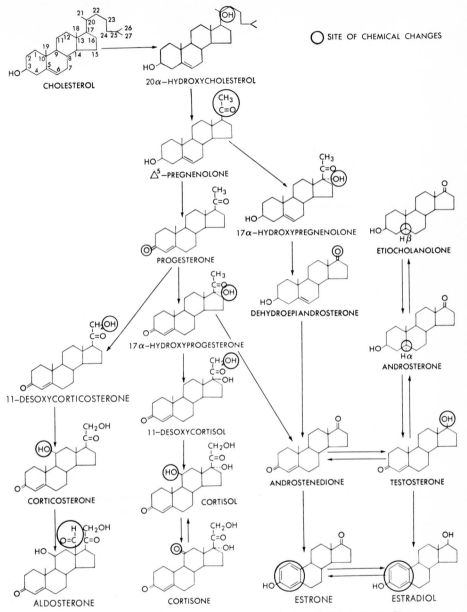

Fig. 12-9.—Biosynthesis of some adrenal steroids. (From Forsham, P.: The Adrenals, Ciba Clinical Symposia, Vol. 15, No. 1, 1963.)

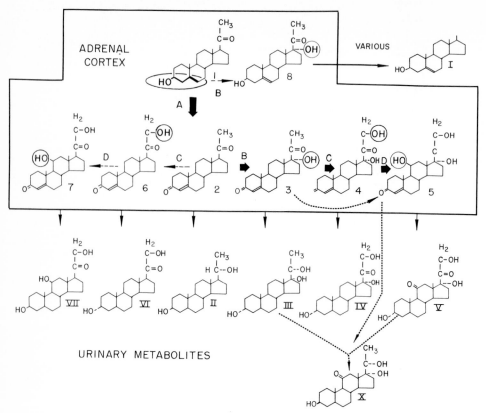

Fig. 12–10.—Biogenesis of cortisol, 5, and secondarily corticosterone, 7, in the adrenal cortex, with the reduced urinary metabolites of these end-products and the intermediate metabolites. The various enzymes are illustrated and their sites of action shown by encircled heavy type: **A,** 3-beta-hydroxysteroid dehydrogenase; **B,** 17-hydroxylase; **C,** 21-hydroxylase; **D,** 11-hydroxylase. The commonest form of the adrenogenital syndrome is characterized by a lack of 21-hydroxylase (C) and hence an accumulation of 17-hydroxyprogesterone (3), with the excretion of large quantities of the latter's reduced metabolite, pregnanetriol (III). (From Bongiovanni, A. M., and Root, A. W.: New England J. Med.: 268:1283, 1963 [Slightly modified].)

action of 3-beta-hydroxysteroid dehydrogenase. This enzymatic molecule is found only rarely in the urine of patients with congenital adrenocortical hyperplasia. However, it is present in normal amounts in patients with adrenogenital syndrome due to adrenocortical tumors. Subsequently progesterone is hydroxylated at carbons 17, 21 and 11, thus being converted into cortisol. Each of these conversions is effected by a separate enzyme. Investigations of steroidal metabolites in patients with adrenogenital syndrome have indicated the faulty cortisol production to be due to a lack, partial or complete, of one or more of the following enzymes: 3-beta-hydroxysteroid dehydrogenase, 11-hydroxylase and 21-hydroxylase. A deficit of the last of these is the cause of the most common form of the disorder.

The specific adrenal androgen or androgens responsible for the virilizing clinical manifestations of congenital adrenal hyperplasia have not been identified. Despite the general elevation of the urinary 17-ketosteroid levels, many investigators regard these metabolites as having insufficient biologic activity to explain the masculinization. However, the fact remains that the

11-desoxy-17-ketosteroids, androsterone and etiocholanolone, dominate the urinary steroidal pattern. Yet both of these 17-ketosteroids possess only a small degree of biologic potency. The possibility of a potent adrenal precursor of these various urinary metabolites has been suggested. Figure 12–11 provides an outline of the adrenal derivation of several of these important 17-ketosteroids. It is apparent that these 17-ketosteroids may originate from certain 21-carbon steroids concerned with cortisol synthesis, as shown in Figure 12–10. Thus, if an overproduction of 17-hydroxyprogesterone occurred, an increased conversion of the latter to androsterone and etiocholanolone would be anticipated. The route of biogenesis to certain urinary 17-ketosteroids is via Δ^4-androstenedione and perhaps testosterone, both of which possess a moderate androgenic activity and would be capable of causing virilization. This particular sequence is applicable to the usual defect of 21-hydroxylase. In a deficiency of 11-hydroxylase the conversion would be directed almost exclusively to etiocholanolone. The deficiency of 3-beta-hydroxysteroid dehydrogenase would lead to an increased excretion of dehydroepiandrosterone and related 17-ketosteroids as shown in Figure 12–11.

Fig. 12–11.—Derivation of important urinary 17-ketosteroids from certain adrenocortical intermediary metabolites. Dehydroepiandrosterone itself appears in the urine to a variable extent. The enzymatic transactions, *A–D*, correspond to those in Figure 12–10. (From Bongiovanni, A. M., and Root, A. W.: New England J. Med. 268:1283, 1963.)

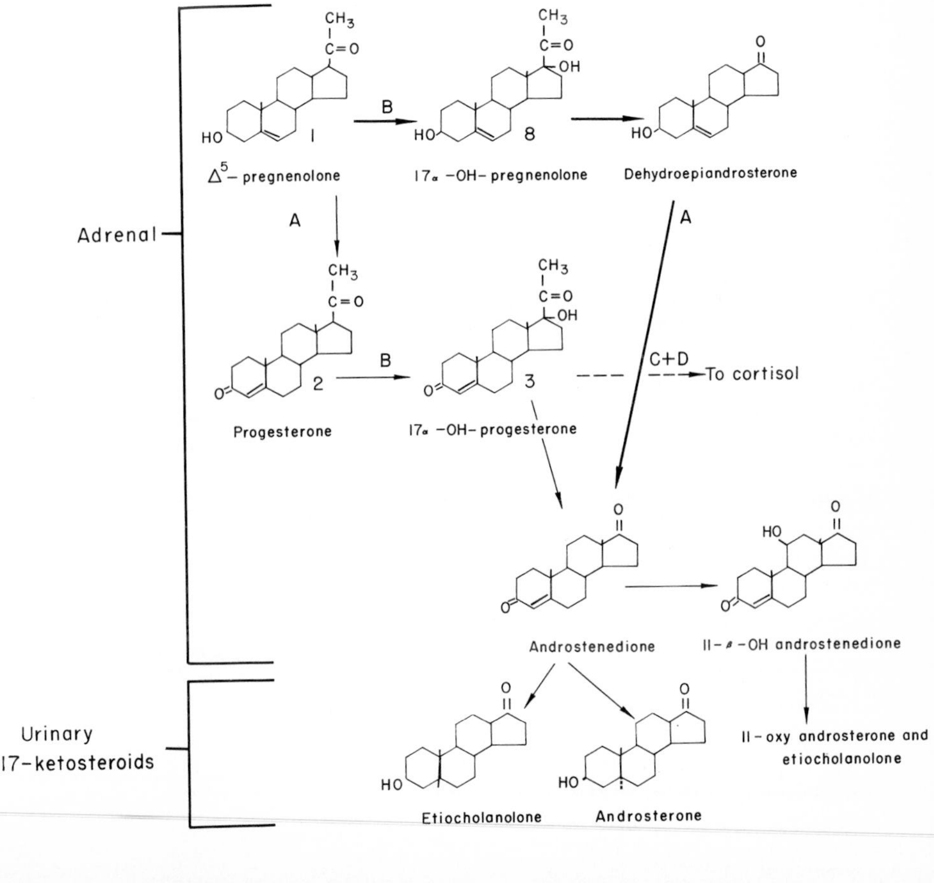

DIAGNOSIS OF ADRENOGENITAL SYNDROME

It is essential to arrive at the correct sex assignment as soon as possible after birth. It should be remembered that the first question of the family and friends concerns the sex of the newborn infant. The anguish of the parents whose offspring cannot be accurately identified is extreme. It is extremely difficult to reverse a faulty decision at any time, but in later life it may be impossible. Furthermore the proper recognition of adrenocortical hyperplasia calls for rapid and precise medical treatment in either sex to forestall the progressive virilization and abnormally rapid growth. The proper tools for correct interpretation and decision are now available and should be applied without hesitation.

Determination of the sex chromatin by buccal or vaginal smear is an accurate guide to the true sex in the adrenogenital syndrome although not necessarily so accurate in other forms of human intersex. In determining the correct sex, radiographic aid may be obtained by the injection of radiopaque dye into the external orifice. In some cases it may be accomplished by urethroscopic examination. It is desirable to solve the problem of proper designation without the necessity for laparotomy, and for further details of these diagnostic procedures the reader is referred to the description by Wilkins.

The diagnosis of congenital adrenal hyperplasia is verified by the finding of elevated urinary levels of 17-ketosteroids and pregnanetriol. The daily output of 17-ketosteroids in urine in the normal child until age 5 is less than 2 mg.; in the presence of adrenal virilizing hyperplasia it will vary between 8 and 20 mg./day, depending on the specific laboratory. In adrenogenital hyperplasia the level tends to be increased to two to four times normal. It is important to remember, however, that during the first week of life the 17-ketosteroid level is normally somewhat higher than those found later, being within the range of 2 and 5 mg./day. Thus, in the infant with adrenogenital syndrome it may not exceed these limits at the first determination. It is important to repeat the test at 2 and 3 weeks of age. A determination of urinary pregnanetriol or 11-ketopregnanetriol should be obtained. *During the first two years of life these steroids are virtually absent; whereas in the adrenogenital syndrome of the common type they are always elevated to diagnostic levels.* These tests are invaluable during the period of infancy as well as during adolescence and adulthood. It is usually unnecessary to measure the plasma levels of pertinent metabolites of cortisol, since they may be within normal range if the patient has compensated for the deficiency by excessive ACTH formation.

In this regard some description of the urinary 17-ketogenic steroids as a measure of cortisol production should be given. Although suitable for the purpose, they lack specificity in their inability to distinguish the metabolites of cortisol from certain "abnormal" metabolites (pregnanetriol and 11-ketopregnanetriol). It would be better for the clinician to utilize a laboratory which measured urinary 17-ketosteroids and pregnanetriol or 11-ketopregnanetriol.

The primary problem in differential diagnosis is distinguishing between a virilizing adrenal tumor and adrenocortical hyperplasia. When virilization first appears after the second year of life, the probability of adrenal tumor increases. If signs and symptoms of adrenal virilizing syndromes are present at birth or shortly thereafter, the cause is almost always adrenal hyperplasia and never tumor. It has been mentioned, however, that occasionally the adrenogenital syndrome due to congenital adrenal hyperplasia does not become apparent until the second or third year of life. This is more often true in the male than in the female. The 17-ketosteroids are increased in both hyperplasia and tumor of the adrenal gland, and although they are more apt to reach extremely high levels in the latter, this is of little help in the average case. If in the adolescent subject the 17-ketosteroids exceed 50 mg./day or in the adult exceed 100 mg./day, the probability of a tumor is extremely high. If the steroids which are identical to or related to dehydroepiandrosterone constitute more than 50 per cent of the total 17-ketosteroids, the possibility of adrenal tumor is increased. Steroids of this variety are precipitated by digitonin and may be detected by a simple technique known as the Allen reaction. Large quantities of pregnanetriol in urine are almost always diagnostic of adrenal hyperplasia. However, at least one case of tumor of the adrenal has been reported in which the pregnanetriol level was elevated. *At the present time, 11-ketopregnanetriol may be considered as the diagnostic urinary steroid in congenital adrenal hyperplasia.*

Jailer suggested the therapeutic test of diminution of urinary 17-ketosteroids following the administration of cortisol or related compounds. It was felt that this was definite proof for adrenal hyperplasia as opposed to neoplasm. In general, this is an accepted therapeutic and diagnostic procedure, but it should be mentioned that in some tumors a modest diminution in the urinary 17-ketosteroids may occur after administration of cortisol; however, experience has shown that there will not be a return to normal as in adrenal hyperplasia. This test of 17-ketosteroid depression by cortisol administration may now be completed within a single day by the fractional collection of four hourly specimens of urine. The test should include two or three controls and at least four specimens after intravenous administration of cortisol hemisuccinate, 2 mg./kg. of body weight as a single dose. Segaloff has described this rapid method for the differential diagnosis of adrenal lesions and noted that the 17-ketosteroid level will drop sharply within two to six hours and remain low for 12 hours or more.

Although the response of the adrenal gland to ACTH stimulation has been proposed as a differential test, the experience of Bongiovanni has been that this is not reliable. The test is based on the hypothesis that a hyperplastic gland will respond by a further increase in the excretion of urinary 17-ketosteroids whereas a neoplasm will not.

An intravenous pyelogram should be made since it may reveal a circumscribed tumor which exerts exogenous pressure on the kidneys. Retroperitoneal air will outline the large adrenal glands of hyperplasia, but technical difficulties do not permit the differential diagnosis of tumor from hyperplasia. A plain film of the abdomen and an intravenous pyelogram are usually recommended.

If a newborn infant with ambiguous genitalia is shown to have female sex chromatin, internal female structures by radiographic studies or laparotomy and elevated levels of 17-ketosteroids and pregnanetriol, particularly 11-ketopregnanetriol, a diagnosis of congenital adrenal hyperplasia may be made. If the urinary steroids are normal for the age of the patient, a virilizing condition of the mother such as an arrhenoblastoma or hilus cell tumor must be sought. In addition, a careful history should be taken to determine whether or not the mother received a progestational steroid during the first 12 weeks of pregnancy.

TREATMENT

After the true sex of the newborn has been determined, it is imperative that the abnormalities of the external female genitalia be corrected. Occasionally internal correction is required when the caudal portion of the müllerian tubercle has failed to canalize and there is no connection with the external genitalia. The ideal time for surgical correction is during the first four years of life but after the first several months postnatally. Since there may be a relative adrenocortical insufficiency during the first few months, there is an increased risk of surgical stress at this time. The infant should be managed with supplementary corticoid therapy before and after surgery. Although the enlarged clitoris has frequently been corrected by partial amputation, it should be emphasized that clitorectomy should be avoided if possible. If hormonal therapy is instituted early, the clitoris frequently diminishes in size and requires no further treatment. The procedure for relocation and recession of the enlarged phallus, with preservation of the gland, has been advised and seems superior to total removal. The reader is referred to the excellent review of Jones and Wilkins for further information regarding the surgical correction of human intersex.

Replacement with cortisol or related steroids is the accepted method of therapy in view of the fundamental biochemical pathogenesis. The dosage of the steroid needed is far less than that necessary in other types of adrenal disease and side reactions are virtually unknown. The prime aims of therapy are: (1) to supply the deficient hormone, (2) to suppress pituitary ACTH secretion and hence adrenal androgens and clinical virilization, (3) to forestall abnormally rapid somatic growth and osseous advance, (4) to permit normal gonadal development, (5) to correct salt and water loss or hypertension and (6) to avoid side reactions of administered steroids in unnecessarily large doses.

Bongiovanni has pointed out the importance of initiating therapy in congenital adrenal hyperplasia as soon as the diagnosis is made. He further emphasizes that the choice of the proper drug is important and advises that compounds be selected which most closely resemble the deficient natural hormone. In this regard, Bongiovanni feels that the newer analogues of cortisone have no place in treatment of this disorder. Furthermore, their pharmacologic design is frequently disadvantageous. It is important to remember that the patient requires not only suppression of adrenal androgens but also the physiologic activity of cortisol itself. Therefore it becomes unreasonable to utilize compounds that are intended to eliminate certain basic actions of the required and deficient substance. Several of the newer compounds actually promote loss of sodium and water and exaggerate the intrinsic problem of the disease process itself. Bongiovanni has suggested that the drugs of choice are cortisone acetate and cortisol (hydrocortisone) for oral or parenteral use.

The dosage needed at the beginning of medical therapy is greater than that subsequently needed for maintenance. In the early period of therapy it is advantageous to administer cortisone acetate or hydrocortisone intramuscularly. During the initial period of therapy, the clinician should attempt to reduce the urinary 17-ketosteroids to a level normal for the age of the patient as quickly as possible. The importance of individualization of therapy is obvious and regulation depends both on the immediate response of the urinary 17-ketosteroids and on the appearance of side effects due to excessive doses. Periodic physical examination and determinations of 17-ketosteroids should be performed. At first it is wise to do these at least once a month but the intervals may be spaced as therapy progresses.

The salt-losing form of adrenogenital syndrome imposes additional and detailed therapeutic demands that must be met promptly. However, it is not the purpose here to enter into specific pediatric endocrinologic problems. The reader is referred to the excellent and complete review by Bongiovanni and Root for this information.

After the administration of therapy in the young child there should be a normal rate of growth and epiphyseal maturation. The excretion of 17-ketosteroids in urine should be kept at a daily level of 2–3 mg. between birth and 5 years of age, 4–8 mg. between 6 and 10 years, and 10–18 mg. thereafter. In the older, previously masculinized female some diminution in the rate of growth of facial hair may be noted. The onset of therapy in these patients will also allow the initiation of ovarian function with subsequent ovulation, menstruation and pregnancy. The masculine habitus, however, may not change appreciably.

Most authorities feel that it is unwise to discontinue the use of glucocorticoids in patients with congenital adrenogenital syndrome. Certainly, it would be unwise in the patient who has the salt-losing variety of the disease. After the patient has obtained an adult growth pattern and is ovulating and menstruating normally, the question arises as to whether cessation of therapy is advisable. There is no doubt that these patients may compensate for their enzymatic lack and secrete adequate cortisol. However, some alteration in ovarian function might be expected. The major objection to discontinuing therapy concerns the possible development of an adrenocortical neoplasm. It is recognized that either a benign or a malignant neoplastic process may result from the unopposed stimulation of the gland by ACTH.

Conception, abortion and full-term pregnancies have been reported in patients with female pseudohermaphroditism secondary to congenital adrenal hyperplasia. In most of these patients no alteration has been necessary in the dosage of steroids throughout pregnancy. However, at the time of delivery, some increase in the dosage regimen has been utilized. The children born of these mothers have been normal, and abnormalities of the genitalia have not been statistically increased. Further, these infants have not demonstrated clinical adrenocortical insufficiency. The current evidence suggests that the index of fertility in the treated female is good and that the incidence of abortion is not increased. Replacement therapy with cortisol should be continued throughout the pregnancy with dosage adjusted to avoid elevations of the urinary 17-ketosteroid level. If the father is heterozygous, it may be anticipated that half the children will have the enzymatic defect. These details should be explained to the prospective parents but complete interdiction of pregnancy is not suggested. In each case the decision should remain with the individuals concerned and should be based on factors other than the disease process itself. If the disease is recognized at birth, the subsequent therapeutic measures allow for complete control and afford the patient no more trouble than that experienced by the patient with diabetes mellitus.

Pituitary and Hypothalamus
Cushing's Disease

Pituitary basophilism in the form of hyperplasia, adenoma or carcinoma may result in the development of a characteristic group of clinical features which include obesity, hirsutism, abdominal striae, plethoric facies and hypertension. Polycythemia and a decreased glucose tolerance may also be present. These features are also present in Cushing's *syndrome* but in the absence of *pituitary basophilism*. It is important to remember that only one or two of the clinical stigmata noted may be present in a patient believed to have typical Cushing's syndrome. It is rare to find all of them in one patient.

The characteristic type of obesity in patients with Cushing's syndrome has been classified as being of centripetal type. The patient's trunk is ponderous and the abdomen protuberant. The arms and legs are thin in comparison to the torso and an accentuation of the dorsal fat pad over the neck gives a characteristic appearance (Fig. 12–12) that has been termed the "buffalo hump." An accentuation of the supraclavicular fat makes the neck appear short and thick. Fat deposition also is prominent over the malar eminences and cheeks, resulting in a typical facial roundness. In addition the corners of the mouth are depressed, causing the so-called "fish-mouth" appearance.

Unlike patients having adrenogenital syndrome with hyperadrenocorticism, patients with Cushing's syndrome demonstrate a marked decrease in muscular strength and the ability to perform work. There is a diminution in the actual mass of muscle tissue of the striated type, probably accounting for the comparatively thin arms and legs.

The degree of hirsutism seen in Cushing's syndrome is much less than that usually associated with adrenogenital syndrome. In the latter there is an extensive growth of coarse hair of the male type. In Cushing's syndrome the hirsutism may be minimal or may consist only of lanugo hair on the sides of the face and the preauricular area. This lanugo hair may also be extensive on the abdomen and back.

The sudden appearance of purple striae in a mature individual or in a young child must be considered as pathognomonic of Cushing's syndrome until proved otherwise. These striae are usually seen on the lateral aspect of the abdomen but may also be present in the axilla. It should be mentioned that striae may be noted on the breasts of the pubescent girl or the adolescent boy with some degree of gynecomastia. Usually the striae in the obese or pregnant patient are pearl gray and not as depressed as those noted in the patient with Cushing's syndrome.

In the patient with adrenogenital syndrome the skin is characteristically coarse and suggests that seen in the adult male. However, in the patient with Cushing's syndrome the skin is quite thin and bruises easily. Areas of ecchymosis are commonly seen and in addition there may be a mild degree of acne. The facial plethora and erythema of the anterior chest wall are additional skin changes.

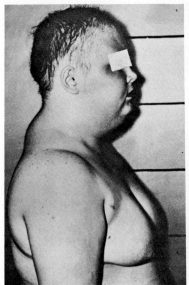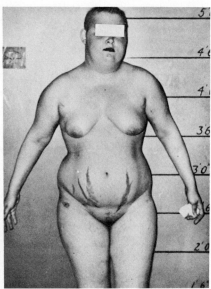

Fig. 12 –12.—Cushing's syndrome. Typical physiognomy of Cushing's syndrome in 20-year-old female. Note the dorsal cervical fat hump, the centripetal obesity and the unusually large striae which radiate toward the pelvic area. (From Kupperman, H. S.: *Human Endocrinology* [Philadelphia: F. A. Davis Company, 1963].)

In Cushing's syndrome there is an increased degree of protein catabolism due to an increased secretion of glucocorticoids from the adrenal cortex. There results a conversion of protein to glucose, but this is accomplished at the expense of destruction or reduction of muscle mass. Thus there is a diminution in muscular strength, and the skin changes described above are probably the result of destruction of the protein matrix of the skin.

Also, in contrast to the patient with adrenogenital syndrome, the clitoris in the patient with Cushing's syndrome is normal. Similar to the patient with adrenogenital syndrome, the patient with Cushing's syndrome demonstrates a secondary amenorrhea. If Cushing's disease occurs before the menarche, menstruation will be delayed until adequate therapy is initiated. Similarly, Cushing's disease prevents the usual preadolescent growth spurt due possibly to the inhibitory effect of excess glucocorticoids on the secretion of hypophyseal growth hormone. Their short stature is similar to that seen in children with precocious sexual maturity. However, if Cushing's syndrome occurs during the prepubescent period and is appropriately managed, a normal growth and developmental period may be anticipated.

Diagnostic Tests.—Laboratory changes seen in Cushing's syndrome include polycythemia, a relative lymphopenia and eosinopenia, diminished glucose tolerance, normal excretion of 17-ketosteroids, normal pregnanetriol and elevation of the 17-hydroxysteroids. Kupperman and associates have shown that, while exogenously administered corticoids significantly decrease glucose tolerance, similar doses of corticoids do not alter the patient's sensitivity to intravenously administered insulin as noted in the insulin tolerance test. Thus the patient with Cushing's syndrome will usually demonstrate a normal insulin tolerance. Kupperman has suggested that corticoids may interfere with glucose utilization but are unable to alter the patient's response to exogenous insulin when there is no excessive glucose load.

Since the cortical excretory product may be only mildly or moderately elevated in Cushing's syndrome, it frequently is necessary to perform specific tests with ACTH or mepyrapone. Inhibitory tests with hydrocortisone may also be necessary to arrive at a specific diagnosis. Thus the provocative and suppressive tests may be of assistance in differentiating between malignant and benign neoplasms.

The mepyrapone (Metopirone, methopyrapone SU-4885) test of pituitary function may also be of value in the differential diagnosis of primary and secondary hypoadrenocorticoidism. The administration of mepyrapone (2-methyl-1-1,2-di-3-pyridyl-1-propanone) determines the ability of the pituitary gland to secrete ACTH. This particular preparation is capable of inhibiting 11-beta-hydroxylase activity and therefore results in a reduction in the adrenal production of cortisol. Since cortisol inhibits ACTH secretion and since mepyrapone causes a reduction in the production of cortisol, the effect of its administration is to increase ACTH secretion, with subsequent stimulation of the adrenal gland. However, since this drug still inhibits the 11-beta-hydroxylation, the resultant effect in intact hypophyseal systems is an increased release of 17-ketosteroids and 17-ketogenic steroids. This is

Fig. 12–13.—**A,** in the normal person, mepyrapone (Metopirone) inhibits 11-beta-hydroxylase activity, producing a reduction in cortisol formation. The resultant increase in ACTH secretion stimulates the adrenal cortex to release 17-ketosteroids and 17-ketogenic steroids. Cortisol continues to be blocked by mepyrapone. **B,** in the patient with pituitary insufficiency the decrease in cortisol formation is unable to effect an increase in ACTH. Therefore there is no change in the 17-ketosteroid excretion. **C,** if, however, ACTH is given with mepyrapone, the normal adrenal will produce an increased excretion of 17-ketosteroids and 17-ketogenic steroids. If the adrenal as well as the pituitary is insufficient, no change will occur.

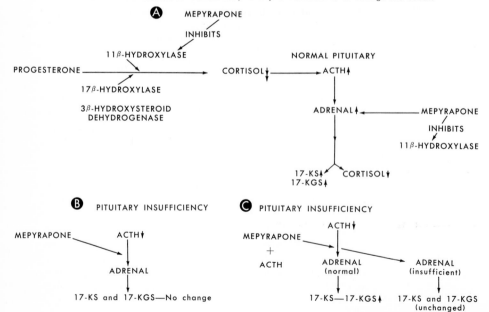

shown diagrammatically in Figure 12–13, *A.* In a patient with poor pituitary reserve, however, the administration of mepyrapone will not result in an increased excretion of 17-ketosteroids and 17-hydroxysteroids. If mepyrapone fails to cause an increase in 17-ketosteroids or 17-ketogenic steroids, the integrity of the adrenal must be tested with an ACTH infusion. If a good adrenal response is effected after ACTH and mepyrapone (as indicated by elevation in 17-ketosteroid and 17-hydroxysteroid excretion), it would imply a good adrenal response but a poor secretion or release of ACTH (Fig. 12–13, *B*). A good response to ACTH together with no response to mepyrapone is seen in patients with selective ACTH deficiency as well as in patients with panhypopituitarism. Failure of response to both agents implies a failure of the adrenal cortex. This is shown in Figure 12–13, *C.*

In the adrenal response test after corticoid suppression, prednisone may be given for one week in daily doses of 20–30 mg. Before and after this week of prednisone therapy, the patient receives a test dose of 40 units of ACTH gel given intramuscularly. Twenty-four-hour urines are collected immediately after each injection. The normal patient will not demonstrate a significant increase in urinary steroids after the second ACTH injection, whereas the patient with Cushing's syndrome due to adrenal hyperplasia will have a marked adrenal response after both ACTH injections.

The ACTH provocative test is accomplished by giving 40 units of ACTH gel intramuscularly and measuring the output in urinary 17-hydroxysteroid. In the patient who has only a moderate elevation in the 17-hydroxysteroid level, the administration of ACTH will result in a marked increase in output, up to 45–50 mg./24 hours or even higher. A marked increase in 17-OH levels after ACTH usually points to hyperplasia, whereas patients with significantly elevated 17-OH levels with a neoplasm of the adrenal cortex fail to show significant and additional increases after ACTH.

The 16-methylated analogue of hydrocortisone, dexamethasone, has been utilized by Liddle to differentiate between hyperplasia and carcinoma of the adrenal. Dexamethasone is not excreted in the urine as a hydroxysteroid and therefore any values obtained represent those due to endogenous steroids. If 0.5 mg. of dexamethasone is given every six hours for eight doses, normal patients will exhibit a complete suppression of 17-hydroxycorticoid excretion. If Cushing's syndrome due to hyperplasia is present, little if any change is noted in the elevated hydroxycorticoid output. But if the dose of dexamethasone is increased to 2 mg. every six hours for eight doses, a definite diminution in the output of 17-hydroxycorticoids will be noted in patients with hyperplasia. Patients with neoplasia of the adrenal gland will not show this suppressive response.

X-ray study of the vertebral column in patients with long-standing Cushing's disease will usually show severe osteoporosis. The osteoporosis is due primarily to the disintegration of protein matrix brought about by the metabolic action of the glucocorticoids. Since the protein matrix of the bone is unable to accept the available calcium, an excess of calcium appears in the urine. Subsequently the intervertebral disks become relatively denser than the decalcified vertebrae, producing a rather characteristic appearance.

Intravenous pyelography and presacral gas insufflation may demonstrate large adrenal tumors. In view of the specific diagnostic tests now available, however, these are not used as routine procedures.

Treatment.—The treatment of Cushing's syndrome has varied over the years according to different concepts regarding the etiology of the disease process. Treatment originally was irradiation of the pituitary gland, and later surgical removal of the pituitary gland was enthusiastically supported. During the past decade the surgical management of Cushing's syndrome has been directed toward bilateral adrenalectomy.

After the diagnosis of Cushing's syndrome has been made, therapeutic management may be approached either medically, surgically or by radiation. While medical therapy has been suggested as a complete and final method of control, it has the disadvantage of possible error. If attempted in patients with neoplasia rather than hyperplasia, valuable time will have been lost. Other disadvantages of medical therapy are that complete remission is rarely if ever achieved and that androgen therapy in the female brings about undesirable virilizing changes.

Surgical therapy usually necessitates bilateral, total adrenalectomy in the case of hyperplasia or excision of the neoplasm when the disease is due to this process. Of course, the radical surgical approach condemns the patient to a lifetime need for replacement therapy. However, until the basic physiology of the disturbances noted in Cushing's syndrome are completely understood, it seems necessary to use this method in most patients.

Radiation therapy has been suggested and is used in various modalities. The pituitary gland itself may be irradiated or yttrium-90 pellets may be inserted into the sella turcica intranasally. Irradiation of the adrenal gland alone as well as irradiation of the pituitary and adrenal glands has been suggested. Certain adverse effects of irradiation have been noted, including alteration in other pituitary tropic activities. Permanent alopecia or hyperemia and telangiectasia may remain at the sites of skin penetration. In some patients given a less intensive course there has been a significant incidence of recurrence. Lawrence and others pointed out the advantages of high-energy therapy over both conventional surgery and x-ray or gamma-ray irradiation. They emphasized the fact that the management of the totally adrenalectomized patient is frequently difficult even with the available replacement steroids. Further, the surgery is not always without some risk. They noted that prolonged remissions after x-ray or gamma-ray therapy have been infrequent and that partial relapse occurs in almost 70 per cent of the patients. They have successfully used proton and alpha-particle beams, generated by the cyclotron, to diminish pituitary gland function. They converted the cyclotron to produce a 900 million electron beam of alpha particles. This beam may be focused to a pinpoint and, so controlled, destroys only part of the hyperactive pituitary and none of the surrounding or intervening tissue. Lawrence and his group have treated three women with Cushing's disease who have now been completely symptom free and apparently cured for over four years.

SIMMONDS' DISEASE

Simmonds' disease, known in the past as hypophyseal cachexia, is characterized by marked asthenia and weakness, extreme weight loss progressing to cachexia, loss or thinning of axillary and pubic hair, a profoundly low basal metabolic rate, diminished or absent urinary excretion of 17-ketosteroids and FSH, amenorrhea and frigidity. In addition, there may be pronounced dryness of the skin, dental caries, sensitivity to cold and anorexia. Psychic changes, usually apathy, depression or somnolence, are frequently associated. Premature or rapid aging occurs, together with progeria. The skin is parchment-like with pallor, thinning and fine wrinkling. Yellow or yellow-brown pigmentation has been described in about one-fourth of the cases.

Serious depression of anterior pituitary function may be produced by benign or malignant tumors, trauma associated with basal skull fracture or infection such as syphilis or tuberculosis. In the original patient described by Simmonds, the pathologic process followed severe puerperal sepsis, and at autopsy the patient was found to have fibrosis of the anterior pituitary gland.

Kupperman recently pointed out that, while Simmonds' disease has been referred to as pituitary cachexia, such a clinical picture does not occur in patients subjected to surgical or radiation hypophysectomy nor does it occur in certain adult patients in whom hypopituitarism develops spontaneously. As more and more patients are observed following complete hypophysectomy, it has become obvious that such patients remain in a static clinical state and do not show evidence of progressive cachexia. Thus, some question has arisen as to the true nature of this disease. At the present time the cachexia previously described in association with Simmonds' disease (as well as the excessive weight gain in Fröhlich's syndrome) are believed to be due to trauma or disease of the midbrain rather than to a specific process involving the adenohypophysis.

Therapeutic measures in the management of patients with so-called Simmonds' disease are the same as those to be outlined for the treatment of Sheehan's syndrome.

SHEEHAN'S SYNDROME

Sheehan of Liverpool in 1937 described a syndrome similar to Simmonds' disease but of lesser magnitude. He described a form of panhypopituitarism due to pituitary necrosis that originates as a consequence of thrombosis or ischemia usually secondary to postpartum hemorrhage. Such necrosis of the adenohypophysis results in destruction of all anterior pituitary functions. It is important to remember, however, that subclinical entities of this syndrome may exist. It has been estimated that if more than 90 per cent of the adenohypophysis is destroyed, typical Sheehan's syndrome will develop.

As a result of the severe hypotension occasionally accompanying the hemorrhagic postpartum state, it has been suggested that vascular spasm arrests both the portal and direct arterial blood supply. Should spasm continue for several hours, necrobiosis of pituitary tissue occurs. The thrombosis noted in the vasculature is believed to be secondary to subsequent blood flow in the infarcted areas after the vascular spasm has been corrected.

Diagnosis.—The diagnosis is suggested by a history of postpartum hemorrhage followed by a postpartum amenorrhea. Increasing lassitude and fatigue develop, together with a total disinterest in the environment and family situation. Many patients are extremely intolerant to extremes of temperature, become anorexic yet only rarely have an appreciable loss in weight. Patients with Sheehan's syndrome do not lactate, and the combination of postpartum hemorrhage and absence of lactation should suggest this diagnosis. It should be mentioned that a similar degree of blood loss in the nonpregnant patient will not be followed by these manifestations of panhypopituitarism. The pituitary gland of the pregnant female with its increased vascularity is extremely sensitive to temporary episodes of vascular insufficiency.

Physical findings in Sheehan's syndrome are rather striking and are due to the diminished adrenal, thyroid and gonadal function. In addition to the absence of axillary and pubic hair, there may also be a diminution in the hair on the lateral aspects of the eyebrows. A generalized thinning of the cephalic hair and a resistance to the effect of permanent waving may also be noted. The skin appears prematurely aged, being dry and coarse, with a definite yellowish tinge. As a result of the severe diminution in estrogen secretion the vaginal mucosa becomes atrophic and the uterus and cervix undergo severe hypoplasia. The only secondary sex organs which remain unaffected are the breasts. This is in contrast to the patient with anorexia nervosa in which breast atrophy does occur. If severe anorexia does occur in a patient with Sheehan's syndrome, severe weight loss and cachexia may supervene. Other findings are hypotension, diminution in heart size and hypoactive tendon reflexes.

The laboratory findings demonstrate a generalized reduction in the secretion of all endocrine glands. Because of decreased thyroid function, a low uptake of radioactive iodine and a low level of serum protein-bound iodine are found. Despite the severe hypothyroidism, the blood cholesterol level is not elevated as it is in patients with primary hypothyroidism. In Sheehan's syndrome there is diminished absorption of glucose from the intestine, preventing the hyperglycemia necessary to elicit the output of insulin from the pancreas. Thus, the oral glucose tolerance test may not show the characteristic findings usually associated with hypopituitarism. Because of the hypoadrenocorticoidism the levels of 17-hydroxycorticoids and 17-ketosteroids in the urine are low. Administration of a provocative dose of 40 units of ACTH gel will cause an increased output of adrenal steroids in the urine. Although these patients have severe degrees of adrenal insufficiency, they do not demonstrate the hyperpigmentation seen in Addison's disease. The excessive pigmentation in the latter disease is due to increased secretion of the melanophore-stimulating hormone and does not occur in Sheehan's syndrome.

The mepyrapone test is useful in differential diagnosis since it will distinguish primary from secondary hypoadrenocorticoidism. Because of the inadequate secretion of pituitary gonadotropins secondary ovarian failure occurs. The ovaries are small and there is a resultant cessation of estrogen secretion. These patients have an atrophic vaginal smear and an atrophic endometrium.

Differential Diagnosis.—The differential diagnosis of Sheehan's syndrome must consider anorexia nervosa, Chiari-Frommel syndrome and Forbes-Albright syndrome.

The most important factor in excluding *anorexia nervosa* is the history of postpartum hemorrhage antedating the severe aversion to food. As a matter of fact, most patients with anorexia nervosa do not give a history of any pregnancies. In contradistinction to patients with Sheehan's syndrome, patients with anorexia nervosa usually show a normal distribution of pubic and axillary hair. Also, the degree of cachexia is much more extreme in anorexia nervosa. Because hypoadrenocorticoidism is a characteristic finding in Sheehan's syndrome, the levels of 17-ketosteroids and 17-hydroxysteroids are low; these metabolites of the adrenal are normal in anorexia nervosa. A flat intravenous glucose tolerance curve is found in both conditions, but the patient with anorexia nervosa will show a normal tolerance for intravenous glucose whereas the patient with Sheehan's syndrome will have hypoglycemia.

Although anorexia nervosa was formerly thought to occur only in women, recent reports have indicated the same process in the male. In general, a loss of 25–30 per cent of the normal weight is necessary for the diagnosis of anorexia nervosa, but in some instances the weight loss may not be of this magnitude. Anorexia nervosa is seen during three specific periods of life. The first is prepuberal, and this group has the best prognosis. The second is during adolescence and patients with this type are the most difficult to cure. The third period is after age 25; while these patients respond better to therapy, the condition is more protracted. Most patients in the adolescent group give a previous history of obesity. Many will acknowledge a definite fear of being overweight but describe themselves as compulsive eaters. Both psychotic and neurotic patients will be discovered in a study of this particular group.

Patients with anorexia nervosa present a disturbance of the body image and are unconcerned about their own emaciation. This serious error in self-appraisal is of diagnostic importance. Such patients also have a disturbed perception of the visceral state; they are unable to recognize hunger or to know when they are fully satiated. In addition, they have a complete lack of autonomy and usually feel ineffective or useless. Most of the patients have been found to come from homes in which food and cooking were of prime importance to the mother, and a "nagging mother" pattern was regularly reported. Most were the only child in the family or came from two-child families.

Anorexia nervosa must be considered a medical emergency. No psychotherapy except simple supportive measures should be offered until the acute physical symptoms have been treated medically and the patient has gained weight.

Chiari-Frommel syndrome must be differentiated from Sheehan's syndrome, particularly since the amenorrhea in both follows pregnancy. Another specific finding is the presence of galactorrhea which is unrelated to nursing in previous pregnancies. These patients are well developed, with normal breasts, pubic and axillary hair and generally good health. Assays of estrogen in urine or vaginal cytology will demonstrate diminished estrogen excretion. The FSH is low and there may be some decrease in glucose tolerance. Although an x-ray of the sella turcica may show slight enlargement, the visual field examination is usually within normal range.

The syndrome is attributed to increased production of prolactin in the adenohypophysis resulting from the disappearance of inhibitory factors in the hypothalamus. The pituitary dysfunction is assumed to cause the galactorrhea. The antigonad action of prolactin gives rise to secondary atrophy of the uterus and ovaries with subsequent amenorrhea. A similar syndrome, but unrelated to pregnancy and having radiologic evidence of pituitary tumor, is usually referred to as the Ahumada-Del Castillo syndrome. Recent studies using mepyrapone as a test of pituitary function have indicated pituitary competence in the Chiari-Frommel syndrome. Such studies emphasize the hypothalamic origin of this disease. The diagnosis may be aided by a prolactin assay (squab or pigeon crop sac method). Although in the original report by Frommel only one of the 28 patients recovered spontaneously, newer methods of therapy which utilize progestational agents or clomiphene citrate have resulted in ovulation and pregnancy.

Persistent amenorrhea following a normal delivery is seen rather frequently by the average practitioner as a persistent exaggeration of the abnormal pituitary-ovary relationship of pregnancy. These patients do not have Chiari-Frommel syndrome, nor do they fit in the classification of Sheehan's syndrome. The administration of progesterone in these patients will result in prompt withdrawal bleeding, and the use of newer progestational agents given in a cyclic manner for two or three months will usually be followed by normal ovulatory menses. Since there is no abnormality of adrenal function, results of assays of 17-ketosteroids and 17-hydroxysteroids are normal. The basal body temperature is monophasic and pregnanediol will not be present to any extent in the urine. The excretion of pregnanetriol in urine is normal.

In the past, the induction of ovulation in patients with Chiari-Frommel syndrome has not met with uniform success. The specificity of diminished secretion of FSH, and probably also LH, has been resistant to most therapeutic regimens. Substitutional therapy in the form of human FSH followed by human chorionic gonadotropin has been successful in a small number of patients. Similarly, the use of clomiphene citrate has resulted in ovulation in a small number of patients. Clomiphene apparently causes release of pituitary gonadotropins although the exact mechanism of action is not well understood. In a few patients we have obtained ovulation and pregnancy by giving clomiphene for 10 consecutive days (100 mg. daily), followed by 10,000 I.U. of HCG (Follutein) 4 days later. Greenblatt and associates reported that a peak in FSH secretions was obtained before changes in estrogens or LH. The rise in estrogen secretion followed the rise in FSH which was followed by a peak in LH level. They found the peak in estrogen secretion to coincide with the probable day of ovulation, which seemed to have occurred about 24 hours after the peak in LH. Greenblatt suggested that the release of gonadotropins and consequent ovulation are achieved either by direct stimulation of the hypothalamico-pituitary axis or by negating the inhibitory influences of estrogens on this axis because of the competitive antiestrogenic action of the drug itself. O. W. Smith, however, has suggested that the primary site of the action of clomiphene is either directly on the enzyme systems involved in ovarian steroidogenesis or as a potentiator of gonadotropins.

Forbes-Albright syndrome is similar to the Chiari-Frommel syndrome and is characterized by *amenorrhea* and persistent lactation. There is a diminished excretion of FSH with a consequent estrogen deficiency. The facies may appear slightly acromegalic and the sella turcica may be normal or just slightly enlarged. The classic osseous and soft tissue changes typical of the acromegalic patient, however, are not seen in Forbes-Albright syndrome. In contradistinction to patients with Sheehan's syndrome, pubic

TABLE 12-1.—DIFFERENTIAL DIAGNOSIS OF DIFFERENT PITUITARY SYNDROMES AND ANOREXIA NERVOSA*

	SHEEHAN'S SYNDROME	ANOREXIA NERVOSA	CHIARI-FROMMEL	FORBES-ALBRIGHT
1. Weight	N	Marked decrease (cachectic)	N to ↑	N to ↑
2. Pubic and axillary hair	0	+	+	+
3. Cephalic hair	Thin	Thin	N	N
4. Hirsutism	0	0	0	0 to +
5. Skin	Very dry—"crinkly"	Dry	N	N
6. Blood pressure	↓	↓	N	N
7. Strength	Weak	Weak	N	N
8. Intolerance to cold	+	+	N	N
9. Breasts size	N	Atrophied	↑	↑
10. Lactation	0	0	+	+
11. Amenorrhea	+	Intermittent but in late stages +	+-Postpartum	+-Primary
12. Progesterone response	0	0	0	0
13. Basal body temperature curve	Monophasic	Monophasic	Monophasic	Monophasic
14. Sella turcica—size	N	N	N to ↑	N to ↑
15. Visual field	N	N	N to ↓	N to ↓
16. Glucose tolerance				
(a) Oral	Flat	Flat	N to ↓	N to ↓
(b) I.V.	Hypoglycemic level	N	N to ↓	N to ↓
17. 17-Ketosteroids	↓	↓	N	N to ↑
18. 17-Hydroxysteroids	↓	Low N	N	N
19. Adrenal response to ACTH	+	+	++	++-+++
20. Protein-bound iodine	↓	↓	N	N
21. Thyroid response to TSH	+	+	++	++
22. Pregnanediol	↓	↓	↓	↓
23. Pregnanetriol	↓	↓	N	N
24. Vaginal smear	Atrophic	Atrophic	Atrophic	Atrophic

N = Normal
0 = Absent
+ = Findings are positive

↓ = Decreased
↑ = Increased

*From Kupperman, H. S.: *Human Endocrinology* (Philadelphia: F. A. Davis Company, 1963), vol. 1.

and axillary hair are present and the cephalic hair is not thinned. There is no evidence of diminished strength or of intolerance to cold and, as mentioned, there is usually persistent lactation. Levels of 17-ketosteroids are normal or slightly elevated and the 17-hydroxysteroids are normal. Enlargement of the sella turcica was present in eight of fifteen patients and in three of these a chromophobe tumor was found at operation. Lactorrhea generally began in the third or fourth decade and lasted as long as twenty-one years. In nine patients the lactorrhea did not follow pregnancy. The major differentiating points in Sheehan's syndrome, anorexia nervosa, Chiari-Frommel syndrome and Forbes-Albright syndrome are shown in Table 12-1.

In the past, the prognosis for subsequent ovulation in patients with Forbes-Albright syndrome has been practically hopeless. No reports have appeared describing the use of clomiphene citrate or human FSH plus HCG in the treatment of this disorder.

Therapy of Sheehan's Syndrome.—The rationale of therapy in Sheehan's syndrome is simply one of replacement or substitution of the hormones normally produced by the endocrine end-organs.

The adequacy of thyroid therapy cannot be ascertained by the usual protein-bound iodine test and therefore the therapeutic regimen must be carefully regulated. To avoid induction of thyroid toxicity with exogenous thyroid, low dosages must be used at the start of therapy. Triiodothyronine in a dose of 5 μg. daily, increasing in increments of 5 μg./day every five days, seems to be a satisfactory approach. The dose is then increased to patient tolerance, usually at the level of 75–100μg. daily. Triiodothyronine achieves its full effect within two to three days and is as rapidly dissipated. Thyroid extract, thyroid globulin and sodium levothyroxine take two to three weeks to achieve their full effect and consequently require two to three weeks to be completely dissipated. Sodium levothyroxine may be used, beginning with a dose of 0.025 mg. and increasing the dose at this increment level at intervals of 14 days until the maximum therapeutic dose is reached. This is usually in the range of 0.2–0.3 mg. daily.

The degree of hypoadrenocorticoidism is combated by the administration of glucocorticoids and mineralocorticoids when this is deemed necessary. These may be administered in the following dosage schemes: hydrocortisone, 10 mg. twice daily; cortisone, 12.5 mg. twice daily; prednisone, 2.5 mg. twice daily; 6-methylprednisolone, 2 mg. twice daily; dexamethasone, 0.375 mg., or pentamethasone, 0.3 mg. twice daily. These doses of glucocorticoids are physiologic and in general do not interfere with the normal defense mechanisms of the body. The secretion of aldosterone from the adrenal cortex is not dependent on the secretion of ACTH. Therefore, in most patients the use of 9-alpha-fluorohydrocortisone is not necessary. If the systolic blood pressure is below 100 mm. Hg, the fluorinated mineralocorticoid may be administered in a dose of 0.1 mg. daily as a maintenance dose.

Estrogen therapy should be given not only for the excellent psychologic effect but also to prevent specific degenerative changes in extragenital organs. A regimen of therapy employing a sequence of estrogen followed by estrogen plus a synthetic progestin seems best. Diethylstilbestrol (0.5 mg. twice daily), ethinyl estradiol (0.05 mg. twice daily), sodium estrone sulfate (1.25 mg. twice daily) or chlorotrianisene (12 mg. twice daily) should be given for 20 consecutive days. During the last five days of this treatment cycle one of the oral synthetic progestational agents should also be given; 10 mg. of norethynodrel, norethindrone or medroxyprogesterone may be utilized for this purpose. The addition of the progestational steroids will permit a cyclic secretory change in the endometrium which will prevent the excessive uterine bleeding occasionally seen when estrogens are used alone. These agents will also prevent the development of endometrial hyperplasia. This same therapeutic plan may be used in patients with Chiari-Frommel syndrome or Forbes-Albright syndrome. The use of clomiphene citrate in a few patients with Sheehan's syndrome has not resulted in subsequent ovulation.

Hirsutism

Hirsutism may be defined as the growth of hair in unusual places or in unusual amounts. As a gynecologic problem it is of great importance as a possible sign of defeminization and virilization. Excess hair may be a symptom of an organic disorder or merely a feature of ethnic background. Whatever its cause, it is disturbing to an estimated 15 per cent of women and merits a systematic diagnostic and therapeutic approach. The various etiologic factors are shown in Table 12-2.

Genetic and *racial factors* establish the limits and predisposition to hair growth in white females. Some facial, abdominal and chest hair may be normal for women from France, Italy, Greece, Spain, parts of Ireland and South America and from Semitic groups in any country. It is sparse in the Mongoloid, Japanese, Chinese, American Indian and intermediate in the people of Great Britain, the Scandinavian countries and Northern Germany.

Hair growth on the mons veneris (pubarche) and axilla appears in the female at the time of menarche and continues to increase until the late teens. When excess hair is racial in origin, it is likely to be heavy not only on areas such as lip, chin and chest (where it is characteristic in the male), but also on the arms, legs and temples. Normally hairy women tend to have a low hairline at the temples, heavy scalp and heavy eyebrows. The coarse hair appearing during puberty on the mons and in the axilla represent a response to androgens secreted by the adrenal cortex (adrenarche) but also possibly from the hilar cells of the ovary. Physiologic hirsutism is normal during the adrenarche of puberty, during pregnancy and during menopause. The excess hair gained during pregnancy is lost during the puerperium. In severe malnutrition, e.g., anorexia nervosa, and occasionally in juvenile myxedema, the arms, legs and back may be covered with fine, soft hair resembling lanugo hair. This growth is not disfiguring, is useful in diagnosis (excluding panhypopituitarism) and disappears on recovery. Also, many normal women have a light down on the cheeks and may become unnecessarily alarmed when they suddenly discover it on looking in a mirror with a tangential source of light. A fine, lanugo-type hair is occasionally seen on the vulva of infants. It does not signify precocity nor does it indicate increased androgen production. Such hair growth does not merit a diagnosis of hirsutism or pubarche. It may be a response to diaper irritants.

TABLE 12-2.—ETIOLOGY OF HIRSUTISM

1. Physiologic–puberty, pregnancy, menopause
2. Genetic–racial, familial, individual predisposition
3. Hypothalamic–stress syndrome
4. Pituitary–Cushing's disease, functioning chromophobe adenomas
5. Adrenal
    a) Hyperplasia
    b) Tumor
6. Ovarian
    a) Polycystic ovarian disease (Stein-Leventhal syndrome)
    b) Hyperthecosis
    c) Tumors
        1) Arrhenoblastoma
        2) Adrenal rest tumors
        3) Hilus cell tumors
        4) Pseudomucinous cystadenoma
7. Intersex problems
    a) Male pseudo-hermaphroditism
    b) Variants in gonadal dysgenesis
8. Iatrogenic
9. Achard-Thiers syndrome

ETIOLOGY

Table 12-2 lists the major causes of hirsutism for the purpose of differential diagnosis. By and large, the most common etiology seen by the gynecologist is due to either a racial, a genetic or a constitutional factor. However, in most large clinics a number of patients will be seen with Stein-Leventhal syndrome or "gray-zone" variants of acquired adrenal hyperplasia. The major etiological factors are: (1) physiological (puberty, pregnancy, menopause) and genetic; (2) hypothalamic-may be initiated by stress situations in which adrenal androgens are increased; (3) pituitary dysfunction, e.g., Cushing's Disease (see p. 598), acromegaly and chromophobe adenomas; (4) adrenal hyperplasia or tumor; (5) ovarian-sclerocystic ovarian syndrome or arrhenoblastoma; (6) intersex problems; (7) iatrogenic.

Benign adrenal tumors, rather than malignant, are more likely to produce either predominantly glucocorticoids (with resultant typical Cushing's syndrome) or predominantly androgens (with virilism). In the former case, the urinary Porter-Silber chromogens are elevated and 17-ketosteroids are not; in the latter there is a pronounced elevation in the urinary 17-ketosteroids. The type of hirsutism in the two conditions is markedly different since the hair in Cushing's syndrome is lanugo-like and that in virilizing tumors is thick and firm. In addition, in the latter state temporal or vertex baldness may occur—a feature of a virilizing syndrome, not of constitutional hairiness. Malignant adrenal tumors may produce a mixture of both clinical syndromes noted above and they may give rise to either small or very great increases of urinary steroid excretion. Acquired adrenal hyperplasia in an adult is almost invariably associated with Cushing's syndrome rather than a virilizing syndrome. Occasionally, however, congenital adrenal hyperplasia is mild and becomes manifested in late childhood or adolescence instead of at birth. (See p. 594.) Patients with congenital adrenal hyperplasia are usually born with malformations of the genitalia attributable to the action of adrenal androgen in fetal life and, in the absence of such a malformation, the appearance of virilism in a prepuberal female should arouse strong suspicion of adrenal tumor.

Sclerocystic ovarian disease (Stein-Leventhal syndrome). (See also p. 416). This is one of the most common diseases associated with hirsutism seen by the gynecologist. It is frequently associated with infrequent or irregular menses and a tendency to obesity. It usually appears after the menarche making its distinction from constitutional hirsutism difficult. The hirsutism in this situation, once established, seldom disappears but there is little, if any, virilism. Occasionally there is a thick and oily skin with acne but clitoral hypertrophy and temporal balding are rarely evident. In addition to obesity, some hypertension and slight glucose intolerance may appear, suggesting an excess of glucocorticoids rather than androgen. The urinary 17-ketosteroids may be in the high normal range but not clearly above it. In general, one may state that hirsute women, as a group, have an average 17-ketosteroid excretion higher than that of normal women of the same age but a single determination in an individual subject is seldom diagnostic. Testosterone, the androgen par excellence, is metabolized to the same end products (androsterone and etiocholanolone) as many normal adrenal steroids and virilizing amounts of it (10 mg. daily) contribute only about 4 mg. to urinary 17-ketosteroid excretion. Table 12–3 lists normal, elevated and lowered values for 17-ketosteroids.

Ovarian tumors. Certain tumors of the ovary in genetically normal women may be regarded, at least functionally, as being composed of testicular tissue. Arrhenoblastomas, which may appear at any time from puberty to menopause, may contain the tubular as well as the interstitial elements of testicular tissue. They may possess the gonadotropin-inhibiting and androgen-producing functions of the testis and may produce slight or pronounced virilism with or without hypogonadotropic amenorrhea. The in vitro production of testosterone by such tumors has been demonstrated. As mentioned above, however, because of the potency of testosterone, the determination of 17-ketosteroids may be normal or only slightly elevated.

Hilar cell tumors of the ovary are composed of cells analogous to, or possibly identical with, Leydig cells of the testis and produce testosterone. These tumors are rare and usually are seen in postmenopausal women.

Other tumors such as adrenal rest (luteomas) or masculinovoblastomas apparently also produce testosterone although they are rare and have not been extensively studied.

In certain rare intersex problems testicular tissue may be present from birth in phenotypic females with certain chromosomal disorders: (1) testicular feminization; (2) XO-XY chromosomal mosaicism; (3) ovotestes; (4) true hermaphroditism. The hirsutism is not a major problem in these entities, merely being a part of the abnormal endocrine profile.

Hirsutism may be due to the administration of certain drugs. The major

TABLE 12-3.—NORMAL, ELEVATED, AND LOWERED VALUES
OF 17-KETOSTEROIDS IN URINE

NORMAL VALUES

Children (before age 8 years)	0 to 0.5 mg./day
Males	8 to 25 mg./day
Females	5 to 14 mg./day

ELEVATED VALUES

Adrenogenital syndrome (hyperplasia, tumor)
Cushing's syndrome (adrenal hyperplasia, carcinoma)
Precocious puberty
Precocious adrenarche
Stein-Leventhal syndrome (normal or slightly elevated)
Stress
ACTH administration

LOWERED VALUES

Adrenal cortical insufficiency (Addison's disease)
Hypopituitarism
Myxedema, severe hyperthyroidism
Male hypogonadism
Gonadal dysgenesis
Malnutrition, starvation, anorexia nervosa
Severe liver disease
Senescence
Chronic disease states
Corticosteroid administration

(From Schneeberg, N. G.: Adrenal cortical factors in infertility, in Behrman, S. J., and Kistner, R. W., [eds.]: *Progress in Infertility* [Boston: Little, Brown and Company, 1968].)

offenders are Dilantin, testosterone, anabolic agents such as Nilevar and Maxibolin and progestins of the norethindrone type (especially if given in high dosage for the treatment of endometriosis). In some individuals, however, even the usual dose used in the oral contraceptives will cause acne and hirsutism.

DIAGNOSIS

A careful history should be taken and genetic, racial and familial tendencies toward excessive hairiness should be noted. In addition, the physiologic changes of puberty, pregnancy, and menopause should be considered and various stress factors or acute anxiety situations evaluated. The following diagnostic procedures will prove helpful in diagnosis: x-ray of the sella turcica, visual fields, ophthalmoscopic examination, and culdoscopy. In addition these laboratory assays should be determined: urinary 17-keto-steroids; total gonadotropins (if the patient is amenorrheic); serum testosterone. If the 17-ketosteroids are elevated, they should be fractionated in an effort to determine whether the elevation is of adrenal or ovarian origin. Adrenal stimulation and suppression tests together with ovarian stimulation and suppression should be done (Table 12–4). If adrenal tumor is suspected intravenous pyelography and retroperitoneal air studies are indicated. A sequence of diagnostic studies is shown in Table 12–5.

Kupperman has suggested that the metopirone test may be utilized with other cross-testing methods to distinguish androgens of adrenal origin from those formed in the ovary. He has found that, following the administration of metopirone to patients in whom the 17-ketosteroids, testosterone and pregnanetriol are normal or elevated as a result of adrenal overactivity, a marked increase in these excretory products occurs in the urine. Since metopirone blocks the hydroxylation processes necessary for the production of cortisol, the augmented release of ACTH effects these changes. Dexamethasone administration produces a marked diminution in these excretory products whereas no change is brought about by Premarin in a dose of 7.5 mg. daily. The administration of dexamethasone and HCG produces very little change.

When metopirone is given to patients whose ovary is responsible for

---

TABLE 12–4.—TECHNIC OF TESTING

1. Obtain baseline urinary 17-ketosteroids
2. Stimulation of adrenal cortex: 25-40 U. ACTH

Day 1	Normal gland	2 fold increase in 17-KS
	Hyperplasia	2-3 fold increase
	Tumor	No effect
Day 2	Normal gland	2 fold increase in 17-KS
	Hyperplasia	3-4 fold increase
	Tumor	no effect

3. Obtain baseline urinary 17-ketosteroids
4. Suppression of adrenal cortex: Dexamethasone, 0.5 mg. every 6 hours, × 3 days.

Normal adrenal	some decrease in 17-KS
Hyperplastic	over 50% decrease
Tumor	no effect.

TABLE 12-5.—Sequence of Diagnostic Procedures Utilized in the
Work-up of the Hirsute Female

1. History and physical examination (including pelvic)
2. Postprandial blood glucose, fasting eosinophil count, protein-bound iodine
3. Glucose tolerance test
4. X-ray of sella turcica, spine, and pelvis; epiphyseal survey (children)
5. Urinary 17-KS and 17-hydroxycorticosteroids; plasma cortisol and diurnal variation
6. Buccal smear for nuclear sex chromatin; karyotype if indicated

17-KS NORMAL	17-KS ELEVATED
a. Culdoscopy, peritoneal pneumography	a. Pregnanetriol determination; fractionation of 17-KS
b. HCG stimulation and stilbestrol suppression tests during adrenal suppression	b. Corticosteroid suppression and ACTH stimulation
c. If a and b are negative, proceed to adrenal studies (next column)	c. Intravenous urogram, retroperitoneal pneumography
d. If adrenal studies are negative and b suggests ovarian origin, consider exploration of ovaries	d. Adrenal exploration if tumor is strongly suspected
e. If ovaries are normal, explore and take biopsy of adrenals	e. If adrenals appear normal at exploration, examine and take biopsy of ovaries; consider wedge resection

(From Schneeberg, N. G.: Adrenal cortical factors in infertility, in Behrman, S. J., and Kistner, R. W., [eds-]: *Progress in Infertility* [Boston: Little, Brown and Company, 1968].)

increased androgen secretion, no change is found in the 17-ketosteroids, testosterone or pregnanetriol. Dexamethasone effects very little change but dexamethasone plus HCG produces a marked increase in these urinary steroids. Premarin causes a diminution of the same steroids as a result of ovarian suppression. (See Table 12-6.)

It should be noted that dehydroepiandrosterone (formed chiefly in the adrenal) is a poor precursor for the formation of testosterone. The latter is usually synthesized from androstenedione (formed chiefly in the ovary) in the liver or peripherally. Metopirone may affect enzyme systems in the adrenal increasing the conversion of dehydroepiandrosterone to androstenedione thus effecting an increased secretion rate of testosterone. This accounts for the elevation in testosterone following the administration of metopirone as noted in Table 12-6 in combined adrenal and ovarian dysfunction.

TABLE 12-6.—Responses of 17-Ketosteroids, Testosterone, and Pregnanetriol
to Various Stimuli

ORIGIN OF ANDROGEN	CONTROL	METOPIRONE	DEXAMETHA-SONE	DEXAMETHA-SONE +HCG	PREMARIN
Ovary	17-KS ↑ Testosterone ↑	Poor	Poor	Excellent ↑	↓ Excellent
Adrenal	17-KS ↑ Testos. ↑ P. triol. ↑	Excellent (2+Increase)	Excellent (Depression)	Poor	Poor
Combined Disease A	17-KS N. or ↑ Testos. N.	Excellent	Poor	Good	Poor
Combined Disease B	17-KS ↑ Testos. N.	Excellent	Poor	Good	Poor

(After Kupperman)

TREATMENT

Unfortunately, in the majority of hairy women, no curable disorder will be discovered. Therefore, treatment should be limited to cosmetic management, such as bleaching of hair or hair removal. Chemical depilatories, usually containing barium or strontium sulfide, are effective in removing hair temporarily. They give off an odor of hydrogen sulfide, which may be objectionable, and may cause skin irritation.

Shaving, cutting, or tweezing hair may be suitable in some cases and, contrary to popular notion, they do not stimulate hair growth. Removal with wax has been especially effective, and new growth of hair is fine-tipped rather than bristly as it is after shaving or after chemical depilation.

The only acceptable method of removing hair permanently is by electrical methods which destroy the hair papilla. There may be a recurrence of 15 to 20 per cent of hair after electrolysis, even with the best technique, but these can be retreated.

X-ray therapy, although effective in removing hair, should not be used because of the long-term sequelae of radiodermatitis and carcinoma.

Pituitary and adrenal tumors are usually managed by surgical extirpation but x-ray therapy for specific pituitary lesions may be indicated. Hirsutism associated with the adrenogenital syndrome or acquired adrenal hyperplasia may be treated by the administration of hydrocortisone or one of its more potent substituents.

Ovarian tumors must be surgically removed but ovarian wedge resection for Stein-Leventhal syndrome is gradually being replaced by more physiologic methods such as clomiphene citrate. In a few patients lack of ovulation and hirsutism is due to both adrenal and ovarian factors. In such patients, the administration of both hydrocortisone and clomiphene is necessary to induce ovulation. Unfortunately, the excess hair does not always disappear and even when it diminishes, it does so over a rather prolonged interval.

BIBLIOGRAPHY

Precocious Puberty

Albright, F., et al.: Syndrome characterized by osteitis fibrosa disseminata, areas of pigmentation and endocrine dysfunction with precocious puberty in females, New England J. Med. 216:727, 1937.
Benedict, P. H.: Endocrine features in Albright's syndrome (fibrous dysplasia of bone), Metabolism 11:30, 1962.
Brown, R. W., and Kistner, R. W.: Gynecological Disorders: Clinical Aspects, in Velardo, J. T. (ed.): *Essentials of Human Reproduction* (New York: Oxford University Press, 1958).
Collipp, P. J., et al.: Constitutional isosexual precocious puberty, Am. J. Dis. Child. 108:399, 1964.
Eberlein, W. R., et al.: Ovarian tumors and cysts associated with sexual precocity: Report of three cases and review of the literature, J. Pediat. 57:484, 1960.
Frantz, A. G., and Robkin, M. T.: Effects of estrogen and sex difference on secretion of human growth hormone, J. Clin. Endocrinol. 25:1470, 1965.
Goodman and Gilman: *The Pharmacological Basis of Therapeutics.* (Ed. 3) (New York: The Macmillan Company, 1965).
Hahn, H. B., Jr., Hayles, A. B., and Albert, A.: Medroxyprogesterone and constitutional precocious puberty, Mayo Clin. Proc. 39:182, 1964.
Jolly, H.: *Sexual Precocity* (Springfield, Ill.: Charles C Thomas, Publisher, 1955).
Kupperman, H. S., and Epstein, J. A.: Medroxyprogesterone acetate in the treatment of constitutional sexual precocity, J. Clin. Endocrinol. 22:456, 1962.
Lacy, C. M.: Idiopathic true precocious puberty: A new approach in therapy. Personal Communication.
Liu, N., Grumbach, M. M., de Napoli, R. A., and Morishima, A.: Prevalence of electroencephalographic abnormalities in idiopathic precocious puberty and premature pubarche: Bearing on pathogenesis and neuroendocrine regulation of puberty, J. Clin. Endocrinol. 25:1296, 1965.

Lloyd, C. W.: Precocious puberty of the female type, J. Clin. Endocrinol. 15:1518, 1955.
Loop, J. W.: Precocious puberty-pneumoencephalography demonstrating a hamartoma in the absence of cerebral symptoms. New England J. Med. 271:409, 1964.
Pedowitz, P.; Felmus, L. B., and Mackles, A.: Precocious pseudopuberty due to ovarian tumors, Obst. & Gynec. Surv. 10:633, 1955.
Sulman, F. G.: The mechanism of the "Push and Pull" principle. II. Endocrine effects of hypothalamic depressants of the phenothiazine group. Arch. internat. pharmacodyn. 118:298, 1959.
Thamdrup, E.: Precocious sexual development—A clinical study of one hundred children. Danish M. Bull. 8:140, Nov., 1961.
Van Wyk, J. J., and Grumbach, M. M.: Syndrome of precocious menstruation and galactorrhea in juvenile hypothyroidism: An example of hormonal overlap in pituitary feedback, J. Pediat. 57:416, 1960.

Amenorrhea

Asherman, J. G.: The myth of tubal and endometrial transplantation, J. Obst. & Gynaec. Brit. Emp. 67:223, 1960.
Becker, K. L.; Hayles, A. B., and Albert, A.: Gonadal dysgenesis due to mosaicism of an X chromosome fragment, Proc. Staff Meet. Mayo Clin. 38:422, 1963.
———; Paris, J., and Albert, A.: Ovarian dysgenesis due to deletion of the X chromosome, Proc. Staff Meet. Mayo Clin. 38:389, 1963.
Bongiovanni, A. M., and Root, A. W.: The adrenogenital syndrome, New England J. Med. 268: 1283, 1963.
de la Chapelle, A.: Cytogenetical and clinical observations in female gonadal dysgenesis, Acta endocrinol. 40 (supp. 65): 1, 1962.
Greenblatt, R. B., et al.: Gynecologic aspects of sexual precocity, Pediat. Clin. North America, pp. 71–93, February, 1958.
Kahana, L., et al.: Endocrine manifestation of intracranial extrasellar lesions, J. Clin. Endocrinol. 22:304, 1962.
Lloyd, C. W.: The Ovaries, in Williams, R. H. (ed.) Textbook of Endocrinology (Philadelphia: W. B. Saunders Company, 1962).
Morris, J. M., and Mahesh, V. B.: Further observations on the syndrome "testicular feminization," Am. J. Obst. & Gynec. 87:731, 1963.
Stein, I. F., and Leventhal, M. L.: Amenorrhea associated with bilateral polycystic ovaries, Am. J. Obst. & Gynec. 29:181, 1935.

Use of Progestins

Kistner, R. W.: The use of progestational agents in obstetrics and gynecology, Clin. Obst. & Gynec. 3:1047, 1960.
———: Treatment of carcinoma in situ of the endometrium, Clin. Obst. & Gynec. 5:116, 1962.
———: Hormonal Management of Endometriosis, in Meigs, J. V., and Sturgis, S. H. (eds.): Progress in Gynecology (New York: Grune & Stratton, Inc., 1963), vol. IV.
———: The Use of Progestins in Obstetrics and Gynecology (Chicago: Year Book Medical Publishers, Inc., 1969).

Dysfunctional Uterine Bleeding

Henriksen, E.: Disorders of the ovulatory phase, Clin. Obst. & Gynec. 2:180, 1959.
Kelley, J. V.: Intravenous estrogen therapy, an assessment, Obst. & Gynec. 17:149, 1961.
Menzer-Benaron, D., and Sturgis, S. H.: Relationship between Emotional and Somatic Factors in Gynecologic Disease, in Meigs, J. V., and Sturgis, S. H. (eds.): Progress in Gynecology (New York: Grune & Stratton, Inc., 1957), vol. III.
Noyes, R. W.: Underdeveloped secretory endometrium, Am. J. Obst. & Gynec. 77:929, 1959.
Salvatore, C. A.: Arterioles of the endometrium in the etiopathogenesis of dysfunctional hemorrhage, J. Internat. Coll. Surgeons 29:599, 1958.

Dysmenorrhea

Chesley, L. C., and Hellman, L. M.: Variations in body weight and salivary sodium in menstrual cycle, Am. J. Obst. & Gynec. 74:582, 1957.
Davis, A.: Alcohol injection for relief of dysmenorrhea, Clin. Obst. & Gynec. 6:754, 1963.
Doyle, J. B.: Paracervical uterine denervation by transection of cervical plexus for relief of dysmenorrhea, Am. J. Obst. & Gynec. 70:1, 1955.
———, and DesRosiers, J. J.: Paracervical uterine denervation for relief of pelvic pain, Clin. Obst. & Gynec. 6:742, 1963.
Fluhmann, C. F.: The Management of Menstrual Disorders (Philadelphia: W. B. Saunders Company, 1956).
———: Dysmenorrhea, Clin. Obst. Gynec. 6:718, 1963.
Goldzieher, J. W.; Henkin, A. E., and Hamblen, E. C.: Characteristics of the normal menstrual cycle, Am. J. Obst. & Gynec. 54:668, 1947.
Greenblatt, R. B.; Hammond, D. O., and Clark, S. L.: Membranous dysmenorrhea: Studies in etiology and treatment, Am. J. Obst. & Gynec. 68:835, 1954.
Ingersoll, F., and Meigs, J. V.: Presacral neurectomy for dysmenorrhea, New England J. Med. 238:357, 1948.

Jacobs, W. M.; Conner, J. S., and Rogers, S. F.: Presacral neurectomy, Am. J. Obst. & Gynec. 85:437, 1963.

Jones, H. W., Jr.: A phase of the autonomic nervous system in obstetrics and gynecology, Obst. & Gynec. Surv. 14:171, 1959.

Kroger, W. S.: Hypnosis for relief of pelvic pain, Clin. Obst. & Gynec. 6:763, 1963.

Landesman, R., et al.: Vascular bed of bulbar conjunctiva in normal menstrual cycle, Am. J. Obst. & Gynec. 66:988, 1953.

Markee, J. E.: The Morphological and Endocrine Basis for Menstrual Bleeding, in Meigs, J. V., and Sturgis, S. H. (eds.): Progress in Gynecology (New York:Grune & Stratton, Inc., 1950), vol. II.

Menaker, J. S., and Powers, K. D.: Management of primary dysmenorrhea, Obst. & Gynec. 20:66, 1962.

Page, E. T.; Kamm, M. L., and Chappell, C. C.: Paracervical block in obstetrics and gynecology, S. Clin. North America 42:927, 1962.

Phelps, B.: Menstruation, in Velardo, J. T. (ed.): Essentials of Human Reproduction: Clinical Aspects, Normal and Abnormal (New York: Oxford University Press, 1958).

Rogers, J.: Menstruation and systemic disease, New England J. Med. 259:676, 721, 770, 1958.

Taylor, H. C., Jr.: Pelvic pain based on a vascular and autonomic nervous system disorder, Am. J. Obst. & Gynec. 67:1177, 1954.

Adrenogenital Syndrome

Allen, W. M.; Hayward, S. J., and Pinto, A.: A color test for dehydroiso-androsterone and closely related steroids of use in the diagnosis of adrenocortical tumors, J. Clin. Endocrinol. 10:54, 1950.

Blackman, S. S., Jr.: Concerning function and origin of reticular zone of adrenal cortex: Hyperplasia and adrenogenital syndrome, Bull. Johns Hopkins Hosp. 78:180, 1946.

Bongiovanni, A. M.: The detection of pregnanediol and pregnanetriol in the urine of patients with adrenal hyperplasia: Suppression with cortisone, Bull. Johns Hopkins Hosp. 92:244, 1953.

———, and Root, A. W.: The adrenogenital syndrome, New England J. Med. 268:1283, 1963.

Childs, B.: Congenital adrenal cortical hyperplasia, J. Clin. Invest. 35:213, 1956.

Eberlein, W. R., and Bongiovanni, A. M.: Pathophysiology of congenital adrenal hyperplasia, Metabolism 9:326, 1960.

Epstein, J. A., and Kupperman, H. S.: Dexamethasone therapy in the adrenogenital syndrome: A comparative study, J. Clin. Endocrinol. 19:1503, 1959.

Forsham, P. H.: The Adrenals, in Williams, R. H. (ed.): Textbook of Endocrinology (3d ed.; Philadelphia: W. B. Saunders Company, 1962).

Gold, E. M.; Kent, J. R., and Forsham, P. H.: Clinical use of a new diagnostic agent methopyrapone (SU-4885) in pituitary and adrenocortical disorders, Ann. Int. Med. 54:175, 1961.

Gross, R. E.: The Surgery of Infancy and Childhood (Philadelphia: W. B. Saunders Company, 1953).

Jailer, J. W.; Gold, J. J., and Wallace, E. Z.: Evaluation of the "cortisone test" as a diagnostic aid in differentiating adrenal hyperplasia from adrenal neoplasia, Am. J. Med. 16:340, 1954.

———, et al.: 17-alpha-hydroxy-progesterone and 21-desoxyhydrocortisone: Their metabolism and possible role in congenital adrenal virilism, J. Clin. Invest. 34:1639, 1955.

Jones, H. W., Jr.; Holman, G. H., and Stempfel, R. S., Jr.: Masculinization of female fetus associated with administration of oral and intramuscular progestins during gestation: Nonadrenal female pseudohermaphroditism, J. Clin. Endocrinol. 18:559, 1958.

———, and Scott, W. W.: Hermaphroditism, Genital Anomalies and Related Endocrine Disorders (Baltimore: Williams & Wilkins Company, 1958).

———, and Wilkins, L.: Genital anomaly associated with pre-natal exposure to progestogens, Fertil. & Steril. 11:148, 1960.

Kupperman, H. S.; Finkler, R., and Burger, J.: Quantitative effect of cortisone upon ketosteroid excretion and clinical picture of the adrenogenital syndrome, J. Clin. Endocrinol. 13:1109, 1953.

Symington, T.: Morphology and secretory cytology of human adrenal cortex, Brit. M. Bull. 18: 117, 1962.

Tanner, J. M.: The development of the female reproductive system during adolescence, Clin. Obst. & Gynec. 3:135, 1960.

Wilkins, L.: The Diagnosis and Treatment of Endocrine Disorders in Childhood and Adolescence (2d ed.; Springfield, Ill.: Charles C Thomas, Publisher, 1960).

Cushing's Syndrome

Kupperman, H. S.: Human Endocrinology: Vol. 2. Cushing's Syndrome (Philadelphia: F. A. Davis Company, 1963), p. 746.

Liddle, G. W.: Test of pituitary-adrenal suppressibility in the diagnosis of Cushing's syndrome, J. Clin. Endocrinol. 20:1259, 1960.

Montgomery, D. A., and Welbourne, R. B.: Cushing's syndrome: A review, Quart. Rev. Surg. Gynec. & Obst. 16:201, 1959.

Soffer, L. J., et al.: Cushing's Syndrome, in Ciba Foundation Colloquia on Endocrinology: Vol. 8. The Human Adrenal Cortex (Boston: Little, Brown & Company, 1955).

Simmonds' Disease and Sheehan's Syndrome

Israel, S. L., and Conston, A. S.: Unrecognized pituitary necrosis (Sheehan's syndrome) as a cause of sudden death, J.A.M.A. 148:189, 1952.
Sheehan, H. L.: Postpartum necrosis of the anterior pituitary, J. Path. & Bact. 45:189, 1937; Irish J. M. Sc. 270:241, 1948.
———, and Stanfield, J. P.: The pathogenesis of postpartum necrosis of the anterior lobe of the pituitary gland, Acta endocrinol. 37:479, 1961.
———, and Summers, V. A.: Syndrome of hypopituitarism, Quart. J. Med. 18:319, 1949.
Smith, C. W., and Howard, R. P.: Variations in endocrine gland function in postpartum pituitary necrosis, J. Clin. Endocrinol. 19:1420, 1959.

Chiari-Frommel Syndrome

Forbes, A. P., *et al.*: Syndrome characterized by galactorrhea, amenorrhea and low urinary FSH: Comparison with acromegaly and normal lactation, J. Clin. Endocrinol. 14:265, 1954.
Frommel, R.: Über puerperale atrophie, Ztschr. Geburtsh. u. Gynäk. 7:305, 1882.
Kaiser, I. H.: Pregnancy following clomiphene-induced ovulation in Chiari-Frommel syndrome, Am. J. Obst. & Gynec. 87:149, 1963.

Hirsutism

Greenblatt, R. B.: *The Hirsute Female* (Springfield, Ill.: Charles C Thomas, Publisher, 1963).
Greenblatt, R. B., and Coniff, R. F.: Hirsutism and the Stein-Leventhal syndrome, Fertil. & Steril. 19:661, 1968.

CHAPTER 13

Steroid Therapy

General Considerations

RAPID ADVANCES in the field of synthetic biochemistry during the past decade have led to the development of an entire group of new substances which are extremely important in the everyday practice of obstetrics and gynecology. These agents are, for the most part, synthetic variations of progesterone, testosterone, estradiol and hydrocortisone. Certain minute variations in structure, together with unfamiliar symbols and designations used by biochemists, have led to confusion in the minds of most practitioners. Since function of these agents may be intimately correlated with structure, it is important that the physician be familiar with the pharmacologic properties of these structural classes.

The steroid hormones comprise one of the most interesting groups of the biologic organic compounds known as *lipids*. Lipids are widely distributed in nature and have a greasy, oily or waxy consistency. They are relatively insoluble in water but are soluble in ether, benzene, acetone and chloroform. Included in the large category of lipids are the sterols, the sex hormones, the adrenal cortical hormones, the bile acids, the provitamins D, the steroidal sapogenins, the cardiac aglycones, the steroidal alkaloids and certain carcinogenic hydrocarbons.

A large number of compounds, including the sex hormones, are derived from a complex organic ring structure known as cyclopentanoperhydrophenanthrene. In this compound there are three rings of six carbons each (phenanthrene) and one ring of five carbon atoms (cyclopentane). Compounds derived from this basic structure are known as *sterids*. However, if one or more hydroxyl groups and a long chain carbon, hydrogen and oxygen are attached at carbon-17, the compound is known as a *sterol* (e.g., cholesterol). When one or more carbonyl (C=O), hydroxyl (OH) and methyl (CH$_3$) groups (any or all) are attached to the cyclopentane or phenanthrene rings, the compound is called a *steroid*. In general there are five basic steroid nuclei (Fig. 13-1) and all of the steroid compounds are derived from one of these parent compounds. They are: *estrane* (18 carbon atoms), the source of the natural estrogens; *androstane* and *etiocholane* (19 carbon atoms), the source of almost all of the natural androgens [these two nuclei differ only in the stereo or optical position of the hydrogen atom extending from carbon atom number 5]; *pregnane* and *allopregnane* (21 carbon

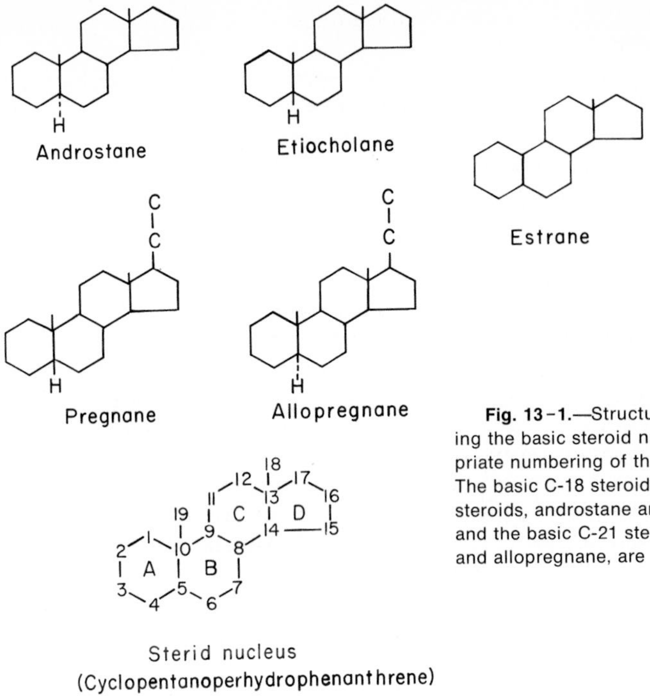

Androstane

Etiocholane

Estrane

Pregnane

Allopregnane

Fig. 13-1.—Structural formula showing the basic steroid nucleus with appropriate numbering of the carbon atoms.
The basic C-18 steroid estrane, C-19
steroids, androstane and etiocholane,
and the basic C-21 steroids, pregnane
and allopregnane, are illustrated.

Sterid nucleus
(Cyclopentanoperhydrophenanthrene)

atoms), the source of progesterone and its derivatives as well as the corticoids. These two nuclei, like androstane and etiocholane, differ only in the
position of the C-5 hydrogen atom.

The common steroids are derivatives of these basic sterid nuclei, the
structural changes being indicated by specific suffixes and symbols. For
example, when the six-carbon ring is "unsaturated," a double bond is inserted in the ring at the point of "desaturation," or, in other words, between
adjacent carbon atoms which have lost one hydrogen atom each. When one
or more double bonds are present in the ring, the suffix *ene* replaces the
ane ending. The symbol Δ indicates the presence of the double bond and a
superscript number its location. Recently steroid chemists have tended to
eliminate the symbol for delta (Δ) and instead the Δ^4 compounds are called
pregn-4-ene-3,20-dione (for progesterone) or androst-4-ene-3,17-dione
(androstenedione). If a hydroxy (OH) group is substituted for a hydrogen,
the suffix *ol* is used together with the number of the carbon to which it is

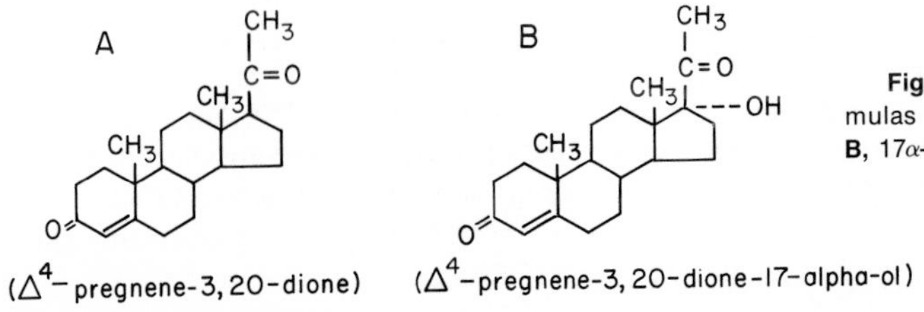

A

CH_3
|
C=O
CH_3
CH_3

B

CH_3
|
C=O
CH_3
---OH
CH_3

Fig. 13-2.—Structural formulas for **A**, progesterone and
B, 17α-hydroxyprogesterone.

(Δ^4-pregnene-3,20-dione)   (Δ^4-pregnene-3,20-dione-17-alpha-ol) added. Substitution by a keto (=O) group is demonstrated by the suffix *one* and its location similarly identified. Thus in Figure 13–2 the structural formula for progesterone is shown. This is basically a C-21 sterid, pregnane. Since there is a double bond in ring A, the term pregnane is changed to pregnene and the position of the double bond is between carbon 4 and carbon 5, thus the expression Δ^4. Two ketone groups are present, one on carbon 3 and another on carbon 20, thus 3,20-*dione* (meaning 2 ketone groups). The proper identification of progesterone is therefore, Δ^4-pregnene-3,20-dione. Figure 13–2 also shows 17α-hydroxyprogesterone.

Since steroids are derived from lipids, they are usually not soluble in aqueous solutions. They are measurable in urine as the result of conjugation with water-soluble sulfate or glucuronide-producing esters. The carbon atom at position 3 uniformly possesses a readily esterified hydroxy group or a ketone group which may be converted into a hydroxy group. A double bond is frequently found between carbons 4 and 5 and this particular structural construction is referred to as an alpha-β-unsaturated-3-ketone group. This configuration is characteristic of physiologically active compounds such as progesterone, testosterone, hydrocortisone and cortisone. When this structural arrangement in the A ring is modified in order to present a 3-hydroxy group for the formation of water-soluble conjugates, the potency of the compound is greatly diminished.

Biosynthesis of Steroids

It is important to realize the relative nonspecific formation of all steroid hormones since they are produced in similar fashion in the testes, the ovary and the adrenal. In the ovary progesterone, androgens and estrogens can be synthesized by the follicle, corpus luteum and stroma. The pathways and the biochemical details of the reaction appear to be remarkably similar. Therefore, in the biosynthesis of estrogens it is necessary to consider the formation of progesterone and androgens in sequence. The biosynthetic pathways indicated are adapted from the chapter by Dr. Kenneth J. Ryan in *Progress in Infertility*. The reader is referred to this book for further detail.

According to Ryan, pregnenolone (pregn-5-ene-3,20-dione) can be considered a pivotal compound from which all other steroids arise. Progesterone was once thought to play this role, but more recent data have indicated the possibility of bypassing progesterone for the formation of estrogens and androgens. Pregnenolone has little apparent endocrine activity. It serves its chief function as precursor for other more active compounds.

Pregnenolone can be synthesized from acetate via cholesterol, 20-hydroxy-cholesterol and 20,22-dihydroxycholesterol (Fig. 13–3). This sequence of steps has been demonstrated in the adrenal, testis, follicle, corpus luteum, and ovarian stroma. The steps between cholesterol and pregnenolone are of particular interest since it is at this level that the primary locus of luteinizing hormone action is being placed. The acetate-to-cholesterol conversion takes place in the soluble and microsomal fractions of the cell while the cholesterol-to-pregnenolone conversion takes place in the mitochondrial fraction.

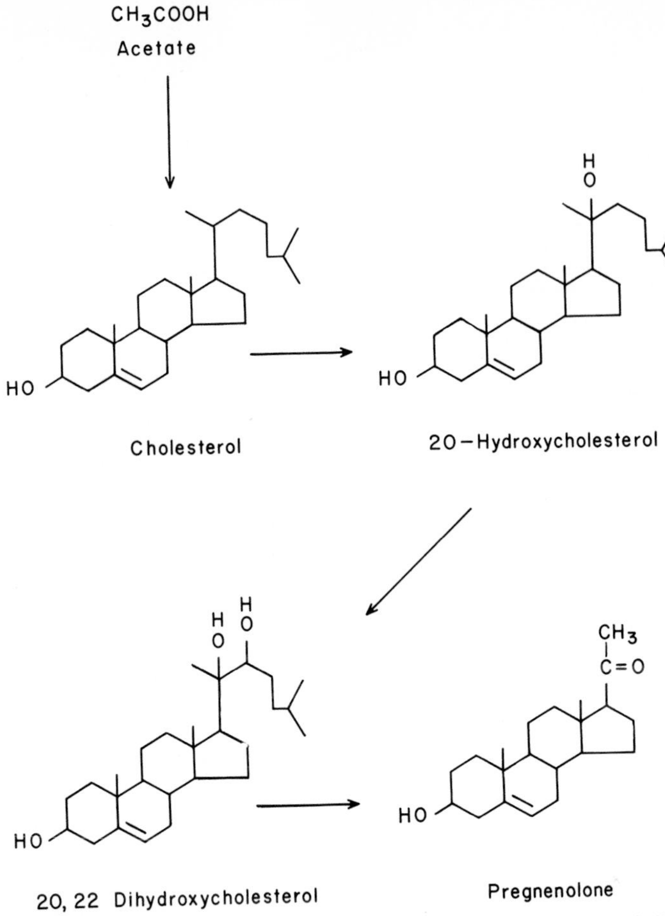

Fig. 13–3.—Conversion of acetate to pregnenolone via cholesterol, 20-hydroxy and 20, 22-dihydroxycholesterol.
(Figs. 13–3 through 13–7 courtesy of Dr. Kenneth J. Ryan.)

The conversion of pregnenolone to progesterone is a facile reaction that occurs in all endocrine tissues and involves a shift of the Δ^5-3β-hydroxyl configuration to the Δ^4-3-ketone of the active luteal principle (Fig. 13–4). The enzyme system is located in the microsomal fraction of the cell and requires a diphosphopyridine nucleotide cofactor.

Progesterone, when formed, can be secreted as such or converted to 20α-hydroxypregn-4-en-3-one (Fig. 13–4), another active progestational principle. The reaction involves the reduction of the 20-ketone of progesterone to the 20α-hydroxyl group of the metabolite.

Another progestationally active metabolite of progesterone, 20β-hydroxypregn-4-en-3-one, has also been demonstrated. This suggests that there may be still other active hormones which have not as yet been identified.

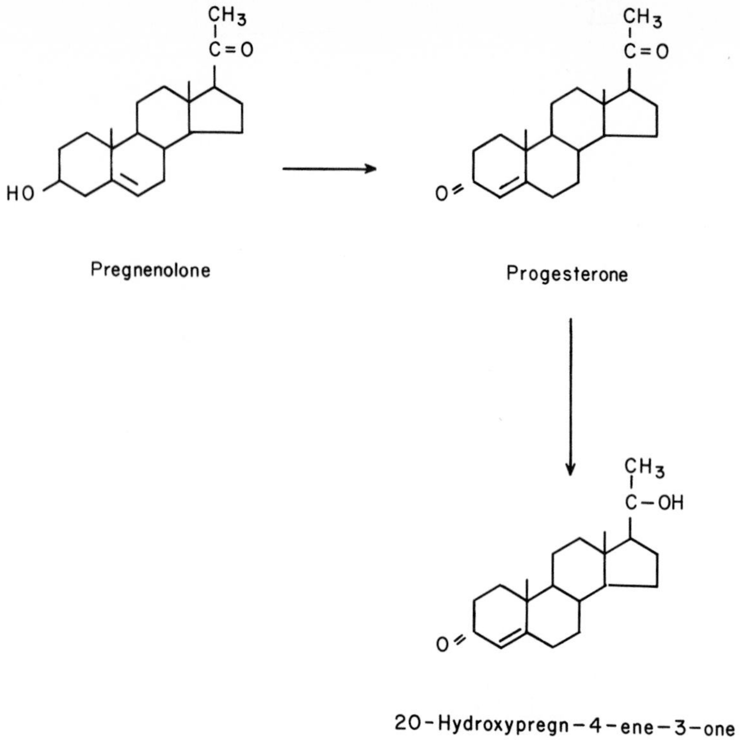

Fig. 13–4.—Conversion of pregnenolone to progesterone and on to 20-hydroxypregn-4-en-3-one.

FORMATION OF ANDROGENS

The "androgens"—androstenedione, testosterone, and dehydroepiandrosterone—can be formed in the testis, adrenal, follicle, corpus luteum, or ovarian stroma by 17-hydroxylation of pregnenolone or progesterone and cleavage of the side chain. There are three possible pathways. The first (progesterone→ 17-hydroxyprogesterone→ androstenedione ⇆ testosterone) seems to be most operative in corpora lutea and granulosa cells (Fig. 13–5), while the other two, (pregnenolone → 17-hydroxypregnenolone → 17-hydroxyprogesterone → androstenedione ⇆ testosterone) and (pregnenolone → 17-hydroxypregnenolone → dehydroepiandrosterone → androstenedione ⇌ testosterone), seem to be most operative in the follicle and theca cells (Fig. 13–6). Dehydroepiandrosterone may also be first converted to androstenediol and thence to testosterone, bypassing androstenedione (Fig. 13–7).

These compounds are considered androgens solely in a chemical sense since only testosterone of the group has significant biological androgenic activity. The other compounds can be converted to testosterone in the endocrine gland or peripherally.

The reactions described for 17-hydroxylation and side-chain cleavage take place in the microsomal fractions of the cell while the dehydrogenase

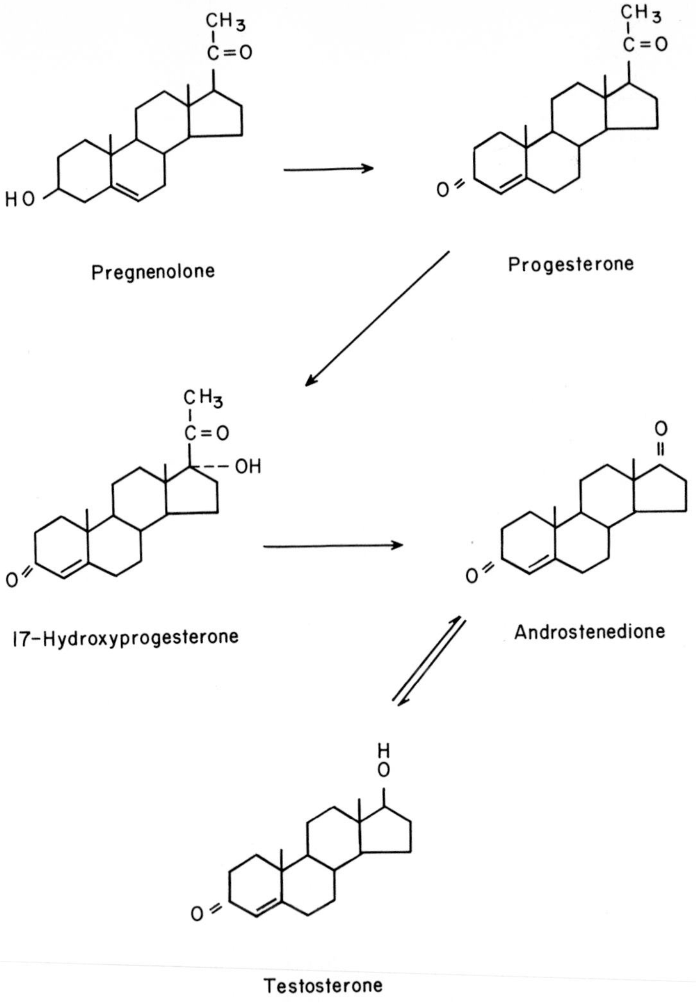

Pregnenolone

Progesterone

17-Hydroxyprogesterone

Androstenedione

Testosterone

Fig. 13-5.—Androgen formation via progesterone.

reactions involved in the testosterone-androstenedione conversion are effected by soluble enzyme systems.

The androstenedione formed can be secreted by the ovary, which probably is the source of this steroid measured in the blood of female subjects. Androstenedione is present in the plasma of female subjects in levels of 0.130–0.145 μg. per 100 ml., twice the level in males. It is therefore a normal metabolite of the ovary whose clinical significance does not become apparent except in cases of hirsutism or polycystic ovary syndrome.

The biologically active androgens of both the adrenal cortex and the testis are grouped under the general term of C-19 steroids. Some of the degradation products of the C-21 steroids, however, are found in the urine classified as C-19 steroids. As seen in Figure 13-1, the basic sterids of the C-19 group are androstane and etiocholane, the nuclei differing only by the

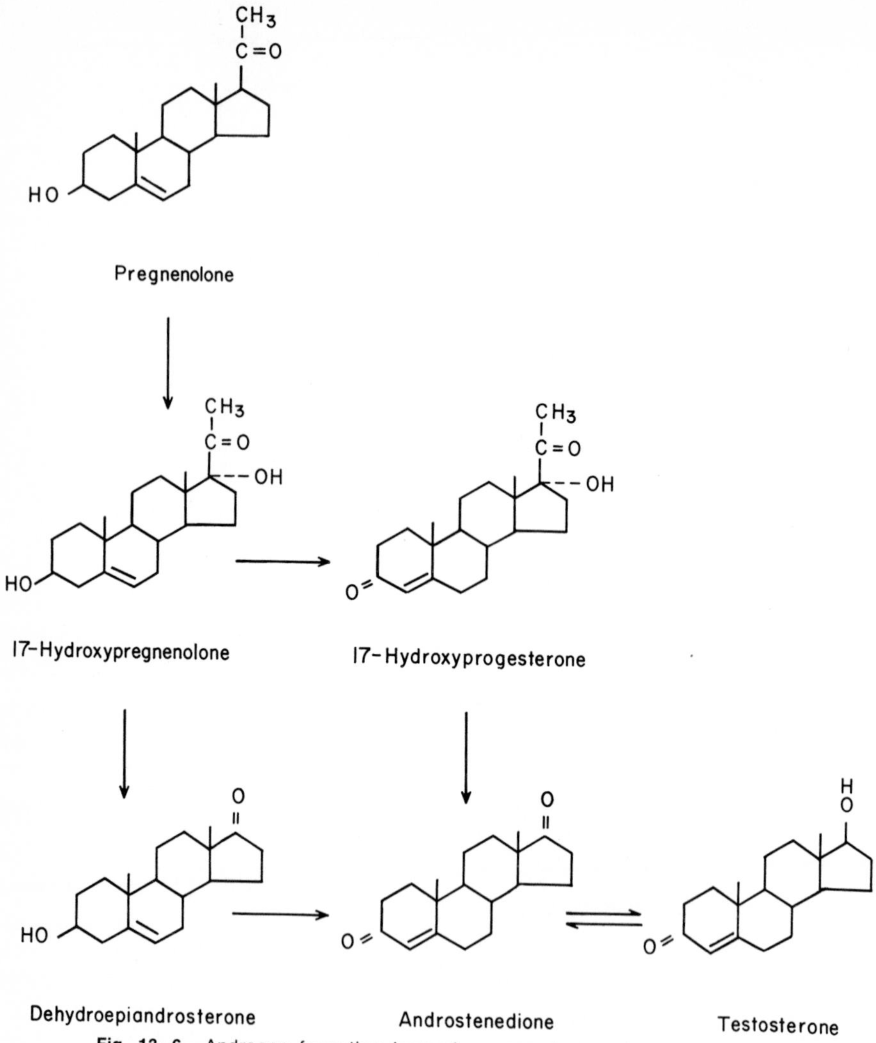

Pregnenolone

17-Hydroxypregnenolone   17-Hydroxyprogesterone

Dehydroepiandrosterone   Androstenedione   Testosterone

Fig. 13-6.—Androgen formation bypassing progesterone via either 17-hydroxyprogesterone or dehydroepiandrosterone.

position of the C-5 hydrogen atom. If a double bond exists in the A ring between carbon atoms 4 and 5, androstane is then termed androstene, and if there are keto groups on carbon atoms 3 and 17 the term dione is added. This compound is then known as androstenedione. Androsterone is a common name for the compound androstane which contains a ketone in the 17 position and a hydroxy radical in the 3 position (Fig. 13-8).

Testosterone is a common name for the natural androgen derived from etiocholane which has a double bond in the 4–5 position in the A ring, a ketone in the 3 position and a hydroxy radical in the 17 position. Testosterone is the only natural androgen of importance which does not possess a ketone group on carbon atom number 17 (Fig. 13-8).

The remainder of the C-19 steroids are named as derivatives of andros-

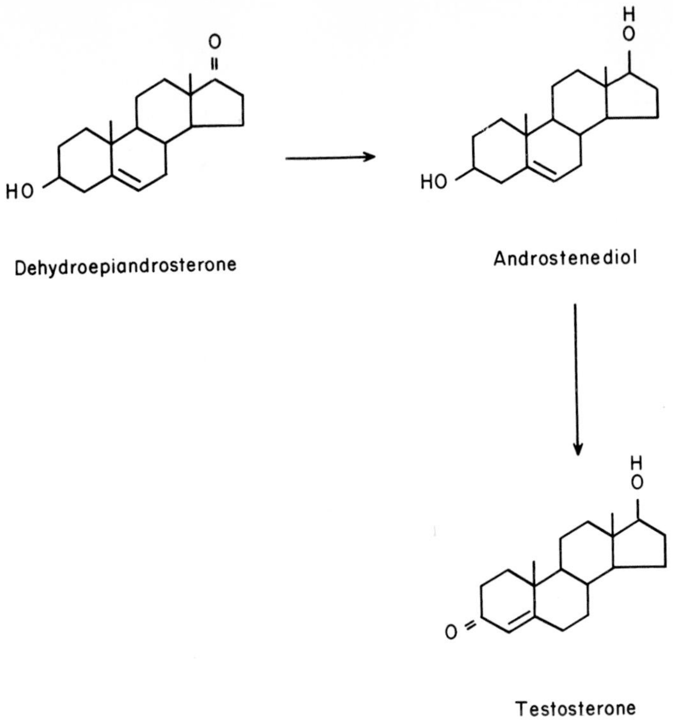

Dehydroepiandrosterone

Androstenediol

Testosterone

Fig. 13-7.—Alternate pathway for testosterone bypassing androstenedione.

terone or of the basic sterid nuclei, androstane and etiocholane. The changes are indicated by specific prefixes *epi* or *iso*. These terms may be used interchangeably and indicate optical, or stereo, isomerism. Thus in the compound illustrated in Figure 13-8, the term *epi* indicates a change in the 3-hydroxy group to the beta position, since the hydroxy group in androsterone is in the alpha position. The term *dehydro* indicates a loss of two atoms of hydrogen from the molecule, resulting in the double bond between these two points. Thus in the structural formula of dehydro-epiandrosterone, this indicates a loss of one atom of hydrogen from carbon atoms 5 and 6, resulting in the double bond between these two points.

Dehydroepiandrosterone, dehydroepiandrosterone sulfate, and Δ^4-androstenedione are the principal androgens secreted by the adrenals. In addition to these, 11β-hydroxy-Δ^4-androstenedione may also be secreted by the adrenals in significant quantities. The ovaries and testes are known to secrete Δ^4-androstenedione. Testosterone is secreted mainly by the testes; its secretion by the ovaries and the adrenal is controversial. The secretion of dehydroepiandrosterone by the ovaries and testes has also been established under pathologic conditions.

The androgens secreted by the adrenals and gonads undergo extensive metabolism in the body before excretion in the urine. The chief areas of metabolism are carbon atoms 3, 4, 5, and 17 of the steroid molecule. Δ^4-Androstenedione undergoes reduction of the double bond in the 4 position to give rise to 5α-and 5β-steroids. The 3-ketone is further reduced mainly to

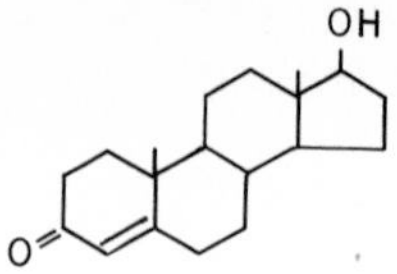

Fig. 13-8.—Basic C-19 steroids testosterone and androsterone and related compounds.

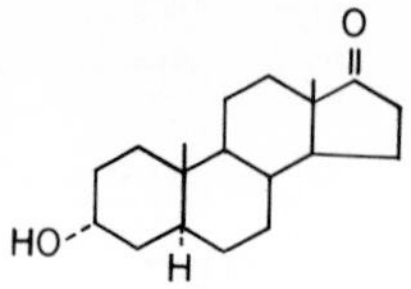

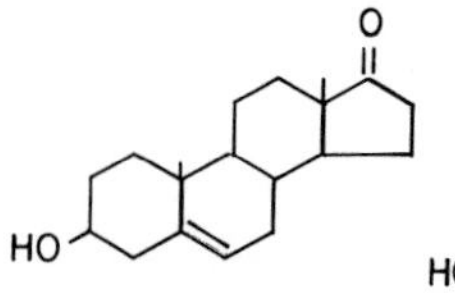

Testosterone   Androsterone

Dehydroepiandrosterone   11-hydroxyandrosterone
or
dehydroisoandrosterone

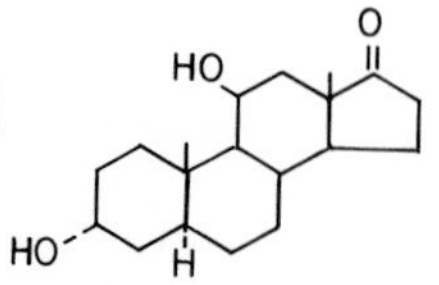

3α-hydroxysteroids but also to a small extent to 3β-hydroxysteroids. Thus the metabolites of Δ^4-androstenedione that occur in the urine in major quantities are androsterone (5α-androstan-3α-ol-17-one) and etiocholanolone (5β-androstan-3α-ol-17-one). Dehydroepiandrosterone sulfate is also converted in part to these metabolites via dehydroepiandrosterone and Δ^4-androstenedione. Oxidation-reduction at carbon 17 also takes place extensively. Thus testosterone may be converted to Δ^4-androstenedione by oxidation of the 17β-hydroxyl to a 17-ketone and then be converted to androsterone and etiocholanolone. These metabolites undergo conjugation in the 3 position and are excreted in the urine as sulfates and glucuronides. The principal 11-deoxy-17-ketosteroids in urine that arise from the metabolism of non-11-oxygenated androgens are dehydroepiandrosterone, androsterone, and etiocholanolone.

Mahesh has emphasized several points regarding the metabolism and excretion of androgens. First, although dehydroepiandrosterone, androsterone, and etiocholanolone are quantitatively important metabolites of androgens, they are by no means the only ones. Several others are present in smaller quantities, and some of them may never have been oxidized in the 17 position or may have been reduced to 17-hydroxy compounds and thus not belong to the group of 17-ketosteroids at all. Second, the formation of Δ^4-androstenedione is not obligatory in the metabolism of androgens. For instance, testosterone may be reduced in ring A prior to oxidation at carbon 17, giving rise to androsterone and etiocholanolone without going through the formation of Δ^4-androstenedione. The same metabolic end products may be formed through several different metabolic pathways. Finally, urinary 17-ketosteroids are not the exclusive metabolites of androgens. Compounds like 11-deoxy-cortisol (Δ^4-pregnene-17α,21-diol-3,20-dione), 17α-hydroxyprogesterone, and 17α-hydroxypregnenolone also serve as precursors to 11-deoxy-17-ketosteroids and cortisol is an important precursor of 11-oxygenated 17-ketosteroids.

According to Ryan, androstenedione, dehydroepiandrosterone, and testosterone are all synthesized in the ovary although only the androstenedione appears to be a major normal secretory product. These compounds are reduced primarily to androsterone and etiocholanolone and can be measured in the urine as 11-deoxy-17-ketosteroids. Several epimeric forms and hydroxylated derivatives are also possible. These reactions are chiefly a result of metabolism in the liver.

The contribution of the ovary to 11-deoxy-17-ketosteroids is ordinarily overshadowed by the adrenal component, but Mahesh and Greenblatt have shown that in the polycystic ovarian syndrome the ovarian products may be measurable especially with adrenal suppression tests. Although the problem of distinguishing between the ovarian and adrenal contributions has not been completely solved, a combination of adrenal suppression and ovarian stimulation and suppression tests may be of value. (See Chapter 7, Stein-Leventhal Syndrome.) For a review of the metabolism of ovarian steroids, the reader is referred to the excellent review by Ryan in *Progress in Infertility*.

The first method suitable for plasma testosterone assay in normal women was described by Finkelstein and associates. All methods involve several chromatographic steps for the purification of the testosterone fraction, and the final quantitation may be done by fluorometric, double isotope, and gas chromatographic methods. Although hirsutism in females can be explained on the basis of elevated plasma testosterone levels in a large number of cases, there appears to be no precise relationship between 17-ketosteroids and physiologically active circulating androgen levels.

The measurement of secretion rates of various androgens has been attempted by Lieberman and associates. Despite the careful experimental design which includes all 11-deoxy-androgens, pathways of metabolism and interconversion of various androgens are numerous.

In summarizing his evaluation of androgen function, Mahesh has stated:

"There is no procedure available that can be adopted on a practical basis for the satisfactory evaluation of androgen function. The need for means of evaluating androgen function is well recognized and this area has been one of active interest and experimentation. It is hoped that with further improvement of experimental techniques and instrumentation and with the advances in knowledge about the secretion, metabolism, and interconversion of androgens, such evaluation can be made more objectively in the future."

For a complete review of the subject of assay methods of androgen, the reader is referred to the chapter by Mahesh in *Progress in Infertility*.

FORMATION OF PROGESTERONE

The C-21 steroids include both the corticoids and progesterone and their derivatives. The former will not be discussed in detail here but it should be remembered that the term corticoids includes those steroids of the adrenal cortex that are involved in carbohydrate and salt and water metabolism. There is one structural feature about the corticoids which separates them from other C-21 compounds. This is the presence of the 17-alpha-ketol group (Fig. 13–9). Specifically, this means that there is a two-carbon atom side chain attached to the number 17 carbon atom. The first of these, the C-20 position, possesses a ketone group whereas the terminal one (C-21) contains a hydroxy group. As will be noted in the structural formula for progesterone, there is no hydroxy group present on the C-21 carbon. In addition, the corticoids differ from progesterone in that the 11 carbon may contain either a ketone or a hydroxy group (except for 11-desoxycorticoste-

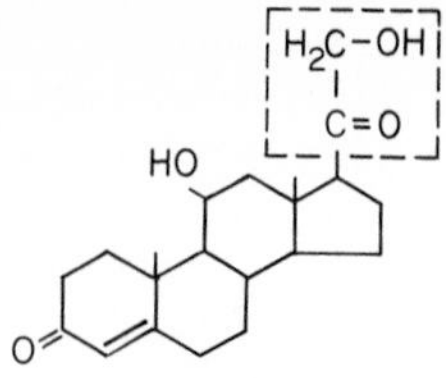

Fig. 13-9.—Basic steroid nucleus of corticosterone, showing the characteristic 17-alpha-ketol group and a hydroxy group on the 11 carbon.

Corticosterone

rone). Figure 13-10 illustrates a scheme for biosynthesis of adrenal steroids (see also Fig. 12-9, p. 591).

The nomenclature in the case of the derivatives of progesterone is based on the use of suffixes such as *ol, one* or *ene* applied to the basic sterid nucleus, pregnane. Progesterone is an arbitrary common name for the naturally occurring steroid and one derivative of progesterone, 17-alpha-hydroxy-progesterone, is named as a variation of the basic molecule.

Progesterone is produced not only by the corpus luteum but by the placenta and by the adrenal cortex as a precursor to the formation of 17-hydroxycorticosterone. The probable route of biosynthesis of progesterone is as follows: Cholesterol may be converted into a 20-hydroxylated cholesterol derivative which in turn is converted into isocaproic acid with the formation of pregnenolone during this reaction. Pregnenolone is one, or possibly the only, primary steroid produced from cholesterol in the formation of other steroids. Pregnenolone is then converted into progesterone. Pregnenolone differs structurally from progesterone in that a hydroxy radical, rather than a ketone, is present in the 3-beta position and a double bond exists in the 5-6 rather than the 4-5 position. (See Fig. 13-6.)

The progesterone (and presumably pregnenolone and 20α-hydroxypregn-4-en-3-one) molecule is ordinarily reduced in the liver to one of the many possible epimeric forms of pregnanediol, pregnenolone or a 16-hydroxy derivative and excreted as such in conjugated forms. The one form of pregnanediol (5β-pregnane-3α, 20α-diol) measured in the conventional urinary assay represents approximately only 20 per cent of the hormone's metabolites but suffices as a clinical guide to its secretion (Fig. 13-11).

Progesterone and pregnenolone can also be 17-hydroxylated and the compounds reduced to form the pregnanetriols which are urinary excretory products. The chief form measured in urine is 5β-pregnane-3α, 17α, 20α-triol, but many epimeric forms are possible (Fig. 13-12).

Pregnanediols and pregnanetriols present in urine can therefore be used

Fig. 13-10.—Diagrammatic representation of the synthesis of hydrocortisone from progesterone via 17-hydroxyprogesterone and 11-desoxycortisol. Note consecutive hydroxylation in the 17-alpha position, then the 21 position to form an alpha-ketol group and finally the 11 position to form hydrocortisone.

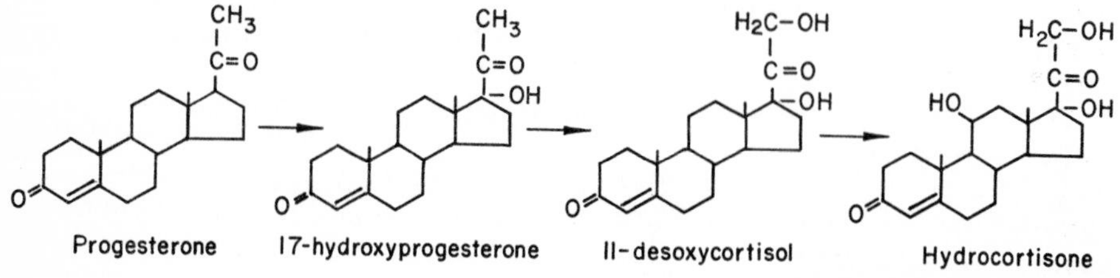

Progesterone   17-hydroxyprogesterone   ll-desoxycortisol   Hydrocortisone

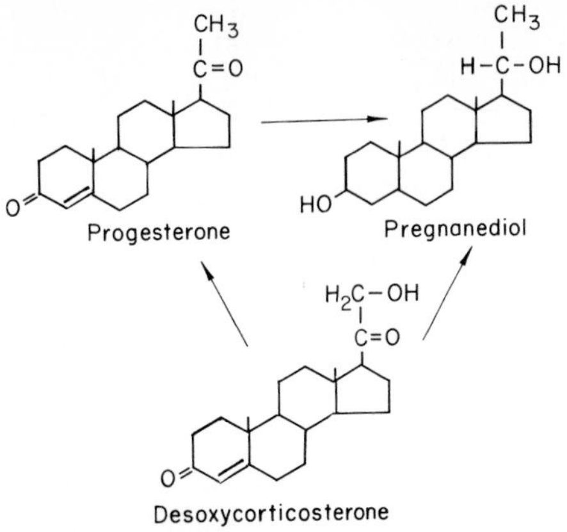

Fig. 13-11.—Schematic representation illustrating that desoxycorticosterone and progesterone may be metabolized to pregnanediol.

as guides to the relative amounts of progesterone secreted and serve as a criterion for corpus luteum function. However, biologic end points (basal body temperature, endometrial biopsy, and vaginal cytology) are cheaper, simpler, and just as reliable. In infertility work, pregnanediol values have been used as guides to the quality of corpus luteum function, and in a predictive sense to the adequacy of the corpus luteum of pregnancy and the placenta during the early months of gestation.

Assay of progesterone and its metabolites is of extreme importance in patients who are unable to become pregnant, or who habitually abort, because of inadequate corpus luteum function. Unfortunately, even if it is possible to measure progesterone in the blood, the effective concentration in the cells of the uterus or placenta is still unknown. Until very recently it was necessary to measure pregnanediol in urine and extrapolate progesterone function from these data—a precarious conclusion, particularly when only 5 to 17 per cent of injected progesterone is recovered in the urine as pregnanediol. Furthermore, at least two, possibly more, progestational hormones besides progesterone are present in the human female. There are other problems involving the adrenal since the stress of surgery or intravenous corticotropin will produce an increase in urinary pregnanediol. This does not occur in adrenalectomized patients.

In addition to these difficulties, little is known about the degree of binding of progesterone to its carrier protein and even less about the conjugated forms of the hormones. Finally, some degree of conversion of precursors to active progesterone may occur in peripheral tissues. If this occurred to a substantial degree, measurement of free or bound progesterone in plasma would have little clinical significance.

The bioassay of plasma materials in general lacks sensitivity although

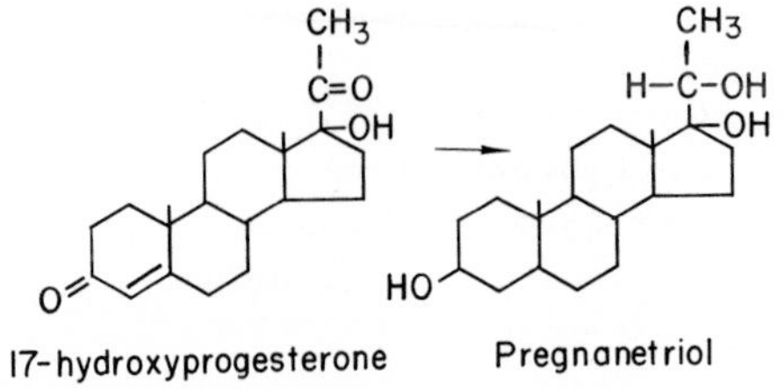

Fig. 13-12.—Schematic representation of 17-hydroxyprogesterone metabolized to pregnanetriol. Note that in pregnanediol hydroxy radicals have replaced the ketones on carbons 3 and 20, whereas in pregnanetriol there is an additional hydroxy radical in the 17-alpha position.

the Hooker-Forbes assay for progesterone is able to detect the *activity* evoked by as little as 0.0002 μg. of progesterone. Unfortunately, large amounts of estrogen in the sample inhibit the reaction but small amounts increase the sensitivity to progesterone. The Hooker-Forbes assay has not been employed extensively and is not available to most clinicians.

All factors considered, the measurement of pregnanediol in urine is still the only practical test for determining progestational activity. But several determinations during the luteal phase of the cycle are mandatory. Urine is usually collected in pools for 2 or 3 days in order to avoid the marked day to day variations. Levels up to 2 mg. per 24 hours are found before ovulation but during the luteal phase of the cycle extreme variations occur. It would be necessary to have almost daily assays to evaluate corpus luteum function properly.

Blood levels of progesterone are still difficult to measure accurately. Woolever found plasma progesterone to vary between zero and 0.53 μg. per 100 ml. of blood during the follicular phase of the cycle and between 0.6 and 2.1 μg. per 100 ml. during the luteal phase (see Fig. 5–11). Production rates may, in the future, be the most accurate method of assessing progestational activity. Dominquez and associates calculated the secretion rate of progesterone as 2.3 to 5.4 mg. per day during the follicular phase and between 22 and 43 mg. during the luteal phase. In ovariectomized females, Little found a production rate of 1.3 mg. per day.

During early pregnancy the problem of establishing normal values has been even more complex. Shearman found a mean excretion of 6.2 mg./day of pregnanediol in urine during the seventh week of pregnancy, rising to 8.2 mg./day during the tenth week. In a study by Robertson and Maxwell, citing 12 patients with threatened abortion, there seemed to be no value in the level of pregnanediol which could predict the outcome of pregnancy, even though eight aborted and four did not. Cox and associates consider a pregnanediol level below 2.9 mg./day to indicate severe deficiency before the eleventh week of pregnancy. In a study of 74 patients with recurrent abortions, Klopper and MacNaughton concluded that a *reduction in hormone production is the effect, rather than the cause, of abortion.*

Plasma progesterone levels during early pregnancy are the equivalent of those found during the luteal phase of the cycle. After the ninth or tenth week of gestation levels begin to rise. Progesterone in uterine venous blood has been found to be 10 times as high as that in the peripheral circulation.

The production rate of progesterone during pregnancy has been calculated at 92 mg./day at 15 weeks, 263 mg./day at 27–31 weeks and 322 mg./day during the third trimester. Dignam has commented that the methods used in these studies may be criticized because precursors other than progesterone may contribute to pregnanediol and thus invalidate the measurement of the production rate.

For a complete review of the problem of progesterone assay methods, the reader is referred to the chapter by Dignam in *Progress in Infertility.* He has concluded: "Hormonal studies have not in general been of value in predicting which pregnant patients might benefit from progestational therapy. Indeed, no one has been able to show convincingly that such therapy improves the situation. Rather, a number of careful reports fail to show any benefit from it."

FORMATION OF ESTROGENS

Estrogens can be readily formed from androstenedione or testosterone via a several-step aromatization reaction which occurs in the microsomal fraction of the cell. The placenta is the most active tissue in this regard, but the reaction also occurs in the adrenal, testis, follicle, granulosa cell, theca, corpus luteum, ovarian stroma, and hilus (Fig. 13–13). There are several pathways possible. Estradiol appears to be derived from testosterone and estrone from androstenedione; although once formed, estradiol and estrone are interconvertible via a soluble steroid dehydrogenase present in many tissues of the body. Estriol may be formed in the ovary or as a peripheral metabolite in the liver and will be considered in the discussion of metabolism of ovarian hormones.

There are three major, naturally occurring estrogens in the human female. They are derived from the basic sterid estrane and are known as estrone, estradiol and estriol. The *one* ending signifies the presence of a single ketone on the molecule at the 17 position, whereas the *diol* ending indicates the presence of two hydroxy groups, one at position 3 and one at position 17. The suffix *triol* indicates the presence of three hydroxy groups at positions 3, 16 and 17. As the degree of oxidation of the molecule increases, the physiologic activity of the compound decreases; thus estradiol is most active, estriol is least active (see Fig. 13–14).

The original experiments of Allen and Doisy showed conclusively that the ovarian follicles and the follicular liquor of the sow were the sources of a hormone that could induce the estrus pattern in the ovariectomized rat that was consistent with that of the intact rat. Because it was thought that the follicular hormone was responsible for the state of estrus, the hormone was named estrogen (from the Greek *oistros*—mad desire, plus *gennan*—to produce).

It has been demonstrated that the follicular fluid contains a wide variety of steroids, that the cells of the follicle can synthesize hormones in vitro, and that stimulation with exogenous gonadotropins produces increase in follicular size and increased production of hormones. The follicular phase of the cycle can be correlated with increased levels of estrogens in urine and during menopause the marked decline in urinary estrogens can be correlated with the absence of follicles. Although the follicle normally produces progesterone, androgens and estrogens, its major secretory product appears to be estradiol. The relative contribution of the granulosa and theca cells within the follicle and the validity of the two-cell theory in endocrine control mechanisms remain to be worked out.

During the last 5 years particular attention has been given to the *production* and *secretion* rates of estrogen rather than a simple quantitation of estrogens in urine or blood. The investigations of Tait, Gurpide and associates, and Barlow have provided clinicians with relatively rapid methods of determining production and secretion rates of estrogen. Utilizing newer techniques, secretion rates for estrogen have been reported in the range of 200–500 *micrograms* (µg.) per day at the ovulatory peak, 60–200 µg. per day during the follicular phase and 150–300 µg. per day during the luteal phase. By comparison, the production rate of progesterone has been estimated at 4 *milligrams* (mg.) during the follicular phase and 30 mg. per day

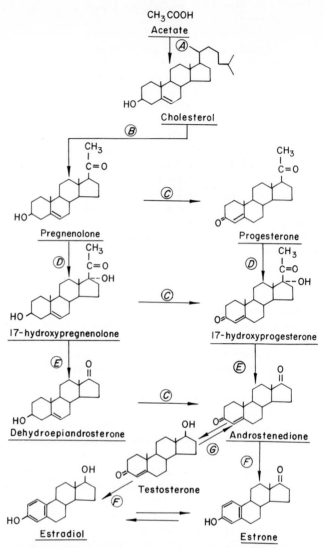

Fig. 13–13.—Possible metabolic pathways for the ovarian biogenesis of estrogens. Letters above arrows denote the following metabolic pathways and the enzyme systems involved:**A,** formation of the sterol nucleus; **B,** cleavage of cholesterol side chain with formation of C-21 steroid; **C,** isomerase reaction with changing of double bond from C-5 to C-4, and dehydrogenation at C-3; 3β-ol dehydrogenases; **D,** 17α-hydroxylation, i.e., introduction of hydroxy radical in alpha position on C-17; **E,** cleavage of side chain, converting C-21 to C-19 steroids; **F,** aromatization, i.e., introduction of double bonds into ring A with conversion of C-19 to C-18 steroids; **G,** 17β-ol dehydrogenase reactions (reversible), i.e., conversion of hydroxy radical in beta position on C-17 to ketone group, or vice versa. (From Smith, O. W., and Ryan, K. J.: Am. J. Obst. & Gynec. 84:141, 1962.)

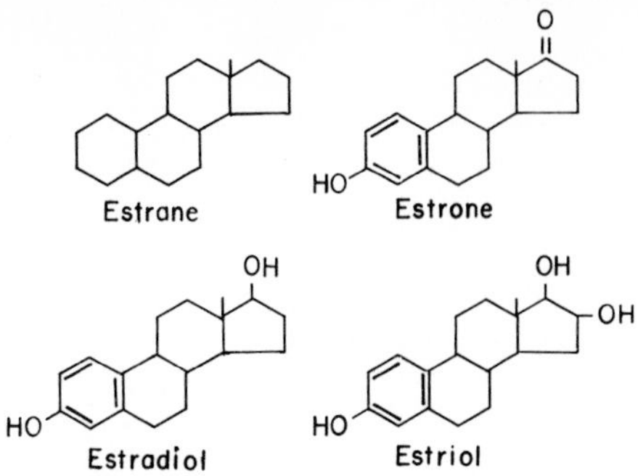

Fig. 13-14.—Structural formulas of the three naturally occurring estrogens, together with the basic steroid nucleus, estrane.

during the luteal phase. The ovary apparently secretes progesterone throughout the cycle and studies made before and after oophorectomy indicate that the contribution of the adrenal is minimal. The production rate of androstenedione is estimated at 3.4 mg. per day, no significant change being noted during the ovarian cycle. Blood levels of androstenedione in the female vary between 0.130 and 0.145 μg. per 100 ml., twice the adult male levels. The production rate of testosterone in women varies from 0.4 to 1.7 mg. per day.

Metabolism of Estrogens.—Because estrogens are usually secreted in such small amounts during the nonpregnant state, assay of their metabolites has been most difficult. The time-honored and well-worn scheme, known by every medical student, was that of estradiol→estrone→estriol. During recent years, however, a fantastic, almost geometric, increase in the number of estrogen metabolites has appeared. Four epimeric estriols and several epimeric ketols are known to contribute to the estrogen pool. Furthermore, estrogens may be hydroxylated at positions 2, 6, 11 and 15, and the two hydroxyl compounds may form methoxy derivatives. If these are multiplied by the three classic estrogens, there is an almost infinite variety of metabolites to be considered, most of them not measured by the conventional urinary assays. Although most of these reactions occur in the liver, estradiol → estrone interconversion and hydroxylation can occur in other tissues.

In most instances ovarian steroids are metabolized to biologically less active substances and the reactions are considered catabolic and detoxifying. Whether estrogen is metabolized while exerting a biologic function has not been established.

How does estrogen exert its specific effects? Experiments by Jensen and Jacobson utilizing tritium labeling of estrogenic steroids, indicated that the uterus, vagina, and pituitary preferentially bound estrogenic hormones such as 17β-estradiol. Other tissues such as liver and muscle did not show such binding but showed concentrations of estrogen proportional to the concentration of this hormone in the blood. These experiments, now confirmed, suggest that the uterus has a limited number of specific binding sites which, at high levels of estrogen, may become saturated.

Several investigators have reported that these receptor sites were quite specific and bound only active estrogens such as 17β-estradiol, hexestrol, and diethylstilbesterol. The receptors did not bind testosterone, cortisol or progesterone. Surprisingly, 17α-estradiol, a weak estrogen, was bound only to a limited extent. Other studies have shown that ethinyl estradiol and norethynodrel (the progestin in Enovid) compete for the same receptor sites as 17β-estradiol.

The bound estrogens are released by proteolytic enzymes but not by nucleases which, together with other evidence, strongly suggest that the receptors are protein, a large protein of about 200,000 molecular weight.

One concept of the action of bound estrogen involves histamine release from uterine cells which, in turn, affects the vasculature of the uterus. Villee, Hagerman and Joel have proposed that a key enzyme, pyridine nucleotide transhydrogenase, is thus activated and accounts for the primary action of estrogen. Talawar and associates have suggested that estrogen increases all ribonucleic acid (RNA) synthesis by inhibiting the action of a protein which suppresses RNA synthesis. Gorski believes that the estrogen receptor is a protein which in some manner influences the synthesis of one, or at most, a few proteins. In any case, it seems likely that the synthesis of RNA and protein are part of the total tissue response to estrogens (and androgens) with little or no information being available concerning progesterone.

Estrogens seem to be metabolized quite rapidly in the human female unless they are esterified, in which case their action may be decidedly prolonged. Approximately 6–10 per cent of injected estrone can be recovered in the urine and feces of the human female, whereas up to 15–30 per cent may be recovered from the injection of estriol. Fecal estrogens have been detected and seem to be derived from the biliary system and in part from direct excretion into the intestines. It has been shown that neither the ovary nor any part of the reproductive system is necessary for the metabolism of estrogens. The inability to recover 100 per cent of the injected estrogen may be due to storage in fat depots independent of the reproductive tract, to an inability to measure completely all the metabolites of the estrogens or to the conversion to certain metabolites that may not be detected by present methods. Estrogens in urine are present in the form of water-soluble glucuronic and sulfuric acid conjugates. There is evidence to indicate that the liver is an important organ in the inactivation of estrogenic substances. This is borne out clinically by the demonstration of a so-called hyperestrin state in patients with cirrhosis, infectious hepatitis and chronic liver disease. Certain experiments indicate that the liver eliminates estrogens from the circulation rather than inactivating them. Therefore, the estrogens may be removed by the liver and excreted into the biliary tract and subsequently into the feces. Inactivation of estrogenic hormones has also been described in the state of inanition as well as in a state of vitamin B complex deficiency.

Measurement of Estrogens

Whereas the concentrations of most other important steroid hormones are measured in milligram quantities, estrogens are present in *microgram* amounts, except during pregnancy. The human female usually synthesizes between 80 and 200 μg. of estrogen per day, with cyclic variations in estrogen production related to the phase of the menstrual cycle. Luteal phase levels are higher than those of the follicular phase and there is an ovulatory peak which usually exceeds 200 μg. per day. The endogenous production rate figures for estrogen are among the lowest for the known steroid hormones and this low production rate is reflected in the low titer in urine and blood.

Prior to 1953 only three estrogens, estrone, estradiol-17β, and estriol were known. During the past 15 years advances in assay technology have disclosed some 20 estrogens. Methods have been described for the measurement of blood or plasma estrogens but the techniques are not sufficiently sensitive or accurate to measure reliably the low levels of circulating estrogens, except during pregnancy. One exception to this is the isotopic method of Svendsen which measures estrone and estradiol with percentage recoveries of about 65 per cent. The method is sensitive and can measure as little as 5 μg. estrone or estradiol per 100 ml. of plasma. A similar isotopic method has been described by Ichii which is even more sensitive, detecting 2 μg. of estrone or estradiol per 100 ml. of plasma.

The chemical methods for the estimation of the classic estrogens in urine are divided into 3 main groups: (a) colorimetric (b) fluorimetric (c) gas chromatographic. Isotopic methods and techniques depending on thin layer chromatography have also been proposed but have been employed on a very limited scale in clinical practice.

There is no doubt that a rapid estrogen assay method is necessary for the practitioner who specializes in infertility and endocrinologic aspects of gynecology. Barlow has commented on this problem as follows:

"Urinary estrogen methods have reached a high degree of sensitivity and specificity, but for clinical usage the practicality of some of them is limited. Using the method developed in our laboratory we are able to measure urinary estrogen excretion accurately down to 0.2 μg. per day for each of the three classic estrogens. The purity of the isolated urinary estrogens is such that the same method is also suited to the determination of secretion and production rates. This method is more time consuming, and therefore less practical, than Brown's for determining estrogens in a large number of specimens. The Brown method is not accurate enough for very low titer urines nor is it suitable for the determination of secretion and production rates. The methods of Preedy and Siiteri achieve the degree of purification required for secretion and production rate determinations but they are more tedious than is our method, without any increase in specificity or sensitivity. Of these methods, Brown's would be the only available chemical assay having the practical convenience required for clinical application on a large scale."

Because of increased clinical demand for a "rapid" estrogen assay several shortened chemical methods have been introduced in which only estrone or estriol is measured. Estrone methods may prove to give a usable index of total estrogen excretion, but as yet there has not been enough experience with them. One such determination could be misleading since the proportion of estrone relative to estradiol-17β, and particularly to estriol, can vary quite widely. At present, such shortened methods may reasonably be applied only when doing serial measurements, as during a course of human gonadotropin treatment (mentioned below). Shortened methods which measure only estriol are not as sensitive as the estrone methods and are best applied in pregnancy since abnormalities of pregnancy are primarily reflected in the estriol levels.

Since the diagnostic usefulness of estrogen assay in the infertility work-up is quite limited and such assay will rarely be required, it would seem important only to have a reliable assay. Whether a chemical or a biologic one would be more reliable under these limited circumstances depends almost entirely on the laboratory facilities and the experience of the personnel doing the measurements. If the laboratory has had extensive experience in bioassay techniques, a biologic method of estrogen measurement should be chosen. If the laboratory has not had a great deal of experience with bioassays, a chemical method would probably be better.

For research purposes there can be little argument with the preference for chemical estrogen methods because of their greater accuracy and reproducibility. Of those available, Brown's is the most practical, and it is applicable to most of the problems found in infertility and clinical research. If, however, the research is to be carried out on patients with low estrogen titers, or if endogenous estrogen production and secretion rates are to be measured, Brown's method is not adequate. In the latter situations Barlow's method or that of Preedy or Siiteri should be used.

Estrogen Therapy

The clinical application of estrogenic substances is predicated on the fact that this hormone has the unique potential of stimulating growth and maintaining the functional adequacy of the genital system in the female. In addition, it acts as a regulator of pituitary gonadotropic secretion and exerts a controlling influence on specific metabolic processes. Thus, the stimulus of estrogen is of prime necessity in the growth of the endometrium and uterus. The ribonucleoprotein and alkaline phosphatase content of the endometrium increases during the proliferative phase of the cycle as a direct effect of estrogen. Proliferation and desquamation of the vaginal epithelium is similarly controlled by this steroid substance, as is the deposition of glycogen in the vaginal epithelial cells. As a result of the development of the vaginal epithelium and the deposition of glycogen, the acidity of the vaginal secretions is maintained. Estrogen also produces growth and proliferation of the endocervical glands with resultant secretion of a thin, watery, mucoid substance necessary for sperm migration through the cervix into the uterus. The epithelium of the oviduct is markedly changed as a result of estrogen stimulation; there is an increase in height with growth and prominence of the ciliated cells as well as enlargement of the secretory cells. Further, there is evidence to indicate that estrogens may have a direct effect on the ovary which may be an increase in the sensitivity of that organ to the action of LH.

Besides the effect of estrogenic substances on the genital tract, important actions on extragenital organs have been described. Estrogen is known to be the major stimulant of epithelial growth in the mammary gland. Its administration to immature or castrated animals in which the mammary gland is still rudimentary causes the epithelium to proliferate and form a duct system with glands identical to those of normal mature animals. The continued administration of large doses of estrogenic substances to normal animals results in epithelial proliferation of various types in the mammary glands, depending on the species or the particular strain of animal utilized. The use of estrogenic substances in both male and female human subjects has provided abundant evidence to confirm the stimulative effect on the mammary epithelium of animals. Exogenous estrogen induces mammary epithelial growth in human female castrates and occasionally results in mastodynia. Bilateral oophorectomy in ovulating females uniformly results in relief of mastodynia associated with cystic disease and in diminution in the size of breast masses. The morphologic pattern of chronic cystic mastitis has never been reported in human or animal experimentation in the absence of estrogen stimulation. Conversely, chronic cystic mastitis has been produced in both human subjects and animals by excessive, prolonged administration of estrogenic substances.

In addition to their effect on the mammary epithelium, estrogens cause increased pigmentation of the mammary areolae. Other effects include increased proliferation of buccal and gingival membranes, inhibition of linear bone growth and acceleration of epiphyseal closure. Whereas progesterone is a natruretic and chloruretic agent, estrogens cause moderate retention of sodium chloride and water. In addition, estrogens are recognized as protein anabolic agents with resultant retention of nitrogen, calcium and phosphorus.

Estrogens impart the "female contour," being responsible for fat deposition in the hips and buttocks, at one time the much sought-after hour-glass figure. Pubic and axillary hair growth occur only in the presence of adequate endogenous estrogen, tempered by adrenal androgen. For example, in the patient with gonadal dysgenesis (Turner's syndrome), karyotype XO, estrogen insufficiency is obvious and pubic and axillary hair is sparse—adrenal androgen here is apparently normal. In the patient with testicular feminization, estrogen is present in normal amounts as evidenced by the feminine body contour and breast development. But the gonad in this condition produces both androgen and estrogen. Since there is a defect in end-organ "appreciation" of androgen, neither pubic nor axillary hair develops.

In addition to the many effects estrogen has on specific end organs and its extra-genital, metabolic properties, its ability to stimulate or suppress the hypothalamus and the subsequent release or inhibition of gonadotropic hormones is perhaps its most important contribution to the maintenance of the ovarian cycle. An oversimplification of the available data indicates that small amounts of estrogen stimulate the hypothalamus to release its specific neuro-hormones whereas large amounts suppress both FSH and LH releasing factors.

Fifteen separate estrogenic steroids have been listed as occurring in the human female. They are estradiol-17-beta, estrone, estriol, 2-methoxyestrone, 18-hydroxyestrone, 6-hydroxyestrone, 16-epiestriol, 2-methoxyestriol, 16-oxoestradiol-17-beta, 16-oxoestrone, 16-alpha-hydroxyestrone, 16-beta-hydroxyestrone, 11-beta-hydroxyestradiol-17-beta, equilenin and estranediol. In regard to therapy in the human female, both naturally occurring and synthetic estrogens are available. We have used both varieties and feel there are specific instances in which one may be superior to another. We have utilized either ethinyl estradiol (Estinyl) or sodium estrone sulfate (Premarin) for most indications. Both of these preparations are orally active, water-soluble estrogens which provide the physiologic and metabolic benefits of natural estrogens. When a long-acting estrogen is desirable we have used estradiol valerate (Delestrogen), prepared from the naturally occurring follicular hormone. This compound is formulated in sesame oil and has a potent and prolonged estrogenic action that lasts approximately two to three weeks after a single intramuscular injection. The synthetic estrogens diethylstilbestrol, chlorotrianisene (Tace) and methallenestril (Vallestril) have been used with success in specific disorders which will be considered in this chapter. (See Fig. 13–15.) In general, the side effects of nausea and other gastrointestinal complaints are more common with the synthetic estrogenic preparations. Chlorotrianisene is a unique preparation in that it is stored in the body fat and is released gradually to provide a smooth, long-lasting response. Unlike other estrogens, chlorotrianisene does not cause pituitary enlargement and causes only minimum adrenal hyperplasia in laboratory test animals.

Although the beneficial effects of estrogenic substances are well known, the fear of malignancy being caused or aggravated by these substances has always worried and disturbed the physician. This unfounded fear has been passed on by many physicians to their patients so that the impression of "hormones" causing cancer is widespread. There is no doubt that the hormones, particularly estrogens, are potent growth-promoting agents. However, there are no data which definitely implicate estrogens in the development of cancer of any organ in the human female. If this correlation did exist, particularly in relationship to the development of mammary carcinoma, the incidence of this disease should have greatly increased during the past three decades. No such increase has been noted, nor has there been a trend to such a change. In genetically susceptible patients it may be assumed that estrogens might be an adjunctive influence in the development of carcinoma of the breast or endometrium, but even proof of this is lacking. It is far less hazardous to employ estrogenic agents intelligently and according to direction than to permit the human female to undergo specific degenerative processes which in themselves may cause premature death.

One of the major indications for the use of estrogens, and also one of the most rewarding uses from the viewpoint of the patient, is gonadal dysgenesis or Turner's syndrome. As noted in Chapter 16, the major difficulties

Fig. 13–15.—Synthetic estrogenic substances.

Hexestrol

Benzestrol

Diethylstilbestrol

Dienestrol

Triphenylethylene

Tri-para-anisylchloroethylene

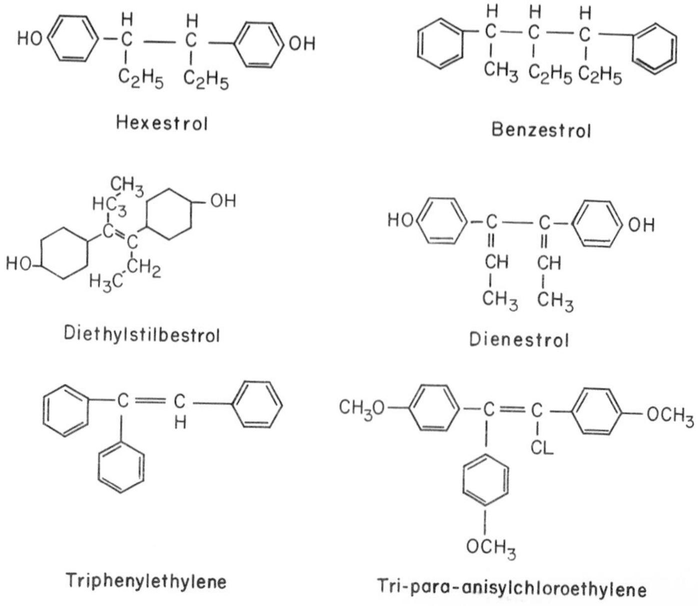

noted by the patient in Turner's syndrome are short stature and failure of sexual development. Since the ovaries are rudimentary, they cannot be stimulated to follicular development or ovulation. Therefore, substitutional therapy is employed. The short stature, being a genetic defect, is not the result of an insufficiency of estrogen and therefore cannot be obviated. However, estrogen should not be employed until linear growth has ceased. Administration before closure of the epiphyses may actually hasten this process and result in diminished stature.

Several regimens of therapy may be utilized. Premarin, 2.5–3.75 mg., may be given orally for 20 consecutive days followed by a 10-day rest period. Withdrawal bleeding will usually occur within two to three days after the cessation of the estrogen. Estinyl, 0.05 mg. twice daily, may be given in a similar manner. Diethylstilbestrol may be given in a dose of 1 mg. daily for 20 days followed by 10 days without therapy. Recently we have used one of the sequential estrogen-progestin oral contraceptive agents in the treatment of patients with gonadal dysgenesis. The *sequence* of estrogen and progestin seems to provide a sharper and more normal menstrual-like flow and prevents the development of endometrial hyperplasia.

The administration of estrogen to these individuals is extremely important, not only for the bleeding it produces, but for the extragenital effects as well. Thus a normal maturation, similar to that of normal pubescence, of primary and secondary sexual organs occurs. Breast development is stimulated, the skin turgor is improved, pubic and axillary hair increase in amount, the vaginal epithelium thickens and the vagina develops to a point which permits normal sexual intercourse. In addition to these direct effects, estrogen therapy prevents premature aging and forestalls the development of osteoporosis and atherosclerosis.

Estrogenic substances have been employed for years in the treatment of gonorrheal vaginitis in children. The thin mucosa of the vagina in the prepubescent female was the cause of the susceptibility of the vagina to invasion by the gonococcus. However, at present, most of the strains of gonococci encountered are susceptible to one of several antibiotics: penicillin, streptomycin, chlortetracycline, oxytetracycline and carbomycin. Treatment with one of these agents over four to five days will usually result in cure. However, in certain patients who are sensitive to these agents, estrogens may be given orally for a period of 20 days. It is desirable that uterine bleeding be avoided and therapy be kept at a minimum so that breast development will not occur and epiphyseal closure will not be hastened.

Estrogen therapy has been utilized in the prepubescent female in an effort to prevent abnormal tallness which might be expected on the basis of a familial trait. The rationale of therapy is based on the fact that estrogens effect premature closure of the epiphyses of long bones and prevent abnormal linear growth. This method of therapy has not been associated with uniform success. A similar situation exists in the prepubescent male in whom androgens are used intentionally to close the epiphyses prematurely. To achieve such an effect in the male, androgenic steroids must be administered in unusually high doses and must be combined with estrogens. In certain instances of short stature in the prepubescent female, estrogens have been administered with the hope that an increase in the growth increment could be obtained before epiphyseal closure. The results of this therapeutic approach have been disappointing.

The uses of estrogens in obstetrics are relatively few. They have been used rather extensively in both threatened and habitual abortion as well as for completion of a "missed" abortion. No statistical evidence is available at present to indicate that either progestational agents or estrogens influence favorably the outcome of pregnancy after regular uterine cramps and bleeding have been established. Further, caution must be exerted to avoid converting an inevitable abortion into a "missed" one by the administration of these agents. Similarly, because of the multiplicity of uncontrolled factors in the maintenance of pregnancy in the human female, it cannot be stated categorically that exogenous estrogens or progestins have improved the salvage rate in patients classified as habitual aborters. Ideally, the treatment of the habitual aborter should begin during the preconceptional period and the reader is referred to Chapter 10 for specific therapeutic regimens.

Despite several reports in the literature indicating the effectiveness of estrogens in facilitating uterine contractility in patients with a missed abortion, present evidence tends to negate this observation. Similarly, there is no evidence that estrogenic substances are capable of inducing therapeutic or criminal abortion.

Estrogens have been used for 25 years to inhibit postpartum lactation and prevent breast engorgement. Use of oral preparations was started on the day following delivery and continued for 10–15 days in a variation of dosage. Breast congestion was noted to follow the early discontinuance of these substances. In many cases the cessation of estrogen therapy was followed by withdrawal uterine bleeding which occasionally was excessive. It is now believed that the oral administration of estrogenic substances cannot compensate rapidly for the sudden depletion of estrogens from the blood stream which occurs during the first few hours post partum. For this reason, most recent reports indicate the superiority of the long-acting estrogenic agents or combinations of estrogen and androgen. Favorable results have been obtained by the use of estradiol valerate (Delestrogen) or a combination of estradiol valerate with testosterone enanthate (Deladumone). Most investigators utilizing these preparations have varied the time of injection, but all give it either during labor or immediately post partum. Apparently, in order to obtain the best subjective results without rebound phenomena, the injection should be given within the first five minutes after the delivery of the placenta.

Dysfunctional uterine bleeding is a term used to describe conditions of abnormal bleeding in which organic lesions of the female genital tract or systemic disease cannot be demonstrated. It occurs most commonly during the initiation and decline of ovarian function and thus is commonly seen during the mid- and late teens. The abnormal bleeding results from an imbalance of various endocrines rather than a deficiency of pituitary or ovarian hormones per se. The commonest cause in this age group is delayed ovulation. As a result, the endometrium is stimulated by constant, although irregular levels of estrogen and endometrial biopsy shows a proliferation or hyperplastic effect.

When hemorrhage from the uterus is of functional origin, oral estrogen therapy in the range of 7.5–12.5 mg. of Premarin a day is usually capable of producing hemostasis within three to five days. Estrogen is the growth hormone of the endometrium and therefore is able to induce a new phase of endometrial growth with proliferation of glands and stroma bringing about arrest of hemorrhage. Intravenous administration of Premarin has been suggested for the rapid correction of uterine hemorrhage, the suggested dosage being 20 mg. and the arrest of bleeding usually occurring within eight hours. We have not had uniform success in treating hemorrhage of this kind with intravenous Premarin but have relied on the use of combined estrogen-progestin preparations as outlined in the subsequent paragraphs.

After the acute hemorrhagic episode has been controlled, withdrawal bleeding will usually occur within three to five days after discontinuing estrogen therapy. The control of subsequent bleeding is brought about by employing a schedule of cyclic estrogen-progestin therapy. Cycles of this variety are usually repeated for six consecutive months, following which they are discontinued. In the majority of patients a return to normal ovulatory function occurs if no other permanent cause of ovulatory suppression is present.

Estrogens have been successfully employed in the treatment of primary dysmenorrhea. Although not a curative plan of therapy, complete relief from pain results in almost all patients. Two regimens may be utilized: 3.75 mg. of Premarin orally daily for 20 days, beginning on the fifth day of the menstrual flow; or Estinyl, 0.05 mg. twice daily, given in the same manner. Either one of these estrogens will suppress ovulation, and cycles of this kind may be kept up for six months. Following this, the patient is allowed to ovulate and menstruate spontaneously for one to three months and then treatment is restarted.

The use of estrogens for the treatment of endometriosis is described in detail in Chapter 8.

Estrogens have not been used primarily for contraception but it is a fact that, by their ability to inhibit ovulation, they are effective for this specific indication. While estrogens are effective and may be used for short-term therapy, their use for long periods is contraindicated on the basis of stimulation of the epithelium of the breast and of the endometrium. In order to limit the incidence of "break-through" bleeding with the various medications now available for oral contraceptive use, an estrogen has been added to each. (See Chapter 15.)

The induction of ovulation by the use of estrogenic substances has not been uniformly successful. Although there is abundant evidence in animals to indicate that estrogen stimulates or facilitates the release of luteinizing hormone from the pituitary, this has not been reproducible in the human female. The method of action is probably mediated through the hypothalamus. Several clinical experiments utilizing estrogens more or less duplicated the animal experiments but did not result in ovulation. Brown, Bradberry and Jungck gave stilbestrol to patients during the fifth to eighth days of the cycle and found a rise in gonadotropin titers. Funnel described a rise in urinary LH in menopausal women following the administration of estrogen, and the observations of Albert indicated that, whereas all doses of estrogen caused an increase in gonadotropin excretion, large doses caused a diminution. Kupperman reported induction of ovulation by the intravenous administration of conjugated estrogens in a specific group of patients.

Estrogenic substances have also been used in the specific deficiency of cervical mucus in the infertile patient. During the normal ovulatory cycle at the acme of estrogen secretion the cervical mucus becomes watery-clear and permits entry and migration of spermatozoa. In patients who have a deficiency of cervical mucus, as evidenced by a poor response to the fern test, small doses of estrogen may be given for a week or 10 days prior to the time of ovulation in order to improve the physical characteristics of cervical mucus.

Estrogens have been suggested as specific therapy in patients who are infertile because of deficient endometrial development during the luteal phase of the cycle. The cause may be inadequate estrogen secretion by the follicle or deficient secretion of both estrogen and progesterone by the corpus luteum. In patients of this type, I have primed the endometrium for three months using one of the sequential oral contraceptives. Following this, I have utilized small doses of estrogen during the proliferative phase of the cycle, e.g., ethinyl estradiol 0.02 mg. followed by an estrogen-progestin combination such as Provest for 7 to 10 days following ovulation.

A specific entity of sclerosis of the endometrium following curettage for incomplete abortion or hydatidiform mole has been described by Asherman. Traumatic intrauterine synechiae have developed in many of these patients so that, although ovulation occurs normally as determined by basal body temperature, bleeding is impossible. In some of these patients, estrogenic substances given in large dosage may cause a regeneration of the endometrium if the basalis has not been completely removed. The long acting preparation Delestrogen seems of particular value for this use since 20–40 mg. may be administered every two to three weeks for a minimum period of six months. Louros has recently suggested the use of a plastic intrauterine device to keep the walls of the uterine cavity from forming synechiae. In addition, a pseudopregnancy with estrogen and progestin or estrogen alone is given for six months.

Another major indication for the use of estrogenic substances occurs following bilateral oophorectomy performed during the childbearing period. This is particularly true in patients who have extensive endometriosis or pelvic inflammatory disease necessitating the complete removal of the internal genitalia during the third or fourth decade of life. All such patients should receive exogenous estrogen and it has been our routine to administer 5 mg. of Delestrogen on the day of surgery and to repeat this five to seven days later. The patient is then placed on a daily dose of either Estinyl, 0.05 mg. daily, or Premarin, 1.25 mg. daily, for at least one year. At the end of this time estrogen administration may be reduced to a similar dose three times weekly or even twice weekly depending on individual response. Estrogens may be given in this dosage indefinitely, or they may be discontinued temporarily and studies of endogenous estrogen production carried out. A simple vaginal smear test may indicate an adequate endogenous secretion of estrogen, presumably from the adrenals. In such patients exogenous estrogens are not necessary. In patients who are unable to produce sufficient endogenous estrogen and who have symptoms of estrogen deficiency, such as hot flashes and vasomotor instability, exogenous estrogens are again given.

Androgen Therapy

Androgens have been used therapeutically by the gynecologist for over 20 years, but unanimity of opinion regarding their use has not been forthcoming. Hamblen has condemned the indiscriminate use of androgens, and since the introduction of potent anabolic steroids without virilizing side effects, the use of androgenic substances for many indications has been greatly curtailed. Although androgens are found regularly in the human female organism, their precise physiologic role is unknown. These androgenic substances are the result of a process of metabolism of the steroids in the adrenal cortex. It is interesting to note, however, that growth of pubic hair in an occasional patient with ovarian dysgenesis will be obtained only if testosterone is added to estrogen.

Before discussing the specific therapeutic indications for the use of androgens, a consideration will be given to the effects of androgen therapy in the female and the side effects which occasionally limit or prohibit its use.

The important effects of androgen therapy in the female are based on inhibition or modification of the effects of estrogen on the usual target organs. In addition, androgenic substances have a decided effect on metabolic processes and the psyche of the individual. The major side effects are amenorrhea, acne, hypertrichosis and a deepening of the voice. The development and severity of these symptoms depend on the total amount of testosterone given. There is a wide range of variability in individuals, patients with a dark complexion and oily skin being much more susceptible to acne than patients with a light complexion and dry skin. The effects are also more likely to be seen if treatment with androgenic substances is prolonged and continuous than if higher doses are given intermittently or for just a short period.

Acne is one of the commonest side effects of the administration of androgens in the female. It is due to an excessive secretion of the sebaceous glands together with a proliferation of their epithelium. As a matter of fact, skin biopsy has been used as a method of assay for the potency of various androgenic substances. In addition to acne, hirsutism may occur, though usually it occurs at a later time and may in certain individuals be rather extensive. Usually the excessive hair growth begins on the face and gradually extends to the arms, legs and finally to the trunk. As with acne, there is a pronounced individual variation and a racial predisposition to the development of hirsutism.

Alopecia of the male type may follow prolonged therapy with androgens. It usually begins as a bilateral receding of the hair over the frontal bones but it may also be associated with a central balding over the occiput. After prolonged therapy the patient may also notice that the voice has become rough or husky. This is due to a hyperemia and thickening of the vocal cords and, unfortunately, is not always reversible after male hormone has been discontinued. Enlargement of the clitoris may occur following prolonged therapy and usually is due to an initial hyperemia. The patient may notice increased sensitivity in the clitoral area which causes a feeling of pressure and burning. If the dose reaches 300 mg. of testosterone per month and if treatment is prolonged, a permanent hypertrophy of the clitoris together with marked turgescence will occur. Finally, as a result of the antiestrogenic effect of the androgen, the breasts may show a diminution in size together with flaccidity.

Other side effects are quite variable and include both stimulation and depression of the central nervous system. In some patients a marked irritability or aggressiveness may be noted. Because of the retention of sodium and chloride, an increased amount of water will be held in the intracellular spaces, with a resultant weight gain. Since androgenic substances are protein anabolic agents the patient may note an additional weight gain due to natural muscle hypertrophy. Many of these side effects can be minimized by using androgens in intermittent fashion or in a dosage under a maximum of 300 mg. monthly. Many patients will use the same measures to control the side effects of androgen that they use when these symptoms occur spontaneously. Thus, the acne may be alleviated by the use of drying agents and sulfur preparations. A good depilatory cream or hydrogen-peroxide bleaching will prevent the unsightliness of excess hair growth. The use of cool compresses and hydrocortisone ointment will minimize clitoral turgescence. Beyond this, the patient should be instructed in a low-sodium diet in which excess calories are avoided. The use of a diuretic agent will aid in the elimination of salt and water.

De Watteville has suggested that androgens may be indicated for the following conditions: osteoporosis or general debility, psychic asthenia or mild depression, mild stress incontinence, menopausal syndrome, dyspareunia, frigidity, functional uterine bleeding, endometriosis, leiomyomata uteri, dysmenorrhea, premenstrual tension, suppression of lactation or postpartum congestion of the breasts, and generalized breast cancer. Many of these conditions can be adequately treated either with estrogenic substances or with the newer progestational steroids. The use of androgens together with estrogens in the treatment of osteoporosis is discussed in Chapter 14. While testosterone may have a definite place in the treatment of the psychic asthenia and mild depression of premenopausal and menopausal women, the use of the newer anabolic steroids which do not have the side effects of virilization appear to be a superior choice at this time.

We have not used androgenic substances in the treatment of functional uterine bleeding, endometriosis, dysmenorrhea or premenstrual tension since the introduction of the newer progestational steroids and the potent diuretic agents. Furthermore, we have had success in estrogen treatment of mild stress incontinence associated with a moderate trigonitis in the premenopausal and menopausal female. The major indications for the use of androgens are the menopausal syndrome in a specific group of patients, dyspareunia in an occasional patient, frigidity, suppression of lactation, mastodynia and generalized breast cancer.

In a small but definite group of patients who have typical symptoms of a menopausal state and who had previously been treated for cancer of the breast or uterine corpus, androgenic substances may be successfully used. Similarly, in a postmenopausal patient, or even a premenopausal one whose uterus contains leiomyomas and who complains of vasomotor symptoms, the use of an androgenic substance is indicated. Such patients may be given 10 mg. of methyl testosterone daily for 20 days of each month. If such a dosage regimen is not deemed adequate, combined treatment of 5 mg. of methyl testosterone and 0.25 mg. of diethylstilbestrol may be substituted. Apparently the combined therapy holds some superiority over the use of androgen alone, due to the combination of synergistic and antagonistic effects. Complete relief from menopausal symptoms may be obtained with lower dosage of each of the components and in this way the undesirable side effects of each hormone are avoided. In patients complaining of dyspareunia due to an atrophic vaginitis, a combination of estrogen and androgen therapy may also be given. It has been shown that the atrophic vaginal epithelium is stimulated by testosterone alone, although this may be due to a conversion of testosterone to estrogen. The dosage just outlined may be used or injections of testosterone propionate (given intermittently during the month to total 250 mg.) may be substituted. Our own choice of therapy is a vaginal cream containing estrogen together with oral use of combined estrogen and androgen. Dyspareunia due to dryness and inflammation of the mucous membrane caused by the postmenopausal state is improved by this therapy.

In patients with postmenopausal frigidity the use of combined estrogen and androgen will produce a hyperemia of the vulva and clitoris, increasing the sensitivity of these organs and greatly improving the response of the female partner during coitus. This medication should be given intermittently and under close observation by the physician since nymphomania in postmenopausal women has been described with prolonged therapy of this type. Frigidity in younger women is most often due to psychic factors and not related to hormonal insufficiency. In these patients androgenic substances are of little therapeutic value.

Functional uterine bleeding has been treated for many years with variations of androgenic substances. The rationale for therapy was derived in part from the direct action of the male hormone and in part from the indirect antiestrogenic effect. The direct effect may be on the pituitary gland, with suppression of gonadotropic substances. This has been proved in animal experimentation and shown in postmenopausal women. Thus, the increased excretion of pituitary gonadotropins in urine in the postmenopausal woman has been shown to be significantly reduced or completely suppressed by treatment with androgens. Secondary ovarian stimulation is negated. However, to accomplish this gonadotropic suppression, large doses of testosterone propionate must be given. These must be of the order of 150 mg. or more each week throughout the entire cycle, and these amounts are, of course, sufficient to produce signs and symptoms of virilization in many women.

Testosterone may have a direct antiestrogenic effect on the target organ, particularly the breast and the endometrium. In this way, the proliferation induced by estrogens is inhibited by adequate amounts of androgen. In patients with recurrent dysfunctional uterine bleeding associated with an anovulatory process and a hyperplastic endometrium, doses of 500–1,000 mg. of testosterone per month will produce marked regressive changes in the endometrium. Hypermenorrhea may be diminished or, in some patients, amenorrhea may result. In certain patients with hypermenorrhea due to submucous leiomyomas, testosterone has proved of value. Although definite proof is lacking, it seems likely that testosterone has a direct effect on the development and function of the coiled arterioles of the endometrium.

Despite the efficacy of testosterone and other androgens in the treatment of dysfunctional uterine bleeding, we have preferred the newer synthetic progestins plus estrogen for this condition. The progestins simulate more closely the normal, rhythmic hormonal stimulation of the endometrium and, of more importance, do not have the undesirable side effects of virilization.

Endometriosis has long been an indication for the use of androgenic substances and remains so at the present time. Numerous case reports indicate that testosterone, even in low doses which do not inhibit ovulation, will provide symptomatic relief from pain and result in objective improvement. Since it is known that prolonged anovulation, whether brought about by estrogens or by combinations of estrogens and progestins, will ameliorate endometriosis, the improvement brought about by androgens is paradoxical. In the doses usually prescribed ovulation persists, and some patients have become pregnant while on androgen therapy. Although reports have been made of objective improvement and diminution in the size of adnexal masses, histologic proof of changes in endometriosis by androgens is lacking. As a matter of fact, Scott and Wharton observed no histologic changes in artificially induced endometriosis in the Rhesus monkey after treatment with testosterone for as long as 27 months.

We have preferred the progestational agents together with estrogens in the hormonal management of endometriosis. This is discussed in detail in Chapter 8.

As previously mentioned, the abnormal uterine bleeding associated with submucous leiomyomas is due to the abnormal endometrium overlying the tumor. The use of androgenic substances in the nonsurgical treatment of leiomyomas makes use of the fact that not only is the endometrium affected by large doses of androgens but effects have been demonstrated on the myometrium as well. The antiestrogenic effect of androgens probably inhibits further growth of leiomyomas, which undoubtedly are due to estrogen stimulation. It has previously been shown that the administration of testosterone to castrated guinea pigs will prevent the development of estrogen-induced leiomyomas in this test animal. In certain patients in whom surgery is not desirable for medical reasons, androgens may be indicated. It may be necessary to produce a moderate degree of virilism, but these symptoms may be minimized by measures previously outlined. In the younger patient, particularly when infertility is a problem, we prefer conservative therapy with myomectomy. The progestational steroids have not proved of particular value in the treatment of hypermenorrhea associated with submucous fibroids. Enovid, probably because of its estrogen content, will occasionally cause enlargement of leiomyomas. We have employed the most androgenic progestins as a temporizing procedure to minimize the hypermenorrhea, until the patient can be prepared for surgery.

Androgenic substances have been used advantageously in the treatment of mastodynia associated with extensive fibrocystic disease of the breast. In this disease process there is extensive, diffuse nodularity, usually in the upper outer quadrants of both breasts. The breasts are often large and occasionally pendulous and they may be extremely painful just before and during the menstrual periods. It is necessary to perform a meticulous examination of the breasts in such patients to be certain that a dominant lump is not present. If such a lump is present, it should be followed through at least one menstrual period to see if it is hormonally regulated. Many such "dominant" lumps will disappear if the patient is examined in the postmenstrual phase; if the lump remains, it must be excised in order to exclude the possibility of malignancy. We have not been in favor of aspiration of a cystic "dominant" lump since it may merely overlie a carcinoma or carcinoma may be present in the cyst wall and simple aspiration would not show tumor cells. After the disease process has been proved conclusively to be benign, hormonal agents may be used to secure relief from recurrent pain.

Several regimens of therapy are available, and choice of the proper one will depend on the degree of pain relief as opposed to the seriousness of undesirable side effects. Methyl testosterone may be given throughout the cycle in a dose of either 5 or 10 mg. daily; if acne occurs 10 mg. may be given every other day. Another method is to use the androgen only in the postovulatory phase, giving 10 mg. daily during the last two weeks of the menstrual cycle. The patient should be cautioned against the excessive use of salt during this time, and occasionally the addition of a diuretic agent is of extreme value. Several authors have suggested the use of testosterone propionate, giving 300–600 mg. in four separate doses during the cycle. The use of testosterone in this fashion may bring about rather remarkable relief and this relief may persist for several months beyond the time of discontinuance. Some patients, especially those with a dark complexion or moderate acne, will not tolerate testosterone in doses of this proportion. They may be treated with Norlutate, 5 mg. daily from day 5 through day 24 of the cycle. Norlutate, being the most androgenic of the available progestational agents, seems to be more effective than the others for this specific disease.

Progestational Therapy

Although the corpus luteum was first described almost 300 years ago by the Dutch anatomist, Regner de Graaf, widespread clinical application of its secretion, progesterone, has only recently become commonplace in the practice of obstetrics and gynecology. Fraenkel in 1910 had proved to the satisfaction of his doubting confreres that the fate of the embryo depended on the functional integrity of the corpus luteum; about the same time Ancel and Bouin demonstrated that the typical progestational changes in the endometrium were produced by the endocrine activity of this same structure. Since the treatment of recurrent abortion and dysfunctional uterine bleeding is still a major problem confronting the practitioner in 1970, these historical observations form the background for the therapeutic schemes outlined in this chapter.

After Corner and Allen isolated a crystalline hormone from the corpora lutea of sows in 1929, progress was rapid. The structural formula was soon determined and Wintersteiner produced the hormone from an inert steroid

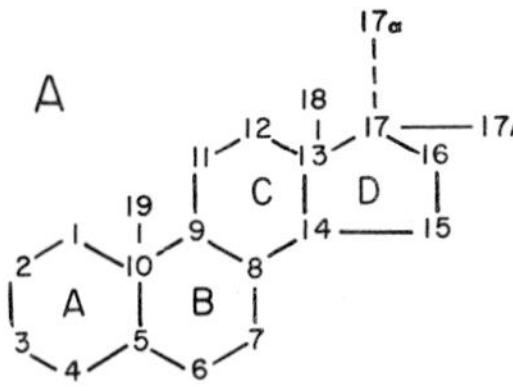

Fig. 13–16.—A, cyclopentanophenanthrene ring, showing numbering of carbons. B, comparative formulas of the naturally occurring steroids; left to right, progesterone, testosterone and estradiol 17-beta.

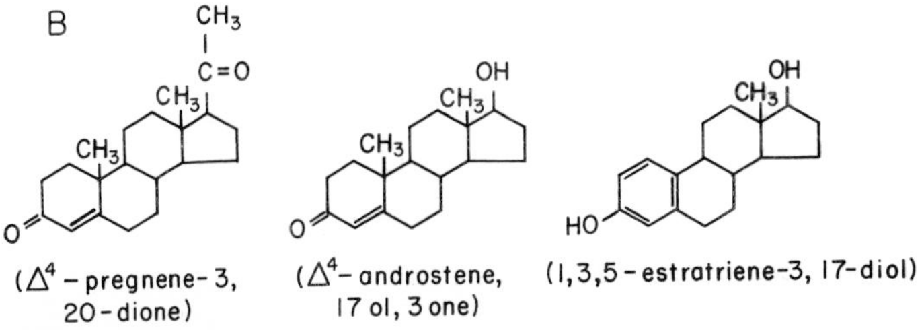

(Δ^4 – pregnene- 3, 20 - dione)   (Δ^4- androstene, 17 ol, 3 one)   (1,3,5 - estratriene-3, 17-diol)

of known composition in 1934. This hormone, called *progesterone* (from the Latin *pro*—in favor of, plus *gestatio*, from *gestare*—to bear), may be looked on biochemically as a "flat" molecule with an anterior surface, a posterior surface and a ketone (=O) group at each end. The progesterone nucleus (Fig. 13–16, *A*) is a saturated derivative composed of three six-membered carbon rings (*A, B, C*) and a five-membered ring (*D*): cyclopentanophenanthrene. Since the progestins to be discussed are substituted progesterones or variants of testosterone, it should be noted that substituents on the anterior surface of the molecule are referred to as "beta" positions whereas those on the posterior surface are designated "alpha" positions. Figure 13–16, *B*, shows the comparative formulas of the three naturally occurring steroids, progesterone, testosterone and estradiol.

Biologic Effect.—It is important to realize the wide spectrum of activity of progesterone since it (or one of the substituted progestins) may be selected for therapy on the basis of one or more of its specific effects. The actions of progesterone are, for the most part, not normally displayed until after estrogen has accomplished its growth effect on the reproductive tract and associated structures. Estrogens are concerned with growth; progesterone with differentiation. In the *vagina* most of the evidence suggests that the peak of vaginal cornification occurs at the time of ovulation. Progesterone causes a diminution of cornified cells and produces cellular clumping. *Cervical mucus* "ferning," a measure of estrogen effect, is negated by the action of progesterone. The *endometrial* changes brought about by progesterone are well known and consist of enlargement and differentiation of the stromal cells to form decidua, stromal edema and tortuous glands with prominent glycogen secretion either in the cells or gland lumina. The *myometrial* response to progesterone is less well understood; but recent work by Csapo indicates that progesterone does have a blocking action on the reactivity of isolated muscle strips to oxytocin and in the pregnant rabbit this appears to be an absolute block. It has also been shown that progesterone, when added to an organ bath in which an isolated uterine segment is suspended, produces an immediate depressant action on the tension developed by the myometrium in response to direct electrical stimulation. *Ovarian* function may be modified by progesterone since large doses, or constant secretion, inhibit LH and ovulation as well as restrict the development of follicles. In the *breasts,* progesterone acts on the initial growth stimulus of the estrogens and induces lobular-alveolar formation. Progesterone causes a rise in the *basal body temperature* of from 0.2 to 0.8 F. degrees during the luteal phase of the cycle which is maintained until the onset of menstruation. Reference to these various biologic effects will be made in comparing the "progestational" qualities of the newer, synthetic progestins.

The progestational agents used in the treatment of endometriosis have been discussed in Chapter 8. The progestational agents used in the latest oral contraceptives are discussed in Chapter 15. Each progestin is a potent steroid and must be used in accordance with recommended dosage and schedule. They are not a panacea for all gynecological disorders, but if used intelligently for specific indications they will give desirable results in most instances. Although these agents possess the same potential for the production of biological effects as progesterone, they have the advantages of increased potency when given orally and increased duration of effect when administered parenterally. Some are more androgenic than others and may cause acne and hirsutism. Thus, selection of a certain progestin for a specific indication is important for optimum benefit.

Proved Indications for the Use of Progestins

Dysfunctional Uterine Bleeding.—This term describes conditions of abnormal bleeding in which organic lesions or systemic disease cannot be demonstrated. The highest incidence is noted in the postmenarchal and premenopausal periods, that is, during the initiation and the decline of ovarian function. Normal menstrual cycles are characterized by proper balances between protein adenohypophyseal gonadotropins and steroid ovarian hormones. Dysfunctional bleeding probably results from an imbalance of these endocrines rather than a deficiency of pituitary or ovarian hormones per se. The endometrial growth pattern in this entity is often deficient in progesterone effect and usually shows a proliferative, hyperplastic or occasionally anaplastic effect. When excessive uterine bleeding is associated with histologically normal, secretory endometrium, the etiology is usually organic in nature.

Endocrine therapy, in order to be effective, must be based on an accurate diagnosis of the underlying hormonal defect. In practically all instances, this is possible if endometrial tissue is obtained at the proper time. An endometrial biopsy or curettage may be utilized, but the tissue obtained on the first day of bleeding is most informative in regard to subsequent therapy. The specific disorders and suggested therapeutic schemes follow.

Amenorrhea.—This is always a symptom and a search must be made for its etiology (see p. 567). Amenorrhea caused by systemic disease, ovarian failure or pituitary tumors cannot be expected to be corrected by substitution therapy with ovarian-like hormones. While diagnostic procedures are being performed, therapy may be instituted with progestins since the response may be most useful in diagnosis. For example, if bleeding occurs after the administration of progesterone, it may be concluded that (1) endogenous estrogen is being produced, (2) a responsive endometrium is present, (3) pituitary gonadotropic activity (FSH) is present and (4) the amenorrhea is not due to pregnancy. If bleeding does not occur after progesterone alone, it is necessary to prove the ability of the endometrium to respond by preliminary estrogen priming followed by progesterone. If artificial cycles are desired, therapy may be prescribed as outlined below and should be continued for at least three and preferably six months. Certain patients with secondary amenorrhea (postpartum type) may revert to a normal cycle after such therapy. There is no good evidence that the progestins cause ovulation in patients with primary amenorrhea.

The following regimens are suggested.

Diagnostic test: Progesterone, 50 mg. intramuscularly (bleeding will occur in two to six days)

Delalutin, 250 mg. intramuscularly (bleeding will occur in eight to 10 days)

Artificial cycles: Use any estrogen-progestin combination in 20–21 day cycles.

Hypomenorrhea.—Although not a frequent problem, most patients dislike scanty periods. Infertility or generalized metabolic disorders may coexist, and specific therapy for such entities should be instituted. This histologic pattern is usually one of "progestational immaturity" if the cycle is of the ovulatory type. Such patients may be treated with an estrogen-progestin combination, preferably containing 100 μg. of estrogen from the fifteenth to the twenty-fifth day and treatment should continue for three successive cycles. If the pattern is of the hypoplastic, anovulatory, inadequate, proliferative type, the estrogen-progestin combination should be given from day 5 to day 25. This will result in bleeding episodes of normal amount and duration.

HYPERMENORRHEA AND POLYMENORRHEA.—These terms are utilized to indicate excessive flow at the time of normally expected periods together with a shortened interval. The menstrual pattern is totally lacking in rhythm and is the type most commonly seen in "anovulatory bleeding." It occurs as a result of rises and falls in serum estrogen without the differentiating effect of progesterone and is seen frequently in patients in their late teens or early twenties who have never established regular ovulation. Since the endometrium may show varying degrees of hyperplasia and occasionally either in situ or invasive carcinoma, thorough curettage is mandatory before beginning substitutional therapy. Attempts should be made, of course, to find the cause of anovulation and correct it, but regulation of cycles and prevention of excessive bleeding may be accomplished even if exact etiologic factors are not discovered. This is believed to be of prophylactic importance because it has been shown that many patients with actual invasive endometrial carcinoma have had prolonged periods of estrogen stimulation proceeding through various phases of cystic and adenomatous endometrial hyperplasia, anaplasia, carcinoma in situ and finally carcinoma. If the patient is seen during an episode of profuse hemorrhage, the hemorrhage may be arrested by one of the following methods and then cyclic progesterone therapy prescribed.

Arrest of hemorrhage may be secured by giving an estrogen-progestin every 12 hours for four days. The patient should be cautioned that a withdrawal flow will occur two to four days after discontinuing the medication. Beginning on the fourth or fifth day of the withdrawal flow, the progestin is reinstituted in a dose of 5 or 10 mg. daily for 20 consecutive days.

If the endometrial biopsy has been of simple, proliferative type, artificial cycles should be continued for at least three months and these may have to be reinstituted as the need arises. If the biopsy has shown hyperplasia or anaplasia, it is deemed advisable by the author to utilize artificial cycles for nine months to one year and then to perform repeat diagnostic curettage.

HYPERMENORRHEA WITH NORMAL CYCLES.—When menstrual flow is excessive or prolonged, a submucous leiomyoma should always be suspected. However, if curettage performed at the time of bleeding reveals histologically normal *secretory* endometrium and organic disease is absent, the etiology of the hypermenorrhea becomes theoretical and is ascribed to "unstable endometrial vasculature." In any event, relief from this distressing problem may be obtained by using an estrogen-progestin combination preferably one containing an androgenic progestin, e.g., Ortho-Novum, Norlestrin, Norinyl, Ovral. These tend to produce very scanty flows even in women who have had previous hypermenorrhea.

If treatment is given only during the week or 10 days before the expected onset of menses, and therefore, without suppression of ovulation, benefit is unlikely to occur. If these methods are not successful, careful search for other causes of excessive bleeding should be assiduously undertaken. Leiomyomas, abnormal pregnancy, polyps, endometritis, adenomyosis or endometriosis may be missed on the first examination but re-evaluation will frequently lead to their discovery.

PREMENSTRUAL STAINING.—Although this entity may be caused by endometrial or endocervical polyps, and rarely by vaginal endometriosis, it is most commonly due to progesterone insufficiency during the latter part of the luteal phase. If an endometrial biopsy done at the time of staining indicates "progestationally immature endometrium," treatment may be instituted utilizing an estrogen-progestin daily from day 18 through day 24, repeated for three consecutive cycles.

Primary Dysmenorrhea.—This common disorder of young females is associated with ovulatory menstrual cycles since relief may be obtained in almost all patients by suppression of ovulation with various steroids. In the past, this has been accomplished with estrogenic substances. The pathophysiology of primary dysmenorrhea is unknown but is believed to be associated with tissue anoxia, sloughing of endometrium and uterine muscle hypermotility. The administration of any estrogen-progestin combination which suppresses ovulation will alleviate menstrual cramps in about 80–90 per cent of patients. This is an unusual finding since, in the past, the addition of progesterone in the last half of an estrogen-induced artificial cycle usually resulted in severe dysmenorrhea. Administration of the newer progestins *throughout* the cycle may affect the sloughing process and myometrial contractility favorably. If the dysmenorrhea is aggravated by the cyclic use of progestational agents, the possibility of endometriosis or adenomyosis is strongly suggested.

Endometriosis.—This disease is frequently seen in women who have long intervals of uninterrupted ovulatory menstruation. It is often associated with infertility and improves during pregnancy. This improvement is believed to be due to a decidual reaction in areas of endometriosis brought about by chorionic estrogen and progesterone and it has been suggested that repeated pregnancies actually prevent or delay the development of the disease. In lieu of pregnancy, in the unmarried or the infertile patient, one of the regimens given here may be used to secure anovulation (pseudopregnancy) for periods varying from nine to 12 months. It should be noted that the progestins are administered constantly and not cyclically. These progestins have also been used before conservative laparotomy for extensive endometriosis since they produce a decidual reaction in areas of advanced endometriosis. The dissection in the region of the cul-de-sac, especially when the rectum is adherent to the posterior aspect of the uterus and cervix, is simplified by this procedure. Medication should be given from six weeks to two months prior to surgery, depending on the extensiveness of the endometriosis. Following a conservative laparotomy, ovulation is inhibited for three to 12 months in order to keep inactive any areas of residual endometriosis (see Chapter 8).

Mastodynia.—Mastodynia is almost always associated with ovulatory cycles and is frequently correlated with the finding of bilateral chronic cystic mastitis. It is generally not seen postmenopausally and it usually disappears following removal of the ovaries. The process is not commonly seen in anovulatory patients with adequate estrogen. Sequential stimulation of the epithelium of the ducts and acini by estrogen followed by progesterone is believed to be the underlying cause. Relief may be obtained by several methods. The patient may be made anovulatory with estrogen alone, but this is not desirable on a long-term basis. Since antiestrogens and androgens have proved successful, progestins having antiestrogenic effect have also been used with beneficial results. Norlutin, 10 mg. daily may be administered from day 5 through day 24 for at least three cycles.

If recurrence of mastodynia occurs or if patients have had several breast resections for fibrocystic disease, I have utilized Depo-Provera for its ability to suppress gonadotropins, lower estrogen and to secure marked amelioration of breast pain. The only untoward side effect is that of hot flashes, occasionally sweats, due to the postmenopausal levels of estrogen that occur subsequent to treatment. Some patients note a minor degree of depression. Both symptoms improve if small amounts of estrogen, e.g., ethinyl estradiol 0.02 mg., are given when needed. This amount of estrogen is also effective if breakthrough or intermittent bleeding occurs. The regimen I have used is as follows: 100 mg. Depo-Provera every 2 weeks for 4 doses; then 200 mg. monthly for 6 to 12 months. The effect of the Depo-Provera is prolonged and some women will not ovulate for 12 to 18 months after therapy has been discontinued. If earlier ovulation is desired, clomiphene citrate is quite effective.

Galactorrhea.—Persistent mammary secretion following delivery may or may not be associated with amenorrhea. Disturbed pituitary function should be investigated, but if a tumor is not found, relief may be obtained by the administration of any estrogen-progestin combination, preferably one containing 100 μg. of estrogen. Clomiphene citrate has been shown to be effective in the induction of ovulation and suppression of galactorrhea of the Chiari-Frommel syndrome (see Chapter 9). Cessation of lactation is presumably due to suppression of prolactin by the progestational agent.

Proposed Indications for the Use of Progestins

Idiopathic Infertility.—This designation is used to describe the situation that exists when complete evaluation of the infertile couple reveals no abnormalities. There is some evidence to suggest that the use of progestins to produce a period of anovulatory cyclic withdrawal bleeding resulted in an increased incidence of subsequent pregnancy in this group. A "pituitary-rebound" phenomenon was postulated as the reason for subsequent implantation and maintenance of pregnancy, but studies by other investigators have not duplicated these results. If deficiencies of pituitary gonadotropins, ovarian steroids or the endometrium could be demonstrated to have been corrected by this regimen, it would seem more logical and attractive.

Inadequate Luteal Phase.—This term describes a deficient state of the endometrium, diagnosed by endometrial biopsy, which is presumably due to diminished secretion, or utilization, of endogenous progesterone. Studies of basal body temperature records and pregnanediol excretion in the urine may corroborate the endometrial picture. Since preparation of the endometrium is necessary for proper implantation of the ovum, treatment with progesterone should be started shortly after ovulation. However, it has seemed advisable to withhold synthetic progestins until day 18 (of a 28-day cycle), rather than to start immediately after ovulation, because of the effect these preparations have on the glandular epithelium of the endometrium. Jones prefers intravaginal progesterone suppositories or intramuscular progesterone to the synthetic progestins because of the altered morphology of the endometrium. The early changes in the glands precisely simulate those brought about by progesterone, but when the drug is continued the glands appear inactive and exhausted. The endometrium should be so "primed" for at least three cycles before initiating planned coitus.

I have utilized the sequential oral contraceptives for three months to prime the endometrium and prevent pregnancy. Following this the patient is instructed to chart her basal body temperature, plan coitus at the time of ovulation, begin the synthetic progestin on day 18 (of a 28-day cycle) and to observe closely a failure in the temperature to drop after 14 to 16 days. If the temperature remains elevated for 18 consecutive days, pregnancy is assumed and Deluteval is initiated in a dose of 500 mg. every week. (See chapter on Habitual Abortion.)

If pregnancy occurs, the following therapeutic problems arise. Should the progestin be continued? Which progestin should be utilized? What dosage should be given? Clear-cut answers are not available to these questions, but the following schemes may be of aid to the practitioner. (1) Progestin therapy may be continued without interruption until such time as it can be determined by a gonadotropin test that pregnancy has occurred. If the test gives a positive result, Deluteval may be continued. (2) In view of recent reports concerning nonadrenal masculinization of female infants born of mothers receiving steroid therapy during early pregnancy, care in the selection of the proper agent is imperative. A known androgenic steroid, such as methyltestosterone, should never be given during early pregnancy and substances similar to it should be avoided. However, there is no valid reason for not giving progesterone or closely allied substances which have minimal androgenic potential.

In a review of 101 such masculinized infants, 34 of the mothers had received ethinyl-testosterone (Pranone), 35 had received 17-alpha-ethinyl-19-nortestosterone (Norlutin) and 15 had received testosterone (or other androgens). These three drugs were thus incriminated in 84 of 101 patients. Ten mothers with virilized babies had received *no* steroidal substances, one had received Enovid, two had received intramuscular progesterone and four had been given diethylstilbestrol. Although, in some animal assays, progesterone has androgenic potential, carefully performed experiments indicate that masculinization of the fetus is not due to the direct action of progesterone itself. One may postulate that mothers of masculinized infants who receive no treatment, or who receive progesterone, may metabolize either endogenous or exogenous progesterone abnormally to form androgens. Diethylstilbestrol may stimulate the fetal adrenal to an increased output of androgens.

Therapeutic Regimens During Pregnancy.—It should be noted that progesterone production by the ovary and placenta has been calculated at about 40–80 mg./day during the first trimester and 160 mg./day during the second. Only a few observations have been made on the production rate of progesterone and most of these were done during the second and third trimesters. Solomon calculated a production rate of 92 mg./day during the 15th week of pregnancy, 263 mg./day at 27–31 weeks and 322 mg./day during the third trimester.

Progesterone, although the ideal replacement therapy, must be given by repeated intramuscular injections and its use is therefore impractical. A suggested regimen during pregnancy is:

> Deluteval 2-X, 2 cc. of the double strength every week until 16 weeks then every 2 weeks until 38 weeks. (Each 1 cc. contains 250 mg. hydroxyprogesterone caproate and 5 mg. estradiol valerate.)

In over 1,300 pregnant diabetic patients treated at the Joslin Clinic in the past 15 years, no virilized babies have been born to mothers receiving large amounts of intramuscular progesterone, Delalutin or Deluteval.

Habitual Abortion.—Because of the multiplicity of uncontrolled factors entering into the maintenance of pregnancy in the human female, it cannot be stated categorically at present that exogenous progesterone has improved the salvage rate in patients classified as habitual aborters. Furthermore, evidence shows that the prognosis for patients who have never had a successful pregnancy (primary habitual aborters) is quite different from that of others (secondary) who intersperse multiple abortions with term gestations. Since the prognosis in the two groups is indisputably different, it follows that one cannot obtain meaningful results in a therapeutic investigation that does not treat these groups separately. Both Goldzieher and Shearman recently reported a higher salvage rate in patients of primary type who received placebo medication than in those who received a synthetic progestin.

If progesterone therapy is to be administered at all, it is best started during the preconceptional stage and then continued as indicated in the preceding paragraphs. In order to avoid waste of time, money and the possibility of fetal malformation, common sense suggests that the use of a progestogen be reserved only for those cases in which *a progestogenic deficiency can be shown to exist and that compounds be utilized which have given the least trouble.*

Since these potent progestogenic agents may prevent the spontaneous expulsion of dead fetus and placenta, a threatened or spontaneous abortion may be converted into a "missed" type. Repeated pelvic examinations and pregnancy tests should be performed during the treatment period. The reader is referred to the chapter on Habitual Abortion for a full account of the subject.

Threatened Abortion.—No statistical evidence is available to indicate that the new progestins influence favorably the outcome of pregnancy after regular uterine cramps and bleeding have been established. Caution must be exerted to avoid converting an inevitable abortion into a "missed" one.

Premature Labor.—Recent evidence is available to show that progesterone, *administered systemically,* in large doses is without evident effect on spontaneous uterine activity or on the uterine response to oxytocin in late human pregnancy. Experiments in which progesterone in oil was administered *intra-amniotically* to human subjects have shown a depression of spontaneous uterine activity for 10–16 hours after administration of the drug. Further studies are necessary to substantiate these findings.

BIBLIOGRAPHY

General References

Allen, E., and Doisy, E. A.: Ovarian hormone: Preliminary reports on its localization, extraction and partial purification and action in test animals, J.A.M.A. 81:819, 1923.
Asherman, J. G.: The myth of tubal and endometrial transplantation, J. Obst. & Gynaec. Brit. Emp. 67:223, 1960.
Dorfman, R. I.: Steroid-hormones in gynecology, a review, Obst. & Gynec. Surv. 18:65, 1963.
——, and Ungar, R.: *Metabolism of Steroid-Hormones* (Minneapolis: Burgess Publishing Co., 1953).
Eckstein, P.: Ovarian Physiology in the Non-Pregnant Female, in Zuckerman, S. (ed.): *The Ovary* (New York: Academic Press, Inc., 1962).
Kistner, R. W.: Habitual abortion: General consideration and management, M. Sc. 5:782, 1959.
——: Infertility: Diagnosis and treatment, M. Sc. 9:161, 1961.
Kupperman, H. F.: The Choice of Drugs in Endocrine Dysfunction, in Modell, W. (ed.): *Drugs of Choice 1960–1961* (St. Louis: C. V. Mosby Company, 1960).
——: *Human Endocrinology* (Philadelphia: F. A. Davis Company, 1963).
Lloyd, C. W.: The Ovaries, in Williams, R. H. (ed.): *Textbook of Endocrinology* (Philadelphia: W. B. Saunders Company, 1962).
Rosenberg, A. P., and Greenblatt, R. B.: A simplified introduction to steroid chemistry for the clinician, J. Am. Geriatrics Soc. 5:486, 1957.
Smith, G. V., and Smith, O. W.: The urinary excretion of estrogenic and gonadotropic hormones during normal menstrual cycles, the period of conception and early pregnancy, New England J. Med. 215:908, 1936.
Smith, O. W., and Smith, G. V.: The influence of diethylstilbestrol on the progress and outcome of pregnancy as based on a comparison of treated and untreated primigravidas, Am. J. Obst. & Gynec. 58:994, 1949.
——, Smith, G. V., and Schiller, S.: Estrogen and progestin metabolism in pregnancy, J. Clin. Endocrinol. 1:461, 1941.
Southam, A. L.: Dysfunctional uterine bleeding in adolescence, Clin. Obst. & Gynec. 3:241, 1960.
Szego, C. M.: Steroid Action and Inter-action in Uterine Metabolism, in Pincus, G. (ed.): *Recent Progress in Hormone Research* (New York: Academic Press, Inc., 1953), vol. VIII.
Turner, H. H.: A syndrome of infantilism, congenital webbed neck and cubitus valgus, Endocrinology 23:566, 1938.
Wilkins, L.: *The Diagnosis and Treatment of Endocrine Disorders in Childhood and Adolescence;* (2d ed.; Springfield, Ill.: Charles C Thomas, Publisher, 1957).
Zander, J.: Steroids in the human ovary, J. Biol. Chem. 232:117, 1958.

Estrogens

Albert, A.: Some Personal Experience with a Clinical Estrogen Assay and Comments on Some of the Material and Thoughts Presented During the Conference, in Paulsen, C. A. (ed.): *Estrogen Assays in Clinical Medicine* (Seattle: University of Washington Press, 1965).
Barlow, J. J.: Estrogens, Assay Methods, in Behrman, S. J., and Kistner, R. W. (eds.): *Progress in Infertility* (Boston: Little, Brown & Company, 1968).
——: A sensitive method of high specificity for determination of urinary estrogens, Ann. Biochem. & Exper. Med. 6:435, 1963.
——: Adrenocortical influences on estrogen metabolism in normal females, J. Clin. Endocrinol. 24:586, 1964.
——, and Emerson, K., Jr.: Adrenocortical stimulation of ovarian estrogen production, Obst. & Gynec. 25:422, 1965.
——, and Logan, C. M.: Estrogen secretion, biosynthesis and metabolism: Their relationship to the menstrual cycle, Steroids 7:309, 1966.
Brown, J. B., and Blair, H. A. F.: A method for the determination of very small amounts of oestrone in human urine, J. Endocrinol. 20:331, 1960.
——, Kellar, R., and Matthew, G. D.: Preliminary observations on urinary oestrogen excretion in certain gynaecological disorders, J. Obst. & Gynaec. Brit. Emp. 66:177, 1959.
Giorgi, E. P.: The determination of steroids in cyst fluid from human polycystic ovaries, J. Endocrinol. 27:225, 1963.
Gurpide, E.; Angers, M.; Van de Wiele, R. L., and Lieberman, S.: Determination of secretory rates of estrogens in pregnant and nonpregnant women, J. Clin. Endocrinol. 22:935, 1962.
Huang, W. Y., and Pearlman, W. H.: The corpus luteum and steroid hormone formation, J. Biol. Chem. 238:1308, 1963.
Loraine, J. A., and Bell, E. T.: Hormone excretion during the normal menstrual cycle, Lancet 1:1340, 1963.
Mahesh, V. B., and Greenblatt, R. B.: The in vivo conversion of dehydroepiandrosterone and androstenedione to testosterone in the human, Acta endocrinol. (Kobenhavn) 41:400, 1962.

————, and Greenblatt, R. B.: Steroid secretions of the normal and polycystic ovary, Recent Prog. Hormone Res. 20:341, 1964.

Ryan, K. J., Biosynthesis of Lipids, in Popjak, G. (ed.): *Proceedings of Fifth International Congress of Biochemistry* (New York: The Macmillan Company, 1963) vol. 7, p. 381.

————: Synthesis of Hormones in the Ovary, in Grady, H. G., and Smith, D. E. (eds.): *The Ovary* (Baltimore: Williams & Wilkins Company, 1963) p. 69.

————, and Petro, Z.: Biosynthesis by human ovarian granulosa and theca cells, J. Clin. Endocrinol. 26:46, 1966.

————, and Smith, O. W.: Biogenesis of steroid hormones in the human ovary, Recent Prog. Hormone Res. 21:367, 1965.

Savard, K.; Marsh, J. M., and Rice, B. F.: Gonadotropins and ovarian steroidogenesis, Recent Prog. Hormone Res. 21:285, 1965.

Short, R. V., and London, D. R.: Defective biosynthesis of ovarian steroids in the Stein-Leventhal syndrome, Brit. Med. J. 1:1724, 1961.

Smith, O. W.: Estrogens in the ovarian fluids of normally menstruating women, Endocrinology 67:698, 1960.

Van de Wiele, R. L.: The Determination of Estrogen Secretion Rates, in Paulsen, C. A. (ed.): *Estrogen Assays in Clinical Medicine* (Seattle: University of Washington Press, 1965).

Zander, J.: Steroids in the human ovary, J. Biol. Chem. 232:117, 1958.

————; Forbes, J. R.; von Munsterman, A. M., and Neher, R.: Δ^4-3-Keto-pregnene-20α ol and Δ^4-3-ketopregnene-20β ol, two naturally occurring metabolites or progesterone, J. Clin. Endocrinol. 18:337, 1958.

Progesterone

Cox, L. W.; Cox, R. I., and Skipper, J. S.: The management of threatened abortion by pregnanediol estimation and vaginal cytology, Australian & New Zealand J. Obst. & Gynaec. 4:160, 1964.

Cox, R. I.: Gas chromatography in the analysis of urinary pregnanediol, J. Chromatogr. 12:242, 1963.

Davis, M. E., and Plotz, E. J.: Hormones in human reproduction: Part II. Further investigation of steroid metabolism in human pregnancy, Am. J. Obst. & Gynec. 76:939, 1958.

Dignam, W. J.: Progestins, Assay Methods, in Behrman, S. J., and Kistner, R. W. (eds.): *Progress in Infertility* (Boston: Little, Brown & Company, 1968).

————; Pion, R. J.; Lamb, E. J., and Simmer, H. H.: Plasma androgens in women, Acta endocrinol. (Kobenhavn) 45:254, 1964.

Dominguez, O. V.; Francois, G. D.; Watanabe, M., and Solomon, S.: Progesterone secretion in man, Program of the 44th Meeting of the Endocrine Society, 1962, p. 17 (Abstract.)

Drosdowsky, M. A.; Dessypris, A.; McNiven, N. L.; Dorfman, R. I., and Gual, C.: A search for progesterone in human urine, Acta endocrinol. (Kobenhavn) 49:553, 1965.

Ejarque, P. M., and Bengtsson, L. P.: Production rate of progesterone in human midpregnancy, Acta endocrinol. (Kobenhavn) 41:521, 1962.

Eton, B., and Short, R. V.: Blood progesterone levels in abnormal pregnancies, J. Obst. & Gynaec. Brit. Emp. 67:785, 1960.

Finkelstein, M.; Forchielli, E., and Dorfman, R. I.: Estimation of testosterone in human plasma, J. Clin. Endocrinol. 21:98, 1961.

Fotherby, K.: Excretion of pregnanetriol during the normal menstrual cycle, Brit. M. J. 1:1545, 1960.

————: The biochemistry of progesterone, Vitamins Hormones (New York) 22:153, 1964.

Futterweit, W.; McNiven, N. L.; Narcus, L.; Lantos, C.; Drosdowsky, M., and Dorfman, R. I.: Gas chromatographic determination of testosterone in human urine, Steroids 1:628, 1963.

Gurpide, E.; MacDonald, P. C.; Chapdelaine, A.; Van de Wiele, R. L., and Lieberman, S.: Studies on the secretion and interconversion of the androgens: II. Methods for estimation of rates of secretion and metabolism from specific activities of urinary metabolites, J. Clin. Endocrinol. 25:1537, 1965.

Hooker, C. W., and Forbes, T. R.: A bioassay for minute amounts of progesterone, Endocrinology 41:158, 1947.

Hughes, H. E.; Loraine, J. A.; Bell, E. T., and Layton, R.: Cytological observations, cervical mucus "ferning" and hormone assays in early pregnancy, Am. J. Obst. & Gynec. 90:1297, 1964.

James, F., and Fotherby, K.: A method for the estimation of 6-oxygenated metabolites of progesterone in urine, Biochem. J. 95:459, 1965.

Jones, G. E. S.; Turner, D.; Sarlos, I. J.; Barnes, A. C., and Cohen, R.: The determination of urinary pregnanediol by gas liquid chromatography, Fertil. & Steril. 13:544, 1962.

Klopper, A. I.: Pregnanediol and Pregnanetriol, in Dorfman, R. I. (ed.): *Methods in Hormone Research* (New York: Academic Press, Inc., 1962) vol. I.

————, and Billewicz, W.: Urinary excretion of oestriol and pregnanediol during normal pregnancy, J. Obst. & Gynaec. Brit. Emp. 70:1024, 1963.

————, and MacNaughton, M.: Hormones in recurrent abortion, J. Obst. & Gynaec. Brit. Emp. 72:1022, 1965.

Little, B.; Tait, J. J.; Black, W. P., and Tait, S. A. S.: The secretion rate and metabolic clearance rate of progesterone 7-H³ in men and ovariectomized women, Program of the 44th Meeting of the Endocrine Society, 1962, p. 7. (Abstract.)

Loraine, J. A., and Bell, E. T.: Hormone excretion during the normal menstrual cycle, Lancet 1:1340, 1963.

Mahesh, V. B.: Evaluation of Androgen Function, in Behrman, S. J., and Kistner, R. W. (eds.): *Progress in Infertility* (Boston: Little, Brown & Company, 1968).

———, and Greenblatt, R. B.: The in vivo conversion of dehydroepiandrosterone and androstenedione to testosterone in the human, Acta endocrinol. (Kobenhavn) 41:400, 1962.

———, and Greenblatt, R. B.: Isolation of dehydroepiandrosterone and 17α-hydroxy-Δ-pregnenolone from the polycystic ovaries of Stein-Leventhal syndrome, J. Clin. Endocrinol. 22:441, 1962.

Riondel, A.; Tait, J. F.; Tait, S. A. S.; Gut, M., and Little, B.: Estimation of progesterone in human peripheral blood using S-thiosemicarbazide, J. Clin. Endocrinol. 25:229, 1965.

Ryan, K. J.: Hormones of the placenta, Am. J. Obst. & Gynec. 84:1695, 1962.

Sandberg, D. H.; Ahmad, N.; Cleveland, W. W., and Savard, K.: Measurement of urinary testosterone by gas-liquid chromatography, Steroids 4:557, 1964.

Shearman, R. P.: Some aspects of the urinary excretion of pregnanediol in pregnancy, J. Obst. & Gynaec. Brit. Emp. 66:1, 1959.

———, and Garrett, W. J.: Double blind study of effect of 17-hydroxyprogesterone caproate on abortion rate, Brit. M. J. 1:292, 1963.

Short, R. V., and Levett, I.: The fluorimetric determination of progesterone in human plasma during pregnancy and the menstrual cycle, J. Endocrinol. 25:239, 1962.

Solomon, S.; Watanabe, M.; Dominguez, O. V.; Gray, M. J.; Meaker, C. I., and Sims, E. A. H.: Progesterone and aldosterone secretion rates in pregnancy, Excerpta Med. (International Congress Series) 51:267, 1962.

Sommerville, I. R.; Pickett, M. T.; Collins, W. P., and Denyer, D. C.: A modified method for the quantitative determination of progesterone in human plasma, Acta endocrinol. (Kobenhavn) 43:101, 1963.

Staub, M. C.; Gaitan, E., and Dingman, J. F.: A simple method for the determination of urinary pregnanediol and pregnanetriol by glass fiber paper chromatography, J. Clin. Endocrinol. 22:87, 1962.

Tait, J. J.: Review: The use of isotopic steroids for the measurement of production rates in vivo, J. Clin. Endocrinol. 23:1285, 1963.

———, and Horton, R.: Some theoretical considerations on the significance of the discrepancy in urinary and blood production rate estimates of steroid hormones, particularly in those of testosterone in young women, Steroids 4:365, 1964.

Van der Molen, H. J.: Determination of plasma progesterone during pregnancy, Clin. chem. acta 8:943, 1963.

———, and Groen, D.: Determination of progesterone in human peripheral blood using gas-liquid chromatography with electron capture detection, J. Clin. Endocrinol. 25:1625, 1965.

Van de Wiele, R. L.; MacDonald, P. C.; Gurpide, E., and Lieberman, S.: Studies on the secretion and interconversion of androgens, Recent Progr. Hormone Res. 19:275, 1963.

Woolever, C. A.: Daily plasma progesterone levels during the menstrual cycle, Am. J. Obst. & Gynec. 85:981, 1963.

———: Progesterone and progesterone therapy in pregnancy, Clin. Obst. & Gynec. 8:565, 1965.

———, and Goldfien, A.: A double-isotope derivative method for plasma progesterone assay, Internat. J. Appl. Radiation & Isotopes 14:163, 1963.

Wotiz, H. H.: Studies in steroid metabolism: XV. The rapid determination of urinary pregnanediol by gas chromatography, Biochim. et biophys. acta 69:415, 1963.

Zander, J.: Progesterone, in Dorfman, R. I. (ed.): *Methods in Hormone Research* (New York: Academic Press, Inc., 1962) vol. I.

Zarrow, M. X.; Neher, G. M.; Lazo-Wasem, E. A., and Salhanick, H. A.: Biological activity of certain progesterone-like compounds as determined by the Hooker-Forbes bioassay, J. Clin. Endocrinol. 17:658, 1957.

CHAPTER 14

The Menopause

Estrogens

THE APPARENT CONCLUSIONS derived from the avalanche of literature on the use of estrogens in the medical and lay press vary widely, depending upon the age, sex and medical background of the reader. The postmenopausal female envisions the return of youth, beauty, vigor and sexual interest subsequent to the administration of estrogens and progestins. The premenopausal female is ecstatic at the thought of preventing the dreaded symptoms of the menopause and the associated physical changes such as facial wrinkles, drooping breasts, muscular weakness and diminished libido. The internist sees the possibility of disease prevention, particularly atherosclerosis and osteoporosis, and the psychiatrist hopes for an improved adjustment to an abrupt and dramatic change in self-concept.

The gynecologist, however, casts a suspicious glance at these fantastic claims. And rightfully so, since those gynecologists who have been using estrogenic substances for 30 years have not seen the extravagant improvements or supposed prophylaxis cited by protagonists of the "feminine forever" school. Rather, they have worried about breast tenderness and masses, the reappearance of uterine fibroids and irregular bleeding. Some, apparently without adequate scientific proof, have associated the administration of estrogens with cancer of the breast and uterus.

The administration of estrogens to postmenopausal, surgically castrated, prematurely menopausal or congenitally deficient (ovarian dysgenesis) females has been practiced by most gynecologists since the availability of potent compounds in the 1930s. The new twist, or variation on a theme, suggests that: (1) all estrogen-deficient females should receive hormonal replacement unless contraindications exist, (2) medication should be continued forever, (3) estrogen therapy should be given constantly instead of in the usual 21-day cycles, (4) dosage should be increased or decreased as dictated precisely by vaginal cytology, (5) estrogen administration should be periodically interrupted by a progestational agent in order to prevent the development of hyperplasia and cancer of the endometrium (the latter sequence necessitates cyclic "withdrawal bleeding"), and (6) the sequential use of progestational agents will diminish the incidence of mammary carcinoma in women receiving constant estrogens. (There is no statistically significant evidence for this.)

These basic tenets are dependent upon three assumptions which are not based on scientific evidence: (1) that all postmenopausal, and many pre-menopausal, women are estrogen-insufficient, (2) that administration of estrogens and progestins to premenopausal females who are still actively menstruating will retard specific aging processes, and (3) that continuous estrogen is necessary to effect these desiderata.

Assays of estrogenic substances in urine or blood (more precise than vaginal cytology) during the first year or so after cessation of menses show values that are not appreciably lower than those of the proliferative phase of the normal cycle. Cytologic examinations during the early menopause, age 45–60 years, have shown an excellent cornification index in almost 25 per cent of patients tested. During the late menopause, age 61–85 years, a high cornification index was found in 5 per cent of patients. Cytologists have criticized the percentage of cornified cells stated as being desirable, as being much higher than that usually seen in the majority of normal females with normal menstrual cycles. Furthermore, most gynecologists object to the recommendation that estrogen levels of the premenopausal woman be increased, and regular bleeding ensured, on the basis of an al-tered maturation index of vaginal cytology. I cannot agree with the direc-tion to treat "primarily and principally the vaginal smear, not the symp-toms."

Premenopausal females having regular ovulatory menstrual cycles, exhibit normal vaginal cytology and normal assays of estrogens and preg-nanediol in urine. Unfortunately, many readers have been misinformed about this age-group. The impropriety of diagnosing early menopause in the presence of normal menstrual function is, on occasion, embarrassingly illustrated by the occurrence of pregnancy. Symptoms should not be as-cribed to estrogen insufficiency on the basis of chronologic age; nor should incipient menopause be diagnosed before the establishment of amenorrhea of some degree.

There is no doubt that when periods become scanty and the cycle is characterized by skips and delays, estrogen insufficiency is present. But too many patients with normal cycles are searching for an answer to their situational problem, hoping that the administration of estrogens and pro-gestins will, at long last, relieve them of their symptoms of anxiety, improve their waning marital relationships and dispel lassitude due to boredom or overwork. The majority of patients in this category describe symptoms of premenstrual tension due to their endogenous estrogen and progesterone, but not due to their insufficiency. As a matter of fact, we have observed drooping breasts, flabby musculature and facial skin dryness with exces-sive wrinkling in numerous women in their early 40s despite normal ovula-tory menses. These changes have even been observed in castrated females who have received estrogen replacement for 20 years or more, and in women having hyperestrogenic states due to granulosa-cell tumors, the-comas or cortical stromal hyperplasia of the ovaries. Undoubtedly such changes are due more to genetic, racial, dietary and climatic factors than to lack of estrogen.

A few gynecologists insist that estrogenic substances be given con-stantly, yet during the reproductive period of her life the human female has a double peak of estrogen secretion during each menstrual cycle. If one insists on the administration of estrogen constantly, in amounts adequate to produce the degree of vaginal cornification desired, the endometrium will eventually become hyperplastic and break-through bleeding will occur. Since many, but not all, carcinomas of the endometrium develop in previously existing areas of hyperplasia, and since a non-hormonally dependent cancer may arise de novo and its bleeding be masked by the assumption that it is due to estrogen hyperplasia, it seems prudent not to produce the hyperplastic process. It has been suggested that the hyperplasia and anaplasia may be prevented by sloughing the abnormal endometrium in cyclic fashion with a progestin, but this produces withdrawal bleeding episodes in postmenopausal women, most of whom are happily rid of this nuisance.

Most gynecologists in the United States do not agree with these suggestions. They prefer to administer estrogenic substances, in 21- to 25-day cycles, to women, regardless of age, who exhibit signs and symptoms of estrogen insufficiency. The only symptoms which disappear with regularity after adequate therapy are those of vasomotor origin, hot flushes and sweats and, for some unknown reason, insomnia. The only sign of estrogen deficiency which uniformly improves is that of senescent vaginitis. If dyspareunia and diminished libido are due to this process, these symptoms will also diminish as clinical improvement occurs.

Atherosclerosis and Myocardial Infarction.—There is evidence now which strongly suggests that the protection against atherosclerosis and myocardial infarction afforded the human female by estrogens is more apparent than real. Even if it is eventually proven that such a relationship exists, recent studies have shown that the addition of certain androgenic progestins may, because of their antiestrogenic effect, negate the benefits of estrogen.

The relationship of prolonged estrogen administration beyond the menopause and the prophylaxis of coronary atherosclerosis has not been solved. Considerable evidence is available to indicate that endogenous ovarian secretion plays a key role in protecting women against clinical atherosclerotic coronary heart disease. It is hoped that analyses of subsequent, controlled series of patients will definitely delineate the effects of exogenous estrogens in this regard.

The dilemma is illustrated by a recent study of 258 women who had bilateral oophorectomy and 283 who had hysterectomy without bilateral oophorectomy before the age of 35. Of these, 155 castrates and 190 controls were available for study at a mean of 17.5 and 16.3 years postoperatively, respectively. In the castrate group there were 6 women with myocardial infarction, 11 with angina pectoris, and 5 with ischemic post-exercise electrocardiograms. The corresponding numbers in the non-castrate group were 6, 22 and 3. The over-all rates for coronary heart disease were 8.2 per cent in the castrate and 8.1 per cent in the non-castrate groups.

Dosage.—The problem of estrogen dosage is similarly confusing. Doses of ethinyl estradiol as low as 0.01 mg. daily produced a fall in serum cholesterol, a rise in phospholipid and a fall in C/P ratio. Other investigators noted similar changes, but found it necessary to use doses of sodium estrone sulfate 2 to 5 times greater than the equivalent of 0.01 mg. of ethinyl estradiol to achieve these effects. In most patients, 1.25 mg. of sodium estrone sulfate was adequate to produce the desired lipid effects, but higher doses (2.5 mg.) were necessary in patients resistant to smaller doses.

The following conclusions may be drawn from the investigative work to date:

1. Bilateral oophorectomy should not be performed as a prophylactic measure in the premenopausal female undergoing hysterectomy for benign disease, or after radical mastectomy if the axillary lymph nodes are negative and the lesion well confined (even when the axillary nodes show cancer, the 5-year survival rate has not been shown to be increased by prophylactic oophorectomy).

2. Exogenous estrogens should be administered if bilateral oophorectomy is necessary for gynecologic disease. This applies to patients having endometriosis, pelvic infection, and invasive carcinoma of the cervix.

3. Long-term estrogens are recommended for postmenopausal women with overt evidence of clinical coronary heart disease and those with other predisposing factors (hypercholesterolemia, hypertension, obesity, cigarette smoking, diabetes, etc.) known to have a higher risk of subsequent overt disease.

OSTEOPOROSIS

There does not seem to be any doubt that the administration of estrogens to postmenopausal women with osteoporosis is the most effective and generally accepted treatment. Therapeutic principles are as follows:

Treatment.—ACTIVITY.—As much as tolerated plus supervised physical therapy.

NUTRITION.—Well-balanced general diet. One quart of skim milk per day for calcium, phosphorus and protein. 400 to 2,000 units of vitamin D per day (1 or 2 multivitamin pills containing vitamin D). Tricalcium phosphate, 3 to 4 500-mg. tablets 3 times per day to supply about 1 G. additional calcium and phosphorus.

HORMONES.—Estrogen-replacement dose or more if tolerated (such as 1.25–2.50 mg. of conjugated estrogens per day for 3 weeks each month) may be given.

After the acute discomfort and associated orthopedic problems are resolved, some form of exercise should be prescribed. The simplest method is to suggest a walk of 1 or 2 miles daily. Most authorities suggest a diet rich in calcium, vitamin D and phosphorus with added calcium, as noted above.

Wallach and Henneman have suggested that estrogen be given in a dose of sodium estrone sulfate, 1.25 mg. daily for 4 weeks followed by a week off treatment. Subsequent cycles are repeated, but the dose of estrogen is then increased to 2.5 mg., then to 5.0 mg. daily. Therapy is continued at the rate of 5 mg. daily, 4 weeks on, 1 week off. This permits regular withdrawal bleeding of the proliferated endometrium and prevents hyperplasia. If bleeding is profuse or irregular, a progestin may be given during the last 10 to 14 days of therapy.

In a series of estrogen-treated patients followed by Gordon for 1,100 patient-years, no cases of cancer of breast, cervix or endometrium were found. In the series of Wallach and Henneman (242 postmenopausal women treated with estrogens for a total of 1,480 patient-years), 7 patients developed cancer of the cervix, uterus or ovary. No patient developed breast cancer. Six of the 7 cancers in this series developed before 1948, during the period when continuous estrogen therapy was being given. Only one cancer occurred in the interval 1948–1958, during which time interrupted cyclic estrogen therapy was used, and this was a carcinoma in situ of the cervix. In the series reported by Gordon, the estrogen was also given in interrupted cycles.

After estrogen therapy for osteoporosis is initiated, it appears desirable that it be continued indefinitely in the same fashion that therapy is continued if once started for vasomotor symptoms. The majority of postmenopausal women, however, do not have distressing symptoms and do not develop symptomatic or proved osteoporosis. It does not appear prudent, at this time, to recommend estrogen therapy for the majority of the population who demonstrate neither signs nor symptoms of estrogen insufficiency. Such a recommendation would certainly bring into focus the troublesome aspects of estrogen therapy, such as mastodynia, gastritis and diarrhea, the nuisance of menstruation and the edema noted in certain individuals with cardiac or renal insufficiency.

Furthermore, it is not known that estrogens will prevent the development of osteoporosis, although certain evidence suggests that this may be so. However, the correlation between menopause and the development of osteoporosis may be spurious, depending on aging rather than lack of estrogen. Thus women experiencing menopause at the age of 30 do not develop osteoporosis for about 28 years, whereas those entering the menopause at 50 develop osteoporosis in only 5–6 years.

As previously mentioned, the view has been expressed that it is medically sound to attempt postponement of the menopause. The desirability of long-term estrogen substitution therapy is attracting even greater attention but, at the moment, the verdict must be held subjudice.

Therapy of the Menopause

The basic concepts of management of the perimenopausal patient include psychotherapy designed to educate, reassure and support; symptomatic therapy, designed to assist the patient through a period of distressing symptomatology; and hormonal therapy, designed to correct estrogen insufficiency.

It is perhaps a cliché to say that "therapeutic nihilism and pessimistic abnegation will serve no useful purpose" in management of the perimenopause. I do not believe that it is unnatural to attempt alleviation of menopausal symptoms or to stave off the forces of attrition associated with the aging process if indeed this is possible. The controversy stems not from teleological considerations, but from our inadequate scientific knowledge of the processes of aging.

PSYCHOTHERAPY

The perimenopausal patient requires a sympathetic hearing. The prescription of a shotgun preparation containing mixtures of hormone, sedative, stimulant, tranquilizer and vitamins is abhorred. Fantasies should be dispelled, phobias dissipated and misconceptions corrected. The physiology of menopause should be explained and the patient should be told which symptoms are due to estrogen insufficiency and which are not. The patient should realize that the perimenopause is not the end of life but the beginning of a new life. New freedoms should be enjoyed, activities in the home and community extended, dormant interests reactivated and unfulfilled ambitions pursued with renewed vigor.

Symptomatic Therapy

Drugs designed to alleviate specific symptoms should be prescribed on a short-term or intermittent basis. The following are the most reliable preparations: Phenobarbital, 30 mg., combined with belladonna, 0.75 mg., given 3 or 4 times daily. Amphetamine-barbiturate compounds are frequently of value. Meprobamate, 400 mg. 4 times daily, may be used advantageously for the relief of psychic and somatic tension states. In certain patients the use of autonomic depressant and spasmolytic agents will afford considerable relief.

The use of hormonal agents during the perimenopause will depend on the state of insufficiency existing and on the length of amenorrhea. Therapy during the premenopause, therefore, will differ from that given during the postmenopause.

Hormonal Regimens During Premenopause

Effective treatment during the premenopausal period, that is, after demonstration of signs or complaints characteristic of estrogen insufficiency, should produce regular but not excessive uterine bleeding, alleviate vasomotor symptoms, retard or prevent the extragenital effects of estrogen insufficiency (arteriosclerosis and osteoporosis), provide adequate conception control, and prevent atrophic changes in the external genitalia necessary for normal and regular sexual function.

This may be accomplished by administration of any sequential estrogen-progestin oral contraceptive. Certain patients will note excessive withdrawal bleeding while taking the sequential agents. This is particularly true in patients who give a history of previous hypermenorrhea. If withdrawal or break-through bleeding is recurrent, a uterine curettage should be done to exclude the possibility of a submucous leiomyoma. Subsequently, these patients should be treated with an estrogen-progestin compound preferably containing 100 μg. of estrogen and a norethindrone progestin.

Treatment of the premenopause is continued until the average age of menopause, that is, about 50–52 years. This is not absolute, however, and if patients request that cyclic withdrawal bleeding be discontinued at the age of 48 or 49, they are then placed on the regimens of estrogen therapy outlined under treatment of the postmenopause. Similarly, certain patients appear younger, both mentally and physically, than their chronological age. If they desire to continue to remain on estrogen-progestin sequential therapy until the age of 54 or 55, I see no reason for not doing so.

Abnormal bleeding, of any type, during the administration of estrogen-progestin sequential agents, should be investigated with the same thoroughness as for abnormal bleeding in patients of this age-group who are not receiving therapy. For minimal break-through bleeding an endometrial biopsy and an endometrial cavity aspiration for cytology are usually adequate. Papanicolaou smears are done annually and examination of the genital organs and breasts every 6 months. Thorough uterine curettage must be done in all patients having recurrent break-through or heavy withdrawal bleeding. An organic cause (leiomyoma, polyp, adenomyosis) is usually found. Patients with previous endometrial hyperplasia or carcinoma in situ who are being treated by cyclic estrogen-progestin therapy should have a curettage every six months.

Therapeutic Regimens During Postmenopause

The postmenopausal state is defined as absence of bleeding for 12 consecutive months after the age of 45. Figure 14–1 illustrates the percentage of women having the menopause in relation to their age. About 30 per cent will have had the menopause by age 45, 60 per cent at age 50, 98 per cent at age 55 and 100 per cent at age 60.

The major clinical problems in therapy of the postmenopause may be summarized as follows:

1. What are the proper indications for estrogen therapy?

2. Which estrogen should be selected and what is the optimum dose regimen?

3. How long should therapy be continued?

4. Are progestins or androgens indicated?

5. What are the contraindications to estrogen therapy?

Although the medical and lay literature abound with indications for the use of estrogenic substances during the postmenopausal era, I utilize the following criteria:

A. The presence of vasomotor symptoms including hot flushes (some patients describe these as cold flushes), hot flashes, sweats and insomnia.

B. Senescent vaginitis and cyto-trigonitis.

C. Post-oophorectomy-hysterectomy.

D. Osteoporosis.

Fig. 14–1.—Graph shows percentage of women reporting having had a menopause, by age at time of survey response.

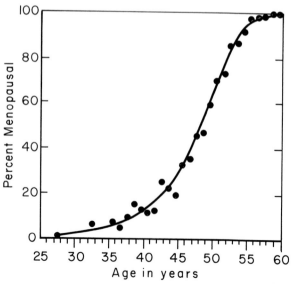

VASOMOTOR SYMPTOMS

Estrogen apparently sensitizes the balance between the diencephalon and the autonomic nervous system. Deprivation of estrogen produces an increased irritability of cutaneous blood-vessels, particularly in the blush areas. The menopausal flush is, therefore, hormonally mediated by way of a disturbance in hypothalamic-autonomic nervous system equilibrium that is reflected clinically in vasomotor instability.

My therapeutic regimen for the relief of vasomotor symptoms in the postmenopausal females is as follows: sodium estrone sulfate (Premarin) 0.625–1.25 mg. or ethinyl estradiol (Estinyl) 0.02–0.05 mg. or diethylstilbestrol 0.25–0.50 mg. (all given daily, orally, in 21- to 25-day cycles).

I have no preference for natural estrogens, except for their improved tolerance, since there is no evidence suggesting any physiologic or pharmacologic difference in action between the natural and synthetic estrogens. An ideal estrogen, not as yet available, would alleviate symptoms, improve signs of insufficiency, retard degenerative changes and not stimulate the epithelium of the breast or endometrium.

At the present time, no therapeutic regimen can guarantee the absence of estrogen-induced bleeding. However, small doses are less likely to result in uterine bleeding and to produce annoying side-effects. Therefore the smallest dose should be used as initial therapy and increases made if necessary on the basis of symptomatic inadequacy. Bleeding is managed as follows:

1. Break-through bleeding—uterine curettage.

2. Withdrawal staining—endometrial biopsy and endometrial aspiration for cytologic examinations.

3. Withdrawal bleeding—if recurrent, uterine curettage.

The incidence of break-through bleeding is low but, since we have discovered early carcinoma in postmenopausal patients having recurrent staining or bleeding during the administration of estrogens, it is a sine qua non indication for curettage. It is not known whether early endometrial cancer will be affected by estrogenic substances so that early bleeding is brought about in an otherwise amenorrheic patient. If this eventually proves to be the case, the administration of estrogens to such patients may be looked upon as a provocative test.

Withdrawal stain occurs in about 1 in 10 patients receiving sodium estrone sulfate (1.25 mg.), ethinyl estradiol 0.05 mg. or diethylstilbestrol 0.05 mg. Biopsy of the endometrium usually shows "proliferative endometrium with stromal necrosis, consistent with estrogen withdrawal." If hyperplasia is found or the endometrial aspiration shows abnormal cytology, a curettage is performed. If the biopsy or curettage shows only proliferative or cystic hyperplastic endometrium, the dose of estrogen is reduced and subsequent bleeding usually does not occur. If adenomatous hyperplasia is found, several courses of estrogen-progestin are given and endometrial sampling repeated at the time of withdrawal bleeding. Menstrual endometrium consistent with progestin effect is then found. Estrogens may then be restarted in the usual cycles, but in a lower dose.

Heavy withdrawal bleeding following the usual doses of estrogen is frequently found to be due to reactivation of a submucous leiomyoma. The diagnosis is usually evident by curettage or hysterography. Subsequent administration of estrogens is usually contraindicated. The gynecologist may then choose to omit hormonal therapy, or to perform a vaginal hysterectomy, and then reinstitute estrogen therapy. In many patients mild vasomotor symptoms can be controlled with the aid of sedatives and autonomic drugs.

I do not advise the use of injectable estrogens for the relief of vasomotor symptoms when the uterus is intact. The length of action is unpredictable and cumulative effect usually results in irregular bleeding. In a very few patients, unable to tolerate or absorb estrogens, the parenteral route is used.

Diminished estrogen is responsible for the atrophic changes occurring in the vagina and vulva which may produce distressing symptoms such as dyspareunia, pruritus and vaginal spotting. The spotting is due to rupture of small capillaries in the areas of telangiectasia seen so frequently in the senile vagina. Since there is no way of being certain that the bleeding is not of uterine origin, a curettage must be performed. Secondary infection of the atrophic vaginal mucosa by trichomonas or pathogenic bacteria is a frequent cause of burning discharge, bleeding, dyspareunia and urinary frequency. The use of vaginal creams containing estrogenic substances may be used to control the atrophic vaginal changes, but many patients find their protracted use distasteful and messy. If there are associated vasomotor symptoms such patients are best treated by oral estrogens as previously indicated.

The base of the bladder and epithelium around the trigone and urethra are responsive to estrogen, and deficiency alters the function of the vesical sphincter and detrusor muscles, resulting in urinary incontinence and dysuria. Oral estrogens should be used to reverse these changes.

Following bilateral oophorectomy there is a rapid drop in the amount of estrogen assayed in the urine. In premenopausal women the mean average approximates 5.0 μg. per 24 hours and in postmenopausal women about 6.3 μg. The mean excretion in a normal ovulating female is 13 μg. at the onset of menstruation, 56 μg. at the time of ovulation and 45 μg. during the luteal phase. We have, therefore, initiated estrogen therapy immediately after surgery and this is continued indefinitely.

Estrogen is given to all women subsequent to hysterectomy and bilateral oophorectomy. Neither endometriosis nor carcinoma of the cervix is a contraindication for estrogen therapy. I have not seen recurrence of endometriosis in these patients if estrogenic substances are given according to the following regimen:

1. Estradiol valerate (Delestrogen) 10 mg. intramuscularly immediately after surgery and repeated five days later.
2. Sodium estrone sulfate (Premarin) 1.25 mg.; ethinyl estradiol (Estinyl) 0.05 mg.; or diethylstilbestrol 0.5 mg. (daily, beginning on 5th postoperative day).

These oral estrogens are given constantly, daily and indefinitely. The dosage may be varied up or down (Premarin 2.5 or 0.625; Estinyl 0.05 twice daily or 0.02; diethylstilbestrol 0.5 twice daily or 0.25) depending upon individual patient tolerance and the appearance of side-effects. Certain patients seem prone to salt and water retention, but note improvement if salt intake is restricted, the dose of estrogen diminished, a diuretic agent prescribed for 2–4 days each week and the estrogen given in 21 to 25-day cycles.

If mastodynia is bothersome, cyclic administration is utilized as above. Certain patients with mastodynia note amelioration of discomfort if methyl testosterone is added to the estrogenic compound. I have utilized sodium estrone sulfate 1.25 mg. plus methyl testosterone 5.0 mg. or ethinyl estradiol 0.02 mg. plus methyl testosterone 5.0 mg. for this purpose, again utilizing 21- to 25-day cycles. Signs of virilization are not usually seen with this total dosage level of 125 mg. methyl testosterone per month. A low-sodium diet and a diuretic agent are employed as adjuvants.

Patients receiving estrogenic therapy of this type after hysterectomy-oophorectomy should have a thorough breast examination every six months. It is not deemed necessary to do routine vaginal cytology for malignancy unless the uterus or adnexae have been removed for premalignant or malignant lesions.

PROGESTERONE

There is no evidence at present that progesterone plays any significant role in the physiology of the menopause, since neither reproduction nor the differentiating effect upon the estrogen-primed endometrium is desirable during the postmenopausal state. Except as noted above in the temporary management of iatrogenic hyperplastic endometrium, the synthetic progestins are not suggested in therapeutic schemes. Furthermore, some of the more androgenic progestins may negate the desired effect of exogenously administered estrogens on extragenital systems.

In rare instances of postmenopausal patients having adenomatous hyperplasia or carcinoma in situ of the endometrium, in whom hysterectomy is contraindicated, potent synthetic progestins such as depo-medroxyprogesterone acetate (Depo-Provera) may be used to produce endometrial atrophy.

The administration of depo-medroxyprogesterone acetate or hydroxyprogesterone caproate (Delalutin) is accepted therapy for metastatic endometrial cancer and results in an objective remission rate of approximately 35 per cent. Specific regimens have been described under endometrial cancer.

There is no statistically significant evidence that the use of synthetic progestins, given in 5- to 10-day courses at intervals of 60 to 90 days to the postmenopausal female, will diminish the incidence of carcinoma of the endometrium made hyperplastic by the constant administration of estrogens. A more physiologic approach is to avoid the development of hyperplasia by intermittent administration of estrogens. Similarly, evidence is not at hand to substantiate the suggestion that mammary cancer will be diminished by interrupting constant estrogen therapy with progestins.

ANDROGEN

Although androgenic substances do inhibit gonadotropin secretion and ameliorate the vasomotor symptoms of spontaneous or surgical menopause, the required dose frequently produces undesirable masculinizing signs and symptoms. I have restricted their use to patients having severe vasomotor symptoms following bilateral oophorectomy in the treatment of mammary or endometrial cancer. However, we have found the administration of depo-medroxyprogesterone acetate (100 mg. every 2 weeks x 4 doses; then 200 mg. per month), to be equally effective.

Many gynecologists do not interdict the use of estrogens in patients who are in good health, without evidence of disease, at least 5 years after surgery for mammary or endometrial cancer. This is particularly true if the lymph nodes have not shown tumor and if the lesion was confined. Most obstetricians permit pregnancy in women of this category, and I can see no difference between the hyper-hormonal state of pregnancy and the use of estrogenic substances given in minimal amounts. One might rationalize that the simultaneous administration of estrogen and androgen or estrogen and progestin would be *less dangerous*, since androgens do effect remissions in mammary cancer and progestins have a similar effect on endometrial malignancy. I have treated numerous patients of this type by both methods and have not noted recurrence of disease.

The use of androgens, given in small amounts (less than 100 mg. per month), has been noted to improve libido, general well-being and appetite in some postmenopausal patients. I have found this to be effective in a few patients, but the majority have not noted significant improvement.

COMBINED ANDROGEN-ESTROGEN

Data are available to support and deny the advantages of combined therapy during the menopause. Such combinations are said to exert an improved protein anabolic effect, increase formation of osteoid tissue in bone and a sense of euphoria, and to restore or improve libido, thus promoting over-all well-being. Similarly, the use of androgens theoretically permits a reduction in the dose of estrogens, resulting in a diminished tendency toward endometrial bleeding.

All these observations may be true, but controlled studies are not available to support the contention. Furthermore, a theoretical objection exists, since the androgen may negate the desired effect of estrogens on the cholesterol-phospholipid ratio, similar to that noted in patients treated with estrogens plus androgenic progestins, thus producing an increased tendency toward coronary vessel atherosclerosis.

I have restricted the estrogen-androgen combinations to patients who note severe mastodynia while receiving estrogens, and to a small group who have been surgically castrated subsequent to mammary carcinoma. The latter seems incongruous, since the oophorectomy was performed to eliminate endogenous estrogen. However, these patients had localized mammary cancers and negative axillary lymph nodes, and were living and well five years after primary therapy. The prophylactic oophorectomy was not indicated, on the basis of present data, and caused distressing side-effects in relatively young and vigorous females. It is disturbing to realize that numerous females, in the age-group 25 to 45, have been subjected to unnecessary surgical or radiation castration on the basis of inadequate statistical data. Instead of prolonging their life-span, injudicious ovarian ablation may have produced premature coronary atherosclerosis and unfortunate demise.

In osteoporosis, and in the absence of solid evidence of the effectiveness of any prophylactic or therapeutic measures, one can only suggest measures that may possibly help and are unlikely to do any harm, such as regular physical activity, adequate calcium intake, and a high protein diet. In patients with impaired absorption of calcium, the addition of vitamin D may be helpful. If the patient's history offers no contraindication, estrogens and androgens may be administered beginning early in the menopause. When such measures are used for the treatment of osteoporosis, it is with the hope that they will halt or slow the progress of the disorder; they are unlikely to reverse it.

BIBLIOGRAPHY

Gordon, G. V.: Osteoporosis. Diagnosis and treatment, Texas J. Med. 57:740, 1961.

Kistner, R. W.: Histological effects of progestins on hyperplasia and carcinoma in situ of the endometrium, Cancer 12:1106, 1959.

————: Treatment of carcinoma in situ of the endometrium, Clin. Obst. & Gynec. 5:1166, 1962.

————, in Greenhill, J. P., (ed.): *Year Book of Obstetrics and Gynecology, 1965–1966* (Chicago: Year Book Medical Publishers), p. 552.

————, Griffiths, C. T., and Craig, J. M.: Use of progestational agents in the management of endometrial cancer, Cancer 18:1563, 1965.

Marmorston, J., Magidson, O., Lewis, J. J., Mehl, J., Moore, F. J., and Berstein, J.: Effect of small doses of estrogen on serum lipids in female patients with myocardial infarction, New England J. Med. 258:583, 1958.

Meisels, A.: The menopause: a cyto-hormonal study, Acta cytol. 10:49, 1966.

Riley, G. M.: Endocrinology of the climacteric, Clin. Obst. & Gynec. 7:432, 1964.

Ritterband, A. B., Jaffe, I. A., Bensen, P. M., Magagna, J. F., and Reed, A.: Gonadal function and the development of coronary heart disease, Circulation, 26:668, 1962.

Robinson, R. W., Higano, N., and Cohen, W. D.: Effects of long-term administration of estrogens on serum lipids of postmenopausal women, New England J. Med. 263:828, 1960.

Wallach, S., and Henneman, P. H.: Prolonged estrogen therapy in postmenopausal women, J.A.M.A. 171, 1637, 1959.

Wilson, R. A., Brevetti, R. E., and Wilson, T. A.: Specific procedures for the elimination of the menopause, West. J. Surg. 71:110, 1963.

————, and Wilson, T. A.: The fate of the nontreated postmenopausal woman: a plea for the maintenance of adequate estrogen from puberty to the grave, J. Am. Geriatrics Soc. 11:347, 1963.

CHAPTER 15

Conception Control

THE WIVES OF North African desert tribesmen mixed gunpowder solution and foam from a camel's mouth and drank the potion. Egyptian women inserted pessaries made from crocodile dung into the vagina or used tampons made from lint soaked in fermented acacia juice. The Chinese fried quicksilver in oil and drank it, or swallowed 14 live tadpoles three days after menstruation. Greek women of the second century made vaginal plugs of wool soaked in sour oil, honey, cedar gum, pomegranate and fig pulp. Others ate the uterus of a female mule. Byzantine women of the sixth century attached a tube containing cat liver to their left foot. In the Middle Ages potions were prepared from willow leaves, iron rust or slag, clay and the kidney of a mule. European brides of the 17th century were instructed to sit on their fingers while riding in their coaches or to place roasted walnuts in the bosom, one for every barren year desired.

These are but a few of the more picturesque methods of "contraception" used in man's efforts to achieve family planning. Obviously, the unwanted child was as much concern to the ancients as to modern man. More successful and more sanitary methods of conception control are now available, based on our knowledge of how conception and pregnancy occur.

The years 1960–1970 might well be termed "the decade of control-conception control," since it was during these years that the results of a previous decade of laboratory, animal and clinical investigation were finally realized. The major unit of control was the development and widespread use of the oral contraceptive. But of almost equal importance was the renaissance of the intra-uterine device, (IUD) a method which does not compete with the estrogen-progestin combination but really should be considered an adjuvant method, one of particular importance in underdeveloped countries or where the "pill" is contraindicated or unacceptable.

The same decade will be remembered for the advances in the induction of ovulation with chemicals such as clomiphene and the production of human gonadotropic substances. Although at present these agents cannot be classified as methods of conception control, subsequent investigation may prove them to be of extreme importance in women who wish to regulate ovulation for this purpose alone.

Methods of contraception utilized prior to 1960 have been diminished by the "pill" and the "IUD" but a brief discussion of each is in order—for historical interest at least.

Condoms

During the 16th century the Italian anatomist Fallopius, for whom the Fallopian tubes are named, devised a linen sheath for the penis, an effective forerunner to the condom. Although Fallopius advised use of the condom to prevent the spread of syphilis, it was not widely accepted. Madame de Sevigne, in a letter to her daughter in 1671, called the condom an "armor against enjoyment and a spider web against danger." Casanova, in his *Memoires,* indicates he used condoms both to prevent venereal disease and to avoid impregnating his women. He was not a fan, however. "I do not care to shut myself up in a piece of dead skin in order to prove I am perfectly alive." Although used extensively in the brothels of the 18th century, the condom could not be manufactured in quantity until vulcanization of rubber was developed about the middle of the 19th century. Today about 700 to 800 million are produced annually in the United States.

The condom, as used today, is a covering for the penis usually made of thin rubber and sometimes previously lubricated. It is designed to capture and hold the seminal fluid, thus preventing its deposition in the vagina and over the cervix. The condom has the added advantage of preventing venereal disease.

There are several objections to the condom. First, it must be applied prior to intercourse. If this application occurs between sexual foreplay and coitus, this frequently annoys both partners. The annoying interlude may cause diminution in erection, particularly in men with borderline impotence. In older males, it frequently diminishes sensation as to make ejaculation difficult and even impossible. The woman may complain of dulled sensation or inability to sense the ejaculatory process. The biggest difficulty with the condom as a contraceptive is that the thin sheath may rupture or loosen, allowing sperm to enter the vagina. Also, pregnancies have resulted from premature ejaculation by the male prior to use of the condom. The average pregnancy rate when condoms are used is 15 per 100 women years —that is, 15 pregnancies will occur each year if 100 couples use the condom as the sole method of protection.

Coitus Interruptus

This is the oldest of the useful methods of contraception. The male withdraws his penis prior to ejaculation. There are several problems, however. Although the numbers of sperm in the fluid ejaculated may total 1 billion, only one is necessary for fertilization. A few sperm are usually present in the lubricating fluids secreted from the penis during sexual excitement. It is possible that several sperm may be on their way to the uterus well before ejaculation. Moreover, a great deal of coital experience and will-power must be employed by the male to enforce this method. The penis must be completely withdrawn, not only from the vagina but from the external genitalia as well. It is a little known fact that pregnancy may occur from ejaculation into or on the labia and, since the female may gain satisfaction from the male's ejaculation against the clitoris, this practice is common. Withdrawal does not, unfortunately, guarantee avoidance of pregnancy. The average pregnancy rate is 16 per 100 women years.

Rhythm Method

The principle here is the avoidance of coitus during the time when the woman may be ovulating. As a practical method of contraception, several difficulties are encountered. There is no way at present, despite extensive research, to determine with any precision when ovulation occurs. One index frequently used is to chart the basal body temperature. A slight dip in temperature is frequently seen at the time of ovulation, and this is followed by a maintained rise after it. The temperature rise is due to the progesterone secreted by the corpus luteum after ovulation. Progesterone is thermogenic, even when given to males, and the maintenance of a temperature rise, followed by a fall just prior to menstruation, is a fairly good index of ovulation. It is not proof, however. Only pregnancy is proof of ovulation.

Even though a woman with a 28-day cycle usually ovulates on the 14th day, a considerable margin of time must be allowed for safety. Under ideal circumstances, intercourse should be avoided from the 11th to the 18th day of each cycle. But even a week's abstinence is no insurance, for sperm may survive for several days, perhaps even longer inside the female genital tract. Pregnancies have been observed to occur after a single coitus seven days prior to apparent ovulation indicated by basal body temperature. If the ovulation is early or late, the risks of pregnancy are greatly compounded.

A simple formula may be used to calculate the fertile period. A woman should record her menstrual cycles for at least one year. The number 18 is subtracted from the number of days in the shortest cycle and 11 is subtracted from the longest cycle. The days in between are considered fertile or unsafe. For example, if the cycle varies between 25 and 32 days, 25 minus 18 equal 7 and 32 minus 11 equal 21. This means that a two week period of abstinence each month, a degree of deprivation unacceptible to most newly married couples whose average frequency of coitus is three to four times weekly. Because of the long life of some sperm, there is still a small risk of pregnancy even if the abstinence is observed. The average pregnancy rate is between 14 and 16 per 100 woman years.

Vaginal Spermicides

These are preparations, marketed as foams, creams or synthetic gels, which are inserted in the vagina against the cervix with a plastic applicator. They act by destroying sperm without harming the delicate vaginal lining. Only one application is required before each night of intercourse. The average pregnancy rate is between 20 and 22 per 100 women years.

Vaginal Diaphragms with Spermicides

The diaphragm was developed over 40 years ago by a European physician and consists of a circular metal spring covered with a fine latex rubber. The spring is flexible along one axis and the entire diaphragm can be compressed and easily passed into the vagina. It is then released in the upper and larger portion of the vagina where it covers the cervix completely. Since the dimensions of the vagina from the area behind the cervix to the pubic bone varies, diaphragms are available in specific sizes. This distance may be measured by vaginal examination, and the proper size prescribed. To increase the effectiveness of the diaphragm, it should be covered with a spermicidal jelly or cream. When the diaphragm is inserted properly, it will completely cover the cervix and cause no discomfort. A properly fitted diaphragm will be unnoticed by the male partner. It should be inserted prior to intercourse and preferably, be removed six to eight hours later, usually the next morning.

A woman using a diaphragm has a 10 to 12 per cent chance of becoming pregnant during the space of one year. Improper insertion, imperfect materials and forgetfulness probably account for most pregnancies.

Intrauterine Contraceptive Devices

The methods described thus far prevent the sperm from reaching the ovum. Intrauterine devices (IUD) utilize a different principle, although the precise mechanism of action is still unknown. IUD's are made of soft, flexible plastic molded into various sizes and shapes. They are inserted into the uterus where they may remain for indefinite periods. Although the original devices were much less effective in conception control than the Pill, newer ones are now available which may afford almost complete protection. In one recent study, a double-coil device was found to be comparable to oral contraceptives. In patients with low motivation for pill taking, such as the indigent population in the United States or in India or China, the double coil may prove to be the method of choice. Another new stainless steel IUD, which looks like a bunch of paper clips strung together, has demonstrated a substantial improvement in effectiveness. Spontaneous expulsions were noted in only 1 per cent of patients, and the need to remove the device occurred in only 5 per cent.

The intrauterine device is not new. It was used in Germany at least 40 years ago, but the method was discontinued because of endometritis and salpingitis. But these early devices were made of metal. Today's plastic devices have alleviated many of the problems. Four major types are available. The spiral is equipped with a small bead-like protuberance which extends out of the cervix into the vagina. The loop is equipped with two small threads which extend into the vagina for identification. The Bow is so called because it resembles a bow tie. The stainless steel ring was used extensively during the early days of clinical research but has fallen into disfavor because of the introduction of newer equipment. These are the Saf-T-Coil and the Majzlin Spring (see Fig. 15–1). Even newer devices known as the "Comet" and the "Butterfly" are now being tested.

Considerable research has been performed in an effort to determine how the devices work. The most logical explanation suggests that the IUD prevents pregnancy by speeding the fertilized egg through the tube. Thus, it arrives in the uterus before the endometrium is prepared for implantation. If this is the correct mechanism of action, the IUDs may be classified as an abortifacient since the fertilized eggs are unable to implant. Since definitions of the beginning of life have varied throughout the centuries, even in the Roman Catholic Church, it is probably more correct to describe the mechanism as "implantation prevention." Recent evidence suggests that the ovum may be delivered to the uterus on time but "toxic" reactions in the endometrial cavity prevent nidation.

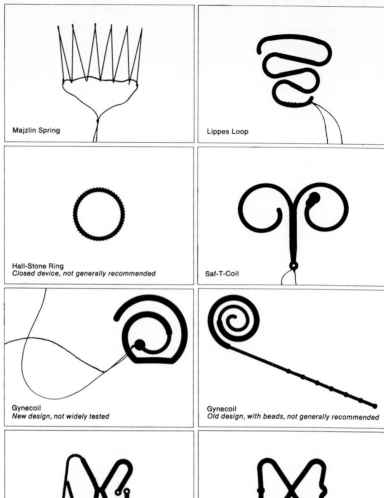

	SPIRAL	DOUBLE COIL	LOOP	BOW	STEEL RING
PREGNANCY	2.5	3.8	4.2	7.6	9.1
EXPULSIONS					
First	23.6	17.9	11.5	1.9	18.3
Subsequent	7.1	3.6	4.5	1.2	4.6
REMOVALS					
Bleeding and/or pain	21.1	21.4	17.5	16.2	11.9
Other medical reasons	11.4	5.6	5.8	6.0	3.5
Planning pregnancy and other personal reasons	8.9	4.8	6.7	6.0	7.6

Fig. 15-1.—Above, types of intrauterine devices. (Courtesy of Planned Parenthood-World Population.) **Below,** data from a study of 27,000 women confirming that explusion is the major drawback of intrauterine devices, particularly during the first two years. Bleeding and pain are the most frequently reported complications. (Courtesy of Dr. Christopher Tietze.)

The IUD is useful in certain women who find mechanical methods too messy and too demanding and in others who are not adequately motivated to use a diaphragm or cream. Some patients have persistent side effects from the Pill. Intrauterine devices are less effective than the Pill and they may produce disturbing symptoms, such as abnormal bleeding and pain.

The bleeding usually consists of intermenstrual spotting but hypermenorrhea has occurred. The exact incidence is unknown but probably occurs more frequently than recorded in most series. In one report of a ward population using a Permaspiral it was found that intermenstrual bleeding occurred uniformly after insertion. This was assumed to be a transient problem, for only 28 of 623 women (4.5 per cent) requested removal because of abnormal bleeding. Obviously enthusiasm for the method was a factor in the low reported incidence of bleeding by these patients since these women had no other choice of effective contraception. In another study using the loop, 96 of 706 devices were removed because of abnormal bleeding but these women had other contraceptive choices. The endometrium in these patients shows focal white cell infiltration of the endometrial stroma, increased edema, and a number of superficial and thin walled vascular channels. Therapeutic methods to stop bleeding have included estrogens, estrogens plus progestins, ascorbic acid, ergotrate and antibiotics. None have been uniformly successful. Furthermore, serious complications have occurred. Perforation of the uterus and pelvic infection have occasionally necessitated hysterectomy in young women.

The intrauterine device should not be used in the presence of uterine fibroids, or if irregular or unexplained bleeding has been noted. Congenital abnormalities of the uterus or infection of the cervix or vagina are contraindications to their insertion. In some instances, the IUD has been placed in a uterus containing an unknown (or known) pregnancy. Abortion usually results and may be followed by infection, peritonitis and sterility. The IUDs are also difficult to insert in a nulliparous woman because the cervix is so small. However, once the device has remained in place for 24 hours, performance in terms of pregnancy rates, expulsions, and removals for reason of comfort proves about the same for women who have borne children and women who have not. This has been the experience of Dr. Christopher Tietze, associate director of the biomedical division of the Population Council.

A major disadvantage of the IUD is the high "fall out" rate. This may go unnoticed. Therefore the patient must examine herself vaginally once weekly to be certain the device is still in place. Spontaneous expulsion of the intrauterine devices is a major clinical problem and the rates vary considerably. The highest rate of expulsion occurs with the permaspiral and the lowest with the bow. Although expulsions usually occur during the first few months after insertion, there is a continuing, albeit low, incidence of recurring loss. Changes in design have been directed toward enlarging the device and increasing its rigidity in order to prevent ejection. This may prove disadvantageous, however, since if the uterus contracts strenuously to eject the foreign body, it will extrude it through the myometrial wall if it cannot force it through the cervix.

Uterine perforations occur infrequently but are major complications. Deaths have been reported to occur in about 1.5/100.000 users per year—approximately the same death rate as that reported in pill users from pul-

TABLE 15-1.—EFFECTIVENESS OF VARIOUS METHODS
OF CONCEPTION CONTROL

METHOD	AVERAGE PREGNANCY RATE (PER 100 WOMEN YEARS)
Douche	37.8
Foam Tablets	22
Jelly alone	20
Coitus Interruptus	16
Condom	14.9
Rhythm	14.4
Diaphragm	12
Intrauterine Devices	3.9
Mini-dose Orals	3.9
Sequential Orals	1.4
Combination Orals	0.2

From Garcia, C. R.: Medical and metabolic effects of oral contraceptives and their implications, Clin. Obst. & Gynec., Vol, II, No. 3, Sept., 1968.

monary and cerebral emboli. Perforation is more likely to occur in post-partum patients, and is more common with the bow than other devices. Insertion should be delayed at least eight to ten weeks after delivery and the physician should utilize a tenaculum on the cervix to straighten the cervico-uterine canal and a sound should be utilized to make certain of uterine position. If the marker on the device cannot be seen at subsequent exams, or the device cannot be felt with a sound, x-rays of the pelvis should be obtained with the uterine cavity visualized with dye. Devices which lie in the peritoneal cavity should be removed to avoid the possibility of bowel obstruction.

The most common major complication of the IUD is unwanted pregnancy. Effectiveness may be correlated with size of the device—the larger the device—the fewer the pregnancies. When pregnancies do occur, the incidence of abortions and ectopic pregnancies is higher than expected. If pregnancy is suspected, the device should be removed because of the high first trimester loss seen with devices in place.

It may be seen from Table 15-1 that the mini-dose oral contraceptives and IUDs have the same degree of effectiveness but each is about 3 times as effective as either the diaphragm or condom. The sequential orals are almost 3 times as effective as the mini-dose orals and IUDs. The combination pill, the bulk of the oral contraceptives now in use, have an effectiveness far exceeding any other method. In terms of theoretical effectiveness, the combination oral contraceptive provides almost 100 per cent protection against pregnancy, the IUD 98 per cent and the diaphragm and condom 85 per cent or more.

There is no doubt that the IUD provides an effective method of contraception and it requires no motivation after insertion if side effects do not occur. (See Table 15-1.) The pregnancy protection rate is less than for oral contraceptives and the complications are much greater than those with traditional forms of mechanical contraception. It seems ideally suited for the patient who cannot or will not use oral contraception and for whom other mechanical methods are unreliable. The IUD, with all of its problems is preferable to an unwanted pregnancy. The device should be sterile and should be inserted by a competent physician who utilizes complete caution, is cognizant of the contraindications, and will remove the device should the occasion arise for doing so.

Oral and Injectable Contraceptives

The young American wife has clearly shown an extraordinary enthusiasm for oral contraception. In a National Fertility Study during the years 1960–1965, Westoff and Ryder reported that 81 per cent of white, non-Catholic women of age 20–24 who were college graduates, were using oral contraceptives. An additional 4 per cent said they may use it in the future. This is indeed an extraordinary level of acceptance for a procedure which was not even available in 1960. It is evident that the Pill, in the few years in which it has been available, has succeeded in transforming the pattern of fertility regulation in the United States. It is already the leading method of contraception among American women. Table 15–2 illustrates the oral contraceptives currently available in the United States and Figures 15–2, 15–3, and 15–4 show the structural formulas for each. There are two major types of oral contraceptives, combined and sequential. The combined agents contain a synthetic progestin and an estrogen; sequential agents utilize estrogen alone for 15 or 16 days followed by a combination of estrogen and progestin for 5 days.

TABLE 15-2.—THE CURRENTLY AVAILABLE ORAL CONTRACEPTIVES COMBINATIONS

DRUG	PROGESTOGEN	MG/TAB	ESTROGEN	MG/TAB	MANUFACTURER
Enovid 5 mg	norethynodrel	5.0	mestranol	.075	Searle
Enovid-E	norethynodrel	2.5	mestranol	.10	Searle
Demulen	ethynodiol diacetate	1.0	mestranol	.05	Searle
Ovulen (21 day, 28 day)	ethynodiol diacetate	1.0	mestranol	.10	Searle
Noriday	norethindrone	1.0	mestranol	.05	Syntex
Norinyl	norethindrone	2.0	mestranol	.10	Syntex
Norinyl-1	norethindrone	1.0	mestranol	.05	Syntex
Norinyl 1+80	norethindrone	1.0	mestranol	.08	Syntex
Norlestrin 1 mg (20-day, 21-day, 28-day, 28 day with iron)	norethindrone acetate	1.0	ethinyl estradiol	.05	Parke-Davis
Norlestrin 2.5 mg (20 day)	norethindrone acetate	2.5	ethinyl estradiol	.05	Parke-Davis
Ortho-Novum 1 mg	norethindrone	1.0	mestranol	.05	Ortho
Ortho-Novum 2 mg.	norethindrone	2.0	mestranol	.10	Ortho
Ortho-Novum 10 mg.	norethindrone	10.0	mestranol	.06	Ortho
Ortho-Novum 1/80-21	norethindrone	1.0	mestranol	.08	Ortho
Ovral	norgestrel	0.5	ethinyl estradiol	.05	Wyeth
SEQUENTIALS					
Oracon	dimethisterone	25.0	ethinyl estradiol	.10	Mead Johnson
Norquen	norethindrone	2.0	mestranol	.08	Syntex
Ortho-Novum SQ	norethindrone	2.0	mestranol	.08	Ortho

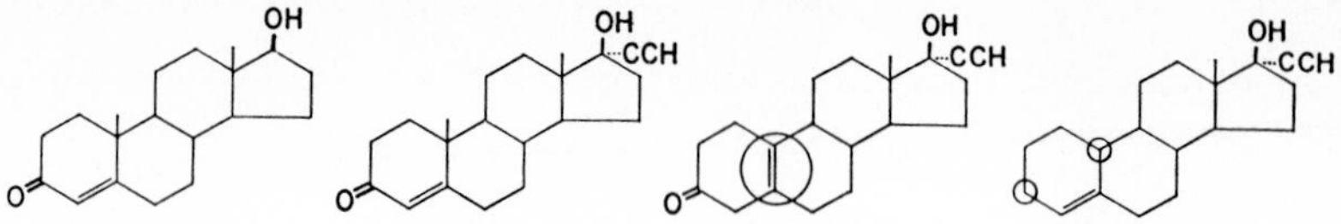

testosterone

ethisterone
(Pranone, Lutocylol)

norethynodrel
(Enovid, Enavid,
Conovid)

lynestrenol (Lyndiol)

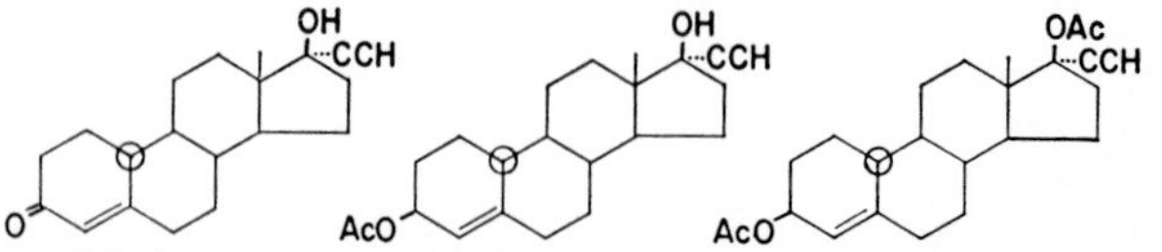

norethindrone
(Norlutin, Ortho-Novum,
Norinyl)

norethindrone acetate
(Norlutate, Norlestrin)

ethynodiol diacetate

Fig. 15-2.—The 19-nor progestins. Ethisterone is structurally the same as testosterone except for the addition of an ethinyl group in the 17-alpha position. Norethynodrel is a 19-nor compound (absent methyl group at position 19) with the ethinyl group at position 17 but with the double bond in the 5,10 position instead of the usual 4,5. Norethindrone is exactly the same but with the double bond in the conventional 4,5 position. Norethindrone with the addition of an acetate in the 3 position has double the potency. The addition of an acetate in the 17 position further increases the potency (ethynodiol diacetate). Lynestrenol is structurally different from norethindrone in one respect, the absence of the oxygen at the 3 position. All other progestational agents have the typical steroid configuration of a double-bond oxygen (ketone) at carbon 3. (From Kistner, R. W., Postgrad. Med. 39:207, 1966.)

Fig. 15-3.—Dimethisterone is similar to ethisterone, but the addition of the methyl group at position 6 increases the potency by six to eight times (this is not a 19-nor compound since the 19-methyl group is present; the ethinyl group is shown at the 17-alpha position). It differs from megestrol in two respects: (1) Megestrol is an acetate ester of hydroxyprogesterone—note the presence of 20 and 21 carbons in the typical configuration (the 17-alpha ketol group); (2) a double bond in the B ring denotes the removal of two hydrogen atoms. Ethynodiol diacetate, by comparison, is a 19-nor compound, more potency being obtained from the addition of acetate at the 3 and 17 positions. Chlormadinone is similar to megestrol, the exceptions being a halogen (chlorine) at the 6 position instead of a methyl group and a "dehydro" B ring. (From Kistner, R. W., Fertil. & Steril. 16:61, 1965.)

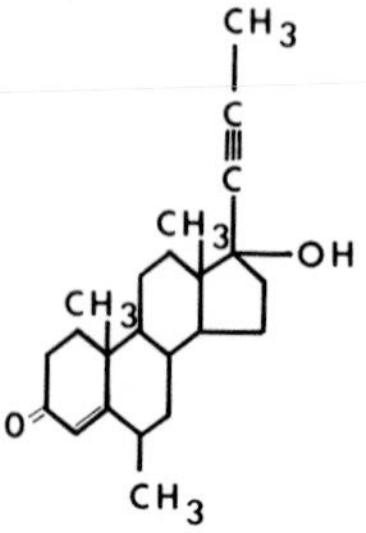

dimethisterone

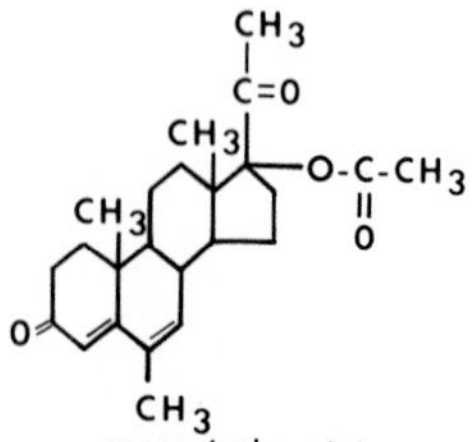

megestrol acetate

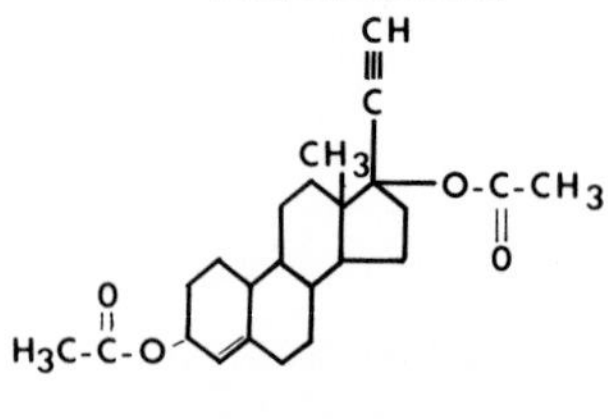

ethynodiol diacetate

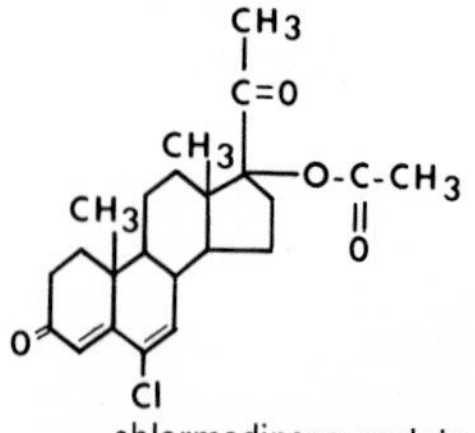

chlormadinone acetate

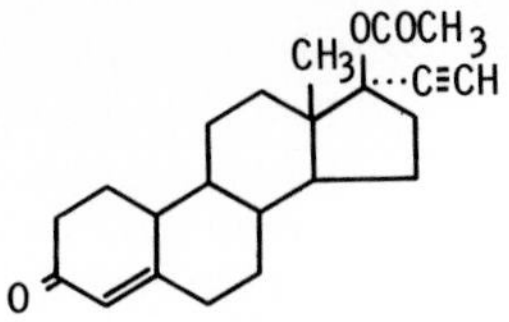

NORETHINDRONE ACETATE

17α-ETHYNYL-19-NORTESTOSTERONE
ACETATE

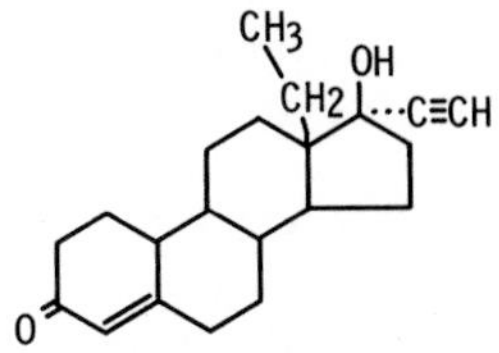

NORGESTREL

dl-13β-ETHYL-17α-ETHYNYL-
17-HYDROXYGON-4-EN-3-ONE

Fig. 15-4.—Structural formulas for norethindrone acetate (Norlestrin) and norgestrel (Ovral). Norgestrel is another 19-norsteroid, similar to norethindrone except for the presence of an ethyl group rather than a methyl group added at the carbon 13 position. Norgestrel is the most potent progestational agent available at the present time and has ten times the potency of norethindrone. (From Kourides, I. A., and Kistner, R. W., Obst. & Gynec. 31:821, 1968.)

Combined Formulations

The Enovid compounds combine a basic progestin, norethynodrel, with varying amounts of mestranol. Norethindrone, or norethindrone acetate, a more androgenic progestin, is used in Ortho-Novum, Norinyl and Norlestrin with varying amounts of mestranol or ethinyl estradiol. Ethynodiol diacetate, used in Ovulen, is a progestin similar to norethindrone acetate but it is less androgenic because of the hydroxyl (OH) configuration instead of the usual ketone (=O) at position 3. Added progestational potency is provided by the addition of a second acetate radical at position 3. The first compound to be made available as an oral progestin was ethinyl testosterone or ethisterone (Pranone). The addition of the ethinyl radical at position 17 converted testosterone, an androgen, into a progestin. Removal of the methyl side chain from position 19 markedly increased the progestational potency and thus these compounds were called 19-nor testosterones. Norethynodrel (in the Enovid compounds) differs by having the double bond in the A ring in the 5-10 position instead of the conventional 4-5 position and thus may be looked upon as an "estrogenic" progestin.

Recently a potent progestin, norgestrel, has been combined with ethinyl estradiol and is marketed under the name of Ovral. This progestin is quite anti-estrogenic and is similar to norethindrone. This 19-nor steroid has mild androgenic activity, about 7.5 per cent of the potency of testosterone proprionate. It differs from norethindrone only by the replacement of the methyl by an ethyl side chain at position 13. (See Figure 15-4.)

The number of available agents affords adequate latitude for selecting an oral contraceptive best suited to a particular patient. Thus, for the patient with an oily skin, acne or a tendency toward hirsutism, an estrogen-dominant progestin, such as norethynodrel, should be selected. For the patient who develops excessive side effects from estrogen (nausea, edema, sore breasts), an androgen-dominant progestin with anti-estrogenic properties is indicated. These include norgestrel and norethindrone. Furthermore, a combination should be selected which contains only 50 μg. of estrogen.

Side-Effects of the Combined Agents.—Estrogen irritates the gastric mucosa and diminishes the rate of sodium excretion by the kidney. These properties are responsible for the side-effects which most commonly cause women to discontinue the medication. In certain women abnormal hepatic function intensifies these side-effects since their levels of circulating estrogen will be high. Such patients complain of nausea (rarely vomiting), edema, generalized bloating, increased tension and headaches. The latter symptoms may be due to slight cerebral edema or to a specific effect of estrogen on the cerebral blood vessels. In women who have a normal amount of endogenous estrogen, it seems prudent to select a progestin-dominant agent. The obviously healthy, robust, full-breasted young women who ovulates and menstruates normally should not be overloaded with estrogen. This is true also of the patient who had had recurrent nausea during pregnancy or hyperemesis gravidarum.

On the other hand, an estrogen-dominant combination is frequently beneficial to the tall, asthenic woman with small breasts and scanty menses. In such individuals the excess estrogen (for her) seems to stimulate feminization, frequently improves libido, increases appetite and weight gain and results in improved well-being.

Estrogens are known stimulants for the growth of uterine leiomyomas and therefore if such lesions are present, the use of an anti-estrogenic progestin is indicated. Similarly, a combination pill, high in estrogen is more likely to stimulate breast growth and increase the discomfort due to fibrocystic disease. A progestin-dominant combination containing only 50 μg. of estrogen will reduce the discomfort due to the growth and edema of mammary tissue seen in women with extensive fibrocystic disease.

The action of the androgenic progestins is antagonistic to that of estrogen and therefore the patient should be carefully evaluated, both historically and physically, before pill selection. The "19-nor" progestins are essentially variants of testosterone and may produce masculinizing effects such as hirsutism, alopecia, acne, hypomenorrhea or even amenorrhea. These agents are protein anabolic and thus may cause increased appetite and excessive weight gain. Progesterone itself may cause lethargy or depression and these same symptoms may be noted in some individuals with the "19-nor" steroids. If symptoms due to the androgenic progestin are excessive, a more estrogen-dominant or sequential oral contraceptive should be substituted.

The solution to the problem of side-effects is obviously that of optimum selection. The answer may not be as simple as changing the estrogen-progestin balance of the medication but in a more precise manipulation of the dosage. The patient may be getting the correct medication, but not enough or too much of it. There are now over twenty compounds available to the physician but only one of these may be ideal for your patient.

The over-all effect of each combined formulation depends on the relative amounts of progestin and estrogen in each tablet, so that a similar effect is achieved by increasing the estrogen or decreasing the progestin content of any product. Thus Enovid-E is considered more estrogenic than Enovid-5 since the estrogen content in the former is increased from 75 to 100 μg. and the progestin is decreased from 5 mg. to 2.5 mg.

The total effect of an oral contraceptive is, of course, complicated by other factors such as the particular progestin used. For example, the 19-norsteroid compounds (norethynodrel, norethindrone and ethynodiol diacetate) are partly metabolized to estrogen thus increasing the estrogenic effect. Norgestrel possesses anti-estrogenic activity. In general, endogenous estrogen production is reduced by oral contraceptives but there is considerable variation in the extent of this reduction and in the metabolism of administered steroids in different individuals. Furthermore, the milligram potency of the two estrogens, mestranol and ethinyl estradiol, are about the same but the potency of the progestins is not related to their milligram dosage.

Newer marketing methods have attempted to simplify administration by having the user take a pill every day for 28 consecutive days (7 placebos or 7 iron tablets following the 21 combined estrogen and progestin). These are available utilizing norethindrone (Noriday), norethindrone acetate (Norlestrin 28 day or 28 day with iron) or ethynodiol diacetate (Ovulen-28). In many of my own patients who have noted side-effects such as headache, insomnia, hot flushes, weakness or depression during the 7-day interval that they are *not* taking the pill, I have used ethinyl estradiol 0.02 mg. daily during these seven days. In almost all instances their symptoms have been relieved. Undoubtedly these side-effects are related to the temporary estrogen insufficiency associated with ovarian inactivity. Because of the high incidence of "breakthrough" bleeding in the norethindrone 1 mg. plus 50 μg. estrogen combinations, additional estrogen has been added, as in Ortho-1-80, indicating that 80 μg. is present instead of the usual 50 μg. Still another plan of recent marketing technic is called the "lunar" scheme in which one tablet is taken for 21 consecutive days starting with the new moon.

Combined formulations have been used by some Catholic physicians to regulate the menstrual cycle so that the rhythm method of conception control may be practiced. In this method, an estrogen-progestin pill is taken from day 16 to day 25 and, in addition, fertile period abstinence is practiced. Since irregular menses are due to irregular ovulation and since the process of ovulation is frequently delayed in such individuals, it seems logical to assume that administration of the agent regularly on day 16 will occasionally result in suppression of ovulation. However, regulation of menses is accomplished, rhythm is practiced and pregnancies usually do not occur.

Failures with norethindrone and its acetate resulting in pregnancy are almost unknown. The same is true for norethynodrel, but, in general, there seems to be fewer failures with strongly progestational agents than with those having more estrogenic effects. The endometrium possibly provides a key to these differences: whereas strongly progestational compounds administered from the fifth day of the cycle allow only minimal proliferative change in the glands and stroma, compounds which are more estrogenic show a longer "early" secretory phase with later appearance of subnuclear vacuoles and more prominent sinusoids.

The mechanism of action of the various combined agents is undoubtedly suppression of ovulation. Corpora lutea have not been observed either by culdoscopy or at laparotomy in women who have been using these agents. Ethinyl estradiol and mestranol diminish FSH but have little or no effect on the midcycle LH peak. The dose of estrogen being used in the sequential agents (.08 mg. of mestranol or .10 mg. of ethinyl estradiol) approximates the amount which will produce ovulation inhibition and contraception for the entire population. Recently the trend has been to reduce the quantity of progestin in combined oral contraceptives, but the amounts of either progestin or estrogen are still sufficient to inhibit ovulation. These combination materials suppress FSH and abolish the midcycle peak of LH without changing the basal secretion of LH. Superficially it would appear that the effects of these agents on pituitary gonadotropins are a result of the individual actions of estrogen and progestin. However, there have been no quantitative studies to rule out synergism or antagonism between estrogen and progestin at the central nervous system (hypothalamus and pituitary) levels. Antagonism operates at the uterine level in that progestational effects are usually dominant on both the endometrium and the cervical mucus. However, if the dose of progestin is too small, the estrogenic effect will prevail.

The consensus of investigators is that over-all effectiveness of combined progestin-estrogen contraception is greater than with sequential therapy. The advantages of multiple antifertility mechanisms versus the single mechanism of ovulation inhibition has been suggested to explain the difference. However, it seems more reasonable that the difference lies with the size of the progestin dose. Since the amounts of progestin used in these combinations are enough to inhibit ovulation, they exceed the daily amount required to produce an antifertility effect for the population.

Thus, the combination estrogen-progestin oral contraceptives provide the most reliable means of birth control presently available, giving virtually 100 per cent protection if the tablets are taken daily for the required number of days in each cycle. Practically all failures result when one or more tablets are missed. But missing one tablet does not mean that pregnancy will occur and it is possible that the safety margin is higher with some products than with others. It is now known that occasional ovulation does occur in women on long term medication, but that other factors such as unfavorable endometrial, tubal and cervical environments contribute to the efficiency of these agents.

A woman's own hormone balance—whether predominantly estrogenic or progestogenic—can be assessed from her history, from symptoms associated with the menstrual cycle and from the physical examination. A rational selection of the proper combination pill may then be made which will secure the desired effect with a minimum of disturbing side effects.

CONTROL BY INJECTIONS

Preliminary clinical trials indicate that monthly injections of a long acting progestin-estrogen compound are a safe and effective method of birth control. A progesterone derivative combined with estradiol enanthate (Deladroxate*) has been administered in this way to more than 500 women in tests conducted in at least six institutions in the United States.

One of the major drawbacks to success with contraceptive methods in many countries is lack of sufficient motivation to take medication daily. There may be sufficient motivation for a monthly injection.

A combination of 150 mg. of progesterone derivative and 10 mg. of estrogen administered by injection on the eighth day of the menstrual cycle consistently inhibits ovulation in most patients. Furthermore, this method results in reasonably consistent cycles which average 27.2 days, with 80 to 90 per cent of the cycles falling within a range of ± 3 days. Only occasionally has the flow been excessive, and undesirable effects have been minimal. After discontinuation of the medication, normal ovulatory cycles have been re-established within 6 to 13 weeks.

Depo-Provera† has been utilized in several clinical studies in a dose of 150 mg. intramuscularly every 3 months. This appears to be an effective contraceptive procedure, although breakthrough bleeding is common.

Preliminary information from studies in which this dose was utilized indicates that the pregnancy rate was 0.5 per cent for 14,000 woman months. Other regimens, utilizing progestins with or without estrogens, have been given monthly or every 6 months. Zanartu, working in Santiago, Chile, has used injections of medroxyprogesterone acetate (Depo-Provera) in a dose of 250 to 300 mg. every 6 months and 200 mg. of nor-ethisterone enanthate every 3 months. Zanartu found that fertility inhibition was as effective as with conventional oral contraceptives and that the intramuscular administration produced no local reactions. Side-effects such as headaches and dizziness were minimal and seldom troublesome enough to necessitate stopping the treatment. The protection obtained with injectable long-acting progestogens is most significant and the risk of forgetfulness, an important factor limiting the effectiveness of oral contraceptives, is obviated.

Particular care has been given to the problem of fertility recovery in subjects who have been under treatment and desire subsequent pregnancy. Fertilization occurs within 3 to 8 months after the last nor-ethisterone acetate injection, and from 6 to 14 months after 250 or 300 mg. of Depo-Provera. Injectable progestogens can usefully be given immediately post partum, before the patients are discharged from the maternity wards, as well as after abortion. They do not interfere with lactation.

SEQUENTIAL FORMULATIONS

C-Quens‡ and Oracon were the first "sequential" oral contraceptives to be marketed. Each product consists of two kinds of tablets. One contains estrogen only and is taken during the first part of the menstrual cycle (for 15 or 16 days, starting on the fifth day). The other tablet contains estrogen

---

*Deladroxate contains 150 mg. of dihydroxyprogesterone acetophenide (Deladroxone) and 10 mg. of estradiol enanthate per cubic centimeter. E. R. Squibb & Sons, N.Y., N.Y.
†Depo-Provera-medroxyprogesterone acetate; 50 mg. per cc. Upjohn Co., Kalamazoo, Michigan.
‡C-Quens has been withdrawn by the manufacturer because the progestin, given during the last 5 days of the cycle, produced benign breast tumors in beagles. The dose administered was 25 times that given to humans; the same dose did not produce breast lesions in monkeys or other primates.

and progestin and is taken for the next five days. The sequential preparations utilize the same estrogenic components as the older products (mestranol in C-Quens, Norquen and Ortho S-Q; ethinyl estradiol in Oracon). The progestin in C-Quens, chlormadinone, and that in Oracon, dimethisterone, have not been used previously as contraceptives. The newer sequential agents are Ortho-Novum SQ, (the first 14 tablets containing 80 μg. of mestranol and the last 6 tablets containing 80 μg. of mestranol plus 2.0 mg. of norethindrone) and Norquen which contains the same estrogen and progestin but is marketed by a different company.

The administration of appropriate amounts of exogenous estrogen effectively inhibits ovulation in the human female. Since the normal menstrual cycle is characterized by secretion of estrogen in the early phase and by secretion of both progesterone and estrogen during the postovulatory phase, the sequential use of estrogen followed by estrogen-progestin seems appropriate because such a regimen simulates, to a certain degree, hormonal secretion and activity.

Although exogenous estrogens, in adequate amounts, will adequately inhibit ovulation, their administration may be associated with undesirable breakthrough bleeding during the latter phase of the cycle. This may be prevented by increasing the dose of estrogen but larger doses frequently cause nausea and breast tenderness. The addition of a progestin to the estrogen during the last few days of the cycle effectively controls this "nuisance" side-effect and produces bleeding similar to that which occurs during a normal cycle. Bleeding usually begins one to three days after discontinuation of the pills. The sequential agents, when properly used, have assured effective oral contraception. However, several observers have suggested that omission of a single sequential tablet is somewhat more likely to result in pregnancy than in the case of combination agents. It has been pointed out that the progestins, in addition to their anti-ovulatory action, may exert other antifertility effects. These include over-maturation of the endometrium which is out of phase with ovulation, should it occur. Glandular atrophy and stromal decidua induced by combination agents may prevent implantation of the fertilized ovum. Furthermore, the progestins effect anti-estrogenic changes in cervical mucus which are not conducive to sperm penetration and motility. It has been pointed out that pregnancies which occur on sequential regimens usually do so when the withdrawal flow is delayed. Pill taking in the ensuing cycle is similarly delayed. Since the estrogen suppression of FSH is absent for seven or more days, and since the peak of LH secretion is not regularly suppressed by sequential agents, conception may occur during the first week of estrogen administration. In recent clinical studies, in which the patient restarts pill taking no later than 7 days after the last estrogen-progestin pill of the previous cycle, pregnancies have not been observed.

One of the major indications for the use of sequential agents is failure of bleeding following withdrawal of the combined contraceptive agents. Patients using the combined estrogen-progestin compounds and experiencing no withdrawal flow should resume the medication five to seven days after it is stopped in order to maintain the pituitary inhibition necessary to prevent follicular maturation. Bleeding usually occurs after the second course of medication. However, if a withdrawal flow does not occur after two or more consecutive cycles of medication, the possibility of pregnancy should be considered. Since progestational agents do not interfere with the detection of human chorionic gonadotropin in the usual pregnancy tests, therapy need not be suspended in order to determine the presence of pregnancy. Some of the progestins display androgenic potential so early recognition of pregnancy is imperative. Although masculinization of female fetuses is probably more theoretical than actual at these lower dose level, it is important nonetheless to discontinue the use of a norethindrone compound should the patient be found to be pregnant.

The major advantage of the sequential method is that it more closely simulates the normal physiology of the menstrual cycle. Another advantage may be in the selectivity of gonadotropin suppression. While the estrogen in the first 16 pills depresses follicular maturation (by partial FSH suppression), the hypothalamic releasing mechanism for LH continues. It may be that the patients who have prolonged amenorrhea after combined agents do so because of interference with the hypothalamic pituitary release of LH. In this way these patients resemble the recent parturient who may have prolonged periods of amenorrhea subsequent to delivery. Certainly the administration of estrogen alone to women for dysmenorrhea or endometriosis has not been associated with prolonged secondary amenorrhea after the estrogen has been discontinued. In any event, the sequential regimen seems to lessen the risk of prolonged anovulation after cessation of therapy.

The sequential program is particularly applicable in women past the age of 35, in whom the increased risk of pregnancy is offset by declining fertility potential. Furthermore, after the woman enters her forties she may note symptoms of estrogen insufficiency, irregular cycles and occasional hypermenorrhea. The sequential agents provide adequate therapy for each of these entities. It should be added, of course, that such irregular and profuse bleeding must be investigated by uterine curettage before proceeding to hormonal therapy. Whether the amount of estrogen present in the sequential pill will aid in the prophylaxis of atherosclerosis, osteoporosis and coronary artery disease is conjectural. In any event, my plan is to administer the estrogen-progestin, in sequence, until the age of 50 or 52, then shift to estrogens alone.

At the opposite end of the age scale there is the problem of the teenager who asks for, or needs, contraceptive control. While many such individuals appear to be physically mature, they may not yet have established their mature endocrine pattern. Thus, they may be vulnerable to dangers of prolonged pituitary suppression. The low dose sequential agents seem to be preferable to the combined pill in this age group. Careful follow up at short intervals is suggested and the patient should be encouraged to discontinue the oral contraceptive at the earliest possible time and to become pregnant.

In return for the apparent reduction in long term risk, the hazard of possible unwanted pregnancy is increased. With the sequential agents, there will be an occasional ovulation, estimated at from 4 to 20 per cent depending upon the dosage. The incidence of pregnancy is said to be on the order of one or two per hundred woman-years. This is higher than that attributed to the combination pills in which the pregnancy rate is between zero and 0.5 per cent. The comparative risks of all methods of conception control is shown in Table 15-1.

Microdose Progestins Alone.—An important new development is the use of a progestin alone taken orally in small daily doses without interruption. The mechanism of action is incompletely understood but ovulation occurs, at least in some cycles, in 30 per cent or more of the subjects. In 26,000 cycles of use, the pregnancy rate was found to be 3.3 per 100 woman years. The only side effect for which significant data is available is breakthrough bleeding which occurred in 18 per cent of all cycles studied. There is as yet insufficient information on potential toxicity, indications for use, or contraindications to the use of continuous low dose progestogens.

A wide variety of progestins are being tested for clinical acceptability with doses ranging from 0.25 to 0.5 mg. of norgestrel or norethindrone. The pill contains no estrogen, thus eliminating all the untoward side-effects of this hormone. According to the April, 1968, report of the British Medical Journal, estrogen, not progestin, was indicted as the culprit responsible for the increased incidence of thromboses and embolism. In the "mini-pro-solo" (small doses of progestin only) pill, we can finally dispose of this major disadvantage of the pill. Moreover, "mini-pro-solo" does not usually interfere with ovulation, thereby eliminating one of the major disadvantages of the current pill. Finally, the system aids the memory problem.

The exact mechanism of action of this everyday progestin pill is unknown. Endocrine studies have shown that most women do ovulate. Only about 22 per cent of those tested have failed to ovulate, probably because of an individual sensitivity to the progestin. Since ovulation occurs, pregnancy is prevented by one or more of the following methods: (1) by changing the cervical mucus to make it unreceptive to sperm; (2) by altering the endometrium both in appearance and function so that a normally fertilized egg will not implant; (3) by speeding the delivery of the fertilized egg through the tube and into the uterus. In animals, estrogen slows the delivery process of eggs to the uterus; synthetic progestins may accelerate it. Since the fertilized egg usually spends about three days in the tube and another three days floating in the cavity of the uterus, it is possible that "early delivery" would result in an inhospitable reception so the egg is cast out in menstruation.

Vaginal Progestin.—Mishell and Lumkin have recently reported on the effectiveness of a progestin-impregnated Silastic* vaginal ring. In two preliminary studies involving a total of 22 women for a total of 11 medicated cycles, 50-400 mg. of medroxyprogesterone acetate (MPA) mixed thoroughly with the Silastic prior to molding of the ring inhibited ovulation for one cycle. Insertion of the MPA-impregnated soft rubber, cylindrical ring, ranging in size from 65–80 mm. in outside diameter, was followed by a "prompt rise in basal temperature as well as . . . an effect on the endometrium and the vagina similar to that observed when the drug is administered intramuscularly." In addition, the MPA inhibits LH release from the pituitary and thus inhibits ovulation at the dosages used. Upon removal of the ring, there was a rapid cessation of drug activity, as demonstrated by a fall in basal temperature and onset of withdrawal bleeding.

This termination of drug activity was usually followed shortly by presumptive evidence of resumption of ovulation which differs from the delay which occurs after stopping MPA injections.

Further studies with the MPA-treated rings are aimed at determining their feasibility as a practical method of contraception. After initial fitting

*Product of Dow-Corning, Inc.

by a physician, the patient can insert these rings herself each month and remove them to allow withdrawal vaginal bleeding.

Long awaited clinical trials utilizing a subcutaneous Silastic capsule have finally been initiated. In Santiago, Chile, 24 mm. Silastic coils filled with megestrol acetate are being implanted in the skin of women's forearms. The advantages are obvious: no calendar watching, no missed pills, no estrogen side-effects. Rudel has reported that each capsule releases about 29 mg. of progestin daily. Of 30 women who received three implants, three became pregnant; but no pregnancies occurred in 35 women who had four capsules implanted during a thirteen-month study. As with constant oral progestins, breakthrough bleeding was the major side-effect occurring in 15 to 20 per cent. An insufficient number of patients has been studied to warrant conclusions regarding effectiveness in the prevention of conception and the incidence of side-effects.

Scommenga has reported the use of crystalline progesterone encased in Silastic capsules placed in standard intrauterine devices in 23 women. It was hoped that progesterone would diminish uterine contractility and lower the expulsion rate of the intrauterine device. However, four women expelled the device and removal was required in four others, two because of endometritis and one because of bleeding.

Estrogens and Non-Steroidal Antifertility Agents

Estrogens in doses considerably larger than those necessary to inhibit ovulation (ethinyl estradiol 1.5–2.0 mg., or diethylstilbesterol 25–50 mg.) have been used to block fertility in women after midcycle coital exposure. The estrogen has been given for short periods up to 6 days during a time corresponding to the period from fertilization to implantation. The data are too preliminary to make a statement as to effectiveness. This has been referred to as postcoital contraception, but in reality, with estrogens, it must be postovulatory. Otherwise, with preovulatory coitus, this would become a high dose estrogen sequential therapy with ovulation inhibition. If estrogen does have a postovulatory contraceptive action, its effect on tubal transport and implantation must be evaluated as these functions may reflect changes in estrogen-progesterone balance.

In 1966, Dr. John Morris and Dr. Gertrude Van Wagenen of the Yale University School of Medicine, reported their studies with the "morning after" pill.

The report described tests performed on several women, most of them rape victims. They were given the familiar synthetic estrogen DES (diethylstilbestrol) for five days after intercourse in doses of 50 to 100 mg. This is two to four times the usual dose, and the patients, quite predictably, exhibited severe nausea and vomiting. None of the patients became pregnant, *presumably* because the estrogen altered the endometrium to prevent the fertilized egg from implanting.

But the size of the dose and the nausea produced were not the principal reservations about this method. The unknown fact is whether any of the patients were indeed pregnant. Medical science has no way of discovering, at this time, whether an egg has been fertilized that soon after intercourse. Dr. Celso Garcia of the University of Pennsylvania made this comment about the "morning after" pill: "One has to consider that very few cycles of observation and very few patients have been reported. We know that in the average fertile couple, there is about a 20 to 25 per cent chance of pregnancy occurring in any given cycle. So the fact that pregnancies have not been demonstrated in these women is not remarkable, and therefore we must not take a premature view that this is an acceptable method of treatment at this time."

SIDE-EFFECTS

From 15 to 35 per cent of patients taking oral contraceptives complain of various undesirable effects. Most of these are similar to the complaints recorded for these patients during their pregnancies. Some of the undesirable effects seem to be related to estrogen alone (nausea, vomiting, breast fullness, mastalgia, vaginal discharge), others to the progestin or the combination of estrogen and progestin (headache, dizziness, depression, apathy, fatigue, pelvic pain, chloasma). As in pregnancy, the incidence of these symptoms diminishes as the number of completed cycles increases. In many instances, the prescription of another estrogen-progestin combination results in a complete remission or great improvement. Chloasma is the most common dermatologic change, but its frequency varies widely. It seems to be more common among patients with olive complexions and also seems to be related to exposure to sunlight. This skin change varies in intensity but regresses after cessation of therapy.

Fluid retention and weight gain are definite problems in some patients. However, they are usually self-limited, and at the end of one year most patients' weights are similar to the pretreatment weights. The protein-anabolic properties of some of the agents may be a factor contributing to an increase of appetite and deposition of muscle mass. Some patients will notice a significant lessening of fluid retention and weight gain following the substitution of a compound containing only 50 μg. of estrogen.

Breakthrough bleeding or spotting occurs with varying incidence in association with all contraceptive regimens but diminishes in succeeding cycles. This "nuisance" side-effect may be managed either by increasing the dosage at the first sign of staining and continuing the medication at the higher level for the remainder of the cycle or by stopping the medication completely and resuming it 5 days later (a new cycle is thereby initiated). There appears to be some evidence that compounds associated with the lowest incidence of breakthrough bleeding are associated with a higher incidence of amenorrhea or failure of withdrawal bleeding. In some reports the incidence of amenorrhea subsequent to withdrawal of the medication has been as high as 40 per cent, suggesting an atrophic effect on the endometrium. If persistent staining or breakthrough bleeding continues beyond the third cycle of treatment, the endometrium should be investigated by biopsy or curettage. In our experience the endometrial cavity and endometrium have been normal in most of these patients. However, occasionally a submucous fibroid, chronic endometritis or an endometrial polyp will be found to explain the abnormal and persistent bleeding.

EFFECTS OF CONTRACEPTIVES ON SUBSEQUENT PREGNANCY

There is no evidence available at the present time to suggest that the incidence of genetic abnormalities is higher among children born to women of similar age who have not taken these compounds. Similarly, the incidence of spontaneous abortion is not increased among patients who become pregnant subsequent to discontinuance of oral contraceptive agents.

There does seem to be evidence, however, that the incidence of spontaneous abortion is somewhat higher in women who become pregnant during the first 3 months after pill cessation—just as occurs if conception occurs within the first 3 months after completion of normal pregnancy. On the basis of these observations, although meager and unsubstantiated, it seems prudent to advise against establishment of pregnancy during the first three months of discontinuation of oral contraceptives.

POSTPARTUM USE OF ORAL CONTRACEPTIVES

Lactation poses 2 major questions: (1) the effect on quality and quantity of breast milk, and (2) the potential effects on the infant if the estrogen or progestin is transmitted through the milk. The answer to the first question is now fairly definite—if oral contraceptive agents taken in current conventional doses are given following initiation of lactation, little if any inhibition is observed clinically. In one controlled study beginning on the 10th day post partum, women receiving estrogen-progestin combinations produced more milk than those given a placebo. This study utilized Lyndiol and milk secretion was determined by weighing the infant before and after each feeding. A slight reduction in "lactation time" from 17.1 months in controls to 15.9 months in users of oral contraceptives was noted in a study utilizing 6 different compounds. While a difference of one or two months may not be important in the United States, in less affluent areas infant nutrition is dependent upon an adequate supply of breast milk.

Thus, the use of an oral contraceptive agent may be started during the postpartum period, but the timing depends to a certain extent on the urgency of the situation. In general, it is recommended that the starting point should be the fifth day after the first spontaneous menstrual period. However, if use of the agent is begun during the third or fourth week post partum, a flow will usually follow within one week after cessation of the medication. If it does not, another 20-day cycle should be initiated. Certain investigators have started giving the compound as early as the fifth or sixth day post partum, as soon as lactation has occurred and nursing has begun. Some of these observers have noted a reduction in milk production, whereas others recorded either no change or an increase. Certainly, if a patient wishes to nurse her infant, therapy should not be started before the appearance of breast milk.

EFFECTS OF CONTRACEPTIVES ON THE MENOPAUSE

There is no statistically valid evidence that oral contraceptive agents either accelerate or delay the onset of the menopause. The effect may be likened to the suppression of ovulation for a long period because of the presence of a granulosa-theca cell tumor or arrhenoblastoma of the ovary. As soon as the tumor is extirpated, ovulation and menstruation are reinstituted. We have given massive doses of Enovid (70 to 80 mg. daily) for two or three years to patients with endometriosis and have not observed an appreciable delay in ovulatory menstrual cycles. As further evidence of the integrity of the total endocrine system, many of these patients have become pregnant during the first two or three ovulatory cycles.

The suggestion that prolonged use of oral contraceptive agents might predispose to ovulation and pregnancy beyond the age of 50 years seems more fanciful than factual. It completely disregards the natural aging process of the ovary and the natural diminution in fertility, even of patients who ovulate regularly, beyond the age of 40 years. Pregnancy after age 56 has not been recorded even in grand multiparas who have ovulated only 15 or 16 times during their lifetimes. It should be remembered that the ova are not simply stored in the ovary during the period of anovulation but undergo a process of follicular development and atresia similar to that noted during pregnancy.

Thyroid and Adrenal Glands

There is no conclusive evidence to indicate an alteration in thyroid or adrenal function in patients taking oral contraceptive agents for long periods. Circulating protein-bound plasma cortisol and iodine increase during the time the compounds are being used, not because of increased function of either the adrenal cortex or the thyroid but simply because of the effect of estrogen on the binding capacity of transcortin and thyroxin-binding globulin. (See Table 15-3.) A similar situation has been noted in patients treated with large doses of estrogen alone, as well as in patients who are pregnant.

Thyroid function may be assessed by means of radioiodine tests, which reflect the kinetics of iodine metabolism. Alternatively, there are tests which depend on the level of thyroid hormone in the blood. This may be measured directly by a PBI determination or indirectly by tests which depend on the uptake of I^{131}-tri-iodothyronine (T3) by the red cells or by a resin.

Estrogen-progestin compounds apparently have no effect on the uptake of radioiodine by the thyroid. The administration of these compounds does, however, alter the total thyroxine concentration in the blood which increases as a result of the increase in thyroxine-binding globulin (TBG). The uptake of I^{131}-T3 by a resin sponge is decreased in this situation. The increase in the PBI is a compensatory process insuring that the concentration of free thyroxine remains constant and that a euthyroid state is maintained. Thus, conventional methods for measuring the level of thyroid hormone in the blood are not applicable as diagnostic tests in women taking oral contraceptives, but it is possible to derive from the PBI and the T3 uptake test a free thyroxine index which can be used for assessing thyroid function in these circumstances.

Tests using ACTH stimulation demonstrate a normal response in the urinary excretion of 17-hydroxycorticoids, 17-ketosteroids, pregnanediol and pregnanetriol in patients receiving oral contraceptives for over 24 months.

Vascular Disturbances

Thrombophlebitis and Pulmonary Embolism

The furor arising from the rash of reports of thromboembolic processes in patients taking oral contraceptives has had salutary effects. First, it has made clinicians more alert to this particular emergency. Second, it has called attention to the appearance of spontaneous thrombophlebitis and pulmonary embolism in women of reproductive age. However, exhaustive efforts of numerous investigators and reviews of the findings by several committees, including those representing and selected by the Food and Drug Administration, had, prior to 1968, failed to show a significant correlation between the appearance of thrombophlebitis, phlebothrombosis and pulmonary embolism and the use of estrogen-progestin combinations.

Two more recent reports appeared in 1968, both from the United Kingdom. These reports indicated a "strong relation" between the use of oral contraceptives and death from pulmonary embolism or cerebral thrombosis in women who did not have conditions which predisposed them to such vascular accidents. The mortality rate per year for users of the Pill between 20 and 34 years of age was estimated at 1.3 per 100,000 and for those aged 35 to 44, 3.4 per 100,000. These figures represent approximately seven times the mortality rate from the same conditions among non-users. (See Table 15-3.)

Death from coronary thrombosis did not appear to be linked to use of the Pill, nor did the risk of thromboembolism seem associated with any particular contraceptive. In another report, the researchers calculated that "the risk of hospital admission for blood clots is about nine times greater in women who use oral contraceptives" than in those who do not.

Several objections to the United Kingdom reports seem obvious. In the latter study the investigators found 399 patients with "phlebitis, thrombophlebitis, thrombosis or embolism in any vein except the cerebral, coronary, hepatic and mesenteric veins; pulmonary embolism or infarction." But they then excluded 338 patients (85 per cent) from the study for a multiplicity of reasons. It is evident, therefore, that something over 75 per cent of the 214 exclusions were probably not taking oral contraceptives at the time of their thromboembolic episodes. If this is true, then only 20 per cent of the valid cases were related to oral contraceptives rather than the

TABLE 15-3.—ESTIMATES OF RISK OF DEATH FROM PULMONARY OR CEREBRAL THROMBOSIS IN USERS AND NON-USERS OF ORAL CONTRACEPTIVES
(Compared with Risk of Death from Certain Other Causes)

CATEGORY AND CAUSE OF DEATH	ANNUAL DEATH RATE/100,000	
	20-34 yrs. of age	35-44 yrs. of age
Healthy Non-Pregnant Women		
Pulmonary or Cerebral Thrombosis		
Users, Oral Contraceptives	1.5*	3.9*
Non-Users, Oral Contraceptives	0.2*	0.5*
Total Female Population		
Cancer	13.7	70.1
Motor Accidents	4.9	3.9
All Causes	60.1	170.5
Maternities†		
Complications of Pregnancy	7.5	13.8
Abortion	5.6	10.4
Complications of Delivery	7.1	26.5
Complications of Puerperium		
Phlebitis, Thrombosis, Embolism	1.3	2.3
Other	1.3	4.6
Total All Maternities	22.8	57.6

*Estimated Death Rate.
†Data from Registrar General for England and Wales for year 1966.
(From Meeker, C. I.: Use of Drugs and Intrauterine Devices for Birth Control. New England J. Med. 280:1058, 1969.)

45 per cent cited by Vessey and Doll. Dr. Louis E. Moses has commented: "Hence, it seems entirely possible that the conclusions reached by them and so readily accepted by the Food and Drug Administration were a product of faulty clinical selection of cases rather than their most elegant statistical evaluation of them."

Another factor of importance is the increasing number of case reports of thromboembolic manifestations occurring in healthy young men and women. Similarly, the incidence of pulmonary embolism has also been shown by many investigators to be significantly higher than hitherto suspected in young, apparently healthy women by isotopic scanning technics.

It is obvious that a Pill user who complains of leg or chest pain will be examined more carefully for thromboembolism than a non-user. In addition, more precise diagnostic measures will be initiated. Should death occur, the pathologist will perform a meticulous search for pulmonary emboli. Leg or chest pains occurring in the non-Pill user are likely to be dismissed unless they are severe or recurrent. Should death occur subsequent to a respiratory infection, a diagnosis of viral pneumonia would probably appear on the death certificate. If an autopsy is performed, and death was due to pulmonary embolism, the embolus would be discovered in only 25 per cent of patients.

If full credence is given to the British findings, Pill users have a sevenfold increased risk of death due to blood clots of the lungs or brain than non-users—and this has been emphasized in press reports. Somewhat less emphasized is the fact that these risks are extremely slight, 1.3 deaths per 100,000 in a woman 20 to 34 years of age, and 3.4 per 100,000 in a woman 35 to 44 years of age. As shown in Table 15–3, a British woman runs a greater risk when she rides in an automobile or crosses the street. Her chances of death from cancer are certainly greater. One physician expresses the degree of risk—and the degree of importance he attaches to the British findings—in this way: "For a woman under age 35, the decision to take the Pill for one year carries about the same hazard as the decision to hop into a car and drive for 12.5 miles." His comparison is based on traffic accident figures from the U.S. National Safety Council.

In 1969 a task force of the Food and Drug Administration's Advisory Council on Obstetrics and Gynecology released its findings of a retrospective study of 175 women aged 15–44 discharged from 43 hospitals after initial attacks of thrombophlebitis, pulmonary embolism or cerebral thrombosis. These patients were matched against 175 hospitalized control patients of the same age without thrombotic conditions. They concluded that users of oral contraceptives had an increased risk of thromboembolism 4.4 times greater than non-users. This committee added that much more research was needed to validate the conclusions of such a limited sample.

The risk of 4.4 noted above is just half of the increased risk in users of oral contraceptives noted in the British report. Furthermore, the study was retrospective and it was necessary to draw on the records of 47 hospitals in five metropolitan areas to assemble a test group of 175 patients. Researchers sifted through the records of almost 3,000 patients admitted for thrombophlebitis, pulmonary embolism or cerebral thrombosis to cull out all patients with a doubtful diagnosis or a possible predisposing illness. In 1970 the Committee on the Safety of Drugs in the United Kingdom reported that thromboembolism risk is doubled with oral contraceptives containing 150 micrograms of estrogen but at 50 micrograms the incidence is 21 per cent below the expected incidence in the general population. It is recommended, therefore, that physicians prescribe preparations containing only 50 micrograms of estrogen whenever possible.

Drill and Calhoun reported the average normal incidence of thrombophlebitis in non-pregnant women of childbearing age to be 1 case per 1,000 women per year based on data from patient visit to physicians. The antepartum incidence of thrombophlebitis is 0.5 cases per 1,000 women per nine months or 0.74 per year. In large-scale studies with users of oral contraceptives, the average incidence was 0.5 cases per 1,000 women per year based on cumulative data of 50,781 woman-years of use. While these studies are prospective, they were not carried out with matched controls.

A prospective report from Puerto Rico failed to reveal any relationship between oral contraceptives and deaths due to pulmonary embolism or coronary disease. The death rate averaged over the eight year study of almost 10,000 women was 5.7 per 10,000 for users of oral contraceptives compared to 6.6 for non-users.

CEREBROVASCULAR ACCIDENTS

Any evidence which suggests that the Pill is related to the development of strokes gives cause for concern. Several reports in the medical literature have merely listed the number of patients who sustained strokes while taking oral contraceptives. British physicians reported eight instances between 1962 and 1965. Another report in the United States listed 17 patients who sustained strokes, four of whom died. In this report, patients had been taking the Pill for one week to three years before the attack occurred. One patient had discontinued the Pill for 10 days and another for five months when the stroke took place.

Such studies are not convincing evidence that strokes are *caused* by the Pill. Again, before such a relationship can be proven statistically, it is mandatory that the incidence of the disease be higher in users than non-users. The above reports list only 25 stroke victims in approximately seven million users. Until recently the incidence of stroke among young, healthy females was thought to be non-existent or negligible. It was not until comparative studies became necessary that the true incidence became known. In that regard, another British study mentions 39 women between the ages of 18 and 45 who had strokes between 1955 and 1965. Of these 39 women, 21 had strokes before 1961 when oral contraceptives were first used, and 18 since then. The study showed that between 1955 and 1960, the number of women in the reproductive age group who had strokes varied from 1 to 5 a year. During the post-Pill years of 1961 to 1965, the number varied between 2 and 4 cases a year.

Any effort to correlate the relationship between cerebrovascular accidents and oral contraceptives must necessarily take into consideration the mortality rate in this disease. Vital statistics listing deaths among women from strokes show that they occur from the first year of life through old age. Among white females between the ages of 15 and 24, the mortality rate from strokes is 1.4 per 100,000 population. Between the ages of 25 and 34, the rate increases to 3.4 per 100,000. From 35 to 44, the rate becomes 10.1 per 100,000. These figures represent spontaneous occurrence of stroke in all women, not in Pill users. By comparison, reports in 1968 by the *British Medical Journal* indicate mortality rates of the Pill from emboli to be: 1.3 per 100,000 between 20 and 34 years of age and 3.4 per 100,000 for those between 35 and 44. In other words, prior to age 35, the incidence of death in both situations is about the same, but after that age a woman's chances of dying from a stroke increase threefold over that of a woman's death due to using the Pill.

It is evident that strokes have always occurred among young, apparently normal, women. However, since these individuals had not been taking any particular medication, specific causes for the strokes were not sought. For the most part, these deaths were thought to be due to congenital abnormalities in the blood vessels of the brain. They probably still are, and if these unfortunate women had been taking aspirin or penicillin, these medications might be indicated as causing the strokes with as much proof as that presented to incriminate the Pill.

Nevertheless, manufacturers of oral contraceptives, desiring to be supercautious, warn that the Pill should not be prescribed for the woman who has a history of stroke. Pregnancy is also contraindicated, but other methods of conception control are advised. Physicians have been warned to discontinue the Pill pending examination of the patient if she complains of sudden partial or complete loss of vision or if there is sudden onset of double vision or migraine headaches. Furthermore, it is suggested that these patients should have ophthalmologic examination. If papilledema or blood vessel disease is observed, the Pill should be stopped.

HYPERTENSION

The sudden appearance of hypertension has been noted in a few users of oral contraceptives. This may be related to the effects of estrogen on the renin angiotensin-aldosterone system with alteration of electrolyte and fluid balance. An individual sensitivity of vascular smooth muscle is probably a basic etiologic factor and such individuals should not use these agents. Garcia reports that 96.8 per cent of 312 subjects in Puerto Rico had normal blood pressure values prior to therapy. Only 17 users disclosed an elevation at any time in the study and no significant increases were observed on serial follow-up relative to long term use.

If hypertension occurs during the administration of oral contraceptives, the medication should be discontinued and diagnostic studies initiated to determine the cause.

MIGRAINE

In a recent survey of members of the American College of Obstetricians and Gynecologists, one third of the physicians had noted migraine attacks in patients using oral contraceptives. A study by three neurologists at Western Reserve Medical School linked stroke-like symptoms with migraine headaches and these in turn with oral contraceptives. The report warned women to stop the Pill promptly if they developed severe migraine, especially if it happened to be accompanied by numbness of the extremities or impaired vision. This report cited only nine patients and did not claim to have established a statistical relationship between strokes, migraine and the Pill. The Western Reserve neurologists also stated that electroencephalograms of the nine patients showed exaggerated brain waves—but that these patterns were *not initiated* by the Pill. Stated simply, this implies that certain patients having a tendency to migraine attacks may have this condition *aggravated,* not caused, by the Pill.

Numerous patients have typical "menstrual" migraine. These attacks occur just prior to the onset of menstruation when the levels of estrogen and progesterone are low, not high. This suggests that the estrogen and progestin in the Pill do not cause migraine attacks since the oral contraceptives substitute approximately normal amounts of each hormone. Furthermore, many women with migraine are appreciably relieved during pregnancy when the estrogen and progesterone levels are extremely high, and similar improvement has been noted in patients treated with the Pill to effect pseudopregnancy. Many patients develop migraine attacks during the days when they are not taking the medication. Thus, it would appear that the effects of estrogen and progestin on migraine conditions reflect an individual sensitivity to these hormones and the attack may be precipitated more by *changing* levels of hormones rather than by the Pill itself.

Nordquist suggests that migraine headaches may be estrogen induced. Evidence to support this theory has not been forthcoming but migraine attacks have been noted in women following injections of estrogen for treatment of the menopause. This has been shown to be dose-related since small doses of estrogen did not induce a migraine attack. Nordquist has also reported that progesterone and the synthetic *progestins protected against migraine* when they were administered in the so-called "minidose." The dose he gave was too small to prevent ovulation, but pregnancy did not occur, presumably because of the progestin's effects on the endometrium and the cervical mucus. In a large number of patients so treated, Nordquist noted a substantial diminution in the incidence of migraine headaches. Combination estrogen and progestin pills did not offer this protection. If the estrogen in the oral contraceptive is the inciting factor, it may be postulated that the use of anti-estrogenic progestins such as norethindrone or norgestrel, given alone, may negate the effect of endogenous estrogen on sensitive neurovascular sites in the cerebral blood vessels.

If the evidence, pro and con, concerning the Pill and migraine attacks has seemed confusing, that is an accurate reflection of the present status. We just don't know. The Hellman Committee in its report to the Food and Drug Administration stated that more studies were necessary before conclusions about the Pill and migraine headaches could be drawn.

HEPATIC EFFECTS

Hepatic function has been thoroughly studied in long-term field trials both in Haiti and in Puerto Rico. Although the incidence of hepatic insufficiency is generally higher in these countries than in the United States, jaundice has not been observed among the women studied. Studies of sulfobromophthalein (Bromsulphalein) excretion and transaminase have shown slight deviations from the normal values, but liver biopsies and other studies of liver function have been within the normal range. Recent studies of patients receiving norethynodrel with mestranol in cycles for suppression of ovulation have indicated a reversible reduction of the hepatic transport maximum for sulfobromophthalein. The relative hepatic storage, however, was unimpaired, and the dye was retained in plasma primarily as a conjugate. The administration of estradiol alone (2.5 mg. a day for ten days) did not alter the transport maximum, the storage, or the percentage of conjugated dye in plasma. These observations suggest that the effect of norethynodrel and mestranol on sulfobromophthalein metabolism is probably related to the progestin that regularly interferes with the transfer of conjugates from the liver cell into the bile. They suggest also that caution should be exercised in the clinical use of these related drugs in children or adults with hereditary, developmental, or acquired defects of hepatic excretory function.

Because of reports that liver dysfunction developed uniformly in postmenopausal women receiving estrogen alone or in combination with progestin, liver function was investigated with transaminase, alkaline phosphatase, thymol turbidity, and cephalin flocculation tests in a group of 36 postmenopausal women with a mean age of 57 years who had received norethynodrel with mestranol for a mean period of 8.7 months. No significant abnormalities were found. Slight abnormalities in cephalin flocculation were noted in six patients, and in another six there was an elevation in alkaline phosphatase of 1 unit. Significant hepatotoxicity from oral estrogen-progestin therapy was not encountered in these subjects.

Alterations in hepatic function associated with jaundice has been reported more frequently during pregnancy and during the administration of estrogens in Chile and the Scandinavian countries. In these countries the genetic importance of this hereditary metabolic disorder has been supported by the experiences of Larsson-Cohn.

Abnormalities in liver function occurring subsequent to the use of oral contraceptives return to normal after the medication is discontinued. A few reports have indicated that a progressive rise in Bromsulphalein (BSP) retention occurs during the first 3 months of use but deterioration does not occur during long term use. In many of my patients receiving 8 to 10 times the usual contraceptive dose for pseudopregnancy in treating endometriosis, the BSP retention has returned to normal after 5 to 6 months of therapy after showing a moderate increase in retention during the first 3 months.

It is not necessary to perform liver function tests prior to initiation of oral contraception if the patient gives no history of jaundice or evidence of liver disease. But these agents are contraindicated if the patient has a history of recurrent jaundice of pregnancy or if an excretory defect, such as that found in the Rotor or Dubin-Johnson syndromes, is present. The development of mild alterations in liver function tests does not necessitate discontinuance of the medication in the absence of jaundice. However, should fever, skin rash, pruritus, arthralgia or dark urine occur, anicteric jaundice should be assumed and the oral contraceptives discontinued.

DIABETES

Wynn has recently reported that about 15 per cent of women taking oral contraceptive agents have a change in carbohydrate metabolism indistinguishable from the effect produced by small doses of exogenous cortisol. This effect, known as "steroid diabetes" occurs as a result of stimulation of the adrenal gland to secrete increased amounts of cortisol and is undoubtedly due to the estrogenic component of the agent. Steroid diabetes may lead to clinical diabetes, but such progression is uncommon unless there is a familial disposition to diabetes mellitus. However, prolonged steroid diabetes is associated with an increased incidence of atherosclerosis and coronary or peripheral vascular disease.

There is no evidence that oral contraceptives produce diabetes, but investigators are concerned about a specific effect of the estrogen-progestin combination which may expose a latent tendency to develop the disease. In one study, 1 user in every 4 utilized blood sugar at a slower rate than normal. It has been known for quite some time that blood sugar levels are elevated in some women during pregnancy. Glycosuria may also appear, but after the pregnancy has been terminated, both the blood and urine tests return to normal. A certain percentage of these women will develop overt diabetes later.

Thus, an important question to be answered is whether the oral contraceptive, if used for prolonged periods, is likely to convert latent diabetes into the active disease. Considerable research on this relationship has already been accomplished, but ironclad conclusions are not available. Spellacy has speculated that "there is a possibility that some women may have developed permanent changes in their sugar metabolism, but we don't know yet whether they will go on to develop true diabetes."

The Hellman Committee, in its report on the safety of oral contraceptives to the Food and Drug Administration, stated that data on the effects of the Pill on sugar metabolism in experimental animals and in women are contradictory. The Committee noted that abnormal glucose tolerance tests have been observed in as many as 40 per cent of women using oral contraceptives. Among women with a family history of diabetes, the abnormal tests were even more frequent. It was also noted that insulin levels were above normal in "supposedly normal" women taking oral contraceptives. This is understandable, since more insulin would be needed for the hyperglycemia. In addition, it is known that some diabetic women require larger amounts of insulin while taking the Pill. The Hellman Committee reported, however, that all of these changes regress after oral contraceptives have been discontinued and are similar to those observed during a normal pregnancy. It is not known whether pregnancy can cause diabetes, although diabetes is more prevalent among women having had numerous pregnancies.

The relationship between oral contraceptives and abnormal glucose tolerance tests may be less a cause for concern than previous reports have indicated. Beck and his co-workers at the University of Colorado concluded that oral contraceptives appeared to be significantly less likely to cause diabetes than a normal pregnancy. They studied 27 women with a family history of diabetes during the latter months of pregnancy and found all glucose tolerance tests to be abnormal. After delivery, all began oral contraceptives and two weeks later they were retested. Abnormal glucose tolerance tests were found in only three patients and these were in a group of 12 classified as having "pregnancy diabetes" when previously tested. After two weeks to six months on the Pill, no additional women showed abnormal glucose tolerance.

Beck suggested that the oral contraceptives alter the glucose tolerance test in a way quite different from that seen in pregnancy or induced by the administration of cortisone-like hormones. Whereas the latter are due to inhibition or retardation of insulin secretion by the pancreas, the oral contraceptives increase the resistance of tissues to insulin so that it cannot function normally—to lower blood sugar. Beck suggests that the oral contraceptives might unmask diabetes in some, but not all, individuals with undetected disease. But pregnancy, or the administration of cortisone, will do a much better job of unmasking.

Dr. Jerome Conn commented, "The question of *possible* adverse effect of oral contraceptive agents on carbohydrate tolerance and the development of diabetes must be kept in proper perspective." It has been shown that a diabetic glucose tolerance curve may be produced in *essentially anyone* with a large enough dose of corticosteroids. This is a far cry from the statement published in the *Lancet* in 1967 that "it may be wise to avoid these drugs (the Pill) in women with known abnormalities of glucose tolerance and possibly also those with a family history of diabetes." According to the work of Beck, pregnancy should also be avoided by patients in this category.

The majority of specialists in obstetrics and gynecology prescribe the Pill for women who are already diabetic. Three-quarters of the physicians polled by the American College of Obstetrics and Gynecologists reported that they give the Pill to diabetic patients. When this is done, the patient should be observed more frequently by the physician managing her diabetes. Increase in the level of blood sugar may necessitate changes of insulin dosage or re-arrangement of diet or both. There is no doubt, however, that the risks associated with use of the Pill do not even approach those due to pregnancy.

The work of Dr. Priscilla White at the Joslin Clinic in Boston is of interest in regard to the effect of hormones and pregnancy on diabetes. For many years, White has treated all pregnant diabetic patients with extremely large doses of estrogen and progesterone. She observed that the use of these hormones materially diminished the high fetal mortality rate usually found in diabetic patients. Since White's patients were classified as "severe" or "very severe" diabetics, her results are all the more remarkable. A few obstetricians have disagreed with Dr. White, feeling that the improved fetal mortality rate was due more to her personal attention and diabetic management than to the hormones. Despite the objection, it is obvious that the tremendous doses of the hormones did not adversely affect the state of the diabetes.

FIBROIDS

The growth of uterine leiomyomas is known to depend on estrogen, usually endogenous—but occasionally exogenous. The majority of reports of enlargement of leiomyomas has occurred in women taking estrogen-progestin combinations constantly, usually for the treatment of endometriosis. They regress in size after therapy is discontinued, similar to the sequence noted during and after normal pregnancy. It is unusual to find significant changes in the size of leiomyomas when combinations utilizing an anti-estrogenic progestin plus only 50 mcg. of estrogen are given in cycle.

The normal secretion rate of endogenous estrogenic substances probably exceeds that given to such patients in pill form and certainly many women develop leiomyomata who are *not* using oral contraceptives.

Goldzieher noted carneous changes in leiomyomas in patients receiving pure progestins in high dosage and I have seen 2 patients who exhibited the same pattern. Both had received Depo-Provera for endometriosis. Patients receiving 2 mg. of norethindrone daily, continuously for 30 to 90 days did not note this change. Wallach states that in the Family Planning Clinic of the University of Pennsylvania, where a substantial number of women have small to medium-sized leiomyomata, no instance of detectable increase in size has been noted. Wallach states further that the presence of small leiomyomata has not been considered a contraindication to hormonal contraception in his Clinic. I am in agreement with this statement and choose to utilize an androgenic progestin plus 50 mg. of estrogen in women harboring small leiomyomas.

Breast Changes

During the early cycles of therapy with oral progestational agents, the incidence of mastalgia associated with fullness and engorgement of the breasts increases. This complaint diminishes rapidly in succeeding cycles. We have noted a diminution in the diffuse nodularity of breast tissue in patients with extensive fibrocystic disease, particularly when norethindrone compounds have been used. Occasionally breast secretion is noted during the cyclic administration of these agents but it is more common during pseudopregnancy or, especially, at the termination of pseudopregnancy. There has been no reported increase in the incidence of fibroadenomas or development of cysts in patients receiving oral contraceptives. It should be emphasized that patients should have a thorough breast examination prior to the initiation of therapy, and any dominant lump should be removed surgically before an oral contraceptive agent is prescribed.

Relation of Oral Contraceptives to Secondary Amenorrhea and Infertility

It has been reported that approximately 65 per cent of women who have taken oral contraceptives became pregnant as desired in the first three months after discontinuance of the agent. However, the incidence of women desiring but unable to accomplish pregnancy in the remaining 35 per cent is unknown. Recently a report of 206 patients noting amenorrhea and infertility after discontinuing oral contraceptives gave factual data in this regard. Undoubtedly there are many more unreported patients with a similar problem, but the number, in relation to the millions of users, is indeed minute. It is assumed, but not proven, that these women are amenorrheic as a result of temporary blockade of pituitary gonadotropic function. Ovarian inactivity with resultant low secretion rates of estrogen and progesterone follows, and the endometrium becomes atrophic. The typical dose, in the patients reported, was 5 mg. of Enovid, and the average duration of therapy was less than one year.

Analysis of the menstrual history of the patients in question, however, reveals that several were treated initially "to regulate cycles," an indication that an oligo-ovulatory status might have been present prior to therapy. Furthermore, patients in the age group reported who are nonusers of oral contraceptives frequently note irregular cycles, prolonged secondary amenorrhea, and infertility. Before concluding that the estrogen-progestin combinations are causally related to these disorders, it would be necessary to show a statistically significant increase in users over non-users. Indeed, secondary infertility is noted by many women who have had a normal first pregnancy, an uncomplicated puerperium, and resumption of normal cyclic menses. In some of these patients, pelvic disorders such as tubal inflammation or endometriosis are etiologic, but in the majority of individuals the precise cause of the infertility is unknown.

Therapy of the anovulatory process following the use of oral contraceptives is said to be unsuccessful. As one investigator stated "what is most disturbing is that some of these women develop severe atrophy of the endometrium and appear to be relatively unresponsive to various types of therapy, including clomiphene citrate." I have not found this to be so in the patients I have seen personally. (These were expected to have post-treatment ovulatory difficulties because of the prolonged use of Depo-Provera for endometriosis recurrent after surgery.) All such patients have had ovulatory menses subsequent to the use of clomiphene or clomiphene-human chorionic gonadotropin (HCG) therapy. As a matter of fact, one of our first treated patients, in 1960, became pregnant after the first course of clomiphene and delivered twins at term.

Patients with oligo-ovulation or secondary amenorrhea occurring subsequent to the use of oral contraceptives should be subjected to a diagnostic evaluation similar to that used for these disorders in nonusers. The physician should not assume a post hoc, ergo propter hoc relationship.

Cancer

Breast.—There is no direct, statistically significant evidence to support the contention that the estrogen or progestin in the oral contraceptive agents initiates carcinoma of the breast, endometrium, or cervix in the human female. Transfer of the data concerning the development of mammary carcinoma in a specific inbred strain of mice by estrogenic substances to the human female is neither logical nor scientifically accurate. In order to duplicate the experiment on a milligram-for-milligram basis in regard to dose and body weight, it would be necessary to administer overwhelming amounts of estrogenic substances to the human female for a period equivalent to one fourth of her natural life. Furthermore, the estrogenic substance in the murine experiment did not initiate mammary carcinoma but merely accelerated the rate at which cancer developed.

If the administration of estrogenic substances, such as diethylstilbesterol, were related to the development of carcinoma of the breast in the human female, it would be logical to assume that the incidence of breast carcinoma had increased. Diethylstilbesterol and other estrogenic substances have been used for over 20 years, yet the incidence of carcinoma of the breast in the human female was the same in 1965 as in 1900. In addition, direct observation of patients receiving estrogenic substances for prolonged periods, either for treatment of osteoporosis or following surgical castration at a young age, actually has revealed a lower incidence of mammary carcinoma in comparison with similar control subjects who did not receive estrogenic therapy.

There is no doubt that women with a family history of mammary cancer are predisposed to the development of this malignancy. This being so, the most important aspect of therapy for these individuals is frequent breast examination and excision of dominant masses. Evidence is not at hand to indicate that such individuals will increase their possibility of developing breast cancer prematurely or at all if they use oral contraceptives.

Garcia and associates have shown that the incidence of physical evidence of chronic cystic mastitis, such as diffuse nodularity, is reduced during the time that oral contraceptives are used. Similarly, cystic mastalgia associated with fibrocystic disease is frequently improved. As of 1966, no cases of mammary carcinoma had been reported among users of oral contraceptives. This proves nothing, however, since the latent period between use of a carcinogen and appearance of the disease may be as long as ten years. Tietze has indicated that a prospective, properly controlled study would necessitate 11,000 women in each group in order to show a five-fold increase in incidence; 85,000 would be needed in each group to show a doubling of the rate. During the years 1956–1967 I did not see one case of breast cancer in users of oral contraceptives at the Boston Hospital for Women Clinic or in my private practice. In 1968, 2 of my patients were found to have localized breast cancer—each had been using oral contraceptives for less than two years.

Cervix.—The relationship of the estrogen-progestin combinations to cervical dysplasia, carcinoma in situ and invasive cancer is presently under intensive and expanded investigation. Several studies, at present incomplete, indicate that there might be an increase in abnormal cytology and biopsies showing carcinoma in situ in women using oral contraceptives. However, one study has been rejected by biostatisticians because of inadequate data regarding predisposing causes. The other study, carried out in a low socio-economic group, matched oral contraceptive users against diaphragm users. Since the *prevalence* of cervical carcinoma is higher in this group of patients anyway (non-white, multiple sexual partners before age 21, increased frequency of coitus prior to age 21), valid conclusions regarding an increased incidence of carcinoma in situ cannot be drawn. Furthermore, it is possible that the use of a diaphragm (preventing penis-cervix contact) might diminish the incidence of cervical neoplasia. The use of oral contraceptives affords the physician an opportunity to screen by vaginal cytology large segments of the population initially, then permits follow-up if the contraceptive prescription is limited to six months. Early reports by Pincus and Tyler indicated a lessened incidence of positive cytology in users than anticipated in an untreated, but similar, population. This might have been suspected since patients with suspicious or positive cytology, or having cervical dysplasia by biopsy, were eliminated from the survey at the beginning of the study. There is no reason to suspect that the oral contraceptives will protect against epithelial abnormalities of the cervix. Recent reports from Puerto Rico indicate that positive cytology does occur. Such data is important since it suggests that oral contraceptives do not mask abnormal cytology.

It is important to differentiate the *incidence* of cervical dysplasia and carcinoma in situ which occurs in users of oral contraceptives from the *prevalence* of these lesions in a similar population. If these agents are used in a low income, non-white, highly fertile population, an increased prevalence of cervical cancer may be anticipated. An increase in incidence of statistical value, according to Tietze, would necessitate a comparative study of 7,500 users and 7,500 matched controls for 1 year if a five-fold rise in incidence is to be detected and 60,000 if a doubling of the rate was desired. In view of these facts, it is not surprising that it has been difficult to set up and effect long-term prospective studies in the United States.

The first long-range prospective study comparing users and non-users of oral contraceptives has recently been reported by Sandmire in a homogeneous group of white middle-class women in Green Bay, Wisconsin. He found 28 cancers of the cervix among 12,000 non-users, a rate of 1 in 428. Six cancers were found in 3,000 Pill users, a rate of 1 in 500. The difference is not statistically significant.

Dr. Paul Younge, chief of the cervical carcinoma in situ clinic at the Boston Hospital for Women, has stated that cancer of the cervix is a preventable disease. The use of oral contraceptive agents makes this goal more realistic since initial screening should detect all degrees of dysplasia and adequate therapy may be instituted.

Endometrium.—Endometrial carcinoma frequently develops in hyperplastic or atypical hyperplastic endometrium (carcinoma in situ). This process has been shown to be related to the continuing secretion of endogenous estrogen without the cyclic differentiating effect of progesterone. I have suggested that carcinoma of the endometrium may be preventable if appropriate therapeutic measures are taken to secure ovulation (and secretion of endogenous progesterone) in younger women and if progestin is supplied cyclically to patients approaching the menopause. We have been able to produce carcinoma of the endometrium in the rabbit by the use of a methylcholanthrene-coated string inserted into one horn of the uterus. The simultaneous administration of progestational agents, however, prevents the development of carcinoma in this laboratory study. Endometrial hyperplasia does not develop in women taking estrogen-progestin combinations. Therefore, I have made the statement that those women who would ordinarily develop endometrial cancer in previously existing hyperplasia will not do so as long as they continue estrogen-progestin combinations.

Contraindications and Cautions in the Use of Oral Contraceptives

The use of oral contraceptive agents is contraindicated (1) when a malignant tumor of the breast or reproductive tract is present or suspected; (2) when epiphyseal closure is incomplete in a young patient; (3) in the presence of hepatic dysfunction; (4) during the immediate postpartum period, and (5) when there is a history of thrombophlebitis or pulmonary embolism. These agents should be used with caution in the presence of cardiac or renal dysfunction. Patients giving a history of depression should be observed closely and the drug discontinued if the depressed state recurs. Unusual visual complaints (scotomata, double vision, photophobia) necessitate thorough opthalmological examination and discontinuance of therapy pending determination of the cause.

I do not prescribe an oral contraceptive agent until a complete physical and pelvic examination has been performed. Furthermore, the history should be sufficiently detailed to determine the presence of previous hepatic disease, a tendency toward or a predisposition to thromboembolic processes, and a familial predisposition to mammary or endometrial cancer. The cervix is visualized at the time of the original examination, and Schiller's test is performed. Erosions and Schiller-positive areas should be managed in accordance with generally accepted gynecological practice. When an oral contraceptive agent is prescribed, the patient is usually seen again in 30 days for the purpose of noting side effects or unusual occurrences. Thereafter, she is seen every six months. Each examination includes palpation of the breasts and abdomen together with a pelvic and rectal examination. The Papanicolaou smear is repeated annually. A prescription for an oral contraceptive is usually limited to six months so that it will not be refilled indefinitely and indiscriminately.

BIBLIOGRAPHY

Ambrus, J. L., *et al.*: Progestational agents and blood coagulation II, Am. J. Obst. & Gynec. 103: 994, 1969.

Beck, P., and Wells, S.: Oral contraceptives and glucose tolerance. Report to the American Diabetes Association, June 1968.

Diczfalusy, E.: Mode of action of contraceptive drugs, Am. J. Obst. & Gynec. 100:136, 1968.

Federal Food and Drug Administration Report on the Oral Contraceptives by the Advisory Committee on Obstetrics and Gynecology, Louis M. Hellman, Chairman, Washington, D.C., August 1, 1966.

Ibid: Second Report, August 1, 1969.

Frieman, D. G.; Suylmoto, J., and Wessler, S.: Frequency of pulmonary thromboembolism in man, New England J. Med. 272:1278, 1965.

Garcia, C. R.: The oral contraceptive—an appraisal and review, Am. J. M. Sc. 253:6, 1967.

———: Medical and metabolic effects of oral contraceptives and their implications, Clin. Obst. & Gynec. 11:669, 1968.

Haba, A. F.; Cuevas, J. O., Pelegrina, I., and Bangdiwala, I.: Deaths among users of oral contraceptives, Obst. & Gynec. 36:597, 1970.

Inman, W. H. W.; Vessey, M. P., Westerholm, B., and Englund, A.: Thromboembolic disease and the steroidal content of oral contraceptives; a report to the Committee on Safety of Drugs, Brit. M. J. 2:203, 1970.

Kistner, R. W.: Oral contraceptives: Safety factors in the prolonged use of progestin-estrogen combinations, Postgrad. Med. 39:207, 362, 1966.

———: Effects of new synthetic progestogens on endometriosis in the human female, Fertil. & Steril. 16:61, 1965.

———: Therapeutic Application of Progestational Compounds in Gynecology, in Marcus, S. L., and Marcus, C. C. (eds.): *Advances in Obstetrics and Gynecology* (Baltimore: Williams & Wilkins, 1966), vol. I.

———: Histological effects of progestins on hyperplasia and carcinoma in situ of the endometrium, Cancer 12:1106, 1959.

———, Griffiths, C. T., and Craig, J. M.: Use of progestational agents in the management of endometrial cancer, Cancer 18:115, 1966.

Ledger, W. J.: The place of intrauterine contraceptive devices in modern clinical practice, Ob/Gyn Digest 37, Nov. 1967.

Martinez-Manautou, J.; Cortez, V.; Giner-Velasquez, J.; Aznar, R.; Cassola, J., and Rudel, H. W.: Low doses of progestogen as an approach to fertility control, Fertil. & Steril. 17:1, 1966.

Meeker, C. I.: Use of drugs and intrauterine devices for birth control, New England J. Med. 280:1058, 1969.

Mishell, D. R., and Lumkin, M. E.: Contraceptive effect of varying doses of progestogen in Silastic vaginal rings, Fertil. & Steril. 21:99, 1970.

Morrell, M. T., and Dunhill, M. S.: The postmortem incidence of pulmonary embolism in a hospital population, Brit. J. Surg. 55:347, 1968.

Peterson, Wm. F.: Personal communication.

Rudel, H. W.: Pharmacology of oral contraceptives, Clin. Obst. & Gynec. 11:3, 1968.

Sharman, A.: Timing of the first ovulation after delivery. Presented at Folkestone Conference on Oral Contraceptives, Folkestone, England, October 15, 1966.

Tietze, C.: Statistical assessment of adverse experiences associated with the use of oral contraceptives, Clin. Obst. & Gynec. 11:698, 1968.

Vessey, M. P., and Doll, R.: Investigation of relation between use of oral contraceptives and thromboembolic disease, Brit. M. J. 2:199, 1968.

Wallach, E. E., and Garcia, C. R.: Emotional factors in oral contraception, Clin. Obst. & Gynec. 11:684. 1968.
———: Breast and reproductive system effects of oral contraceptives, Clin. Obst. & Gynec. 11: 645, 1968.
Westoff, C. F., and Ryder, N. B.: Experience with oral contraception in the United States, 1960–1965, Clin. Obst. & Gynec. 11:734, 1968.
Whitelaw, M. J.; Nola, V. F., and Kalman, C. F.: Irregular menses, amenorrhea and infertility following synthetic progestational agents, J.A.M.A. 195:780, 1966.
Willson, J. R.; Ledger, W. J., Bollinger, C. C., and Andros, G. J.: The Margulies intrauterine contraceptive device, Am. J. Obst. & Gynec. 92:62, 1965.
Wiseman, H.: Clinical management of complaints associated with the use of oral contraception, Clin. Obst. & Gynec. 11:3, 1968.
World Health Organization Technical Report Series No. 386: Hormonal steroids in contraception, Geneva, 1968.
Wynn, V.: Metabolic effects of ethynodiol diacetate. Presented at Folkestone Conference on Oral Contraceptives, Folkestone, England, October 15, 1966.

ADDENDUM

Surgical Sterilization

The use of sterilizing procedures is increasing in most countries. In a recent survey in the United States it was found that, among white couples where the wife was between 18 and 39, 10 per cent had had a sterilizing operation. Six out of 10 had vasectomies or tubal ligation and 4 had sterilizing operations in the course of gynecologic treatment. In the United Kingdom and the United States tubal ligation is performed more commonly than vasectomy.

Vasectomy is simple, safe and effective but has the mild disadvantage of not being immediately effective. In contrast to tubal ligation it involves no measurable risk to life, it carries a reasonable chance of reversibility and it can be done as an outpatient procedure. When a normal, stable, happy couple requests sterilization, vasectomy is preferable to tubal ligation. Emotionally, however, it is difficult for men to avoid equating vasectomy with castration.

Tubal ligation, partial excision or total salpingectomy, is the commonest and most acceptable sterilizing procedure in women. There has been a recent trend to combine tubal ligation with operations on the pelvic floor. However, the tubes are not always easily accessible and postoperative bleeding may be troublesome. Many gynecologists prefer vaginal hysterectomy to that of vaginal tubal ligation as the optimum method of surgical sterilization. The disadvantage of postligation dysfunctional uterine bleeding is prevented and, of course, cervical and uterine malignancy is obviated.

Probably the most common method of sterilization in the female at present is via laparoscopy. In this procedure the proximal portion of the oviduct is coagulated and excised using diathermy. Complications have been minimal, but bowel injuries have been reported and uncontrolled bleeding occasionally necessitates laparotomy. Pregnancy has been recorded after subtotal hysterectomy and no sterilizing procedure is 100 per cent effective. The failure rate of tubal ligation varies from 0.4 to 2.8 per cent and there is an increased risk of ectopic gestation due to damage of the endosalpinx.

CHAPTER 16

Cytogenetics

General Considerations

ALTHOUGH ALMOST ONE hundred years have elapsed since Balbiani described the division of intracellular bodies which he called "batonnets étroits" (thin little sticks), a correlation between these "coloured bodies" or, as we now know them, chromosomes, and abnormalities in development did not appear until 1959. During this year the chromosomal errors associated with three well-known clinical syndromes, Down's, Turner's and Klinefelter's, were described. During the last ten years, over 130 different chromosomal errors have been described in man. In addition to the three previously recognized syndromes, four new ones have been described. Two are the result of the presence of an extra chromosome while in the other two chromosomal material is lacking or deleted.

In 1970, Caspersson and associates described a new method of identification of human chromosomes by DNA-binding fluorescent agents which simplify identification of previously described syndromes and will result in the discovery or elucidation of manifold new syndromes. Caspersson showed that human metaphase chromosomes from blood cultures, treated with quinacrine mustard (QM), show a banded pattern of fluorescence, which, in the chromosomes with the most strongly fluorescent regions (3, 13-15, Y), was found to be constant and reproducible. This pattern appeared to be so characteristic that it could be used for chromosome identification.

The sphere of interest of human cytogenetics in relation to human development concerns four general areas: (1) primary amenorrhea and female infertility, (2) certain mental disorders in both female and male, (3) male infertility, and (4) congenital defects which may be life-threatening and are usually associated with mental retardation.

In 1956, Tijo and Levan, utilizing tissue cultures obtained from human embryos, demonstrated that the diploid chromosome number for men was 46 and not 48 as was previously believed. The introduction of improved technics made it possible to count chromosomes accurately and by 1960 several investigators had prepared diagrams (idiograms) of the human chromosome complement. Because of individual variations in terminology a conference was held in Denver, Colorado, to establish a standard nomenclature for human chromosomes. As a result of this conference, it was agreed that the non-sex chromosomes (autosomes) should be numbered 1 to 22 according to their descending order of length. The sex chromosomes (gonosomes) were termed X and Y. In addition, further specific identification was based on size, position of the centromere and other morphologic features.

In 1963 a second conference was held in London to further delineate chromosomal differentiation. A lettering system (A to G) was adopted for the 7 groups of autosomes and finally, in 1966, further refinements were added. The letter p designated the short arm and q the long arm of the chromosome; a plus (+) sign indicated additional chromosomal material and a minus (−) sign indicated loss of material; the chromosomal number was to be followed by the sex chromosomal complex; for example, 46, XX being the normal female and 46, XY the normal male; a diagonal was to be used to separate the karyotype designations in those individuals who have more than one chromosome constitution (mosaicism); for example, XO/XY.

A human cell nucleus with 23 pairs or 46 single chromosomes is said to be *diploid* (G, *diplous*, double plus *eidos*, resemblance); if only one member of each pair is present, or 23 chromosomes, it is said to be *haploid* (G. *haplous*, simple plus *eidos*, resemblance). Cells with chromosome numbers in the diploid range, but not exactly 46, are termed *aneuploid* (G. *an*, without plus *eu*, well, plus, *plasso*, formed). Cells with multiples of the haploid number (69, 92, etc.) are spoken of as *polyploid* (G, *poly*, many, plus *plasso*, formed).

Polyploidy occurs naturally in all plants, but, except in the liver and uterus, it is rare in human beings. Haploid, diploid or polyploid states may be essentially normal because the full complement of chromosomes is present. Even though the gene products are formed in varying amounts in the various forms of polyploidy, they are in a balanced or proportional condition. However, various forms of aneuploidy involving chromosome additions or, even more striking, deletions, seem to disorganize cell metabolism. In man, homologous chromosomes may occasionally be present in triplicate, a condition known as *trisomy*, but except for the sex chromosomes they are almost never absent or lacking one member of a pair. Autosomal trisomy and polyploidy are common in abortuses.

Chromosomes, except when preparing for cell division, are not distinguishable with standard cytologic technics. At the time cell division approaches, the chromosomes condense and become discrete. Division of somatic cells is termed *mitosis*, but division of germ cells is called *meiosis*.

Clarification of Turner's and Klinefelter's syndromes together with an improved understanding of other intersex problems was simplified by the observations of Barr and Bertram in 1949. They showed a characteristic chromatin mass as a satellite structure near the nucleolus in the nerve cells of female cats. In the human subject they found a similar sex difference in cells obtained from sympathetic ganglia. The same observations were later made on biopsies of skin and on cells of the vaginal and buccal mucosa.

A typical example of the chromatin mass is shown in Figure 16–1.

In the female, *Barr bodies* may be seen in from 20 to 90 per cent of freshly desquamated epithelial cells, whereas this finding is rare in the adult male, occurring in only 1 to 3 per cent of the cells.

It was originally suggested that the appearance of the sex-chromatin mass depended on the presence of the XX chromosome pair. Specifically,

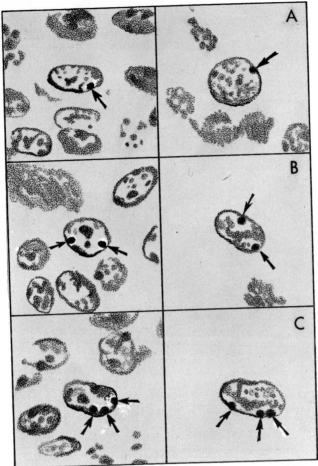

Fig. 16-1.—Sex-chromatin masses in cells of human skin *(left)* and buccal mucosa *(right)*. **A,** normal female XX. **B,** Klinefelter's syndrome with mental deficiency; XXXY. **C,** eunuch with micro-orchism and mental deficiency; XXXXY. (After Sohval, A. R.: Am. J. Med. 31:397, 1961, and Barr, M. L., and Carr, D. H.: Canad, M.A.J. 83:979, 1960.)

the mass was thought to be formed by fusion of heterochromatic portions of two X chromosomes. Its absence from male nuclei was attributed to the lack of sufficient chromosomal material in the Y chromosome to contribute to the formation of an adequately sized chromocenter.

However, on the basis of data derived from simultaneous studies of the sex chromatin and chromosome constitution by Sohval and others, it now appears that the Barr body is probably derived from a single X chromosome. In addition, with rare exceptions, there appears to be an exact relationship between the sex-chromatin pattern and the number of X chromosomes. The maximum number of Barr bodies per nucleus is one less than the maximum number of X chromosomes present. This relationship is also true in instances of *sex-chromosome mosaicism* (the coexistence of cells with dissimilar sex-chromosomal constitutions), which results in corresponding *sex-chromatin mosaicism.* In such cases, different sex-chromatin patterns may be found in different tissues of the same individual. The importance of the Barr body is obvious from the fact that it is the only histologic marker of genetic sex in mammalian species and is independent of age, illness, hormonal status or prior therapy. The Barr body count is lower in the newborn female but it rises to normal in a few days. Certain antibiotics and cortisone may also lower the count.

The findings of Jost are of extreme importance in the consideration of cytogenetics and intersex problems. Jost has shown that removal of the male gonad in the intrauterine fetus will result in the development of female genital ducts and female external genitalia. The obverse is not true, however, so that developmental growth of the ducts and external genitalia apparently will always be along female lines unless diverted by the presence of a male gonad.

Chromatin-Negative Nuclei.—This finding is most often indicative of an XO or XY sex-chromosome complex. In the field of gynecology, the most common example of chromatin negative nuclei is that of Turner's syndrome, 45, XO. While sex-chromatin negativity and an XY complement are the predominant findings in normal males, they are encountered also in male pseudohermaphroditism. This is of considerable diagnostic importance in the phenotypic female and in patients whose external genitalia are not sexually ambiguous (hypospadias or cryptorchism may be the only visible manifestation), so that the somatic appearance is entirely masculine. A normal XY karyotype has also been reported in several chromatin-negative males exhibiting the male counterpart of Turner's syndrome, that is, multiple congenital anomalies of the type frequently found in females with Turner's syndrome. These individuals usually have cryptorchism or other testicular defects.

Chromatin-negative nuclei and an XY complex have been reported in certain patients with Klinefelter's syndrome, as well as in some with hypospadias and small testes, often with gynecomastia and hypogonadism. Abnormal sex karyotypes are found occasionally in chromatin-negative males. These have been an XYY or an unusual XY complex in which the Y chromosome is abnormally long or is partially deleted. XYY is approximately as frequent as XXY in neonates. An XO complement has been described in two chromatin-negative intersex children with intra-abdominal testes and malformed genitalia who were both raised as males.

Chromatin-Positive Nuclei.—This observation in males or females signifies the presence of at least two X chromosomes (an occasional XO sex-chromosome complex in skin cultures of certain chromatin-positive phenotypic females with Turner's syndrome is an exception and may be due to mosaicism such as XO/XX). Chromatin-positive nuclei in phenotypic males, occurring in 3/1,000 live births, may be associated with a variety of sex-chromosome complexes or may indicate merely marked virilization of a normal female (e.g., infants with congenital adrenal hyperplasia). Most often the Barr bodies are encountered singly and the sex chromosomes are XXY or XXY/XY. Chromatin-positive males usually have Klinefelter's syndrome in adulthood. They are also likely to manifest mental deficiency in about 25 per cent of cases. The XXY complex has also been found in association with an autosomal aberration such as 21-trisomy in mongolism. Other abnormal sex chromosome constitutions, such as XXY/XX, XXYY and XXY/XXXY, have been reported in chromatin-positive patients with Klinefelter's syndrome.

Chromatin-positive nuclei containing multiple sex-chromatin masses have been found in mentally retarded phenotypic males as well as in females (48/XXXX, 47/XXX). Chromatin-2-positive nuclei containing duplicated Barr bodies (Fig. 16-1, *B*) have been demonstrated in phenotypic males with Klinefelter's syndrome and an XXXY sex-chromosome complex and in patients with an XXXY/XY mosaic. Chromatin-3-positive nuclei containing triple Barr bodies (Fig. 16-1, *C*) have been found in association with XXXXY, XXXY/XXXXY and XXXY/XXXXY/XXXXXY mosaicism. Each of the two adult subjects had micro-orchism with maldescent. The three boys' testes were small and entirely devoid of spermatogonia. All five individuals were mentally defective.

Chromosome Patterns; Gametogenesis

The second major development has been the remarkable advances in chromosome cell culture techniques and classification. For a detailed analysis of the techniques involved, the reader is referred to the reviews of Hirschhorn and Cooper, Sohval, and Griboff and Lawrence. They prepared cell cultures obtained from peripheral blood, skin or bone marrow and prepared a karyotype of each individual. To do this, photographs of the individual chromosomes are simply enlarged and then carefully cut from the enlargement and paired to provide a matched set (Fig. 16-2). These are arranged and numbered in order of diminishing size. In the normal male there are 22 pairs of nonsex chromosomes known as autosomes. In addition, there is one large and one small chromosome. These are the sex chromosomes, X and Y respectively. In the female there are also 22 pairs of autosomes but the two large or X chromosomes constitute a matched homologous pair. Typical chromosome patterns of the normal female and the normal male are shown in Figure 16-3.

Each chromosome has a characteristic appearance and shows a constriction at a point where the two chromatids join the process of division. This constriction area is termed a centromere and the location of the centromere together with the length of the arms on either side and the over-all length of the chromosome itself are distinguishing features which permit easy identification and subsequent pairing (Fig. 16-4). A normal diploid cell is one containing 46 chromosomes. By a process of meiosis a haploid cell is formed which contains one chromosome of each of the 23 pairs of chromosomes. Thus, at the time of fertilization the zygote is formed by the union of the ovum and the sperm, each of which contains one chromosome of each of the 23 pairs of chromosomes. The resultant zygote therefore is a diploid cell formed from two haploid cells (sperm and ovum) and possesses the diploid number of chromosomes, 46. In the female this is made up of 23 matched pairs, whereas in the male it is made up of 22 pairs plus the X and Y chromosomes. Normal gametogenesis and nondisjunction gametogenesis are shown in Figure 16-5.

In the process of meiosis (Fig. 16-6) each chromosome in the nucleus is arranged next to its homologue by the process known as synapsis. Each of these chromosomes subsequently splits longitudinally, forming two chro-

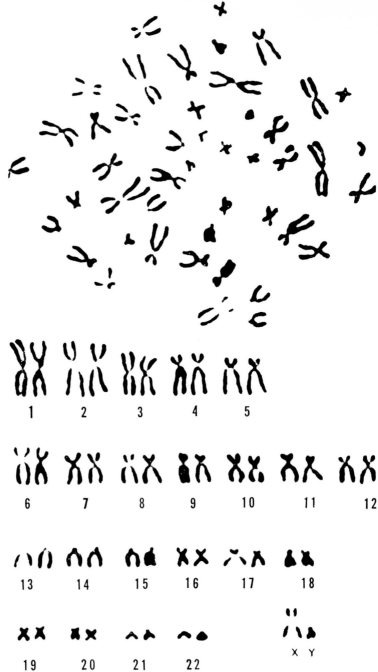

Fig. 16-2.—*Above,* chromosomes of a dividing human cell seen at metaphase. *Below,* karyotype prepared from these chromosomes is that of normal human male containing 22 pairs of autosomes and an XY sex-chromosome complex. (From Barr, M. L., and Carr, D. H.: Canad, M.A.J. 83:979, 1960.)

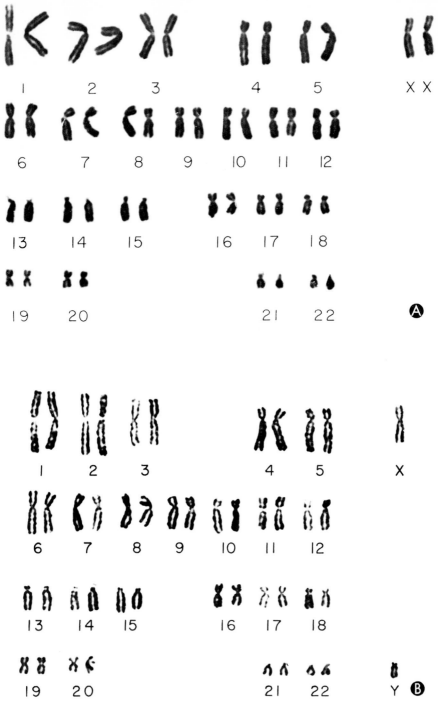

Fig. 16-3.—A, normal female chromosome pattern, showing XX. **B,** normal male chromosome pattern, showing XY. (From Hirschhorn, K., and Cooper, L. C.: Am. J. Med. 31:442, 1961.)

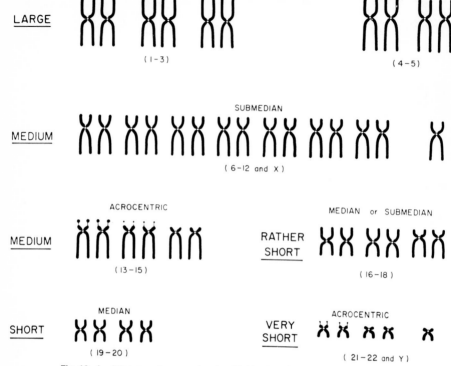

Fig. 16–4.—Idiogram of a normal male with 22 pairs of autosomes and XY sex-chromosome constitution. Chromosomes are arranged in seven groups according to length and centromere position. Classification is a slight modification, after Patau, of the international system of nomenclature adopted in Denver. (From Sohval, A. R.: Fertil. & Steril. 14:180, 1963.)

matids. The result is a four-strand formation known as a tetrad. The new arrangement of genetic material occurs at this tetrad stage as a result of crossing-over between chromatids of homologous chromosomes. Members of chromosome pairs are then separated toward opposite poles, the process known as disjunction, and as a result, when the first meiotic division occurs, two cells are produced, each of which contains one member of each of the 23 pairs of chromosomes in the form of a pair of chromatids. During the second meiotic division, however, the two chromatids which make up the chromosome are separated and then enter separate cells. Thus, each primary germ cell eventually forms four cells, each containing the haploid number of chromosomes. In the female, three of these cells deteriorate into polar bodies while the fourth becomes a fertilizable ovum (see Fig. 16–5). In the male, however, all four gametes persist as spermatozoa. The first meiotic division is a reductional division (Fig. 16–5) whereas the second is essentially a mitotic division.

Fig. 16–5.—Diagrams illustrating the formation of normal gametes and the types of gametes resulting from nondisjunction involving the sex chromosomes. Predicted results from matings involving such abnormal gametes with normal gametes from the opposite sex are shown below. (Figs. 16–5 to 16–7 and 16–9 from Hirschhorn, K., and Cooper, L. C.: Am. J. Med. 31:442, 1961.)

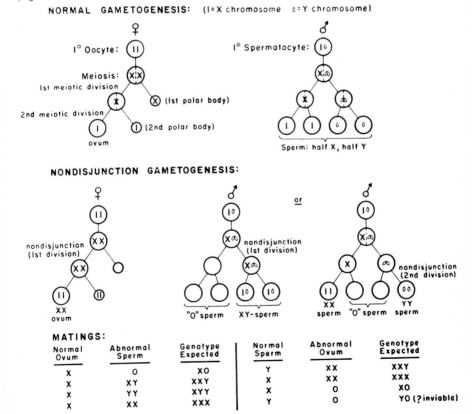

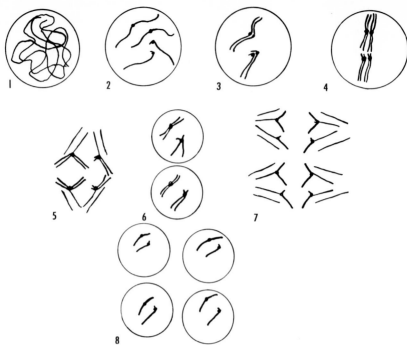

Fig. 16-6.—Meiosis. **1,** nucleus of primary gametocyte in prophase, leptotene stage. **2,** pachytene stage. Individual chromosomes are discernible. **3,** synapsis. Members of each chromosome pair are associated. **4,** diplotene stage. Members of chromosome pairs are seen to be reduplicated. Paired homologues (bivalents) are arranged around equator of cell, nuclear membrane disappears, meiotic spindle appears. **5,** diakinesis. Members of chromosome pairs are separated toward opposite poles (disjunction). **6,** completion of first meiotic division. Two cells are now present, each with half the diploid number of chromosomes present as divalents. **7,** second meiotic division. Pairs of chromatids comprising each chromosome are separated (disjunction). **8,** completion of second meiotic division. There are four cells, each carrying the haploid number of chromosomes.

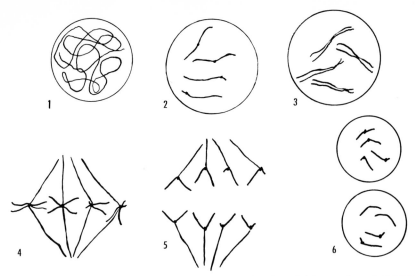

Fig. 16-7.—Mitosis. **1,** early prophase of somatic cell nucleus. **2,** later prophase. Individual chromosomes are apparent. **3,** late prophase—early metaphase. Each chromosome is redupli-cated. **4,** metaphase. Nuclear membrane disappears, chromosomes are arranged on mitotic spindle, no association of homologous chromosomes. **5,** anaphase. Two chromatids com-prising each chromosome are drawn to opposite poles. **6,** completion of mitosis. Two cells each containing the diploid number of chromosomes are present.

Subsequent development is essentially by the process of mitosis and the chromosome number of each cell remains constant (Figs. 16-7 and 16-8). Synapsis does not occur in the process of mitosis and after the chromo-somes are arranged centrally in the nucleus, the chromatids of each chro-mosome are directly separated, thus producing two cells, each with the normal diploid number.

The process of disjunction has been mentioned in the discussion of meiosis. An alteration in this process in which there is a failure of a pair of homologous chromosomes to separate during one of the two meiotic divi-sions or during the process of mitosis is known as nondisjunction. Involve-ment of the sex chromosomes by the process of nondisjunction will result in migration of both chromosomes to the same nuclear pole (Fig. 16-9). An ovum of this structure could therefore contain either two XX chromosomes or no sex chromosomes whatsoever. In a similar manner, if nondisjunction occurs during spermatogenesis, migration of both chromosomes to the same nuclear pole will result in either a sperm with no sex chromosomes or one with both an X and a Y chromosome (XY). The various chromosomal combinations resulting from nondisjunction are illustrated in Figure 16-10. As a result of these combinations it is evident that the XO pattern found in Turner's syndrome may be produced from nondisjunction occur-ring during either spermatogenesis or oogenesis. Thus the union of an X-bearing sperm and an ovum without sex chromosomes would produce the XO pattern as would the junction of an ovum with an X chromosome

NUCLEAR DIVISION

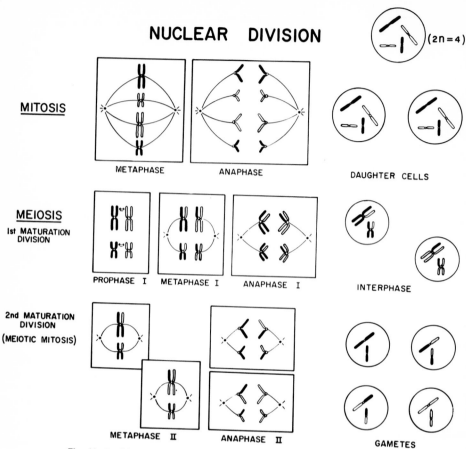

Fig. 16-8.—Distinguishing features of mitotic and meiotic nuclear division. Each parent cell contains two pairs of chromosomes, the dark and light members of each pair derived from the father and mother, respectively. During metaphase of *mitosis*, each chromosome is re-duplicated and arranged separately on the equatorial plate. During anaphase the longitudinal halves separate and pass to opposite poles. Daughter cells are thus produced with chromosomal constitution identical to that of the parent cell. In the first *meiotic* division during metaphase (labeled *I*), the reduplicated members of each homologous pair are together in synapsis on the equatorial plate. Exchange of chromosomal material has previously occurred during prophase. During anaphase, whole reduplicated chromosomes of each pair diverge poleward to produce daughter cells containing half the diploid number. Metaphase of meiosis, second division *(II)*, is essentially mitotic, resulting in gametes containing the haploid number of chromosomes but with varying compositions of parentally derived chromosome material. (From Sohval, A. R.: Am. J. Med. 31:397, 1961.)

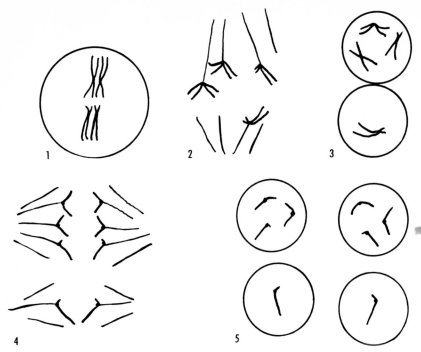

Fig. 16–9.—Meiotic nondisjunction. **1**, diplotene stage, meiotic metaphase. Synapsed pairs of homologous chromosomes. **2**, nondisjunction at first meiotic division. Both members of one synapsed pair are drawn to the same pole instead of being separated. **3**, completion of first meiotic division. One cell contains both members of one chromosome pair; the other lacks any member of that pair. **4**, second meiotic division. **5**, completion of second division. Half the gametes contain one more than the haploid number of chromosomes while half contain one less.

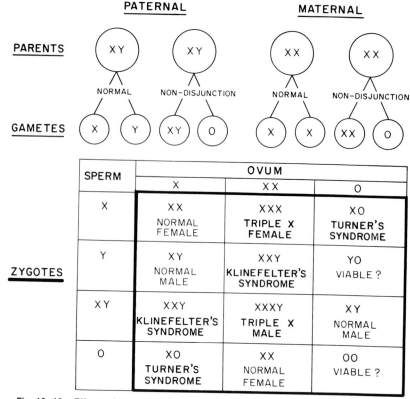

Fig. 16-10.—Effects of nondisjunction occurring during gametogenesis in either or both sexes. The various zygotic possibilities show how (1) Klinefelter's or Turner's syndrome may result from nondisjunction during spermatogenesis or oogenesis; (2) the XXX female can be the product of nondisjunction occurring only during oogenesis, and (3) the XXX male may be due to nondisjunction in both parents. (From Sohval, A. R.: Am. J. Med. 31:397, 1961.)

combined with a sperm bearing no sex chromosomes. Since the Y chromosome is regarded as bearing male-determining genes, the fetal gonad will not develop into a testis in its absence. Similarly, the presence of two X chromosomes seems to be necessary for proper differentiation of the primordial gonad into an ovary. In Turner's syndrome, despite the appearance of the individual, the lack of the Y chromosome prevents the development of the testis. In the absence of the second X chromosome the fetal gonad remains feminine but demonstrates lack of proper differentiation. The development of the duct system, including the oviducts and uterus, represents the type of development described by Jost in the absence of a fetal testicular hormone. Since the rudimentary gonad may not secrete estrogen, the endometrium does not develop and primary amenorrhea exists. The lack of development of mammary tissue similarly reflects the presence of primary ovarian failure. Some XO patients do produce estrogen and have bleeding episodes.

Chromosomal Abnormalities

GONADAL DYSGENESIS (TURNER'S SYNDROME)

Twenty years ago Henry Turner described a syndrome occurring in young females which had the following clinical features: sexual infantilism, short stature, primary amenorrhea, webbing of the neck and cubitus valgus. Laboratory assays revealed very high levels of gonadotropins excreted in urine but extremely low levels of estrogens. Culdoscopy or laparotomy showed that ovarian tissue was either absent or existed only as rudimentary streaks along the lateral aspect of the pelvic peritoneum where the ovary would ordinarily be expected to be found. As more and more patients with this clinical picture were described, the name *Turner's syndrome* became an accepted description. Subsequently the disease was termed *ovarian agenesis* and this later was changed to a more appropriate description, *gonadal dysgenesis.*

Although patients with gonadal dysgenesis are usually seen by the gynecologist because of primary amenorrhea, the presence of one or more congenital abnormalities may cause the parent to seek medical consultation for the child at an earlier age. The most common congenital abnormalities noted in this syndrome are webbing of the neck, cubitus valgus, ptosis, strabismus, nystagmus and cardiac abnormalities such as coarctation of the aorta. The sexual infantilism and diminished breast tissue are quite obvious, and there is usually retardation of linear growth, the average height of these individuals being about 54 or 55 in. (Fig. 16–11). The areolae are widely spaced and underdeveloped and the chest is described as "shield-type." Abnormalities of bone development may also be seen, such as protuberance of the sternum, high palate, rarefaction of bones of the extremities, idiopathic hypertension and delayed closure of epiphyses.

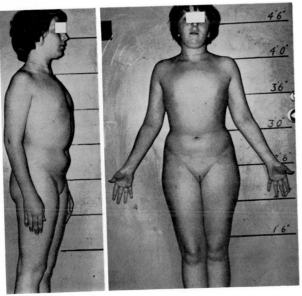

Fig. 16–11.—Turner's syndrome in a 16-year-old apparent female with primary amenorrhea. 17-Ketosteroid and 17-hydroxysteroid values were normal but the FSH was 105 m.u.u. Chromatin pattern negative, castrate vaginal smear, absent pubic hair. There is mild cubitus valgus but no webbing of the neck. (From Kupperman, H. S.: *Human Endocrinology* [Philadelphia: F. A. Davis Company, 1963].)

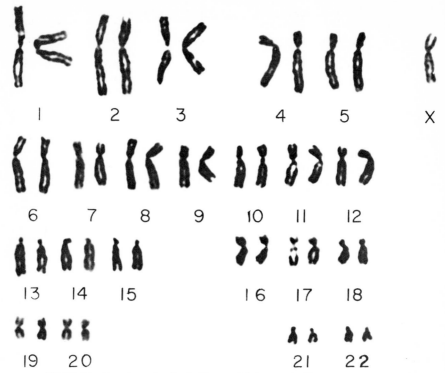

Fig. 16-12.—Karyotype of patient with gonadal dysgenesis. There are 44 autosomes and a single X chromosome. (From Hirschhorn, K., and Cooper, L. C.: Am. J. Med. 31:442, 1961.)

In some cases mental retardation and deafness have been described. I have recently seen one patient with congenital blindness and severe nystagmus. The diagnosis should be suspected in any patient with primary amenorrhea, particularly if there are diminished stature and failure of sexual development. We have routinely performed culdoscopy in such patients in order to verify the diagnosis, since the rudimentary ovarian streak is easily identified. In addition, the characteristic XO cytogenetic pattern (Fig. 16-12) together with the high level of gonadotropins and the low level of estrogens in urine will serve to corroborate the diagnosis. To avoid delay in proper diagnosis, every patient with primary amenorrhea should have a sex-chromatin determination (by buccal mucosal smear), and the chromosomes should be examined if possible.

Although the diminished stature is believed due to a genetic defect, estrogen should not be used prematurely as substitutional therapy because of the possibility of causing early epiphyseal closure. Figures 16-13 and 16-14 illustrate a variant of gonadal dysgenesis due to fragmentation of an X chromosome, in which diminished stature is absent.

Although extra X chromosomes in females do not usually affect physical development or fertility, absence of a sex chromosome is more serious. By far the majority of zygotes with only one X chromosome are aborted. Those infants who reach term have an increased perinatal mortality due to congenital heart defects such as coarctation of the aorta or aortic stenosis.

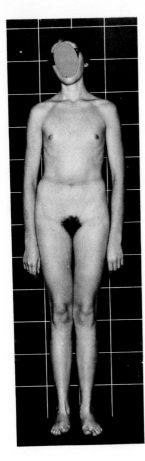

Fig. 16-13.—Female, aged 22, with primary amenorrhea. Note eunuchoid appearance, with long extremities and wide, large feet. Height is 69½ in.; the breasts are prepuberal with infantile areolae and nipples. The 17-ketosteroid excretion was 7.6 mg./24 hours, the pituitary gonadotropins 31 R.U./24 hours and estimated bone age 14 years. The buccal smear was chromatin negative but a small mass of chromatin was seen apposed to the nuclear membrane in 4 per cent of the cells. This patient represents the fourth reported case of a chromosomal constitution consisting of an X chromosome and a fragment of an X chromosome. (From Becker, K.: Proc. Staff Meet. Mayo Clin. 38:389, Aug. 28, 1963.)

Even if the infant survives, certain congenital anomalies exist which may affect every body system. About 90 per cent of 45,X females have skeletal abnormalities. These may not be serious but aid in diagnosis. The most common findings are shortening of the fourth metacarpal and metatarsal bones and deformed medial tibial condyle. Abnormalities of the urinary system are found in 50 to 60 per cent of individuals with horseshoe kidney being the most serious. Disorders of the lymphatic system are extremely common and the webbing of the neck and laxity of the skin of the newborn may be the result of resorption of fluid from these hygromas. The incidence of mental retardation may not be increased over the usual incidence and is estimated to occur in about 15 per cent of 45,X individuals.

Primary ovarian failure is the most common charactertistic of females with only one X chromosome. Only one fertile female with this disorder has been described. The germ cells are present in the embryonic gonad but they usually disappear or are severely depleted at the time of birth. Biopsies of gonadal streaks in infancy and in young adults show degeneration of interstitial tissue with fibrosis. A similar situation prevails in Klinefelter's syndrome.

Mosaicism in patients with the 45,X syndrome occurs frequently but the

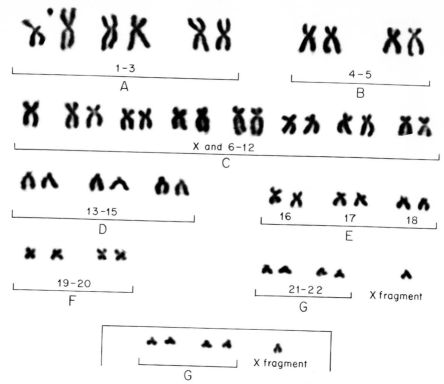

Fig. 16-14.—Karyotype of patient in Figure 16-13 consisted of 46 chromosomes. Only one complete X chromosome was present, evidenced by an unpaired medium-sized metacentric chromosome, and there was an additional small acrocentric chromosome of the G group. Chromosomal constitution was interpreted as consisting of 44 autosomes plus one X chromosome and a fragment of a chromosome which appeared to correspond to the short arms of an X chromosome. (From Becker, K.: Proc. Staff Meet. Mayo Clin. 38:389, Aug. 28, 1963.)

percentage and distribution of the different genotypes vary and thus may affect ovulatory function and fertility. Thus fertility may occur in women with a normal cell line, 46,XX, but who have a basic 46,X genotype. Such a combination of 45,X/46,XX mosaicism may certainly exist in many apparently normal women. Occasionally the X chromosome in the 46 cell line is abnormal, the long arm being duplicated while the short arm is absent (isochromosome Xqi). The X may lack part of the short arm (p−), part of the long arm (q−), or part of both with the result being a so-called ring chromosome (r). It should be noted that cells with one normal and one abnormal X chromosome does not alter the development from that found in women lacking an entire X chromosome.

The phenotype of individuals with an XO/XY chromosome mosaicism may be that of a male pseudohermaphrodite or it may be indistinguishable from one with the 45,X anomaly. Rarely the phenotype is that of a "male" Turner's syndrome or a true hermaphrodite. Since this mosaic is really a combination of the sterile female (45,X) and a normal male (46,XY), these phenotypic variations are readily understandable.

Patients with Turner's syndrome are permanently sterile because follicular development and ovulation cannot occur. However, substitutional therapy should be given since excellent cosmetic and metabolic improvement follows the administration of estrogenic substances. Since the introduction of sequential estrogen-progestin preparations for oral contraception, I have utilized these compounds in place of cyclic estrogens alone. Two patients with Turner's syndrome have been reported to have developed carcinoma of the endometrium following prolonged usage of estrogenic substances given daily and constantly rather than in cycles. Therapy should be withheld until it is determined that growth is no longer occurring. Therapy with cyclic estrogen or estrogens plus progestins should be continued as long as the normal menstrual periods occur in most individuals. The use of estrogenic preparations prevents the premature development of degenerative diseases and also delays the premature aging commonly associated with persistent estrogen deficit. The extragenital effects of estrogen are of equal importance since the incidence of cardiovascular and coronary heart disease has been shown to be statistically increased in patients who have had bilateral oophorectomy at a young age and have not received replacement estrogen therapy. The psychologic effects of sexual maturation are of extreme importance and cyclic estrogen should therefore be initiated about age 14 or 15. Indeed, some of these individuals show a striking response in the development of breast tissue and become quite feminine in appearance.

According to the recent observations of Josso, gonadoblastomas occur exclusively in patients with gonadal dysgenesis. The tumors contain primitive germ cells similar to those found in early stages of maturation of the fetal testis and ovary. The patients reported were phenotypically dissimilar, one having growth failure and pubertal virilization and the other stunted growth but lacking in pubertal development. However, both demonstrated 46,XY/45,X mosaicism. The tumor was associated with abnormal testicular tissue in the first patient and undifferentiated fibrous tissue in the second. The external phenotype in the former patient was male but in the latter it was female. Both had normal uterine and vaginal development. It is known that the risk of malignant tumors developing in the dysgenetic gonad of patients with testicular feminization (see p. 731) is high and these individuals have a 46,XY chromosomal complement. Thus when mosaicism of the 46,XY/45,X type is found in patients with Turner's syndrome, consideration should be given to gonadal extirpation. There is no evidence that the gonads of the 45,X(XO) individual should be removed.

Federman has pointed out that the term, gonadal dysgenesis, is generally used as being synonymous with Turner's syndrome but some investigators restrict the term to patients with a streak gonad and a normal phenotype. Others include any dysgenetic development of the gonad, such as Klinefelter's syndrome or true hermaphroditism, in an all-inclusive fashion. Specific chromosomal arrangements do not, per se, induce the streak gonad. It is due to a failure of the primitive germ cells to migrate from the endoderm to the primitive gonad.

The differentiation of the bipotential gonad is thus arrested and since it lacks the inducing capacity of the male testis, the development of the müllerian ducts and the external genitalia proceed according to female schedule. Gonads of this type lack the potential for estrogen production and subsequent breast development and growth of pubic hair is absent or markedly reduced. The variation in amount of pubic hair in patients with Turner's syndrome is, however, related more to differences in the adrenal secretion of androgen and estrogen than to lack of ovarian estrogen.

Federman has summarized the clinical-cytogenetic correlations as follows: "(1) Short stature and congenital anomalies are more frequent and more severe in the 45/X (XO) patients. Patients with isochromosomes for the long arm of the X show slightly fewer anomalies. These features are thus probably due to monosomy for genes on the short arm of the X. (2) The long arm of the X is necessary for normal ovarian development but less crucial for normal growth and the prevention of anomalies. (3) Mosaicism produces a semiquantitative but not precisely correlated blend of the features of the different stems present. (4) Although a tendency to thyroid auto-immunity is generally distributed among patients with gonadal dysgenesis, the specific occurrence of Hashimoto's thyroiditis is certainly concentrated in and may be specific to patients with an iso-X chromosome. (5) There is evidence that there is genetic information for linear growth, deutan color vision, and the $X_g{}^a$ blood group on the short arm of the X chromosome."

Seminiferous Tubule Dysgenesis (Klinefelter's Syndrome)

Cytogenetic studies of patients with the clinical syndrome of hyalinization of the seminiferous tubules, small testes and elevated urinary gonadotropin values have disclosed the fact that these patients have an extra chromosome, a total of 47, with an XXY configuration (Fig. 16-15). As noted in Figure 16-10, Klinefelter's syndrome may result from a process of nondisjunction which permits the union of an XY sperm with an X-bearing ovum. The same process may result from a union of an XX ovum and a Y sperm. However, this is not absolute and some patients with a chromatin-negative pattern have been described. These patients have a normal chromosomal complement with an XY constitution. The probable explanation of the XY Klinefelter patient is an insufficiency of the male-determining genes on the Y chromosome. Yet the presence of the Y chromosome is sufficient to cause the development of a testis which during fetal development secretes adequate testicular hormone to produce the male phenotype. Gynecomastia (Fig. 16-16) and mental deficiency are quite common but are not necessary findings in Klinefelter's syndrome.

The only invariable feature of Klinefelter's syndrome is testicular atrophy and azospermia or severe oligospermia although many other features have been described: eunuchoid body appearance, diminished body and facial hair, gynecomastia, normal penis, increased pituitary gonadotropins and mental retardation. The development of internal and external genitalia are thoroughly male and recognition prior to the onset of puberty is unusual since there are no abnormal stigmata of an endocrine disorder. Puberty may be delayed but after it occurs the scrotum enlarges, the penis elongates and pubic hair appears. Penile erection is possible as is ejaculation of sperm-free seminal fluid. Somatic structure varies from normal or asthenic to definitely feminine with increased girdle or general obesity. Most patients have normal or slightly increased height with an

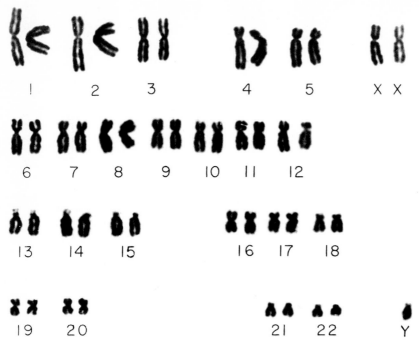

1	2	3	4	5	X X	

6	7	8	9	10	11	12

13	14	15	16	17	18

19	20	21	22	Y

Fig. 16–15.—Karyotype of patient with Klinefelter's syndrome. The most common abnormality is shown here, a complement of 47 chromosomes, 22 pairs of autosomes, an eighth pair of medium-sized metacentrics and an unmatched, short, acrocentric chromosome. The constitution is thus 47/XXY. The Y chromosome apparently determines the testis, which must be hormonally adequate in utero, since the genital ducts and external genitalia are unequivocally masculine. The second X accounts for the presence of the Barr body and is in some way inimical to the functioning of the tubular portion of the testis. It may also be responsible for the mental deficiency so often associated with this syndrome. (From Hirschhorn, K., and Cooper, L. C.: Am. J. Med. 31:442, 1961.)

increase in pubis to sole distance. Federman has pointed out that chronic pulmonary disease such as asthma, emphysema or bronchiectasis seem to occur with increased incidence and there is some evidence that these patients may be inclined to the development of malignant disease. The I.Q. is usually reduced and thyroid function is depressed. Federman believes that a valuable diagnostic clue lies in the behavior and personality of patients with Klinefelter's syndrome. He has stated that these men are usually of limited intelligence and ambition, with poor "sticking" qualities—a tendency to stray from challenge but with a rambling talkativeness.

Elevation of pituitary gonadotropins and testicular biopsy indicate that the basic pathology is gonadal in origin. However, in most biopsies of testicular tissue the Leydig cells are normal or even hyperplastic and are in sharp contrast with the hyalinized seminiferous tubules. The 17-ketosteroids, mostly of adrenal origin, are normal but levels of testosterone in plasma are diminished. Furthermore, stimulation of the Leydig cells by exogenous chorionic gonadotropin is diminished and therefore the hyperplasia of these cells may simply represent a compensatory effect of gonadotropic stimulation.

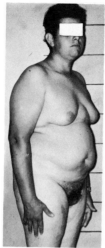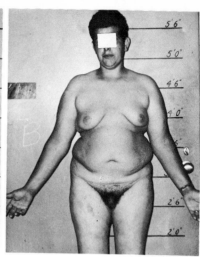

Fig. 16-16.—Klinefelter syndrome in 33-year-old chromatin-positive patient. Weight was 213 lb. and height 67½ in. The small external genitalia and female fat distribution are typical. Note extreme gynecomastia and sparsity of body hair. (From Kupperman, H. S.: *Human Endocrinology* [Philadelphia: F. A. Davis Company, 1963].)

Although at least 15 chromosomal variants have been described in association with Klinefelter's syndrome, the basic karyotypic abnormality is the presence of an extra sex chromosome. The complement of chromosomes is 47,XXY. Carr has described the other chromosomal variations as follows: (1) XXY cells may be present with a normal male cell line (46,XY); these individuals are fertile. (2) An increase in the number of X chromosomes increases the risk of mental retardation. (3) With 4 X chromosomes and a Y (49,XXXXY) skeletal abnormalities are invariably found and undescended testes or ambiguous external genitalia are common. In summary, all patients with Klinefelter's syndrome have at least an XXY pattern in some cells but karyotypes such as 48/XXXY, 48/XXYY, 49/XXXXY and 49/XXXYY have been described.

Evidence available at present indicates that Klinefelter's syndrome affects 1 in 400 live-born males. The incidence of chromatin positive males among mental defectives is about 10 per 1,000 and surveys of penal institutions have shown an increase over what is expected in the general population. Chromatin positive males have also been found with increased frequency in fertility clinics and it has been suggested that over 10 per cent of aspermic males are chromatin positive. It is obvious, therefore, that the incidence of Klinefelter's syndrome in the general population is much above the expected per cent and there is no doubt that it contributes substantially to mental retardation, male infertility and abnormal social behavior.

TRIPLE-X CHROMOSOME PATTERN

Another chromosomal combination resulting from nondisjunction may be noted in Figure 16-10. In this condition, union of an X-bearing sperm and an XX ovum results in the formation of a triple-X female. Several patients who had this triple-X pattern have been reported to have had regular menstrual periods and have been fertile. In an analysis of 16 reported cases, 10 patients gave a history of normal menses, three had noted irregular menstrual periods and three had secondary amenorrhea. The sex-chromatin pattern in these patients has been shown to be positive and in most of the cells from buccal mucosal scrapings two nuclear chromatin bodies have been described. There is a high incidence of this two-chromatin cellular mass in the nuclei in members of this group and in addition the number of "drumstick" polymorphonuclear leukocytes seems increased. In the fertile group of patients with an XXX constitution the oocytes produced would be either X or XX sex chromosomes. Therefore the progeny might include certain individuals with either an XXX or an XXY constitution. However, reports to date indicate normal offspring.

Tetra-X Chromosome Pattern

Only four patients with 48/XXXX chromosomal abnormality have been reported. The small number may be due to the fact that the abnormalities accompanying the failure of the chromosomes to separate after synapsis are, on the whole, not too striking. The following clinical findings have been noted: conductive deafness, myopia, congenital cataracts, narrowed field of vision, retinal abnormalities and mental retardation. In one recently reported case the gynecologic examination was normal and the growth of pubic hair was of female distribution. However, breast development was poor and the patient menstruated only two to three times yearly.

XXXY Pattern

As shown in Figure 16-10, the union of an ovum containing an XX chromosome with an XY sperm would result in a XXX-male or XXXY configuration. Similarly, nondisjunction at both the first and second meiotic divisions would result in an XXX ovum which, combined with a Y sperm, would give this same chromosomal pattern. These individuals have a male phenotype with certain of the features of Klinefelter's syndrome but the idiogram will show a total of 48 chromosomes.

Mosaicism

Mosaicism has been defined as the presence of genetically dissimilar cells in adjacent tissues of a particular person. In this situation the somatic cells contain sex-chromosome complements of more than one type. This process is in general due to divisional errors such as nondisjunction or simple loss of an X or Y chromosome, occurring singly or in sequence. Such errors may occur during the first mitosis of the zygote or at a later cleavage division of the developing embryo, or during both processes. For example, several patients with ovarian dysgenesis have been shown to have a mosaic pattern of the XO/XX type. Although, in general, patients with Turner's syndrome have a chromatin-negative buccal smear, in these individuals the smear may be chromatin positive. Several patients have been reported with XX/XO mosaicism, and chromosome counts showed half XO cells and half XX cells. These individuals may have primary amenorrhea and sexual infantilism together with physical underdevelopment and sparse pubic hair. They are chromatin positive but the usual congenital abnormalities are not present. XO/XX mosaic patients may be an important, albeit rare, group presenting with secondary amenorrhea.

TRANSLOCATION

Chromosomes may become fragmented during the course of either a meiosis, or a mitosis, and fragments may become joined to other fragmented chromosomes (Figs. 16-17 and 16-18). This process, termed translocation, may be the cause of true hermaphrodism, although translocation involving sex chromosomes is extremely rare. Individuals of this type possess both testicular and ovarian tissue and exhibit ambiguous external genitalia, e.g., "males" with hypospadias and cryptorchism and "females" with fused labia and enlarged clitoris. Occasionally an ovotestis with or without a testis and ovary may be present. Griboff and Lawrence studied 25 patients of this type and noted that 19 were chromatin positive and six were chromatin negative. They suggested that the chromatin-positive, true hermaphrodites are the result of translocation of sex-determining genes on the Y chromosome to the X chromosome during spermatogenesis. In the chromatin-negative, true hermaphrodites they suggest that there

Fig. 16-17.—Mechanisms of reciprocal translocation. *Top,* reciprocal translocation involving the exchange of parts of nonhomologous chromosomes early in prophase. *Center,* reciprocal translocation altering the morphology and composition of two pairs of homologous chromosomes at metaphase. The resulting dissimilarity is a potential source of error in the identification of individual chromosomes during karyotype analysis. *Bottom,* the mechanism of centric fusion, a special type of reciprocal translocation involving nonhomologous acrocentric chromosomes. Breakage close to the centromere occurs in the short arm of one chromosome and in the long arm of the other. Of the two newly produced chromosomes, one is necessarily a minute fragment which is usually lost in a subsequent cell division. (From Sohval, A. R.: Am. J. Med. 31:297, 1961.)

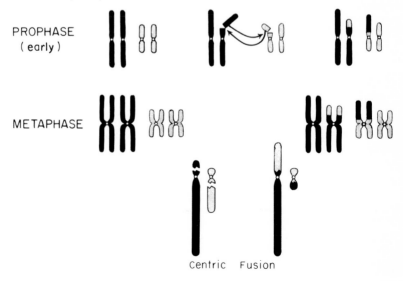

PROPHASE
(early)

METAPHASE

Centric   Fusion

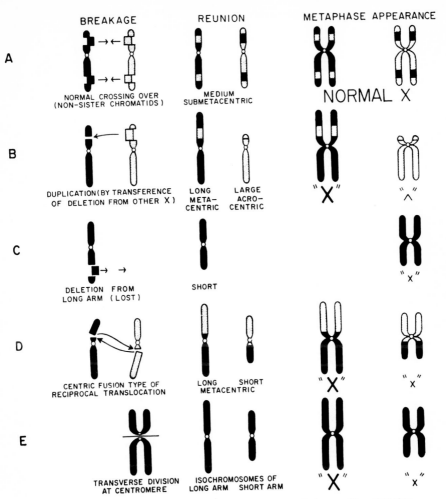

Fig. 16-18.—Mechanisms of translocation producing structural abnormalities of X chromosome through improper reunion after breakage. Abnormally large metacentric X chromosomes are designated "**X**." Small X's are represented as "∧" or "x," depending on location of centromere. Black chromosome is derived from one parent, light from the other. (From Sohval, A. R.: Fertil. & Steril. 14:180, 1963.)

is a translocation of sex-determining genes from the X chromosome to the Y chromosome.

DELETION

Occasionally, fragmentation results in loss of a chromosome fragment that fails to translocate. The remaining fragment of the chromosome with its centromere will survive but will be deficient in those genes contained in the lost fragment. This is a process known as deletion. Figure 16-19 illustrates chromosome movement in normal cell division, nondisjunction and

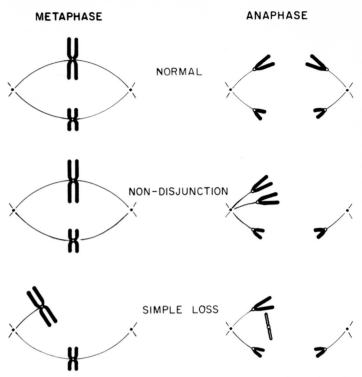

Fig. 16–19.—Chromosome movement in cell division. *Top,* during normal metaphase the longitudinally doubled chromosomes are arranged in the midline equatorial plate. A chromosomal fiber extends in opposite directions from the centromere of each chromosome to the opposite centrioles. In anaphase the halves (chromatids) separate and are known as daughter chromosomes. They migrate to opposite poles of the cell, presumably being drawn there by their respective centromeres. *Center,* nondisjunction is characterized by failure of daughter cells to separate (disjoin) during anaphase. Instead, both migrate to the same pole of the anaphase nucleus. As a result, one daughter cell receives an extra chromosome while the other becomes deficient in this chromosome. *Bottom,* simple loss of a chromosome is occasionally due to failure of a metaphase chromosome to become oriented on the equatorial plate. The centromere of one but not of the other member of a pair of chromatids is effective in drawing its daughter chromosome toward the pole of the anaphase nucleus. The daughter chromosome with the inactive centromere fails to migrate to the nucleus of either daughter cell. It remains in the cytoplasm where it eventually disintegrates. (From Sohval, A. R.: Am. J. Med. 31:397, 1961.)

deletion. In some patients, primary amenorrhea may result from chromosome deletion. For example, Jacobs reported a patient with primary amenorrhea whose idiogram showed 46 chromosomes with 44 autosomes and two X chromosomes. One of the X chromosomes was short and partially deleted and was probably responsible for the amenorrhea. Griboff and Lawrence have postulated that faulty ovarian development may result from deletion of sex genes of one of the X chromosomes. In another patient reported by Harnden and Stewart, study of the chromatin mass was negative and the patient had an XY karyotype, not the XO that would be expected in typical Turner's syndrome. This patient had gonadal dysgenesis but was tall, thin and sexually infantile. She did not have the other stigmata of

Turner's syndrome. The authors suggested that chromosomal deletion was the cause of this particular abnormality.

Other patients with primary amenorrhea, short stature and elevated levels of gonadotropins in urine have been studied and found to be chromatin positive. Though study of the chromosomes revealed 44 autosomes and two X chromosomes, one X chromosome was considerably longer than the other and had a median centromere unlike the usual X chromosome. Three cases of this particular grouping were reported by Fraccaro. He suggested that the abnormal chromosome developed by a splitting of the centromere in an incorrect manner at the time of the second meiotic division. This *isochromosome* is due to transverse rather than longitudinal division through the upper margin of the centromere.

THE XY FEMALE

Still another group of patients who have primary amenorrhea with a feminine appearance have been found to have intra-abdominal, inguinal or labial testes. These patients have been grouped in the past under a general heading of male pseudohermaphroditism, feminizing-testis type. Figure 16–20 illustrates an example of this syndrome. The testes in these individuals actually secrete estrogen and therefore bring about development of the secondary sex characteristics at adolescence. The breasts may be normally developed but axillary and pubic hair is scant or absent. While the external genitalia are normally female, there is minimal development of the labia minora, and the vagina consists of a blind pouch. The clitoris is not usually enlarged. The uterus is absent, but rudimentary oviducts may be present.

Patients with the syndrome of testicular feminization are chromatin negative and have a 46/XY karyotype which cannot be distinguished from that of the normal male. This disorder is a hereditary disturbance of sexual differentiation with transmission via the mother. In this particular group, it has been suggested that there is a mutation of sex genes on the X chromosome which is capable of modifying the action of the Y-chromosome sex genes. Because of fetal end-organ insensitivity, the development of the external genitalia is female but the müllerian ducts are usually absent or are very rudimentary. An enzymatic defect in the synthesis of testicular hormones in the testis may stimulate the development of secondary sex characteristics after puberty. Wilkins found an end-organ insensitivity to androgen in these patients. Since there is a rather high incidence of malignancy in these testes, they should be removed after puberty, and following orchiectomy substitutional estrogenic therapy should be administered.

Carr has stated that thirteen per cent of all women with primary amenorrhea have a normal male chromosome constitution, 46,XY. Although these patients have been classified into four categories, three present similar features and include cases of male pseudohermaphroditism, mixed gonadal dysgenesis, and pure gonadal dysgenesis or agenesis.

The most clearly defined syndrome in females of XY chromosome configuration is that of testicular feminization. The testis in these individuals is similar to those found in cryptorchid males and in the prepuberal patient it is similar to the male gonad found prior to puberty. After puberty immature tubular development occurs and the tubules are lined by imma-

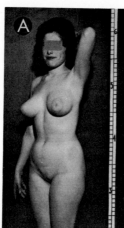

Fig. 16–20.—Testicular feminization. **A,** 18-year-old apparent female with primary amenorrhea, minimal sexual hair, large breasts and areolae but small nipples. FSH before surgery: over 13, less than 52 m.u.u.; 17-ketosteroids, 21 mg./24 hours; 17-ketogenic steroids, 5.5 mg./24 hours; pregnanetriol, 1.2 mg./24 hours. **B,** gonads and rudimentary uterine structures removed from patient in *A.* Note nodular appearance of the gonad.

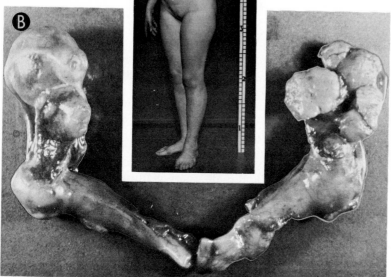

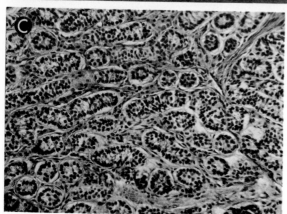

C, photomicrograph of gonad. Immature testicular tubules are lined principally by primitive germ cells with some Sertoli cells present. There is a marked resemblance to the fetal testis. (From Morris, J. M., and Mahesh, V. B.: Am. J. Obst. & Gynec. 87:731, 1963.) *(Continued.)*

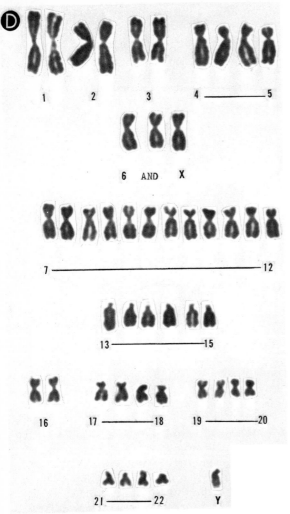

Fig. 16–20 *(cont.).*—**D,** karyotype of a patient with testicular feminization. It is a typical 46,XY distribution.

ture germ cells and Sertoli cells. Spermatogenesis is absent. There is a sparse scattering of Leydig cells but occasionally they are clumped around the hilar area. Primordial follicles and developing follicles are not seen.

Van Wyk demonstrated that patients with testicular feminization produce testosterone, and that the plasma half-life and pathways of testosterone are normal. He also showed that testosterone is converted to estrogen at a normal rate and that estrogen levels are not adequate to explain inhibition of testosterone. The resistance at the cellular level to normal amounts of testosterone, and lack of virilization, has been explained on the basis of a deficiency of dihydrotestosterone. Wilson and collaborators have shown that dihydrotestosterone is probably *the* effective peripheral androgen, at least in certain tissues. They showed that labeled testosterone is rapidly converted to reduction products by the nuclei of target tissues. Dihydrotestosterone has a higher affinity than testosterone for the nuclear protein and thus is the dominant steroid in androgen-sensitive cells. The conversion of testosterone to 5 alpha-dihydrotestosterone is brought about by a 5-alpha reductase enzyme, which has been shown to be present in both nuclei and cytoplasm of male accessory organs. Although dihydrotestosterone has been determined in human peripheral plasma by Ito and Horton, diminished levels have not, as yet, been reported in patients with testicular feminization. However, several patients with this syndrome have been given dihydrotestosterone and seemed unresponsive.

Morris and Mahesh recently reviewed the world literature on testicular feminization and presented four patients studied cytogenetically and biochemically. They concluded:

1. The name "testicular feminization" is in part a misnomer since the basic defect appears to be related to an interference with the mechanism of androgen action.

2. It should be differentiated from incomplete forms of the syndrome which show some degree of clitoridean enlargement and unpredictable secondary sex characteristics. In one such case, deficient androgen production and a normal response to exogenous androgen were noted.

3. An element of gonadal dysgenesis may be present since the gonads of this syndrome differ morphologically from the undescended testis of the male.

4. Peripheral and gonadal blood steroid determinations as well as incubation studies indicate that there may be a quantitative, but no qualitative, defect in hormone production. Dehydroepiandrosterone production, both free and as the sulfate, is exceptionally high, but androstenedione, testosterone, estradiol and estrone values appear to lie in ranges between those produced by the ovary and the testis.

5. The nonaction of androgen plus the presence of testicular, müllerian-inhibiting factor would appear to account for the fetal development. The non-action of androgen plus testicular estrogens is offered as an explanation for the type of secondary sex characteristics encountered.

The other three variations of the XY female have a common chromosome complex, variable internal and external genitalia, a predisposition to gonadal tumors together with an inheritance pattern of some degree. In male pseudohermaphroditism there is a combination of masculinization with female, internal genitalia. Patients with mixed gonadal dysgenesis demonstrate the features of a male pseudohermaphrodite but one gonad is a testis and the other consists of a mere streak of tissue. Both gonads are streaks in pure gonadal dysgenesis even though they may contain testicular tissue on occasion. The risk of malignant change in the dysgenetic gonad or testis in these syndromes seems to be higher than in testicular feminization where the incidence is about 4 per cent.

MONGOLISM (21-TRISOMY)

Because of the rather high incidence of congenital mental deficiency in patients with specific chromosomal defects, it was not unexpected to find a similar defect in the condition known as mongolism. Studies of blood and buccal smears in mongoloids demonstrated that the males were chromatin negative and the females chromatin positive. However, when chromosomal methods were utilized in both sexes, the chromosomal complement was found to be 47, instead of 46 (Fig. 16–21). Because there is an extra number 21 chromosome in all cells in patients with mongolism the name *21-trisomy* has been adopted. Probably the great majority of cases developed as a simple process of "nondisjunction" in the mother's ovary. As mentioned before, during the normal reduction division the chromosomes pair and divide equally, one of each pair to the nucleus of the ovum, one to the nucleus of the first polar body. In a nondisjunction division, one chromosome goes astray, so that two arrive in one nucleus and none in the other nucleus. If the ovum chances to collect an extra 21 chromosome in this way and is fertilized, the offspring carries the extra 21 and is a mongol. If the extra 21 goes into the polar body, the ovum carries none, and after fertilization the zygote has only the one 21 derived from the spermatozoa, which is insufficient for survival. Since reduction-division in the ovary is a rather long drawn-out affair, lasting from before birth to near the time of liberation of the ovum, it is not surprising to find that nondisjunctions increase in frequency with age. It is because of this fact that mongoloid children are so often the offspring of elderly mothers.

The overall incidence of Down's syndrome is about 1 in every 600 births but this varies with maternal age. Penrose calculated that the incidence in women under age 29 is only 1 in 2,000 whereas after age 45 it is 1 in 50. During the first year of life the mortality rate approximates 40 per cent. Many affected individuals do reach adult life and several women with Down's syndrome have borne children. Sixteen offspring have been studied and the syndrome occurred in six of these.

Fig. 16–21.—Karyotype of a patient with mongolism. The diploid number of chromosomes is 47, due to the extra 21 chromosome. (From Hirschhorn, K., and Cooper, L. C.: Am. J. Med. 31:442, 1961.)

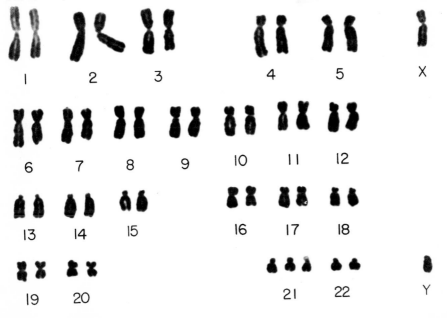

Although most mongols appear as isolated events, there is a slight tendency to familial occurrence. This is of much greater importance in mongols born of young mothers. In such cases, a factor other than ordinary nondisjunction is present. In a study of familial mongolism by Penrose and Polani, it was found that three main aberrants of familial mongolism existed. (1) If mongols have children, half of these children will be mongols. (2) Certain families have an inherited tendency to nondisjunction of chromosomes. (3) In certain cases there is a translocation process.

In the translocation mongol the extra 21 chromosome is not free but is attached, by a process of translocation, to another chromosome. Obviously, since it does not appear on the idiogram as a separate chromosome, these patients appear to have the normal 46 chromosomes. One of the parents, usually the mother, is a carrier. As a carrier, she apparently has only 45 chromosomes, one of the 21 group being attached to another chromosome. Since she herself has the material for a normal chromosome set, she is not herself abnormal. She may transmit the double translocation chromosome to her offspring, who may be normal, carriers or mongols. The practical aspect of the chromosomal abnormality of mongolism is important. If a young woman with a mongol child seeks advice regarding the prospect of further children being affected with this disease, the physician is frequently hard pressed to answer accurately. However, if translocation can be eliminated by chromosome studies, the patient may be reassured that the risk is not much more than the ordinary risk of chance alone. The likelihood of having a Down's child is about 11 per cent when the mother is the carrier; when the father is the carrier it is about $2\frac{1}{2}$ per cent.

Mosaicism may exist in Down's syndrome since some patients will be found to have a normal cell line in addition to cells which are trisomic for the 21 chromosome. In others the long arm of the extra chromosome may be deleted. However, the phenotype of typical Down's syndrome is not necessarily changed in patients with mosaicism and it may vary from normal to severe abnormality. Huang and associates have indicated that over 95 per cent of patients with Down's syndrome have the usual variety of trisomy-21 and another 2 per cent have trisomy-21/normal mosaicism.

The G group chromosomes, 21 and 22, cannot be differentiated on pure morphologic grounds. Autoradiographic studies of the DNA replication pattern have also failed to distinguish these two chromosome pairs. However, several patients have been reported to have an extra G chromosome without the clinical picture of Down's syndrome. In the absence of meiotic studies, these patients have been considered to have either trisomy 22, an extra, structurally abnormal D chromosome, or the aneuploid products of reciprocal translocations. Caspersson and associates reported a method of distinguishing between 21 and 22 by the quinacrine mustard (QM) fluorescence pattern. Earlier studies of the QM fluorescence pattern have shown that the G chromosomes can easily be distinguished in the normal cells. One pair generally demonstrates much brighter fluorescence than the other and it has a prominent band in its long arm. Caspersson suggested that the brightly fluorescing G chromosome occurring in triplicate in patients with Down's syndrome should be referred to as number 21. In one patient studied, one chromosome 21 showed brightly fluorescing satellites. The presence of this marker provides an opportunity for family studies to determine whether the extra chromosome is of maternal or paternal origin.

EDWARD'S SYNDROME (18-TRISOMY)

This unusual syndrome occurs in about 1 of every 5,000 births and is characterized by severe mental retardation and abnormalities in almost all major systems. Gross brain abnormalities are frequent, particularly absence of the cerebellum and corpus callosum. The infant is usually born at term but the placenta is small and the birth weight is reduced. A single umbilical artery is found in over 80 per cent of infants with trisomy-18. The mortality rate is higher than that of Down's syndrome with the mean age at death being near 10 weeks. The mean age of mothers is somewhat increased but not to the degree seen in Down's syndrome and transmission via a chromosome translocation in a parent is apparently rare.

BARTHOLIN-PATAU SYNDROME (13-TRISOMY)

This unusual syndrome was first described by Bartholin in 1657 but the etiology was not clarified until 1960. The perinatal mortality is high, only 14 per cent of those affected living over one year. Brain defects are common particularly absence of the olfactory tracts and bulbs. Holotelencephaly (entire absence of the structures derived from the prosencephalon) is a common finding and mental retardation in survivors is severe.

The incidence of 13-trisomy varies between 1 in 5,000 and 1 in 15,000. The birth weight of the infant is diminished and a single umbilical artery is a common finding. The maternal age of women giving birth to infants with 13-trisomy is increased but it is not as advanced as that seen in Down's syndrome. Bartholin-Patau syndrome may result from transmission of a translocation in a carrier patient but the apparent risk is quite small.

DELETION SYNDROMES

The well-defined syndromes previously described are associated with absence or extra sex chromosomes or extra autosomes of the 13, 18 or 21 group. There are two other syndromes which occur in the human which are due to loss of chromatin material. The more popularly known disorder is called the "maladie du cri du chat" (cat-cry disease) and is due to loss of material from the short arm of a chromosome in group B, usually number 5 (5p-). These infants have a characteristic high-pitched cry, a low birth weight, mental retardation, microcephaly, anti-Mongoloid slant of the eyes with low set ears, transverse palmar crease and underdeveloped mandible. In addition, congenital heart disease is found in over 25 per cent of the patients and, as in 18-trisomy, there is a significant excess of females.

The other autosomal anomaly syndrome is due to deletion of material from the long arm of chromosome 18 and is known only as "18q- syndrome." The phenotypic characteristics include mental retardation, microcephaly, retracted face and prominent chin, tapered fingers, deep voice, abnormal genitalia, hypertelorism of the eyes, atresia or narrowing of the external auditory meatus, atrophy of the optic disc, nystagmus, epicanthus, diminished stature, hypotonia and congenital heart disease. The mean birth weight is diminished but the abnormalities are not incompatible with life. Both the "cri du chat" and "18q-" syndromes are compatible with development into adult life and may, therefore, be found among inmates of institutions for the mentally retarded. Neither is associated with increased age of the mother, in contrast to the situation in the three trisomy syndromes.

SPONTANEOUS ABORTIONS

Although chromosomal abnormalities are said to occur in approximately 1 in every 200 live births, a great many more undoubtedly are present in early abortuses. Fortunately only about 10 per cent of zygotes with chromosomal disorders survive and result in live born infants. Numerous studies of chromosomes in spontaneous abortions have been published and the incidence of derangement varies from 8 to 40 per cent with a mean of 21 per cent. The principal abnormalities are due to trisomy, X-monosomy (45,X), and polyploidy. Among the latter are triploidy (69 chromosomes) and tetraploidy (92 chromosomes).

Studies of abortuses have shown that autosomal trisomy is the most frequently described. The extra chromosome may be found in any group but the smaller pairs are more commonly involved. Trisomy of groups G and D are more frequent in abortuses of older women but trisomy-16 (Group E) is not age dependent. Although monosomy (absence of an autosome) rarely occurs in liveborn infants, X-monosomy (XO) is a frequent occurrence and is responsible for 20 to 25 per cent of all chromosomal anomalies found in abortuses. Carr has calculated that only 2 to 3 per cent of XO zygotes reach term, are liveborn and ultimately are found to have Turner's syndrome.

About 5 per cent of all spontaneous abortions are due to the presence of extra sets of chromosomes in which the normal germ cell complement of 23 chromosomes is tripled (triploidy,69) or quadrupled (tetraploidy,92). Triploidy occurs more frequently than tetraploidy and both have mosaic variations. Almost half of triploid abortuses have shown recognizable embryonic material and about a third have shown macerated embryos. A striking feature of the triploid abortus syndrome is the hydatidiform degeneration of placental villi. Triploidy has been noted in about 70 per cent of placentas showing hydatidiform changes but in only 13 per cent of abortuses in which the diagnosis was hydatidiform mole. A predominance of the normal female karyotype has been noted in molar pregnancies.

Polyploidy has been observed with increased incidence in abortuses of women who became pregnant within six months of stopping oral contraceptives but the anomalies were not compatible with live birth. However, there is no evidence at present that the overall incidence of spontaneous abortion is increased in women who become pregnant shortly after pill discontinuation. Such an increase might be expected if the estrogen-progestin combination used had produced endometrial atrophy. Maintenance of a more normal endometrial morphology by sequential oral contraceptives would be less likely to result in atrophic glands and stroma and, therefore, would be less likely to produce implantation disorders.

Although the number of cases studied is relatively small, there is insufficient evidence to indict chromosomal abnormalities as the cause of repeated spontaneous abortions. However, in such couples one of the parents is frequently found to be a carrier of a chromosomal abnormality in which, at the time of meiosis, translocation may occur and gametes lacking varying amount of chromosomal material are formed.

MISCELLANEOUS ABNORMALITIES

The Stein-Leventhal syndrome has recently been shown to have an hereditary basis and is probably an autosomal dominant condition. Certain other diseases of the skin and connective tissue occasionally affect the female genitalia which may be classified as autosomal dominant disorders. These include ovarian dysgerminoma, vulvar leiomyomata and hereditary telangiectasia. Other disorders of gynecologic interest are autosomal recessive in type and result from homozygous expression of a mutant gene. These include the adrenogenital syndrome, one form of gonadal dysgenesis without aneuploidy (46,XX) and at least one variation of transverse vaginal septum.

Anencephaly may be considered to be an autosomal recessive condition with an empiric probability of recurrence of a subsequent sibling of 1 in 30. However, the presence of a recessive gene in a specific family establishes a risk of 1 in 4. Hydrocephaly may be due to an autosomal or an X-linked recessive trait. The risk of recurrence in a sibling is said to be about 1 in 100.

Hypermenorrhea may occasionally be due to hereditary bleeding disorders which occur as autosomal recessive syndromes. These include prothrombin deficiency, Factor VII and X deficiency, thrombopathic thrombocytopenia and thrombasthenia. Minot-von Willebrand disease is an autosomal dominant inherited condition.

A galaxy of other gynecologic abnormalities occur as autosomal recessive conditions. These include the Laurence-Moon-Biedl and Werner syndromes (hypogonadism), Bowen's syndrome (enlarged clitoris), Gorlin's syndrome (hypoplasia of labia majora), Fraser's syndrome (fusion of labia, enlarged clitoris, bicornuate uterus, malformed oviducts) and leprechaunism (ovarian cysts with clitoral and mammary hypertrophy).

Supernumerary breasts may be inherited as a simple dominant trait and inverted nipples may be the result of single gene mutations. Congenital uterine abnormalites may result from deleterious environmental factors although multifactorial inheritance must be considered. The most likely explanation of those cases due to genetic factors is that the gene is present in the transmitting individuals but either penetrance (ability of a gene to be expressed if present) is absent or expressivity (the degree of manifestation) is mild.

Lynch and associates have called attention to the possibility of an hereditary cancer predisposition. A familial tendency has been noted in breast and endometrial cancer and, according to Simpson and Christakos, the etiology of this syndrome is compatible with that of a single mutant gene of low penetrance and varying expressivity. Ovarian tumors, particularly of the granulosa cell variety, have been reported with increased frequency in women with Peutz-Jeghers syndrome (gastrointestinal polyps with melanosis of lips, oral mucosa and digits), an autosomal dominant disease.

Studies by various investigators have shown that irregular chromosome numbers (aneuploidy) are found in practically all metaphase spreads obtained from squamous-cell carcinoma of the cervix and from a variety of malignant tumors. The findings in adenocarcinoma of the endometrium are not so clear cut. Tseng and Jones reported finding aneuploid cells in all of seven adenocarcinomas of the endometrium but in some cases the presence of diploid cells with apparently normal karyotypes was a rather striking finding. Wagner, Richart and Terner described a diploid or tetraploid DNA-distribution in the cells of cystic glandular hyperplasia of the endometrium which was indistinguishable from that of normal proliferative endometrium. The same diploid or tetraploid DNA distribution was found in 8 of 10 patients with adenomatous hyperplasia but the other two had an aneuploid DNA-distribution pattern which was similar to that found in invasive endometrial adenocarcinoma. These investigators found aneuploid DNA-distribution patterns in all specimens of adenocarcinoma and therefore concluded: "Since every group of precursor lesions in other organs studied by microspectrophotometry have been reported to have aneuploid DNA-distribution patterns, the results of this study suggest that most of the lesions now diagnosed as precursors of endometrial carcinoma either deviate from the pattern of other epithelia or that the morphologic criteria which traditionally are used in the diagnosis of these lesions are insufficiently precise." I would choose the latter conclusion since clinical studies have indicated that only about 10 to 12 per cent of patients with atypical adenomatous endometrial hyperplasia progress to invasive carcinoma. This incidence approximates the 20 per cent of hyperplasia which were found to have aneuploid DNA-distribution patterns and suggests that only these individuals are "cancer prone."

Chronic lymphatic leukemia has given no evidence of chromosomal anomaly but the acute leukemias vary a great deal. Some demonstrate no change, whereas in others there is a great deal of change. In chronic myeloid leukemia a highly specific lesion is present in almost every case. This was first noted by Nowell and Hungerford of Philadelphia and therefore it is called the Philadelphia chromosome, abbreviated as Ph[1]. The Philadelphia chromosome appears as a G chromosome lacking approximately half its long arm. Although originally identified as number 21, Caspersson and associates, using quinacrine mustard fluorescence patterns, state: "The Philadelphia chromosome is number 22 with a deletion—although a translocation cannot be excluded with certainty. It seems as though the chromosome breakage had occurred in the fluorescent region of the long arm of chromosome number 22, making it analogous to our findings in the cri du chat syndrome."

In leukemia the anomaly is different from other chromosomal aberrations in that only the leukemic cells are affected. Some traumatic process, possibly x-ray, presumably damages a white blood cell precursor or, precisely, a specific chromosome of the precursor to cause rapid multiplication of the cell. This damaged chromosome transmits the trait to its numerous offspring. This is about the most direct evidence to support the idea that x-rays produce cancer.

It is interesting to note that leukemia is a common cause of death in mongolism and that G chromosomes are involved in both diseases. This correlation is not absolute, since the leukemia of mongolism is an acute leukemia and does not show the Philadelphia chromosome. It may be possible that leukemia can complicate any chromosomal anomaly whether or not the 21 chromosome is involved. An association with radiation has been demonstrated by Tough and associates. They noted that doses of x-ray to the spine used in the treatment of spondylitis cause a surprisingly large shower of chromosomal anomalies. It has also been shown that therapy with radioactive iodine may produce the same situation.

Prophylaxis

Congenital anomalies, physical maldevelopment and twenty thousand new cases of mental retardation each year are undoubtedly related to chromosomal abnormalities. Almost half of these children die each year. How can these tragedies be prevented? Clear cut answers are not as yet possible although suggestions for prophylaxis are at hand.

The commonest autosomal defect, Down's syndrome, is markedly increased in women over the age of forty. The same is true for syndromes of the 13 and 18-trisomy variety. Prohylaxis is simple: advise completion of pregnancies prior to age thirty five. But increased age does not seem to be a factor in the 45,X anomaly, in the deletion syndromes or in the commonest trisomy found in abortions (trisomy-16). How may these disorders be prevented?

Certain drugs, viruses and radiation are known causes of chromosome damage. Therefore, it is advisable to know at the earliest possible moment that pregnancy has occurred so that all medications known to have a deleterious effect on chromosomes may be avoided. Similarly, radiation, particularly fluoroscopy and therapeutic radiation, should not be utilized during the early stages of pregnancy and diagnostic x-rays should be kept to an absolute minimum. Animals have a mechanism which insures the impregnation of "fresh" eggs but the human female does not. Since "old" eggs have a propensity for abnormal chromosomal development, it seems obvious that methods for early fertilization be provided.

A correlation between radiation and Down's syndrome has been suggested. Epidemics of hepatitis and rubella have indicated the serious effects of certain viruses on chromosome integrity. Certain autoimmune disease states, particularly an increase of thyroid autoantibodies, have been indicted in Down's syndrome and gonadal dysgenesis. The relative hormonal insufficiency of women during the fourth decade of life may lead to prolonged aging of the ova either by delaying follicular release, by slowing transport or by impeding implantation.

Since an increase in polyploid abortuses has been noted when pregnancy occurs soon after discontinuation of oral contraceptives, it might be prudent to advise against early post-pill conception. An irregularity and elevation of luteinizing hormone has been noted during the months after discontinuation of oral contraceptives although a definitive correlation between this observation and chromosomal abnormalities has not been proved. Hydatidiform degeneration of placental villi is associated with triploidy in 70 per cent of patients studied, and both of these conditions have been noted to occur with increased frequency in women in whom pregnancy occurred shortly after they stopped oral contraceptives.

An increase in the incidence of monozygotic twinning has been reported in the families of patients with Turner's syndrome and a similar increase in

TABLE 16-1.—Etiologic Factors in Chromosomal Aneuploidy

Predisposing Factor	Trisomy	45,X(XO)	Polyploidy
Increased maternal age	Yes	No	No
Radiation exposure	Yes	?	?
Virus infection (hepatitis)	Conflicting	?	?
Thyroid antibodies (maternal)	Yes	Conflicting	?
Genetic causes	Some evidence	?	?
Chromosomal factors	Yes	?	?
Post oral contraceptive	No	No	Yes

From: Carr, D. H. Chromosomal errors and development. Am. J. Obst. & Gynec. 104: 327, 1969.

dizygotic twinning has been noted in the families of patients with Klinefelter's syndrome. The significance of these observations is unknown. Carr has summarized the relationship of etiologic factors to chromosomal aneuploidy in Table 16-1.

The gynecologist, obstetrician and pediatrician may, in the near future, be able to render immediate neonatal therapy to certain treatable disorders or interrupt other pregnancies when treatment is not available or is ineffective. The procedure of amniocentesis permits accurate antenatal chromosomal diagnosis. Amniocentesis in Rh disease proved that fetal diagnosis was both possible and clinically useful. Subsequently fetal cells, obtained by centrifugation of amniotic fluid have been used for sex determination by noting the presence or absence of a Barr body. The presence of a Barr body indicates the presence of a female fetus in utero and its absence (except in the case of an XO genotype) indicates a male. This observation is of clinical importance in the management of pregnancies where the mother is a known carrier of hemophilia or muscular dystrophy, both sex-linked hereditary disorders.

Much more information has been obtained in regard to hereditary defects by culturing the primary cells obtained at the time of amniocentesis and performing subsequent karyotypes. Observations of chromosomes have been used in patients where the possibility of Down's syndrome existed and these studies have resulted in the delivery of mongoloid fetuses by therapeutic abortion. But the potential of this procedure is limited by the fact that in Down's syndrome the ratio of non-inherited (21-trisomy) to inherited (D/G translocation) cases approximates 50 to 1. Thus there is little chance of chromosome analysis being done unless suspicion is already stimulated by the previous reproductive history or age of the mother.

The most fertile field for prenatal diagnosis by amniocentesis involves biochemical methods to study cultured cells. One of these methods employs a phenomenon of metachromasia in which certain cell abnormalities induce a pink color in the cytoplasm after the addition of toluidine blue O stain. Metachromasia is manifested in a multitude of hereditary "storage diseases" as well as in cystic fibrosis.

Positive identification of the carrier state has been achieved in a number of inherited metabolic disorders by Dr. B. Shannon Danes. Staining of skin fibroblast cultures reveals cytoplasmic inclusions which reflect the underlying chemical abnormality in Hurler's syndrome, cystic fibrosis and Gaucher's disease. Danes has pointed out that metachromasia is not a test

TABLE 16-2.—FAMILIAL METABOLIC DISORDERS DEMONSTRABLE IN TISSUE CULTURE

Acatalasemia	Cystathioninuria
Chediak-Higashi syndrome	Pompe's disease
Citrullinemia	Homocystinuria
Cystic fibrosis	Refsum's disease
Cystinosis	Galactosemia
Gaucher's disease	Mucopolysaccharidoses
Marfan's syndrome	Lesch-Nyhan syndrome
Orotic aciduria	Branched chain ketonuria
Sphingomyelinosis	Glucose-6-phosphate
(Niemann-Pick variants)	dehydrogenase deficiency

From: Dancis, J. The prenatal detection of hereditary defects. Hospital Practice, 4:37, 1969.

for the presence of specific abnormal substances within cells; for example, lipids and mucopolysaccaharides. It results from the presence of almost any normal or abnormal large molecule when stored within the cell. She has suggested that the most immediate and practical application of her work is in the field of genetic counseling. Table 16-2 lists the various disorders which can be diagnosed postnatally in tissue culture and therefore are potential candidates for detection in utero. A marked reduction in the occurrence of these genetic diseases becomes a definite possibility as a result of these studies. However, the tissue culture test is time-consuming (6 weeks) and expensive and is not yet acceptable for mass screening. Danes has attempted to expedite the procedure by culturing leukocytes from peripheral blood and she has observed the same metachromasia in both patients and carriers that had been observed in skin fibroblasts. This procedure can be completed in 5 days and, if it proves reliable, opens a wide vista for prophylaxis of genetic disease.

Clinical Aspects of Chromosome Determinations

From a practical and purely clinical standpoint, there are certain conditions in which chromosome counts should be routinely performed. These include primary amenorrhea in women, aspermia in men, marked defects in stature and a failure of secondary sex characteristics to develop. Obviously, patients in whom structural defects of the genitalia are noted should also have chromosome counts. As mentioned, many cases of myelogenous leukemia are of genetic origin and the chromosome counts seem to be related to prognosis. Those genetic diseases easily diagnosed clinically (for example, mongolism) need not be referred routinely for chromosome counts. However, the parents of a child with mongolism should have chromosome determinations since this may alter their plans for future children.

Carr has suggested the following indications for sex chromatin study:

1. Male infertility.
2. Shortness of stature in girls.
3. Primary amenorrhea.
4. Ambiguous external genitalia.
5. Mental retardation and/or psychosis.

He has listed the following indications for chromosome analysis:

1. Abnormal sex chromatin findings.
2. To confirm the diagnosis of chromosomal syndromes.

3. Parents with a history of varied terminations of pregnancy (normal, abnormal and aborted).
4. Single interphalangeal crease on one or both fifth fingers.
5. Unexplained failure to thrive.
6. Aggressive, antisocial behavior in tall males.
7. Familial Down's syndrome.
8. Parents under 30 at time of birth of a child with Down's syndrome.
9. Chronic myeloid leukemia.

The clinician may easily identify XY chromosomes of sexual determination without an expensive chromosomal idiogram. A smear of the buccal mucosa may be obtained, fixed in the same fashion as an ordinary Papanicolaou smear and sent to a cytologic laboratory. The cytologist will then be able to report the absence of chromatin bodies (chromatin negative) or the presence of one, two or three bodies (chromatin positive). A simple rule of thumb is that the number of X chromosomes any individual possesses is one more than the number of chromatin bodies in the nuclei of his or her cells. Reference to Table 16–3 will enable the clinician to diagnose the major deviations in sexual development. Not all cases of Klinefelter's syndrome have one chromatin body in the nucleus. However, the presence of one chromatin body plus the male body build always indicates Klinefelter's syndrome. In a similar manner, not all patients with Turner's

TABLE 16–3.—SUMMARY OF CHROMOSOME FINDINGS IN VARIOUS CLINICAL STATES*

CLINICAL STATE	SEX CHROMATIN	CHROMOSOME CONSTITUTION
Normal male	−	(46) XY
Normal female	+	(46) XX
Pseudohermaphroditism		
Male	−	(46) XY
Female	+	(46) XX
True hermaphroditism	+	(46) XX
	−	(46) XY
Klinefelter's syndrome	+	(47) XXY, (47/46) XXY/XX, (48) XXYY
	−	(46) XY, (47/46) XXY/XY
Turner's syndrome	−	(45) XO, (45/46) XO/XX
	+	(45) XO, (45/46) XO/XX, (46) XX
"Pure" gonadal dysgenesis	−	(46) XY
"Atypical" gonadal dysgenesis	±†	(46) Xx
	−	(45) XO
Poly-X conditions		
Female phenotype		
Fertility or premature menopause	+	(47) XXX
Primary amenorrhea	+	(47/45) XXX/XO
Male phenotype		
Microorchidism	+	(48) XXXY, (48/49) XXXY/XXXXY
Mongolism		(47) with trisomy for no. 21
		(46) with Trisomy and monosomy or translocation
Multiple congenital anomalies‡		(47) with trisomy for various autosomes
		(49) XXY with triple trisomy
		(69) XXY, complete trisomy
		(45) with centric fusion
Leukemia‡		Abnormal satellites
Radiation effects		Abnormal numbers and forms
		Abnormal forms and numbers

*From Hirschhorn, K., and Cooper, L. C.: Am. J. Med. 31:442, 1961.
†Sex-chromatin bodies (small) in 7 per cent of buccal smear nuclei.
‡Chromosome abnormalities in some but not all instances.

syndrome are XO, but all patients with this clinical pattern will have Turner's syndrome.

If there is doubt about sex of the infant at birth, various tests such as the chromatin pattern, endocrinological evaluation and laparotomy may help decide how the individual should be raised. However, even these procedures can lead to mistakes and, in general, the best single guide is the state of the external sex organs. Mistakes will be minimized if information is objectively obtained and analyzed in terms of current knowledge and experience. For example, an infant with XY chromosomes whose phallus is poorly developed as well as hypospadiac can never become a satisfactory male. It is better to convert the child to neuter gender and rear as a female, every effort being exerted to accentuate femininity by removing cryptorchid testes and phallus and later administering exogenous estrogens. One of the basic principles to be remembered is that femininity approaches the neuter state. Therefore it is simpler to make an intersex individual appear female than male. Treatment should be based on a wide interpretation of sex and not on any one criterion such as chromosome counts, sex-chromatin pattern, the histologic appearance of the gonad or the nature of the genital ducts. The final question to be answered is: Will the individual adapt better as a male or as a female?

Recent evidence has shown the fallacy of simple counting of chromosomes of a small number of cells as a complete analysis of the individual carrier type. Harnden has emphasized that chromosome number should not be regarded as constant throughout the body, since in a large sample at least 5 per cent of individuals will have a count above or below the modal number of 46. This variability may be among tissues in different parts of the body or among cells in adjacent areas. In addition, abnormal counts increase with age and it has been discovered that an elderly female may normally lack as much as 12 per cent of her original X chromosomes. An elderly man similarly shows a tendency to lose the Y chromosome. Great care must be exercised, therefore, in making the diagnosis of chromosome mosaicism in the older individual. Harnden routinely counts 30 cells and analyzes all of these. When it is practical, more than one tissue should be examined and, if necessary, the number of cells counted and analyzed should be increased to 50 or 100. Exacting studies of the chromosomes of a large number of apparently normal persons have shown a heteromorphic number 16 chromosome. In a study of over 300 subjects by Harnden three types of chromosome arrangements have been identified. These are a deletion in chromosome number 16, an apparent absence of the short arm of one of the 13–15 group and a lengthened short arm of the 21–22 group. Each of these patterns has been seen in 1–2 per cent of the subjects.

Szulman has studied the chromosomes obtained from both therapeutic and spontaneous abortuses at the Boston Lying-in Hospital. He found that the karyotypes of cells of the chorion mirrored those of the skin of the fetus and has used this tissue for analysis. He succeeded in culturing cells in 15 of 17 therapeutic abortions and all had karyotypes within normal range. In spontaneous abortions, however, 60 per cent showed abnormal karyotypes. Early death of the ovum was due, in his series, to complete triplication of the chromosomes (not just the 21 chromosome as in mongolism) or XO configuration. Since XO combinations of the type seen in Turner's syndrome and XXY combinations of the type seen in Klinefelter's syndrome are the result of disjunction, there should be an equal number of both such individuals. Actually, there is a great preponderance of patients with Klinefelter's syndrome. Szulman feels that this is the result of intrauterine death of the fetus having XO configuration.

Triplication of the genome (that is, triple chromosomes of both autosomes and sex chromosomes) is incompatible with life in the human being although it has been reported in certain animal species. Triplication of the genum may be induced in mammals experimentally, but growth does not progress beyond the first half of gestation. Triplication of the genum has been found by Szulman both in macerated fetuses and in the vesicles of hydatidiform moles. Other abortions may be due to a YO chromosomal pattern.

BIBLIOGRAPHY

Barr, M. L., and Bertram, E. G.: A morphologic distinction between neurones of the male and female, and the behavior of the nucleolar satellite during accelerated nucleoprotein synthesis, Nature (London) 163:676, 1949.
———, and Carr, D. H.: Sex chromatin, sex chromosomes and sex anomalies, Canad. M.A.J. 83:979, 1960.
Benirschke, K.: Cytogenetic Abnormalities in Reproduction, in Behrman. S. J., and Kistner, R. W. (eds.): *Progress in Infertility* (Boston: Little, Brown & Company, 1968), p. 817.
Carr, D. H.: Chromosomal errors and development, Am. J. Obst. & Gynec. 104:327, 1969.
———; Barr, M. L., and Plunkett, E. R.: An XXXX sex chromosome complex in two mentally defective females, Canadian M. Assn. J. 84:131, 1961.
Caspersson, T.; Gahrton, G., Lindsten, J., and Zech, L.: Identification of the Philadelphia chromosome as a number 22 by quinacrine-mustard fluorescence analysis. Exper. Cell Res. 61:240, 1970.
Caspersson, T.; Hulten, M., Lindsten, J., and Zech, L.: Distinction between extra G-like chromosomes by quinacrine-mustard fluorescent analysis, Exper. Cell Res. 61:242, 1970.
Caspersson, T.; Zech, L., and Johansson, C.: Differential binding of alkylating fluorochromes in human chromosomes, Exper. Cell Res. 60:315, 1970.
Dancis, J.: The prenatal detection of hereditary defects, Hospital Practice, 4:37, 1969.
Danes, B. S.: Cell cultures and genetic disease, Hospital Practice, 4:88, 1969.
Edwards, J. H., *et al.*: A new trisomic syndrome, Lancet 1:787, 1960.
Federman, D. A.: *Abnormal Sexual Development* (Philadelphia: W. B. Saunders Company, 1967).
Finley, W. H.; Finley, S. C.; Hardy, J. P., and McKinnon, T.: Down's syndrome in mother and child, Obst. & Gynec. 32:200, 1968.
Ford, C. E.: Human cytogenetics: Its present place and future possibilities, Am. J. Human Genet. 12:104, 1960.
———, *et al.*: The chromosomes in a patient showing both mongolism and the Klinefelter's syndrome, Lancet 1:709, 1959.
Fraccaro, M.; Gemzell, G. A., and Lindsten, J.: Plasma level of growth hormone and chromosome complement in 4 patients with gonadal dysgenesis (Turner's syndrome), Acta endocrinol, 34:496, 1960.
Fraser, J., *et al.*: A case of XXXXY Klinefelter's syndrome, Lancet 2:1064, 1961.
Fraser, J. H., *et al.*: The XXX syndrome: Frequency among mental defectives and fertility, Lancet 2:626, 1960.
Greenblatt, R. B.; Carmona, N., and Higdun, L.: Gonadal dysgenesis with androgenic manifestations in the tall eunuchoid female, J. Clin. Endocrinol. 16:235, 1956.
Griboff, S. I., and Lawrence, R.: The chromosomal etiology of congenital gonadal defects, Am. J. Med. 30:544, 1961.
Grumbach, M. M., and Barr, M. L.: Cytologic tests of chromosomal sex in relation to sexual anomalies in man, Recent Prog. Hormone Res. 14:255, 1958.
Hamerton, J. L., *et al.*: Differential diagnosis of Down's syndrome (mongolism) through male and female translocation carriers, Lancet 2:956, 1961.
Harnden, D. G.: Paper presented at the 2d International Conference on Congenital Malformations, New York City, August 8, 1963.
Hirschhorn, K., and Cooper, H. L.: Chromosomal aberrations in human disease: A review of the status of cytogenetics in medicine, Am. J. Med. 31:442, 1961.
Jacobs, P. A., and Strong, J. A.: A case of human intersexuality having a possible XXY sex-determining mechanism, Nature (London) 183:302, 1959.

———, *et al.:* Evidence for the existence of the human "super female," Lancet 2:423, 1959.

———, *et al.:* Chromosomal sex in the syndrome of testicular feminization, Lancet 2:591, 1959.

———, *et al.:* Abnormalities involving the X chromosomes in women, Lancet 1:1213. 1960.

———, *et al.:* Cytogenetic studies in primary amenorrhea, Lancet 1:1183, 1961.

Johnston, A. W., *et al.:* The triple X syndrome: Clinical, pathological and chromosomal studies in 3 mentally retarded cases, Brit. M. J. 2:1047, 1961.

Jost, A.: Problems of fetal endocrinology: The gonadal and hypophyseal hormones, Recent Prog. Hormone Res. 8:379, 1953.

Klinefelter, H. F., Jr.; Reifenstein, E. C., Jr., and Albright, F.: Syndrome characterized by gynecomastia, aspermatogenesis with a-Leydigism, and increased excretion of follicle-stimulating hormone, J. Clin. Endocrinol. 2:615, 1942.

Lennox, B.: Human chromosomes: Some recent developments and an amazingly progressive field, "What's New" (Abbott Laboratories), No. 229, Winter, 1962, p. 12.

Lynch, H. T.: *Hereditary Factors in Carcinoma* (New York: Springer-Verlag, 1967).

Morris, J. M., and Mahesh, V. B.: Further observations on the syndrome "testicular feminization," Am. J. Obst. & Gynec. 87:731, 1963.

Nelson, W. O.: Sex differences in human nuclei with particular reference to the Klinefelter syndrome, gonadal agenesis and other types of hermaphroditism, Acta endocrinol. 23:227, 1956.

Patanelli, D. J., and Nelson, W. O.: Sex chromatin and chromosomes in man, Postgrad Med. 29:3, 1961.

Patau, K.: Chromosome identification and the Denver report, Lancet 1:933, 1961.

Rogers, J.: Chromosomal Aberrations and Gonadal Defects, in *Endocrine and Metabolic Aspects of Gynecology* (Philadelphia: W. B. Saunders Company, 1963).

Simpson, J. L., and Christakos, A. C.: Hereditary factors in obstetrics and gynecology, Obst. & Gynec. Surv. 24:580, 1969.

Sohval, A. R.: Recent progress in human chromosome analysis and its relation to the sex chromatin, Am. J. Med. 31:397, 1961.

———: Sex chromosomes in male infertility, Fertil. & Steril. 14:180, 1963.

Stewart, J. S.: Medullary gonadal dysgenesis (Chromatin-positive Klinefelter's syndrome), Lancet 1:1176, 1959.

———, *et al.:* Klinefelter's syndrome: Clinical and hormonal aspects, Quart, J. Med. 28:561,1959.

Szulman, A. E.: Significance of Chromosomal Abnormalities in Spontaneous Abortions, in Behrman, S. J., and Kistner, R. W. (eds.): *Progress in Infertility* (Boston: Little, Brown & Company, 1968), p. 847.

Tijo, J. H., and Levan, A.: The chromosome number of man, Hereditas 42:1, 1956.

Tseng, P. Y., and Jones, H. W.: Chromosome constitution of carcinoma of the endometrium, Obst. & Gynec. 33:741, 1969.

Tough, I., *et al.:* X-ray induced chromosome damage in man, Lancet 2:849, 1960.

———, *et al.:* Cytogenetic studies in chronic myeloid leukemia and acute leukemia associated with mongolism, Lancet 1:411, 1961.

Turner, H.: A syndrome of infantilism, congenital webbed neck and cubitus valgus, Endocrinology 23:566, 1938.

Wagner, D., Richard, R. M., and Terner, J. Y.: Desoxyribonucleic acid content of presumed precursors of endometrial carcinoma, Cancer 20:2067, 1967.

Wilkins, L.: *The Diagnosis and Treatment of Endocrine Disorders in Childhood and Adolescence* (2d ed.; Springfield, Ill.: Charles C Thomas, Publisher, 1957).

———, and Fleischmann, W.: Ovarian agenesis: Pathology, associated clinical symptoms and bearing on the theories of sex differentiation, J. Clin. Endocrinol. 4:357, 1944.

Index

A

ABDOMEN
  examination, 6
  in tubal ectopic pregnancy, 305-306
ABNORMALITIES (*see* Anomalies)
ABORTION
  habitual (*see below*)
  hormone production reduction and, 631
  infection after, 217-220
    treatment, 218-220
  Pergonal HMG and, 490
  spontaneous, and chromosomes, 738-739
  threatened, progestins in, 654
ABORTION, HABITUAL, 500-526
  anatomic defects in, 517-525
  chronic disease and, 503-504
  drugs contraindicated in early pregnancy, 515-517
  estrogen in, 508-509
    deficiency, 513
  etiologic factors, 500-502
  gonadotropin in, chorionic, 506-507
  hormonal aspects of, 505-517
  hypothalamic insufficiency and, 513
  immunologic factors in, 504-505
  incompetent cervical os, 517-519
    repair, 518-519
  luteal phase inadequacy in, 511-513
    diagnosis, 511-513
    treatment, 513
  management, 502-525
  nutritional disorders and, 503-504
  pituitary insufficiency and, 513
  progesterone in, 509-511
    deficiency, 513-515
  progestins in, 654
  psychosomatic aspects of, 502-503
  thyroid in, 507-508
ABSCESS: appendiceal, 340
ACETATE: conversion to pregnenolone, 621
ACTINOMYCIN D: in chorioadenoma destruens, 540
ADENOACANTHOMA, 436
ADENOCARCINOMA
  cervix, 147, 167-168
  endometrium, 260
  uterine corpus, 257-272
    diagnosis, 265-267
    grade III, 269
    medroxyprogesterone acetate in, 269
    pathogenesis, 263-265
    pathology, 258-263
    symptomatology, 265-267
    treatment, 267-272
ADENOMA
  (*See also* Chorioadenoma, Cystadenocarcinoma, Cystadenofibroma, Cystadenoma)

endometrial hyperplasia and, 250
ADENOMATOID TUMOR: of oviduct, 315
ADENOMYOSIS, 432
  uterine corpus, 221-226
    diagnosis, 221-222
    hysterography of, 222
    microscopic appearance, 223-225
    pathology, 222-225
    pathology, correlation of symptoms with, 225
    treatment, 225-226
ADRENAL (S)
  cortex
    biogenesis of cortisol and corticosterone in, 592
    hyperfunction, and sexual precocity, 553-556
    rest tumor, 406
    stimulation tests, 423
    suppression studies, 422-423
  hyperplasia, congenital, and 11-keto-pregnanetriol, 595
  in infertility, 494-495
  menstrual cycle and, 210
  oral contraception and, 690
  rest tumor, 405-407
    cortical, 406
  steroids, biosynthesis of, 591
  tumors, 405-407
    benign, and hirsutism, 610
    sexual precocity and, 553
ADRENOGENITAL SYNDROME, 588-598
  classic, 589
  diagnosis, 594-596
  treatment, 596-598
AGE AND CERVICAL CANCER, 133
  carcinoma, 134
AGENESIS: ovarian, 719
ALBRIGHT'S SYNDROME: and sexual precocity, 556
ALKERAN (*see* Melphalan)
ALKYLATING AGENTS: response to, in ovarian carcinoma, 377
ALLERGY: causing pruritus vulvae, 50
ALLOPREGNANE, 618-619
ALOPECIA: and adrenal rest tumor, 407
17-ALPHA-HYDROXYPROGESTERONE CAPROATE: in endometrial hyperplasia, 253
AMENORRHEA
  evaluation of patient with, 567-569
  Forbes-Albright syndrome and, 606-607
  primary, 560-563
    Turner's syndrome and, 719-721
  production method, diagram showing, 546
  progestins in, 649
  secondary, 563-566
    basal body temperature graph in, 488
    hypogonadism causing, hypogonadotropic, 565

oral contraception and, 699-700
treatment, 569-573
 AMPICILLIN: in salpingitis, puerperal and postabortal, 296
ANALGESIA: endometriosis and observation, 445
ANAPLASIA
in chorioadenoma destruens, 538
in hydatidiform mole, 530
ANDROGEN
formation, 622-627
ovulation suppression and, 446
postmenopause and, 667-669
therapy, 642-647
ANDROSTANE, 618-619
ANDROSTERONE, 626
ANENCEPHALY: and genetics, 739
ANEUPLOIDY, 706
etiologic factors in, 742
ANOMALIES
chromosome, 719-741
prophylaxis, 741-743
clitoris, 28-29
urethra, 29
vagina, 75-76
vulva, 27-29
ANOREXIA NERVOSA: differential diagnosis, 604
ANTIFERTILITY AGENTS (see Contraception)
APPENDICEAL ABSCESS, 340
"ARIAS-STELLA" REACTION, 308
AROMATIZATION, 420
ARRHENOBLASTOMA, 387-389
atypical, 387
cells in
columnar, 387
cuboidal, 387
epithelioid, 388
spindle-shaped, 388
sarcomatoid, 387, 388
typical tubular, 387
undifferentiated, 387, 388
ARTERIES: hypogastric, 178
ATHEROSCLEROSIS: and estrogen, 660
ATRESIA: follicular, 330-331
AUTOSOMES, 710

B

BARR BODIES, 706
BARTHOLIN GLAND: carcinoma, 65
BARTHOLIN-PATAU SYNDROME, 737
BASOPHILISM: pituitary, 598
BENEMID: in gonorrhea, 292
BENZESTROL, 638
11-BETA-HYDROXYLASE: cortisol and mepyrapone, 600
BIOGENESIS: of cortisol and corticosterone, 592
BIOPSY
cervix, 117-119
cone, 136
technique, 118-119
Younge forceps for, 118-119
endometrial, in infertility 467-469
Duncan curet for, 468
interpretation, 469
technique, 469
BIOSYNTHESIS OF STEROIDS, 591
studies, 420-422
BIRTH CONTROL (see Contraception)
BLADDER: peritoneum and hysterectomy, 236

BLEEDING (see Hemorrhage)
BLOOD
dyscrasias, vulvar changes in, 30-31
examination in tubal ectopic pregnancy, 306
menstrual cycle and, 212
pressure, in tubal ectopic pregnancy, 305
supply of uterine corpus, 177-181
"BLUEBERRY" NODULE: in vagina, 95
BOWEL
large-bowel contents in cystic teratoma, 400
obstruction complicating endometriosis, 456
BRACHYRADIUM THERAPY
inverse square law in, 154
length of linear source in, 155
BREAST(S)
cancer, and oral contraception, 700-701
changes with oral contraception, 699
examination, 5
progesterone and, 648
supernumerary, and genetics, 739
BRENNER TUMOR, 409-411

C

CALL-EXNER BODIES: in granulosa-theca cell tumors, 380
CANCER
(See also Carcinoma and specific cancers)
breast, and oral contraception, 700-701
cervix, 124-168
age and, 133
cytodiagnosis, 142-143
death rates, 125
detection, 141-144
incidence rates, 125
invasive (see below)
oral contraception and, 701-702
precancer, 127-141
social factors and, 126
cervix, invasive, 145-168
advanced, 166-167
brachyradium therapy, 154-155
clinical staging, 148-151
clinical staging after surgery, 163
diagnosis, 151-152
diagnosis, differential, 151-152
histologic grading, 147-148
pathology, 145-148
pregnancy and, 164-165
procidentia and, 164-166
prophylaxis, 152
radiation therapy, 153-160
recurrent, 166-167
spinal cell, 147
spindle cell, 147
spread, methods of, 149-151
surgery, 160-164
symptoms, 151-152
transitional cell, 147
treatment, 152-164
treatment, curative, 152-153
endometrium, and oral contraception, 702
genetics and, 739
metastases (see Metastases)
oral contraception and, 700-702
ovary, secondary, from pelvic organs, 416
oviduct, 315-321
precancer (see Precancer)
uterine corpus, 257-276

CANCER (*cont.*)
  vagina, 96-101
  vulva, 58-67
CANDIDA ALBICANS: as seen in wet smear, 84
CARCINOMA
  (*See also* Cancer and specific carcinomas)
  Bartholin's gland, 65
  breast, metastatic to ovary, 415
  cervix
    age and, 134
    cytodiagnosis, 142-143
    detection, 141-144
    in situ (*see below*)
    squamous cell, 124-127
    squamous cell, epidemiology, 125-127
    squamous cell, grade I, 146
    squamous cell, pathologic diagnosis, 125
  cervix, in situ, 129-141
    cellular morphology, 131
    diagnosis, 134-136
    diagnosis, cone biopsy for, 136
    early stromal invasion in, 137-141
    exfoliated cells, 131
    gland involvement, 130, 132
    pregnancy and, 141
    surface stratification and differentiation
      in, 132
    treatment, 136-137
  clear cell, 408
  embryonic cell, 408
  endometrioid, 363-365
  in endometriosis, diagnosis, 437
  endometrium, 259
    histogenesis, 253
    in situ, 254
    in situ, and progestational agents, 256
    primary, contrasted with ovarian endome-
      trioid carcinoma, 365
  metastases (*see* Metastases)
  ovary, 365-378
    chemotherapy, 373-378
    chlorambucil in, 374-375
    classification, 368
    cyclophosphamide in, 375
    detection, 366-367
    diagnosis, 366-367
    melphalan in, 375-376
    nitrogen mustard in, 374
    prevention, 366
    prognosis, factors in, 367-369
    prognosis, grade of carcinoma and, 369
    prognosis, stage of carcinoma and, 368
    radioresponsiveness, 372-373
    response to alkylating agents, 377
    survival curves, 364
    survival curves and surgical resection,
      371
    survival rates, 372
    Thio-tepa in, 376
    treatment, 369-378
  oviduct, primary, 315-319
    alveolar medullary, 317
    alveolar papillary, 317, 318
    diagnosis, 316-317
    metastatic to peritubal lymphatic, 319
    mucosa in, 318
    papillary, 317, 318
    papillary-alveolar, 317, 318
    pathology, 317-319
    treatment, 319

  pancreas, metastatic to ovary, 416
  sigmoid, 342
  uterus
    corpus, clinical staging, 261
    corpus, in situ, 253-257
    fundus, 259
    lymphatic spread, 262
  vagina, 96-101
    in situ, 95-96
    lymphatic spread, 99
    primary, 96-100
    primary, procidentia and, 97
    primary, treatment, 98-100
    secondary, 100-101
  vulva, 60-65
    basal cell, 65-66
    histologic appearance, 62
    in situ, 49-50
    lymphatic spread, 64
    ulceration in, 61
CASTRATION: in endometriosis surgery, 454
CAUTERIZATION OF CERVIX, 119-121
  electric cautery used, 120
  technique, 120-121
CECUM: redundant or distended, and ovarian
  lesion diagnosis, 340
CELLS
  in arrhenoblastoma (*see* Arrhenoblastoma,
    cells in)
  basal cell carcinoma of vulva, 65-66
  clear cell carcinoma, 408
  division, 730
  embryonic cell carcinoma, 408
  germ cell tumors, 392-405
  granulosa, luteinized granulosa cell tumor
    and precocious puberty, 554
  hilus cell tumor, 411-412
    hirsutism and, 611
  picket, of mucinous cystoma, 359
  spinal, in cervical cancer, 147
  spindle, in cervical cancer, 147
  theca (*see* Granulosa-theca cell tumors)
  transitional, in cervical cancer, 147
CEPHALOTHIN: in salpingitis, puerperal and
  postabortal, 296
CEREBROVASCULAR ACCIDENTS: and oral contraception, 693-694
CEREBRUM
  lesions, and premature menstruation, 551-
    553
  thrombosis, and oral contraception, 691
CERVICAL GANGLION OF FRANKENHÄUSER, 181
CERVICITIS
  acute, 115
  chronic, 88, 116
CERVIX, 103-171
  adenocarcinoma, 147, 167-168
  anatomy, 104-105
  biopsy (*see* Biopsy, cervix)
  cancer (*see* Cancer)
  carcinoma (*see* Carcinoma)
  cauterization (*see* Cauterization of cervix)
  condyloma acuminata, 123
  dysplasia, 127-129
  embryology, 103-104
  endocervix (*see* Endocervix)
  epithelization, squamous, 114
  eversion, postpartum, 111
  exocervix, normal, 107
  frontal section, 105

histologic portio, 106
histologic zones, 106
histology, 105-109
hyperkeratosis, 117
incompetent os, 517-519
    repair, 518-519
infertility and, 474-476
inflammation, 114-117
keratinization, 116-117
leukoplakia, 117
metaplasia, squamous, 112-114
mucus, "ferning," 648
papilloma, 122-124
pathologic alterations, 114-117
physiology, 109-110
    alterations, 110-114
polyps, 121-122
precancer, 127-141
smears, technique, 144
surgery, diagnostic and minor, 117-121
transitional zone, 107
tumors
    benign, 121-124
    detection, 141-144
visualization in dysfunctional uterine bleed-
    ing, 574
CHANCRE: soft, vulva in, 36
CHANCROID: vulva in, 36
CHEMICAL IRRITANTS: causing pruritus vul-
    vae, 50-51
CHEST: roentgenography of metastases, 271
CHIARI-FROMMEL SYNDROME: differential di-
    agnosis, 605-606
CHILDBED FEVER (see Salpingitis, puerperal
    and postabortal)
CHLORAMBUCIL
    ovarian carcinoma and, 374-375
    structural formula, 375
CHLORAMPHENICOL: in puerperal and posta-
    bortal salpingitis, 296
CHLORMADINONE, 678
"CHOCOLATE CYST," 432
CHOLESTEROL, 621
CHORIOADENOMA DESTRUENS, 528, 538-541
    actinomycin D in, 540
    methotrexate in, 538-540
    myometrium in, 538
CHORIOCARCINOMA, 528, 541-543
    primary, 402-403
CHORIOMA, 528
CHORIONEPITHELIOMA: true, 528
CHORIONIC GONADOTROPIN (see Gonadotropin,
    chorionic)
CHROMATIN
    -negative nuclei, 708
    -positive nuclei, 708-709
    sex-, mosaicism, 707
CHROMOSOMES
    abnormalities, 719-741
        prophylaxis, 741-743
    abortion and, spontaneous, 738-739
    deletion, 729-731
        syndromes, 737-738
    determinations, clinical aspects of, 743-746
    mosaicism (see Mosaicism)
    movement in cell division, 730
    nondisjunction, 713
    patterns, 709-718
        normal female, 711
        normal male, 711

sex, mosaicism, 707
summary of findings in various clinical
    states, 744
tetra-X, 727
translocation, 728-729
triple-X, 726-727
trisomy (see Trisomy)
XXXY, 707, 727
XXXXY, 707
XY female, 731-734
CIRCULATORY DISTURBANCES: vulvar changes
    in, 31
CLAMP
    Kelly, in hysterectomy, 237
    Kocher, in hysterectomy, 240-241
CLITORIS
    anatomy, 24-26
    histology, 24-26
    malformations, 28-29
CLOMID (see Clomiphene)
CLOMIPHENE
    contraindicated in ovarian cyst, 486
    formula, structural, 483
    in ovulation induction, 483-487
    possible action sites, 425
    Stein-Leventhal syndrome and, 424-427
COITUS
    interruptus, 671
    vulvar injuries due to, 32
COLPOCELE, 91
COLPOTOMY: in tubal ectopic pregnancy, 307
CONCEPTION CONTROL (see Contraception)
CONDOMS, 671
CONDYLOMATA
    acuminata
        cervix, 123
        vulva, 55
    lata, of vulva, due to syphilis, 33
CONNECTIVE TISSUE TUMORS: of ovary, 412-
    414
CONTRACEPTION, 670-704
    coitus interruptus, 671
    condoms, 671
    effectiveness of various methods, 676
    estrogen and, 687-690
    injectable, 677-687
    intrauterine devices (IUD), 673-677
        complications of, 674
        types, 674
    non-steroidal agents, 687-690
    oral, 677-687
        adrenals and, 690
        amenorrhea and, secondary, 699-700
        breast changes with, 699
        cancer and, 700-702
        cerebrovascular accidents and, 693-694
        combinations currently available, 677
        combined formulations, 679-682
        combined formulations, side-effects, 680-
            682
        contraindications and cautions with, 702-
            703
        diabetes mellitus and, 696-698
        effects on subsequent pregnancy, 688-689
        embolism and, pulmonary, 690-693
        fibroids and, 698-699
        hepatic effects, 695-696
        hypertension and, 694
        infertility and, 699-700
        menopause and, 689-690

CONTRACEPTION (*cont.*)
 migraine and, 694-695
 postpartum use, 689
 progestin alone, microdose, 685-686
 sequential formulations, 683-687
 side effects, 680-682, 688
 thrombophlebitis and, 690-693
 thyroid and, 690
 vascular disturbances and, 690-699
 rhythm method, 672
 vagina
  diaphragms, 672-673
  progestins in, 686-687
  spermicides, 672-673
CORD: rete, 325
CORNUA: of uterine corpus, 173
CORONA RADIATA, 287, 328
CORPUS
 albicans cyst, 348
 luteum
  (*See also* Luteal phase inadequacy)
  cyst, 326
  estrogen and, 190
  formation, 329-331
  full development stage, 330
  hematoma, 347
  mature, high power of, 348
  progesterone and, 190
  proliferative stage, 330
  regression stage, 330
  vascularization stage, 330
 uterine (*see* Uterus, corpus)
CORTICAL STROMAL HYPERPLASIA, 384-385
CORTICOSTEROIDS (*see* Steroids)
CORTICOSTERONE, 628
 biogenesis of, 592
CORTISOL
 biogenesis of, 592
 formation, and mepyrapone, 600
CRANIAL TRAUMA: sexual precocity after, 552-
  553
CRI UTERINE, 576
CULDOCENTESIS: in tubal ectopic pregnancy,
  307
CULDOSCOPY
 in infertility, 472-474
  technique, 473
 in tubal ectopic pregnancy, 307
CUMULUS OOPHORUS, 287, 328
CURET: Duncan, for endometrial biopsy, 468
CURETTAGE
 in dysfunctional uterine bleeding, technique, 575-578
 in endometrial hyperplasia, basal body temperature records after, 484
 in tubal ectopic pregnancy, 307-308
CUSHING'S SYNDROME, 598-602
 diagnostic tests in, 599-601
 infertility and, 494-495
 physiognomy of, typical, 599
 treatment, 602
CYCLOPENTANOPERHYDROPHENANTHRENE,
  619
CYCLOPENTANOPHENANTHRENE RING, 647
CYCLOPHOSPHAMIDE
 ovarian carcinoma and, 375
 structural formula, 375
CYST
 "chocolate," 432
 corpus albicans, 348

corpus luteum, 326
dermoid (*see* Teratoma, cystic)
endometrial hyperplasia and, 249
Gartner duct, prolapse, 94
germinal inclusion, 357
graafian follicle origin, non-neoplastic, 344-
  347
luteinized follicle, 346
ovarian
 clomiphene contraindicated in, 486
 complications of, 336
sclerocystic ovarian disease (*see* Stein-
  Leventhal syndrome)
structure from normally ruptured follicle,
  347-349
teratoma and (*see* Teratoma, cystic)
urachal, 343
vagina, inclusion, 94-95
CYSTADENOCARCINOMA, 355-361
 mucinous, 361
 serous
  low grade, 356
  papillary serous, 355, 356
CYSTADENOFIBROMA, 361-363
CYSTADENOMA
 mucinous, 355-361
 serous, 353-355
CYSTOCELE, 89, 90
CYSTOMA, 349-363
 germinal epithelial origin, 349-363
 mucinous, 360
  dermoid cyst and, 400
  early, 357
  picket cell of, 359
 simple serous, 351-352
  epithelium in, 352
CYTODIAGNOSIS: of cervical cancer, 142-143
CYTOGENETICS, 705-747
 general considerations, 705-709
CYTOLOGY: VAGINAL, 78-79
CYTOXAN (*see* Cyclophosphamide)

D

DEHYDROEPIANDROSTERONE, 593, 624
DELALUTIN: in endometrial hyperplasia, 253
DELAYED MENARCHE (*see* Menarche, delayed)
DELUTEVAL 2X: dosage in endometriosis, 450
DEPO-PROVERA
 in endometrial hyperplasia, 253
 in endometriosis, 450
DERMATOSES OF VULVA
 dry scaly, 52-53
 exudative, 51-52
DERMOID CYST (*see* Teratoma, cystic)
DESOXYCORTICOSTERONE: metabolism, 629
11-DESOXYCORTISOL, 628
DIABETES MELLITUS
 menstrual cycle and, 211
 oral contraception and, 696-698
 vulvar changes in, 30
 vulvitis in, 30
DIAPHRAGMS: vaginal, 672-673
DIENESTROL, 638
DIETHYLSTILBESTROL, 638
DIMETHISTERONE, 678
DIPLOID, 706
DISCUS PROLIGERUS, 287, 328
DIVERTICULITIS: sigmoid, 342

DOWN'S SYNDROME, 734-737
  karyotype in, 735
DRUG SENSITIVITIES: causing pruritus vulvae, 50
DUNCAN CURET: for endometrial biopsy, 468
DYE STUDY: intrauterine, in hydatidiform mole, 532
DYSCRASIAS: blood, vulvar changes in, 30-31
DYSGENESIS
  gonadal (see Turner's syndrome)
  seminiferous tubule (seeKlinefelter's syndrome)
DYSGERMINOMA, 392-396
  diagnosis, 392-395
  lymphocytes in, 393-394
  treatment, 395-396
DYSMENORRHEA, 584-588
  etiology, 585-586
  primary, progestins in, 651
  symptomatology, 585
  treatment, 586-588
DYSPLASIA: cervix, 127-129

E

ECTOPIC
  kidney, 343
  pregnancy (see Pregnancy, ectopic)
EDEMA
  stroma, and endometrial dating, 208
  vulva
    granuloma inguinale causing, 38
    neurodermatitis and, 54
EDWARD'S SYNDROME, 737
ELECTRIC CAUTERY: for cervical cauterization, 120
EMBOLISM: pulmonary, and oral contraception, 690-693
EMBRYO: schematic representation to show anatomic relations of genital tubercle, 18
EMBRYONIC CELL CARCINOMA, 408
ENCEPHALITIS: sexual precocity after, 552
ENDOCERVIX
  histologic, 107-108
  hyperplasia, 113
  normal, 108
  polyps, 121
ENDOCRINE DISORDERS, 545-617
ENDOLYMPHATIC STROMAL MYOSIS, 242-243
ENDOMETRIOID CARCINOMA, 363-365
ENDOMETRIOMA, 432
ENDOMETRIOSIS, 432-457
  analgesia and observation, 445
  carcinoma in, diagnosis, 437
  clinical features, 441-443
  complications, 455-456
  definitions concerning, 432
  diagnosis, 443-444
  ethinyl estradiol in, 449
  histogenesis, 432-435
  hydroureter due to, 440
  incidence, 441
  infertility and, 442-443, 494
  "menstrual," 95
  in menstrual phase, 448
  norethynodrel in, 449
  ovulation suppression in, 446-451
    androgens, 446

  dosage regimens, 450
  estrogens, 446
  norethynodrel and ethinyl estradiol, 447
  progestins, 446-451
  progestins, choice of, 448
  progestins, contraindications, 448, 450
  pathogenesis, 433
  pathology, 435-440
  progestins in, 446-451, 651
  proliferating function in, 432
  proliferating growth in, 432
  prophylaxis, 444-445
  of sigmoid, into lumen, 439
  sites, common, 436
  surgery, 451-455
    castration in, 454
    conservative, 452-454
    extirpative, 454-455
  symptoms, 441-442
  treatment, 444-455
  of uterosacral ligament, 437
ENDOMETRITIS, 217
ENDOMETRIUM
  adenocarcinoma, 260
  anatomy, 177
  biopsy (see Biopsy, endometrial)
  cancer, and oral contraception, 702
  carcinoma (see Carcinoma)
  dating, 194-208
    menstrual phase, 194
  dating, proliferative phase, 194-198
    early, 194-195, 196
    late, 195, 198
    middle, 195, 197
  dating, secretory phase, 194, 199-208
    15th day, 199
    16th day, 199, 200
    17th day, 199, 201
    18th day, 199, 202
    19th day, 199
    20th day, 199, 203
    21st day, 199
    22nd day, 199, 204
    23rd day, 199, 205
    24th day, 199, 206
    25th day, 199, 207
    26th, 27th, and 28th days, 199
  hyperplasia (see Hyperplasia, endometrial)
  inflammation and infertility, 477-478
  irregular shedding, 582
  polyps, 244-247
    management, 246-247
  proliferative changes in menstruation, 187, 194-198
  sarcoma, stromal, 274
  tuberculosis, 299
  tumors, mixed mesodermal, 275-276
"ENDOSALPINGIOMA," 354
ENDOXAN (see Cyclophosphamide)
ENOVID: dosage in endometriosis, 450
ENTEROCELE, 90, 91
ENZYMATIC SEQUENCES: in ovarian steroidogenesis, 421
EPITHELIUM
  in cystoma, simple serous, 352
  germinal, origin of cystoma from, 349-363
  ovary, surface, in newborn, 328
  oviduct (see Oviduct, epithelium)
  vaginal, photomicrograph, 74
EPITHELIZATION: squamous, of cervix, 114

EPOOPHORON, 331
ESTRADIOL
17-beta, formula, 647
ethinyl, in endometriosis, 449
ovulation suppression, 447
excretion, and menstrual cycle, 189
formula, structural, 633
levels, during menstrual cycle, 190
production in pregnancy and trophoblastic disease, 533
ESTRANE, 618-619
formula, structural, 633
ESTRIOL
excretion, and menstrual cycle, 189
formula, structural, 633
production in pregnancy and trophoblastic disease, 533
ESTROGEN
in abortion, habitual, 508-509, 513
deficiency of estrogen, 513
atherosclerosis and, 660
contraception and, 687-690
corpus luteum secretion of, 190
formation, 631-634
formula, structural, 633
measurement, 634-636
in micrograms, 634
menopause and, 658-662
menstruation and, 189
metabolism, 633-634
possible pathways, 632
myocardial infarction and, 660
osteoporosis and, 661-662
ovulation suppression and, 446
postmenopause and, 668-669
production, 631
-progestin combinations to induce pseudopregnancy, 450
secretion, 631
rates in micrograms, 631
synthetic substances, 638
therapy, 636-642
dosage problems, 660-661
ESTROGENIC SUBSTANCE, 186
ESTRONE
excretion, and menstrual cycle, 189
formula, structural, 633
levels, during menstrual cycle, 190
ETHINYL ESTRADIOL IN ENDOMETRIOSIS, 449
ovulation suppression, 447
ETHISTERONE, 678
ETHYNODIOL DIACETATE, 678
ETIOCHOLANE, 618-619
EUNUCH: with micro-orchism and mental deficiency, 707
EXAMINATION
abdomen, 6
breast, 5
pelvic, 7-16
in dysfunctional uterine bleeding, 574
internal, 12-14
internal, method of beginning, 12
internal, palpation of adnexal areas, 14
position for, 8
speculum insertion, 9
in tubal ectopic pregnancy, 306
physical, 5-7
instruments and supplies for, 11
vaginorectal, combined, 15

EXOCERVIX: normal, 107

F

FALLOPIAN TUBES (see Oviduct)
FARRE-WALDEYER LINE: and ovarian anatomy, 325
Feminization, testicular, 732-733
karyotype in, 733
FERN TEST TECHNIQUE, 109-110
"FERNING:" of cervical mucus, 648
FERTILE DAY, 482
FERTILITY
(See also Infertility)
control (see Contraception)
after ectopic pregnancy, 310-311
FEVER, CHILDBED (see Salpingitis, puerperal and postabortal)
FIBERS: of uterine corpus, 181
FIBROIDS: and oral contraception, 698-699
FIBROMA
cystadenofibroma, 361-363
ovary, 412-413
vulva, 57-58
FIBROMYOMA: of uterine corpus, 228
FIBROSARCOMA
ovarii mucocellulare carcinomatodes, 414
ovary, 414
FIMBRIOPLASTY: prostheses for, 479
FLETCHER-SUIT AFTERLOAD APPLICATOR, 157
FOLLICLE
atresia, 330-331
cyst, luteinized, 346
graafian (see Graafian follicle)
normally ruptured, cystic structure from, 347-349
-stimulating hormone, 186
FOLLICULAR ATRESIA, 330-331
FORBES-ALBRIGHT SYNDROME: differential diagnosis, 606-607
FORCEPS
for collection of seminal fluid from endocervical canal, 467
Younge, 118
FSH, 186
FUNDUS (see Uterus, fundus)
FUNGOUS VULVITIS, 40-42

G

GALACTORRHEA
production method, diagram showing, 546
progestins in, 652
GAMETES, 713
GAMETOGENESIS, 709-718
nondisjunction during, 718
GANGLION OF FRANKENHÄUSER, 181
GARTNER DUCT CYST: prolapse, 94
GENITAL SYSTEM: undifferentiated, schematic drawing, 21
GENITALIA
external
development from undifferentiated state, 19
female, 23
female
differentiated, schematic drawing, 21
external, 23
GERM CELL TUMORS, 392-405

GERMINAL
  epithelium origin of cystoma, 349-363
  inclusion cyst, 357
GLAND
  ducts, periurethral, anatomy, 27
  endocrine *(see specific glands)*
  mitoses, 199
  nuclei, pseudostratification of, 199, 208
  vulvovaginal, anatomy, 26-27
GONADAL
  dysgenesis *(see* Turner's syndrome)
  stromal tumors, 378-392
GONADOTROPIN, CHORIONIC
  abortion and, habitual, 506-507
  human, levels in pregnancy, 534
  tests, in hydatidiform mole, 532-533
GONADOTROPIN, HUMAN MENOPAUSAL, 487-491
  Ortho, 487
  Pergonal, 487
    abortion and, 490-491
    administration, 489-491
    adverse reactions to, 490
    dosage, 489-491
GONORRHEA, 288-294
  Benemid in, 292
  diagnosis, differential, 292
  oviduct in, 288-294
  penicillin in, 292
  symptomatology, 290-292
  treatment, 292-294
  vaginitis and, 88-89
  Vibramycin in, 293
  vulva in, 35-36
GRAAFIAN FOLLICLE
  maturing, 345
  origin of non-neoplastic cyst, 344-347
GRANULOMA INGUINALE, VULVA IN, 37-38
  edema, 38
GRANULOMATOUS   SALPINGITIS: nontuberculous, 303
GRANULOSA
  luteinized granulosa cell tumor and sexual
    precocity, 554
  -theca cell tumors, 378-386
    cylindroid pattern, 380
    diagnosis, differential, 381-382
    folliculoid pattern, 380
    folliculoid pattern, Call-Exner bodies in,
      380
    sarcomatoid pattern, 380
    treatment, 382-383
GYNANDROBLASTOMA, 389-392
GYNECOLOGY: intimacy of, 1

H

HAPLOID, 706
HEART DISEASE: coronary, and estrogen, 661
HEMATOMA
  corpus luteum, 347
  rectus muscle, 343
HEMORRHAGE
  uterine, dysfunctional, 573-584
    acyclic pattern, 573
    bleeding associated with ovulation, 578
    constant bleeding, 582-584
    cyclic pattern, 573
    definition, 573

    examination in, pelvic, 574
    examination in, physical, 573-578
    history, 573-578
    intermittent bleeding, 582-584
    irregular shedding of endometrium, 582
    normal bleeding at less than usual in-
      tervals, 579-580
    normal bleeding at more than usual in-
      tervals, 580
    premenstrual staining, 578-579, 651
    profuse or prolonged bleeding at normal
      intervals, 580-582
    progestins in, 649, 651
    uterine curettage technique in, 575-578
    visualization of cervix in, 574
  uterine, functional, definition, 573
  vaginal, abnormal, in tubal ectopic pregnan-
    cy, 305
HERPES
  progenitalis, 51-52
  zoster, 52
HEXESTROL, 638
HIDRADENOMA: vulva, 58-59
HILUS, 324
  cell tumor, 411-412
  hirsutism and, 611
HIRSUTISM, 608-614
  adrenal rest tumor and, 407
  diagnosis, 612-613
    sequence of diagnostic procedures in
      work-up, 613
  etiology, 609-612
  genetic factors in, 609
  racial factors in, 609
  testing technic in, 612
  treatment, 614
HISTOLOGIC
  endocervix, 107-108
  portio, 106
  zones, of cervix, 106
HISTORY, 2-5
HN$_2$ *(see* Nitrogen mustard)
HORMONES
  abortion and
    habitual, 505-517
    reduced hormone production, 630
  excretion during menstrual cycle, 192
  follicle-stimulating, 186
  luteinizing, 186
  luteotropic, suppression by hypothalamic-
    inhibiting factor, 546
  menstruation and, 186-194
  osteoporosis and, 661-662
  in premenopause, 663-664
HPL: levels in pregnancy, 534
HYDATIDIFORM MOLE, 527-537
  chemotherapy, prophylactic, 537
  clinical signs in pregnancy, 531
  diagnosis, 531-535
  epithelial hyperplasia and anaplasia in, 530
  follow-up, 535-537
  gonadotropin tests in, chorionic, 532-533
  intrauterine dye study, 532
  pathologic ovum in, 529
  pregnancy tests and, 536
  treatment, 535
  villi of, typical, 529
HYDROCORTISONE: synthesis, 628
HYDROPS

HYDROPS (*cont.*)
  folliculi, 346
  tubae profluens, in oviduct carcinoma, 316
HYDROURETER: due to endometriosis, 440
17-HYDROXYPROGESTERONE, 624, 628
  metabolized to pregnanetriol, 629
17c-HYDROXYPROGESTERONE: structural formula, 619
HYMEN
  anatomy, 26
  imperforate, 27
  malformations, 27-28
HYPERKERATOSIS
  cervix, 117
  vulva and
    in neurodermatitis, 54
    in Paget's disease, 67
HYPERMENORRHEA, 580-582
  genetics and, 739
  progestins in, 650-651
HYPERNEPHROMA: mesometanephroma resembling, 408
HYPERPLASIA
  adrenal, congenital, and 11-ketopregnanetriol, 595
  endocervix, 113
  endometrial, 247-253
    adenomatous, 250
    curettage for, basal body temperature records after, 484
    cystic, 249
    histologic patterns, 248-251
    management, 251-253
    pathology, 247-251
    progestational agents and, 256
    symptomatology, 251
  in hydatidiform mole, 530
  stromal, cortical, 384-385
HYPERTENSION: and oral contraception, 694
HYPERTHECOSIS SYNDROME, 386
HYPOGASTRIC
  artery, 178
  plexus, 181
HYPOGONADISM
  delayed menarche and, 558-559
  hypogonadotropic, causing secondary amenorrhea, 565
HYPOGONADOTROPISM: and delayed menarche, 558
HYPOMENORRHEA: progestins in, 649-650
HYPOTHALAMUS
  disorders, 598-608
  -inhibiting factor, 546
  insufficiency, and habitual abortion, 513
  lesion causing sexual precocity, 552
  -releasing factor, 546
HYSTERECTOMY, SIMPLE TOTAL, 235-242
  bladder peritoneum and, 236
  clamps in
    Kelly, 237
    Kocher, 240-241
  entering vagina, 239
  hemostasis in, 235-236
  ligaments, 236
  ovaries in, 242
  position for, 235
  technique, 235-242
  treatment of vagina, 239-242
  vessels and, 236-239

HYSTEROGRAPHY: adenomyosis of uterine corpus, 222
HYSTEROSALPINGOGRAPHY, 471-472

I

IDIOGRAM, 712
IMMUNOLOGIC FACTORS: in habitual abortion, 504-505
IMPLANTATION: tubal, intrauterine prostheses for, 480-481
INCOMPETENT CERVICAL OS, 517-519
  repair, 518-519
INFARCTION: myocardial, and estrogen, 660
INFERTILITY, 458-499
  (*See also* Fertility)
  adrenal factors in, 494-495
  cervical factor in, 474-476
  endometrial inflammation and, 477-478
  endometriosis and, 442-443, 494
  female partner
    culdoscopy, 472-474
    culdoscopy, technique, 473
    diagnostic procedures, minimal, 465
    endometrial biopsy (*see* Biopsy, endometrial)
    etiologic classification of factors, 461
    forceps for collection of seminal fluid from endocervical canal, 467
    hysterosalpingography, 471-472
    laparoscopy, 472-474
    postcoital test (*see* Postcoital test)
    study of, 464-474
    tubal insufflation (*see* Insufflation, tubal)
  fimbrioplasty, prostheses for, 479
  general considerations, 458-460
  idiopathic, progestins in, 652
  male partner
    diagnostic procedures, minimal, 462
    etiologic classification of factors, 461
    positive therapy for, 463-464
    semen analysis, 462-463
    study of, 461-464
  management, clinical, 460-497
  oral contraception and, 699-700
  ovarian factor in, 482-494
  oviduct in
    closure, 478
    midsegment reconstruction, 479
    salpingolysis in, 479
    salpingoplasty in, 479
  thyroid factors in, 495-497
  tubal factor in, 478-482
  tuboplasty in, 479
  uterine factor in, 476-478
INFLAMMATION
  endometrium, and infertility, 477-478
  oviduct, 288-303
  pelvis, 289
INJECTABLE CONTRACEPTION, 677-687
INJURY (*see* Trauma)
INSUFFLATION, TUBAL, 469-471
  apparatus for, 470
  evaluation, 470-471
  technique, 469-470
INTESTINAL OBSTRUCTION: complicating endometriosis, 455-456
INTIMACY: of gynecology, 1
INTRAUTERINE CONTRACEPTIVE DEVICES (*see*

Contraception, intrauterine devices)
INVASIVE MOLE (*see* Chorioadenoma destruens)
INVERSE SQUARE LAW: in brachyradium therapy, 154
IRRADIATION (*see* Radiation)
ISOCHROMOSOME, 731
ISONICOTINIC ACID HYDRAZIDE: in tuberculosis of oviduct, 299
ISTHMUS: of uterus, 105, 173
IUD (*see* Contraception, intrauterine devices)

K

KANAMYCIN: in puerperal and postabortal salpingitis, 296
KARYOTYPE, 710
in Klinefelter's syndrome, 725
in mongolism, 735
in testicular feminization, 733
in Turner's syndrome, 720, 722
KELLY CLAMP: in hysterectomy, 237
KERATINIZATION: cervix, 116-117
11-KETOPREGNANETRIOL: and congenital adrenal hyperplasia, 595
17-KETOSTEROIDS
derivation of, 593
response to various stimuli, 613
urinary values, normal, elevated, and lowered, 611
KIDNEY: ectopic, 343
KLINEFELTER'S SYNDROME, 724-726
karyotype in, 725
mental deficiency and, 707
KOCHER CLAMP: in hysterectomy, 240-241
KRAUROSIS
-leukoplakia complex, 43-50
simple, 44
histologic changes in, 45
KRUKENBERG'S TUMOR, 414-416

L

LABIA
majora
anatomy, 20-23
histology, 20-23
histology, photomicrograph, 22
minora
anatomy, 23-24
histology, 23-24
histology, photomicrograph, 25
LABOR: premature, and progestins, 654
LACERATIONS OF PERINEUM, 91-92
complete, 93
LACTOGEN: human placental, levels in pregnancy, 534
LAPAROSCOPY: in infertility, 472-474
LAW: inverse square, in brachyradium therapy, 154
LEIOMYOMA
intraligamentous, and ovarian lesion diagnosis, 343
uterine corpus, 226-242
classification by location, 227
diagnosis, 231-232
hysterectomy in, 235-242
intramural, 227

myomectomy in, 233-235
pathology, 228-230
submucous, 227
subserous, 227
symptomatology, 230
treatment, 232-242
typical structure of, 229
LEIOMYOSARCOMA: of uterine corpus, 228, 230, 273
LEUKEMIA: and genetics, 740-741
LEUKERAN (*see* Chlorambucil)
LEUKOPARAKERATOSIS, 116
LEUKOPLAKIA
cervix, 117
histologic changes in, 48
-kraurosis complex, 43-50
vulva, 47-49
LEUKORRHEA, 79-89
LH, 186
LICHEN
planus, of vulva, 52-53
sclerosus et atrophicus
histologic appearance, 46
vulva, 45-47
LIGAMENT
uterosacral, endometriosis of, 437
uterus (*see* Uterus, corpus, ligaments)
LIPIDS, 618
LIPOMA: vulva, 56-57
LIQUOR FOLLICULI, 328
LIVER
menstrual cycle and, 210-211
oral contraception and, 695-696
LUNG EMBOLISM: and oral contraception, 690-693
LUTEAL PHASE INADEQUACY
habitual abortion and (*see* Abortion, habitual, luteal phase inadequacy)
progestins in, 652-653
LUTEINIZED
follicle cyst, 346
granulosa cell tumor, and sexual precocity, 554
LUTEINIZING HORMONE, 186
LUTEOMA, 386
LUTEOTROPIC
hormone, suppression by hypothalamic-inhibiting factor, 546
-inhibiting factor, 546
LUTEOTROPIN, 546
LYMPHATIC SPREAD OF CARCINOMA
uterus, 262
vagina, 99
vulva, 64
LYMPHATIC SUPPLY: of uterine corpus, 181-182
LYMPHOCYTES: in dysgerminoma, 393-394
LYMPHOGRANULOMA INGUINALE: vulva in, 37
LYMPHOPATHIA VENEREUM: vulva in, 37
LYNDIOL: dosage in endometriosis, 450
LYNESTRENOL, 678

M

MALFORMATIONS (*see* Anomalies)
MALIGNANCY (*see* Cancer)
MASTODYNIA: progestins in, 651-652
MECHLORETHAMINE (*see* Nitrogen mustard)

MEDROXYPROGESTERONE
  acetate, in uterine adenocarcinoma, 269
  in endometrial hyperplasia, 253
MEGESTROL, 678
MEIG'S SYNDROME: and thecoma, 384
MEIOSIS, 714
  nuclear division, 716
MELANOMA: vulva, 66
MELPHALAN
  ovarian carcinoma and, 375-376
  structural formula, 376
MENARCHE, 183
  delayed, 556-559
    constitutional, 557-558
    hypogonadism and, 558-559
    hypogonadotropism and, 558
  sexual precocity and, constitutional, 549
MENINGITIS: sexual precocity after, 552
MENOPAUSAL GONADOTROPIN (see Gonadotropin, human menopausal)
MENOPAUSE, 658-669
  effects of oral contraception on, 689-690
  estrogen and, 658-662
  postmenopause (see Postmenopause)
  premenopause, hormonal regimens during,
    663-664
  psychotherapy of, 662-663
  therapy, 662
    symptomatic, 663
MENSES (see Menstruation)
MENSTRUAL CYCLE, 186
  adrenals and, 210
  blood and, 212
  diabetes mellitus and, 211
  liver and, 210-211
  nervous system and, 211-212
  psyche and, 212
  skin and, 212
  systemic changes associated with, 208-212
  thyroid and, 209-210
"MENSTRUAL" ENDOMETRIOSIS, 95
MENSTRUATION, 3-4, 183-212
  absent, 559-573
  cycle (see Menstrual cycle)
  delayed (see Menarche, delayed)
  endometrial proliferative changes in, 187
  endometrium dating (see Endometrium,
    dating)
  hormonal aspects of, 186-194
  pain of, 3
  premature, 546-556
  premature, constitutional, 546, 548-551
    diagnosis, 548-550
    symptomatology, 548-550
    treatment, 550-551
  premature, organic, 546, 551-556
    adrenal tumors and, 553
    adrenocortical hyperfunction and, 553-
      556
    Albright's syndrome and, 556
    cerebral lesions and, 551-553
    luteinized granulosa cell tumor in, 554
    ovarian tumors and, 553-556
  premenstrual staining, 578-579
    progestins in, 651
  scant, 559-573
MENTAL DEFICIENCY
  eunuch with micro-orchism and, 707
  Klinefelter's syndrome and, 707

MEPYRAPONE: and cortisol, 600
MER-25
  formula, structural, 483
  in ovulation induction, 483-487
  possible action sites, 425
MESODERMAL TUMORS: mixed, of endometri-
  um, 275-276
MESOMETANEPHRIC REST TUMOR, 407-409
MESOMETANEPHROMA, 408
"MESONEPHROMA OVARII" OF SCHILLER, 408
MESOSALPINX, 175
MESOVARIUM, 323, 326
METABOLIC DISORDERS: familial, 743
METAPHASE, 710
METAPLASIA: squamous, of cervix, 112-114
METASTASES
  chest, roentgenography of, 271
  ovary, 414-416
  to oviduct, 320
    from pancreatic carcinoma, 320
  oviduct carcinoma, to peritubal lymphatics,
    319
METHOTREXATE: in chorioadenoma destruens,
  538-540
METOPIRONE: and cortisol, 600
METROPATHIA HEMORRHAGICA: definition, 573
MICRO-ORCHISM: of eunuch, and mental defi-
  ciency, 707
MIGRAINE
  oral contraception and, 694-695
  progestins protecting against, 695
MITOSIS, 706, 715
  gland, 199
  nondisjunction, 717
  nuclear division, 716
MOLE
  hydatidiform (see Hydatidiform mole)
  invasive (see Chorioadenoma destruens)
MONGOLISM, 734-737
  karyotype in, 735
MONILIASIS, 83-86
  treatment, 85-86
  vulva, 41
MONS VENERIS: anatomy, 26
MOSAICISM, 727-728
  sex-chromatin, 707
  sex-chromosome, 707
MOTOR FIBERS: of uterine corpus, 181
MRL-41 (see Clomiphene)
MUCUS: cervical "ferning," 648
MUSCLE: rectus, hematoma, 343
MUSTARGEN (see Nitrogen mustard)
MYOCARDIAL INFARCTION: and estrogen, 660
MYOMA: "parasitic," 226
MYOMECTOMY: technique, 233-235
MYOMETRIUM
  anatomy, 177
  in chorioadenoma destruens, 538
  progesterone and, 648
MYOSIS: endolymphatic stromal, 242-243

N

NEOPLASMS (see Cancer, Tumors)
NERVE SUPPLY
  of uterus, 180, 181
  of vulva, 24
NERVOUS SYSTEM: and menstrual cycle, 211-
  212

NEURODERMATITIS: of vulva, 39, 53-55
NEWBORN: ovarian surface epithelium in, 328
NIPPLE: inverted, and genetics, 739
NITROGEN MUSTARD
  alkylation of X receptor site by, 373
  ovarian carcinoma and, 374
NONDISJUNCTION, 713
  during gametogenesis, 718
  mitosis, 717
NORETHINDRONE, 678
  acetate (Norlestrin)
    dosage in endometriosis, 450
    structural formula, 679
NORETHYNODREL, 678
  in endometriosis, 449
  ovulation suppression, 447
NORGESTREL (OVRAL)
  dosage in endometriosis, 450
  structural formula, 679
NORINYL: dosage in endometriosis, 450
NORLESTRIN (see Norethindrone acetate)
19-NOR PROGESTINS, 678
NUCLEI
  chromatin-negative, 708
  chromatin-positive, 708-709
  division, mitotic and meiotic, 716
NUTRITION
  disorders, and habitual abortion, 503-504
  in osteoporosis, 661

O

OBSTETRIC INJURIES: vulva, 32
OLIGOMENORRHEA, 559-560
OOPHORECTOMY: bilateral, and estrogens, 661
OOPHOROMA FOLLICULARE, 409
ORAL CONTRACEPTION (see Contraception, oral)
ORTHO HMG, 487
ORTHO-NOVUM: dosage in endometriosis, 450
Os, incompetent cervical os, 517-519
  repair, 518-519
OSTEOPOROSIS, 661-662
  activity and, 661
  hormones in, 661-662
  nutrition in, 661
  treatment, 661-662
OVA: pathologic, with hydatid change, 529
OVARIOGENESIS: stages of, 324
OVARY, 323-431
  agenesis, 719
  anatomy, 325-328
  cancer, secondary, from pelvic organs, 416
  carcinoma (see Carcinoma)
  cyst
    clomiphene contraindicated in, 486
    complications of, 336
  embryology, 323-325
  epithelium, surface, in newborn, 328
  fibers of, transverse, 328
  fibroma, 412-413
  fibrosarcoma, 414
  function, and progesterone, 648
  histology, 328-329
  hysterectomy and, simple total, 242
  in infertility, 482-494
  parenchymatous zone, 328
  postmenopausal, 331

resection, wedge, and ovulation induction, 491-494
sclerocystic disease (see Stein-Leventhal syndrome)
steroidogenesis
  clomiphene and MER-25, 425
  enzymatic sequences in, 421
  stimulation tests, 423
  suppression studies, 422-423
  tumors, 331-349
    classification, 332-333
    diagnosis, 337-339
    diagnosis, differential, 339-344
    germ cell, 392-405
    gonadal stromal, 378-392
    granulosa-theca cell (see Granulosa-theca cell tumors)
    hirsutism and, 611
    histogenesis, 349, 351
    incidence, 333-335
    metastatic, 414-416
    mucinous, incidence of malignancy, 353
    nonintrinsic connective tissue, 412-414
    rest (see Rest tumors)
    serous, incidence of malignancy, 353
    sexual precocity and, 553-556
    signs, physical, 337
    symptoms, 335-337
OVIDUCT, 281-322
  ampullar portion, 281-282
    senescent, 284
  anatomy, 281-285
  cancer, 315-321
  carcinoma (see Carcinoma)
  closed, and infertility, 478
  correlation of structure and function, 286-288
  embryology, 285-286
  epithelium
    proliferative phase, 283
    secretory phase, 283
  histology, 281-285
  implantation, intrauterine prostheses for, 480-481
  infertility and, 478-482
  inflammation, 288-303
  infundibular portion, 281-282
  insufflation (see Insufflation, tubal)
  interstitial portion, 281-282
  isthmic portion, 281-282
  midsegment reconstruction in infertility, 479
  normal, 282
  plicae, 284
  pregnancy in (see Pregnancy, ectopic, tubal)
  sarcoma, 320
  senescent, 284
  talc on, reaction to, 304
  tuberculosis (see Tuberculosis)
  tumors, benign, 314-315
    adenomatoid, 315
OVRAL (see Norgestrel)
OVULATION, 329-331
  bleeding associated with, 578
  induction, 482-494
    clomiphene in, 483-487
    gonadotropin in (see Gonadotropin, human menopausal)
  suppression, and endometriosis, 446-451

OVULATION (*cont.*)
wedge resection of ovary and, 491-494
OXYURIASIS, 51

P

PAGET'S DISEASE: vulva in, 66-67
PAIN
of menstruation, 3
in tubal ectopic pregnancy, 304-305
PANCREAS: carcinoma metastatic to oviduct, 320
PAPILLOMA
cervix, 122-124
vulva, 55-56
PARA-AMINOSALICYLIC ACID: in oviduct tuberculosis, 299
PARAKERATOSIS, 117
Paget's disease of vulva and, 67
PARAOOPHORON, 331
PARASITES: vulvar, 51
"PARASITIC" MYOMA, 226
PAS: in oviduct tuberculosis, 299
PEDICULOSIS PUBIS, 51
PELVIS
examination (*see* Examination)
inflammation, 289
normal, sagittal section, 174
plexus, 181
PEMPHIGUS
true, 52
vulgaris, 52
PENICILLIN
in gonorrhea, 292
in salpingitis, puerperal and postabortal, 296
PERGONAL HMG (*see* Gonadotropin, human menopausal, Pergonal)
PERIMETRIUM: anatomy, 177
PERINEAL LACERATIONS, 91-92
complete, 93
PERIURETHRAL GLAND DUCTS: anatomy, 27
PESSARY: Smith-Hodge, in uterine retrodisplacement, 216-217
PHENYLALANINE MUSTARD (*see* Melphalan)
PICKET CELL: of mucinous cystoma, 359
PITUITARY
basophilism, 598
disorders, 598-608
insufficiency, and habitual abortion, 513
syndromes, differential diagnosis, 607
PLEXUS
hypogastric, 181
pelvic, 181
POLYMENORRHEA, 579
progestins in, 650
POLYMYXIN-B: in puerperal and postabortal salpingitis, 296
POLYP(S)
cervix, 121-122
endocervix, 121
endometrial, 244-247
management, 246-247
POLYPLOID, 706
POSTABORTAL SALPINGITIS (*see* Salpingitis, puerperal and postabortal)
POSTCOITAL TEST, 467
interpretation, 467
technique, 467

POSTENCEPHALITIC STATES: and sexual precocity, 552
POSTMENOPAUSE
androgen and, 667-669
estrogen and, 668-669
ovary, 331
progesterone and, 667
therapeutic regimens during, 664-669
vasomotor symptoms of, 665-667
POSTPARTUM USE: of oral contraceptives, 689
PRECANCER
cervix, 127-141
uterine corpus, 253-257
PRECOCITY, SEXUAL (*see* Menstruation, premature)
PREGNANCY
cervical cancer during, 164-165
cervical carcinoma in situ and, 141
combined intrauterine and extrauterine, 311
early, drugs contraindicated in, and habitual abortion, 515-517
ectopic, fertility after, 310-311
ectopic, tubal, 304-310
abdomen in, 305-306
anatomic sites of, 308
biologic tests for pregnancy in, 306-307
blood pressure in, 305
colpotomy in, 307
culdocentesis in, 307
culdoscopy in, 307
curettage in, uterine, 307-308
diagnosis, 304-308
examination, anesthesia used, 307
examination, blood, 306
examination, physical, 305-306
pain in, 304-305
pulse rate in, 305
signs of pregnancy, 305
signs, presenting, 304-305
symptoms of pregnancy, 305
symptoms, presenting, 304-305
temperature in, 305
treatment, 308-310
vaginal bleeding in, 305
effects of oral contraception on, 688-689
estradiol production in, 533
estriol production in, 533
estrogen concentrations during, blood, 509
gonadotropin concentration during, chorionic, 506, 534
lactogen levels in, human placental, 534
molar (*see* Hydatidiform mole)
progestin therapy during, 653-654
tests
ectopic pregnancy and, 306-307
hydatidiform mole and, 536
PREGNANE, 618-619
PREGNANEDIOL, 629
PREGNANETRIOL
17-hydroxyprogesterone metabolized to, 629
response to various stimuli, 613
PREGNENOLONE
acetate conversion to, 621
conversion to progesterone, 622
PREMALIGNANCY (*see* Precancer)
PREMATURE LABOR: progestins in, 654
PREMATURE MENSTRUATION (*see* Menstruation, premature)
PREMENOPAUSE: hormone therapy of, 663-664
PREMENSTRUAL STAINING, 578-579

progestins in, 651
PROBENECID: in gonorrhea, 292
PROCIDENTIA
    cervical cancer complicating, 165-166
    vaginal carcinoma and, 97
PROGESTATIONAL AGENTS
    endometrial hyperplasia and carcinoma in
        situ, 256
    therapy with, 647-654
PROGESTERONE
    in abortion, habitual, 509-511
        deficiency of progesterone, 513-515
    androgen formation via, 623
    biologic effect of, 648-649
    corpus luteum secretion of, 190
    deficiency, in habitual abortion, 513-515
    discussion of term, 648
    formation, 627-630
    formula, 647
        structural, 619
    hydrocortisone synthesis from, 628
    levels during menstrual cycle, 191
    menstruation and, 189, 191
    metabolism, 629
    postmenopause and, 667
    pregnenolone conversion to, 622
    production in milligrams, 631
PROGESTINS
    in endometriosis
        choice of progestin, 448
        contraindications, 448, 450
    -estrogen combinations to induce pseudo-
        pregnancy, 450
    indications
        proposed, 652-654
        proved, 649-652
    microdose, for oral contraception, 685-686
    migraine and, 695
    19-nor, 678
    ovulation suppression and, 446-451
    vaginal, for contraception, 686-687
PROLACTIN, 546
PROSTHESES
    in fimbrioplasty, 479
    intrauterine, for tubal implantation, 480-
        481
PRURITUS VULVAE, 38-51
    allergies causing, 50
    bacteria causing, 42-43
    chemical irritants causing, 50-51
    diagnosis, 40
    drug sensitivities causing, 50
    etiology, 40
        local, 40-50
        systemic, 50-51
    fungous causing, 40-42
    kraurosis-leukoplakia complex and, 43-50
    treatment, 40
    trichomoniasis causing, 40
PSEUDOMYXOMA PERITONEI, 360
PSEUDOPOLYMENORRHEA, 578
PSEUDOPREGNANCY
    in adenomyosis of uterine corpus, 225
    progestin-estrogen combinations to induce,
        450
PSEUDOPUBERTY, 553
PSEUDOSTRATIFICATION: of gland nuclei, 199,
    208
PSORIASIS: vulva, 53
PSYCHE: and menstrual cycle, 212

PSYCHOSOMATIC ASPECTS: of habitual abor-
    tion, 502-503
PSYCHOTHERAPY: of menopause, 662-663
PUBARCHE, 546
PUERPERAL SALPINGITIS (see Salpingitis)
PULSE RATE: in tubal ectopic pregnancy, 305

R

RADIATION
    diagnosis, of metastases to chest, 271
    injuries of vulva, 32
    radioresponsiveness in ovarian carcinoma,
        372-373
    therapy of invasive cervical cancer, 153-160
RADIOLOGY (see Radiation)
RADIUM SYSTEMS: in cervical cancer, 156
RECTOCELE, 90, 91
RECTUM: vaginorectal examination, com-
    bined, 15
RECTUS MUSCLE: hematoma, 343
RESECTION: wedge, of ovary, in infertility,
    491-494
REST TUMORS, 405-412
    adrenal, 405-407
        cortex, 406
    congenital, 405-412
    mesometanephric, 407-409
RETE
    cords, 325
    ovarii, 324, 329
RETRODISPLACEMENT (see Uterus, corpus, ret-
    rodisplacement)
RETROVERSION (see Uterus, corpus, retrodis-
    placement)
RHYTHM METHOD, 672
ROENTGENOGRAPHY (see Radiation)
RUPTURE: normal follicle, cystic structure
    from, 347-349

S

SALPINGITIS
    acute, 290
    granulomatous nontuberculous, 303
    isthmica nodosa, 311-314
        diagnosis, 313-314
        treatment, 314
    physiologic, 301-303
    puerperal and postabortal, 294-296
        ampicillin in, 296
        cephalothin in, 296
        chloramphenicol in, 296
        kanamycin in, 296
        penicillin in, 296
        polymyxin-B in, 296
        symptomatology, 294-295
        treatment, 295-296
SALPINGOLYSIS: in infertility, 479
SALPINGOPLASTY: in infertility, 479
SARCOLYSIN (see Melphalan)
SARCOMA
    endometrial stromal, 274
    fibrosarcoma (see Fibrosarcoma)
    oviduct, 320
    uterine corpus, 272-276
    vagina, 101
    vulva, 66
SCABIES: vulvar, 51

SCLEROCYSTIC OVARIAN DISEASE (*see* Stein-Leventhal syndrome)
SEMINIFEROUS TUBULE DYSGENESIS (*see* Klinefelter's syndrome)
SENILE
vaginitis, 87-88
vulvitis, 43
SENSORY FIBERS: of uterine corpus, 181
SEX
-chromatin mosaicism, 707
-chromosome mosaicism, 707
SEXUAL PRECOCITY (*see* Menstruation, premature)
SHEDDING: irregular, of endometrium, 582
SHEEHAN'S SYNDROME, 603-608
diagnosis, 603-604
differential, 604-607
therapy, 607-608
SIGMOID
carcinoma, 342
diverticulitis, 342
endometriosis of, into lumen, 439
redundant, and ovarian lesion diagnosis, 340
SIMMONDS' DISEASE, 602-603
SKENE'S GLAND, 27
SKIN
diseases, of vulva, 51-55
menstrual cycle and, 212
SMEARS: vaginal and cervical, technique, 144
SMITH-HODGE PESSARY: in uterine retrodisplacement, 216-217
SOCIAL FACTORS: in cervical cancer, 126
SPECULUM INSERTION: for pelvic examination, 9
SPERMICIDES: vaginal, 672-673
SPINAL CELL CERVICAL CANCER, 147
SPINDLE CELL CERVICAL CANCER, 147
SPINNBARKEIT, 109
STAINING, PREMENSTRUAL, 578-579
progestins in, 651
STEIN-LEVENTHAL SYNDROME, 416-427
clomiphene and, 424-427
diagnostic measures, 422
etiology, 419-420
heredity and, 739
hirsutism and, 610-611
ovaries in, 417-418
bisection, 417
gross appearance, 417
high-power view, 418
low-power view, 418
stimulation tests and, adrenocortical and ovarian, 423
suppression studies and, adrenocortical and ovarian, 422-423
treatment, 423-427
wedge resection of ovary in, 491-494
STERIDS, 618
nucleus, 619
STEROID(s), 187, 618-657
biosynthesis, 620-636
adrenal steroids, 591
studies of, 420-422
definition, 618
general considerations, 618-620
nucleus, structural formula, 619
STEROIDOGENESIS, OVARIAN
clomiphene and MER-25, 425
enzymatic sequences in, 421

STEROL, 618
STREPTOMYCIN: in oviduct tuberculosis, 299
STROMA
cervical carcinoma in situ and, 137-141
cortical stromal hyerplasia, 384-385
edema, and endometrial dating, 208
endolymphatic, myosis, 242-243
gonadal stromal tumors, 378-392
vaginal, photomicrograph, 74
STRUMA OVARII, 401-402
SYPHILIS
condylomata lata of vulva due to, 33
vulva in, 33-35

T

TALC: on oviduct, reaction to, 304
TEARS OF PERINEUM, 91-92
complete, 93
TEMPERATURE
basal body
graph in secondary amenorrhea, 488
progesterone and, 648
records after curettage for endometrial hyperplasia, 484
in tubal ectopic pregnancy, 305
TERATOCARCINOMA, 404-405
TERATOMA
benign cystic, 396-402
diagnosis, 396-398
interior of, 397
large, 397
large-bowel contents in, 400
lining of, 399
pathology, 398-400
struma ovarii, 401-402
thyroid tissue in, 401-402
treatment, 400-401
malignant, 403-404
TESTICULAR FEMINIZATION, 732-733
karyotype in, 733
TESTOSTERONE, 626
formula, 647
pathway, 625
response to various stimuli, 613
TETRA-X CHROMOSOME PATTERN, 727
THECA
cell tumors (*see* Granulosa-theca cell tumors)
externa, 186, 329
interna, 186, 329
THECOMA, 383-386
Meig's syndrome and, 384
THELARCHE, 546
THIO-TEPA
ovarian carcinoma and, 376
structural formula, 376
THROMBOPHLEBITIS: and oral contraception, 690-693
THYROID
in abortion, habitual, 507-508
in infertility, 495-497
menstrual cycle and, 209-210
oral contraception and, 690
tissue in cystic teratoma, 401-402
TRANSITIONAL
cell cervical cancer, 147
zone of cervix, 107
TRANSLOCATION, 728-729
TRAUMA

cranial, sexual precocity after, 552-553
vulva (*see* Vulva, injuries)
TRICHOMONADS: seen in wet smear, 81
TRICHOMONIASIS, 80-83
  pruritus vulvae due to, 40
  treatment, 81-83
TRIETHYLENE THIOPHOSPHORAMIDE (*see* Thiotepa)
TRI-PARA-ANISYLCHLOROETHYLENE, 638
TRIPHENYLETHYLENE, 638
TRIPLE-X CHROMOSOME PATTERN, 726-727
TRISOMY, 706
  13-, 737
  18-, 737
  21-, 734-737
    karyotype in, 735
TROPHOBLASTIC DISEASE, 527-544
TUBERCULOSIS
  endometrial, 299
  oviduct, 296-301
    diagnosis, 298
    isonicotinic acid hydrazide in, 299
    para-aminosalicylic acid in, 299
    pathology, 297-298
    streptomycin in, 299
    treatment, 299-301
  uterine corpus, 220
TUBES (*see* Oviduct)
TUBOPLASTY: in infertility, 479
TUMORS
  adrenal, benign, and hirsutism, 610
  Brenner, 409-411
  cancer (*see* Cancer)
  cervix
    benign, 121-124
    detection, 141-144
  endometrium, mixed mesodermal, 275-276
  hilus cell, 411-412
    hirsutism and, 611
  Krukenberg's, 414-416
  luteinized granulosa cell, and sexual precocity, 554
  ovary (*see* Ovary)
  oviduct, benign, 314-315
    adenomatoid, 315
  uterus, corpus, 220-253
  vagina
    benign, 93-95
    premalignant, 95-96
  vulva, benign, 55-58
TUNICA ALBUGINEA, 324
TURNER'S SYNDROME, 719-724
  amenorrhea in, primary, 719-721
  karyotype in, 720, 722

U

ULCER: and vulvar carcinoma, 61
URACHAL CYST, 343
UREMIA: vulvar changes in, 30
URETHRA
  malformations, 29
  meatus, anatomy, 26
URETHROCELE, 89-90
UTEROSACRAL LIGAMENT: endometriosis of, 437
UTERUS
  arcuate, 522
  bicornuate, 182
    complete, 522

operation for, 521
    partial, 522
  bleeding (*see* Hemorrhage, uterine)
  carcinoma (*see* Carcinoma)
  cervix (*see* Cervix)
  contraceptive devices in (*see* Contraception, intrauterine devices)
  corpus (*see below*)
  cri uterine, 576
  curettage (*see* Curettage)
  didelphys, 182, 522
  double, 76
  dye study in hydatidiform mole, 532
  fundus, 173
    carcinoma, 259
  hemorrhage (*see* Hemorrhage, uterine)
  infertility and, 476-478
  isthmus, 105, 173
  maldevelopment
    Jones classification, 520-523
    nonobstructive, 522
  prostheses for tubal implantation, 480-481
  septate, 522
    duplex, 182
    repair technique, 523-525
  unicornis, 182, 520, 522
UTERUS, CORPUS, 172-279
  adenocarcinoma (*see* Adenocarcinoma)
  adenomyosis (*see* Adenomyosis)
  anatomy, 173-182
  blood supply of, 177-181
  cancer, 257-276
  carcinoma (*see* Carcinoma, uterus, corpus)
  cornua of, 173
  embryology, 182-183
  fibers
    motor, 181
    sensory, 181
  fibromyoma of, 228
  frontal section, 105
  infections, 217-220
    postabortal, 217-220
    postabortal, treatment, 218-220
  leiomyoma (*see* Leiomyoma)
  leiomyosarcoma, 228, 230, 273
  ligaments
    broad, 174-175
    cardinal, 175
    infundibulopelvic, 175
    relaxation, 214
    round, 175
  luteum (*see* Corpus, luteum)
  lymphatic supply, 181-182
  nerve supply, 180, 181
  retrodisplacement, 212-217
    pathologic physiology, 214-215
    primary, 213
    secondary, 214
    Smith-Hodge pessary in, 216-217
    symptomatology, 215-216
    treatment, 216-217
  sarcoma, 272-276
  structure, 177
  tuberculosis, 220
  tumors, benign, 220-253

V

VACUOLATION: basal, in endometrium, 208
VAGINA, 70-102

VAGINA (*cont.*)
    anatomic relations of, 73
    anatomy, 72-75
    "blueberry" nodule in, 95
    cancer, 96-101
    carcinoma (*see* Carcinoma, vagina)
    cyst, inclusion, 94-95
    cytology, 78-79
    diaphragms in, 672-673
    double, 76, 182
    embryology, 70-72
    entering, in hysterectomy, 239
    epithelium, photomicrograph, 74
    hemorrhage, abnormal, in tubal ectopic
        pregnancy, 305
    histology, 72-75
    lower, formation of, 71
    malformations, 75-76
        Jones classification, 520-523
    physiologic alterations, 76-79
    progesterone and, 648
    progestins in, for contraception, 686-687
    relaxation, 89-93
        treatment, 92-93
    sarcoma, 101
    smears, technique, 144
    spermicides in, 672-673
    stroma, photomicrograph, 74
    treatment, in hysterectomy, 239-242
    tumors
        benign, 93-95
        premalignant, 95-96
    upper, formation of, 71
    vaginorectal examination, combined, 15
VAGINITIS
    gonorrheal, 88-89
    nonspecific, 86-87
    senescent, 87-88
VASOMOTOR   SYMPTOMS: postmenopausal,
    665-667
VENEREAL DISEASES: vulvar changes in, 33-38
VESSELS
    disturbances, and oral contraception, 690-
    699
    uterine, and hysterectomy, 236-239
VESTIBULE, ANATOMY, 26
    bulbs, 26
VESTIGIAL REMNANTS, 331
VIBRAMYCIN: in gonorrhea, 293
VITAMIN DEFICIENCIES: vulvar changes in, 31
VULVA, 17-69
    anatomy, 20-27
    in blood dyscrasias, 30
    cancer, 58-67
    carcinoma (*see* Carcinoma, vulva)
    in circulatory disturbances, 31
    condylomata
        acuminata, 55
        lata, due to syphilis, 33
    in diabetes, 30
    edema, due to granuloma inguinale, 38

    embryology, 18-20
    fibroma, 57-58
    hidradenoma, 58, 59
    histology, 20-27
    injuries, 31-32
        accidental, 31-32
        coital, 32
        obstetric, 32
        x-ray, 32
    kraurosis of, simple, 44
    leukoplakia, 47-49
    lichen sclerosus et atrophicus of, 45-47
    lipoma, 56-57
    malformations, 27-29
    melanoma, 66
    moniliasis, 41
    nerve supply, 24
    neurodermatitis, 39, 53-55
    normal, in multiparity, 10
    in Paget's disease, 66-67
    papilloma, 55-56
    physiologic alterations, 30-31
    pruritus (*see* Pruritus vulvae)
    sarcoma, 66
    skin diseases, 51-55
    tumors, benign, 55-58
    in uremia, 30
    venereal diseases and, 33-38
    in vitamin deficiencies, 31
VULVITIS
    bacterial, nonspecific, 42
    contact, 43
    diabetic, 30
    fungous, 40-42
    moniliasis, 41
    nonspecific, 39, 42
    senile, 43
VULVOVAGINAL GLAND: anatomy, 26-27

W

WEDGE RESECTION: of ovary, for infertility,
    491-494

X

X-RAY (*see* Radiation)
XXXXY MOSAICISM, 707
XXXY MOSAICISM, 707, 727
XY FEMALE, 731-734

Y

YOUNGE FORCEPS, 118

Z

ZONA PELLUCIDA, 329
ZOSTER: vulva, 52